How to Use This Saunders Nursing Survival Guide

This book presents need-to-know information on pharmacology in a complete, easy-to-learn format to help you master one of the most difficult subjects in nursing.

These headings walk you through each chapter:

What You WILL LEARN An introductory list of checkpoints to outline what is covered in each chapter.

What It IS A "short and sweet" section devoted to the de the topic.

What You NEED TO KNOW The essential information an a discussion of why they are important.

What You DO Nursing interventions that apply everything you learned in the What You NEED TO KNOW section.

Do You UNDERSTAND? Various activities and exercises (with answers) so you may review and make sure you understand each topic.

Technical terms (and common hospital terms) are given easy-to-understand explanations, and, if you're likely to hear something referred to in a certain way in the hospital setting, we've highlighted the term in color.

These icons punctuate the text:

 Highlights the most important points to study or use in the clinical atmosphere.

 Alerts you to urgent information about dangerous conditions and how to avoid them.

 Points out age-related variations in signs and symptoms, nursing interventions, and patient teaching.

 Clues you in to possible variations related to a patient's cultural background.

 Instructs you to head to the Internet for additional resources.

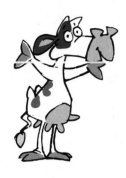

Tell Us What YOU Think

The *Saunders Nursing Survival Guide* series has been created with the help of student feedback to serve your nursing review needs. In order to continue this tradition we invite you to voice your opinion. A website has been created to allow you the opportunity to Tell Us What YOU Think. Please go to the website SNSGSurvey.elsevier.com and help us continue to provide you with student-focused and friendly review activities. Your ideas will be used to create new and fun ways for students like you to learn and review the difficult topics they face throughout their nursing education.

Go to: SNSGSurvey.elsevier.com and Tell Us What YOU Think.

Saunders
Nursing Survival Guide
Pharmacology

Second Edition

Linda E. McCuistion, PhD, RN, ANP, CNS
Professor, Division of Nursing
Our Lady of Holy Cross College
New Orleans, Louisiana

Kathleen Jo Gutierrez, PhD, RN, ANP, CNS
Independent Practice, Internal Medicine
Littleton, Colorado;
Associate Professor
University of Colorado Health Sciences Center
Denver, Colorado

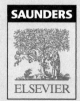

SAUNDERS

ELSEVIER

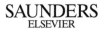

11830 Westline Industrial Drive
St. Louis, Missouri 63146

SAUNDERS NURSING SURVIVAL GUIDE: PHARMACOLOGY

ISBN-13: 978-1-4160-2935-9
ISBN-10: 1-4160-2935-4

NOTICE

Pharmacology is an ever-changing field. Standard safety precautions must be followed, but as new research and clinical experience broaden our knowledge, changes in treatment and drug therapy may become necessary or appropriate. Readers are advised to check the most current product information provided by the manufacturer of each drug to be administered to verify the recommended dose, the method and duration of administration, and contraindications. It is the responsibility of the licensed prescriber, relying on experience and knowledge of the patient, to determine dosages and the best treatment for each individual patient. Neither the publisher nor the author assumes any liability for any injury and/or damage to persons or property arising from this publication.

ISBN-13: 978-1-4160-2935-9
ISBN-10: 1-4160-2935-4

Acquisitions Editor: Catherine Jackson
Developmental Editor: Amanda Sunderman Politte
Editorial Assistant: Heather Bays
Publishing Services Manager: John Rogers
Project Manager: Helen Hudlin
Designer: Jyotika Shroff
Cover Art Illustrator: Chris Sharp, GraphCom Corporation

Working together to grow libraries in developing countries

www.elsevier.com | www.bookaid.org | www.sabre.org

ELSEVIER   **BOOK AID** International   **Sabre Foundation**

Printed in the United States of America

Last digit is the print number: 9 8 7 6 5 4 3 2 1

About the Authors

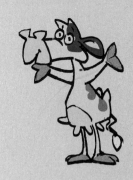

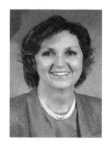

Dr. Linda E. McCuistion is a professor in the Division of Nursing at Our Lady of Holy Cross College. Dr. McCuistion is licensed as an advanced practice nurse and has 35 years of nursing experience, including acute care and home health nursing. She is a past advisory board member, consultant, and reviewer of a software preparation company for the state licensure examination. Dr. McCuistion has served as coordinator for the Graduate Plus Internship program for new nursing graduates to ease their transition into the workforce. Dr. McCuistion has served as a legal nurse consultant and as a member of a medical review panel and is past advisory board member of a school for surgical technicians. She has served as a consultant to improve the quality of nursing care and to assist in the preparation for accreditation of acute care facilities. Dr. McCuistion is past president, vice-president, and faculty advisor of the Sigma Theta Tau International Honor Society in Nursing, Xi Psi chapter-at-large, as well as past associate editor of the *NODNA Times,* which is the New Orleans District Nurses' Association newsletter. Dr. McCuistion was chosen as a Great One Hundred Nurse by the New Orleans District Nurses' Association in 1993. She has lectured regionally and nationally on a variety of nursing topics and has published articles in nursing journals and written chapters in several nursing books. Dr. McCuistion has been listed in "Who's Who Empowering Executives and Professionals."

Dr. Kathleen Jo Gutierrez completed an Associate degree in nursing from the Community College of Denver, a Bachelor of Science degree in nursing from Metropolitan State College of Denver, and a Master of Science degree from the University of Colorado at Denver Health Sciences Center. She also completed a post-master's program as an adult nurse practitioner through Beth El College in Colorado Springs. Her interest

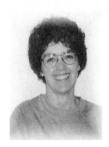

in education and professional development led her to a Doctoral degree in education from the University of Denver.

Dr. Gutierrez is a primary health care provider in the Denver area. In the 20 years before entering private practice, she was an Associate Professor of Nursing at Regis University in Denver and is presently an Associate Professor with the University of Colorado at Denver Health Sciences Center.

In addition to her work on *Saunders Nursing Survival Guide: Pathophysiology,* second edition, Dr. Gutierrez is the author and editor of *Pharmacotherapeutics: Clinical Reasoning in Practice, Pharmacotherapeutics: Clinical Decision-Making in Nursing,* and *Pharmacology for Nursing Practice.*

Dr. Gutierrez is named in "Who's Who in American Nursing," "Who's Who in American Education," "Who's Who in Medicine and Health Care," and most recently "Who's Who in American Women." She is board certified as both an adult nurse practitioner and medical-surgical clinical nurse specialist. She is a member of the American Nurses Association, the National Organization of Nurse Practitioner Faculties, the American Academy of Nurse Practitioners, the American Association of Diabetic Educators, and Sigma Theta Tau, the International Honor Society of Nursing.

Contributors to the First Edition

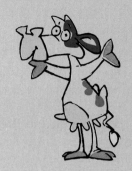

Marie M. Adorno, APRN, MN, CNS
Assistant Professor of Nursing
Our Lady of Holy Cross College
New Orleans, Louisiana

**Deborah S. Anderson, RPh, PharmD,
     BS (Pharm.)**
Clinical Pharmacist, Internal Medicine
Ochsner Foundation Hospital
Clinical Assistant Professor, Pharmacy Practice
Xavier University of Louisiana College of Pharmacy
Adjunct Faculty, Nursing Practitioner Program
Loyola University of New Orleans
City College, School of Nursing
New Orleans, Louisiana

Joanne M. Bullard, BSN, MN, APRN
Assistant Professor of Nursing
Our Lady of Holy Cross College
New Orleans, Louisiana

Jennifer S. Couvillon, MSN, RN, BSN
Instructor of Nursing
Adult Health, Critical Care
Louisiana State University Health Sciences
     Center School of Nursing
New Orleans, Louisiana

Lynn J. Drummond, MSN, BS, RN
Nurse Educator and Clinical Manager
Community Health Agency
Southfield, Michigan

Pamela B. Egan, MN, RN,C-FNP, C-ANP, CS
Family Nurse Practitioner
Covington Family Health Clinic
Covington, Louisiana
Owner and President
Egan Healthcare Services
Home Health, Medical Equipment, Pharmacy
Metairie, LaPlace, Covington, and Plaquemine
     Parish, Louisiana

Kathleen Jo Gutierrez, PhD, RN, ANP, CNS
Independent Practice, Internal Medicine
Littleton, Colorado
Affiliate Faculty
Regis University
Denver, Colorado

Annette M. Knobloch, RN, BSN, MPH, LCCE
Associate Professor of Nursing
William Carey College
New Orleans, Louisiana

Linda Eilee Schmidt McCuistion, PhD, RN
Professor, Division of Nursing
Our Lady of Holy Cross College
New Orleans, Louisiana

Karen K. Mullins, BSN
Charge Nurse Med-Surg
Med-Surg Nursing
Dukes Memorial Hospital
Peru, Indiana

Mary Ann Nemcek, DNS, RN
Assistant Professor of Nursing
Loyola University
New Orleans, Louisiana
Continuing Education Coordinator
Home Care Services
Egan Health Care Services
Metairie, Louisiana

Phyllis G. Peterson, RN, MN, AOCN
Assistant Professor
Division of Nursing
Our Lady of Holy Cross College
New Orleans, Louisiana

Susan S. Rick, DNS, RN, CNS
Assistant Professor of Nursing
Louisiana State University Health Sciences Center
New Orleans, Louisiana

Jennifer C. Robinson, MSN, RN
Instructor of Nursing
Southeastern Louisiana University
Hammond, Louisiana

Linda J. Rubino, MSN
Assistant Administrator
Egan Health Care
Metairie, Louisiana

Eileen H. Stoll, MSN, RN, CCRN
Assistant Professor
Division of Nursing
Our Lady of Holy Cross College
New Orleans, Louisiana

Annette Walton, RN, BSN
Renaissance Home Health Care
Southfield, Michigan

Contributor

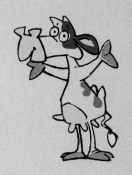

Phyllis G. Peterson, RN, MN, AOCN
Assistant Professor
Division of Nursing
Our Lady of Holy Cross College
New Orleans, Louisiana

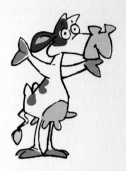

Reviewers

Tabitha T. Garrison, RN, BS, BSN, MSN
James Madison University
Harrisonburg, Virginia

Nancy L. McCartney, RN
O.H.S.U. ENT/Neuro
Portland, Oregon

Lori Theodore, RN, ADN
South Lake Hospital, Progressive Care Unit
Clermont, Florida

Preface

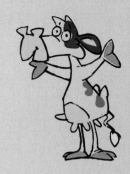

An understanding of pharmacologic concepts provides a solid foundation for the nurse to administer drugs, provide patient teaching, monitor desired body responses and drug effects, and intervene to make drug therapy more tolerable by managing adverse effects. It is important for the nurse to be aware of pharmacologic and biologic entities, such as mechanisms of action, appropriate use, toxicities, drug interactions, and nursing responsibilities.

Patient teaching is of prime importance for the nurse in the management of drug therapy. It may involve informal teaching such as the monitoring of vital signs, deciding whether to take a drug with food, and determining the duration of drug treatment; or patient teaching may involve formal classes that teach drug self-administration. Detailed and enthusiastic patient teaching on the part of the nurse enhances patient compliance and adherence to a prescribed regimen.

This book is one in a series created in response to input from nursing students. Focus groups held at the National Student Nurses' Association convention identified helpful methods to achieve mastery of new information. Their responses were used to design the basic structure and approach behind the *Saunders Nursing Survival Guide* series. In addition, throughout the development of this book, student nurses met to evaluate and critique its content and progress.

The drug information in this book is presented in a manner that promotes a clear understanding of drug actions and body responses. Because there are literally thousands of drugs, it is impossible to memorize all specific information for each drug. This book organizes drugs with similar characteristics into classifications or families to help the learner assimilate the information. Great care has been taken to organize the drug information into an easily understandable format.

We include many features in the margins to help the reader focus on the most important information needed to succeed in the classroom and in the clinical setting. TAKE HOME POINTS are composed of both study tips for classroom tests and "pearls of wisdom" to assist you in caring for patients. These are drawn from our many years of combined academic and clinical experience. Content marked with a **Caution icon** ▽ is vital and usually involves nursing actions that may have life-threatening consequences or significantly affect patient outcomes. The **Lifespan icon** 🐢 and the **Culture icon** ☯ highlight variations in treatment that may be necessary for specific age or ethnic groups. A **Web Links icon** 🖥 will direct you to sites on the Internet that give more detailed information on a given topic. Each of these icons will specifically help you focus on real-world patient care, the nursing process, and positive patient outcomes.

We also use consistent headings that emphasize specific nursing actions. **"What You WILL LEARN"** provides a list of the concepts to be learned in that chapter. **"What It IS"** describes the action and use of the drugs in a given classification. Most drug classification discussions include a box that focuses on the most common drugs in the category, highlighting prototype drugs in color. **"What You NEED TO KNOW"** summarizes contraindications and precautions, drug interactions, and adverse effects of the drug classification. **"What You DO"** includes bulleted lists of nursing interventions and responsibilities because, as professionals, we are responsible for providing expert, comprehensive care for our patients. Finally, **"Do You UNDERSTAND?"** provides questions and exercises that are both entertaining and useful to reinforce the topic's concepts. This five-step approach provides you with information and helps you learn how to apply it in the clinical setting.

We hope this book will make a difficult topic easier and will provide you with new insights and understanding about drug classes and their uses. Share the knowledge you gain with others, and most of all, use this information to make a positive difference in the lives of your patients.

Linda E. McCuistion, PhD, RN, ANP, CNS
Katheen Jo Gutierrez, PhD, RN, ANP, CNS

This book is dedicated to my family and friends as well as all nursing students and faculty who endured Hurricane Katrina and continue to pursue their dreams.
— Linda E. McCuistion

To my husband and soul-mate, Pat, who stands beside me through thick and thin, maintains our home, nourishes me, and helps me to keep my sanity—
I don't know what I would do without you.

To my daughter, Pam, and son-in-law, Brad, whose ability to be forthright and honest helps keep my life in perspective, especially through life's challenges.

And to our son, Michael, who even in his physical absence, remains the most honest, compassionate, devoted, nonjudgmental individual I have ever known.
— Kathleen Jo Gutierrez

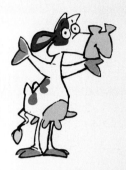

Acknowledgments

I would like to express my deep appreciation to Dr. Gerald DeLuca and Sister Bernardine Hill who have helped me develop my writing style with their expert guidance. A special thanks is extended to my family and friends for their support, encouragement, and advice: Dr. Robert Ekas, Jr., Patricia Smart, Myra Wood, and Phyllis Peterson. To these people I offer my sincere appreciation. My thanks and appreciation to Robin Carter, Amanda Politte, Catherine Jackson, Heather Bays, and Kathleen Gutierrez for their patience and expertise.

— *Linda E. McCuistion*

No author writes a book alone. Thanks to Linda McCuistion for the opportunity to once again participate in this project and to the students, nurse educators, and health care providers for their collaboration over a number of years. Continued thanks to the staff and editors at Elsevier for their patience and understanding, continually sound advice, marketing savvy, and most importantly, friendship. These wonderful people have once again made an important contribution to helping nursing resources come to fruition.

— *Kathleen Jo Gutierrez*

Contents

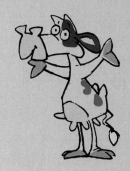

Drug Concepts

What You WILL LEARN

After reading this chapter, you will know how to do the following:

✔ Compare the pharmacokinetic phase with the pharmacodynamic phase of drug action.

✔ Recall the three principles of drug action.

✔ Discuss the major factors influencing the four phases of pharmacokinetics.

✔ Describe the major factors influencing the site of drug action and drug-reception interactions.

✔ Contrast agonist drugs with antagonist drugs.

✔ Compare predictable and unpredictable adverse drug effects.

This chapter presents the basic principles of pharmacology upon which drug therapy (pharmacotherapeutics) is based. **Pharmacotherapeutics** is the use of drugs to alleviate the signs and symptoms of disease, delay disease progression, cure a disease, or facilitate nondrug interventions. Whenever a drug is used, the benefits of its use should be greater than the risks of side effects. All aspects of the use of a drug must be considered.

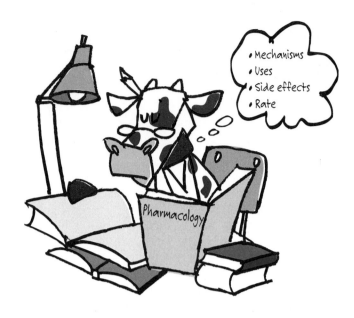

Mechanisms
• Uses
• Side effects
• Rate

Pharmacology is the study of the mechanism of action, uses, side effects, and fate of drugs in the body. In other words, it is the study of what biologically active compounds do in the body (**pharmacodynamics**) and how the body reacts to them (**pharmacokinetics**). There are thousands of drugs and hundreds of facts about each of them. Memorizing facts is unnecessary if you learn to predict the behavior of each drug based on a few facts and an understanding of the principles of pharmacology.

Most drugs are synthetic in origin; they are discovered in the laboratory. A few are still obtained from natural sources. Any drug can have a chemical name, a **generic name,** and a **brand** or **trade name.** All drugs available by prescription and many over-the-counter (OTC) drugs have a generic name. The generic name of a drug is suggested by the manufacturer and accepted by the appropriate national or international committee. Manufacturers use brand names to describe their specific drugs.

There are three important principles about drug action to remember:

Principle 1: Drugs modify existing functions within the body; they do not create new function.

Principle 2: No drug has a single action.

Principle 3: Drug effects are determined by the drug's interaction with the body.

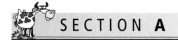

SECTION A

PHARMACOKINETICS

Pharmacokinetics describes the fate of a drug—that is, *what the body does to a drug.* This process includes four components: absorption, distribution, metabolism, and excretion.

What You NEED TO KNOW

Absorption

For a drug to produce a pharmacologic effect, it must be **absorbed,** that is, transferred from its site of administration (e.g., gastrointestinal tract, muscle, skin) into the bloodstream. Factors that influence the rate and extent of drug absorption into the circulation include the dosage formulation (e.g., capsule, tablet, solution, suppository), route of administration (e.g., oral, parenteral, rectal, topical), patient age, pregnancy, and disease states. The rate at which drugs are absorbed determines the onset of effects. In turn, the amount of drug absorbed determines the intensity of effects.

In many cases, drug absorption follows the same pathways as those of nutrients: passive and facilitated diffusion, active transport, and pinocytosis. These pathways allow drugs to penetrate cell membranes to create physiologic effects.

Both drug-related and patient-related factors influence drug absorption. Drug-related factors that influence absorption include ionization state, molecular weight, solubility, and the drug's formulation (e.g., solution versus tablet). Small, nonionized, lipid-soluble drugs pass through cell membranes most readily. Patient-related factors influencing absorption depend on the route of administration. For example, the presence of food in the gastrointestinal (GI) tract, stomach acidity, and blood flow to the GI tract influence the absorption of orally administered drugs.

Distribution

Following absorption, drugs are distributed via the circulation to plasma and tissue-binding sites and then to the site of action and the organs of excretion. As with drug absorption, several factors influence drug distribution. These factors include blood flow, plasma protein binding, tissue binding, and solubility. The distribution of a drug is faster in tissues that are well perfused, such as the kidneys, heart, liver, and brain. The distribution of a drug to poorly perfused tissues, such as muscle and body fat, is slower.

Most drugs are bound to plasma proteins for distribution to sites of action. The binding of drugs to plasma proteins, such as albumin, reduces the amount of "free" drug (i.e., that part of the drug not bound to proteins) in the blood. Free drug molecules reach equilibrium between the blood and tissues. Thus a decrease in free drug in the serum translates to a decrease in the amount of drug that enters a given tissue or organ.

For a drug to enter an organ, it must permeate all membranes that separate the organ from the site of drug administration. For example, benzodiazepines (a psychoactive class of drugs) are very lipophilic, which means they readily cross the intestinal wall, capillary walls, and blood-brain barrier. Because of this characteristic, they distribute rapidly to the brain and are useful in treating anxiety and seizures. However, they are slowly released from fat stores. Thus an overweight or obese person may remain sedated for a longer period than a lean person who received the same dose of the drug. In contrast, some antibiotics pass from the intestine into the bloodstream but cannot pass into the brain. The placental membranes prevent fetal exposure to some drugs but allow the passage of others. Tetracycline antibiotics, heavy metals (e.g., lead), and environmental pollutants (e.g., fluoride) are stored in bones and teeth.

Metabolism

The body attempts to rid itself of foreign substances, such as drugs, chemicals, and toxins, regardless of whether these substances are therapeutic or harmful. Most drugs are metabolized before they are lost from the body. The term *metabolism* often refers to the process of making a drug more polar (more or less electrically charged) and water-soluble. A polar drug is one that carries a positive or negative electrical charge. Therefore metabolism is the processing and breaking down of drugs by body enzymes and chemical transformation.

TAKE HOME POINTS

- The movement of a drug by one or more transport mechanisms is influenced by the electrical charge (polarity) of the cell membrane and by the charge on the drug molecule.
- Small, nonionized (uncharged) drug molecules are lipid-soluble and readily cross cell membranes.
- Large, ionized (charged) drug molecules are water-soluble and do not readily cross cell membranes.

Although the metabolic processes most often result in drug inactivation and excretion, it is wrong to assume that a drug metabolite will be less active or more easily excreted than the parent drug. Metabolic reactions can transform an active drug into a less-active or inactive form. A **prodrug,** one that is inactive or less-active when administered, can be transformed into a more active drug form through two basic reactions.

Drug metabolism reactions have been broadly classified into phase 1 and phase 2 reactions. In phase 1 reactions, drugs are oxidized or reduced to a more polar form to permit excretion. During phase 2 reactions, a large chemical group is attached to the drug molecule, rendering the drug more water-soluble and facilitating excretion of the metabolite from the body. Drugs undergoing phase 2 reactions may have already undergone phase 1 transformation.

The live's microsomal enzyme system, known as the **cytochrome P_{450} system,** is responsible for much of the metabolism of many drugs, although selective other tissues, including the intestines, also metabolize drugs. Cytochrome P_{450} is an enzyme located in the endoplasmic reticulum of liver cells. Cytochrome P_{450} enzymes can be induced (increased in activity) or their activity inhibited (decreased in activity) by a number of drugs or chemicals. Both smoking and drinking induce the cytochrome P_{450} enzymes. This speeds up the metabolism of a number of drugs. In some cases, the result is a lower-than-expected drug concentration, leading to reduced therapeutic effects. Most drug interactions today are the result of cytochrome P_{450} induction or inhibition activities. Genetic factors that influence enzyme levels account for some of the differences we see in drug metabolism.

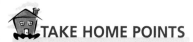

TAKE HOME POINTS

The cytochrome P_{450} enzyme 3A4 is responsible for the metabolism of more than 50% of clinically prescribed drugs metabolized by the liver. Examples of drugs metabolized by this system include acetaminophen, lovastatin, macrolide antibiotics, progesterone, estrogen, and diazepam.

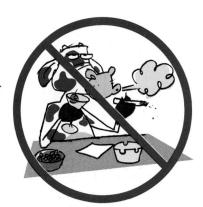

Smoking and drinking defeats the drug's delivery.

Elimination

Drug elimination refers to the movement of a drug or its metabolites from the tissues back into the circulation and then to the organs of elimination. The primary organs of drug elimination are the kidneys. Involved to a lesser degree are the GI tract, respiratory system, sweat, saliva, tears, and breast milk.

Renal elimination of drugs involves both filtration and secretion. Filtration occurs at the glomerulus of the kidney; secretion occurs along the renal tubules. Because drugs, their metabolites, and toxins are concentrated in the kidneys, the kidneys are frequently the site of toxicity. Undesirable symptoms in a patient with kidney failure may be due to drug accumulation rather than to the disease process itself.

Drugs eliminated through the feces may be concentrated in the bile before entering the intestine. In some cases, these drugs are reabsorbed into the portal bloodstream as they move through the intestines. This cycle is known as **enterohepatic circulation.**

Volatile drugs, those that exist in gas or vapors, are eliminated through the lungs. This route is only of importance for general anesthetics. Inhaled anesthetics are administered and lost through the lungs, providing for easily controlled anesthesia by adjusting the concentration of the drug in the inhaled gas mixture.

The term **half-life** describes the relationship between drug volume in the body and clearance. It is the time required by the body to metabolize and decrease the original plasma concentration of a drug by one-half. Half-life is a useful measurement in that it reflects the time required to attain 50% of steady state.

Let's use an example. A single 1000-mg dose of a drug with a half-life of 4 hours is administered. The total amount of drug in the body decreases by half to 500 mg after 4 hours, to 250 mg after 8 hours, to 125 mg after 12 hours, and to 62.5 mg after 16 hours. The drug amount will continue to decrease accordingly with each subsequent half-life until gone from the body.

Owing to long half-lives, certain drugs may accumulate, posing an increased risk for toxicity. Patients with renal or liver disease ordinarily have increased drug half-lives. By understanding the concept of half-life, the nurse can appreciate why some drugs are administered daily, some twice a day, and others four times a day. The shorter the half-life, the more frequent the dosing; the longer the half-life, the less frequently the drug is administered.

Clearance (CL) reflects the integrity of glomerular filtration and is measured through serum or urine creatinine clearance measurements. Assuming 100% bioavailability and steady state, a therapeutic drug range is reached when the rate of drug elimination equals the rate of drug administration. However, because drug elimination takes place through the kidneys, lungs, liver, and other structures, it is important to remember the additive characteristic of clearance: CL kidneys + CL liver + CL other = CL systemic. If any of these structures are faulty, drug clearance is decreased and accumulation is possible.

TAKE HOME POINTS

It takes approximately four half-lives to reach steady state and, likewise, another four half-lives to effectively eliminate the drug from the body.

What You DO

Nursing Responsibilities

- Learn definitions and processes involved in drug therapy.
- Know that pharmacokinetics is more than just the memorization of processes. It involves a sound understanding of absorption, distribution, metabolism, and elimination and the factors that influence each of the processes.
- Recognize that drugs with a long half-life may accumulate, posing an increased risk for toxicity.
- Realize that undesirable symptoms in a patient with kidney failure may be due to drug accumulation rather than to the disease process itself.
- Recognize that although there are other enzyme systems involved in drug metabolism, the cytochrome P_{450} enzyme 3A4 is responsible for the liver metabolism of more than 50% of clinically prescribed drugs.
- Know that only unbound drug molecules are free to act at the site of action. Bound drug molecules do not exert a pharmacologic effect.

Do You UNDERSTAND?

DIRECTIONS: **Indicate in the space provided whether the statement is** *true* **or** *false.* **If the answer is false, correct the statement to make it true (using the margin space).**

- _____ 1. Pharmacokinetics is what the body does to the drug.
- _____ 2. Absorption of a drug is defined as the movement of the drug from the stomach to the bloodstream.
- _____ 3. The process of metabolism makes a drug more polar and water-soluble so that it may be eliminated.
- _____ 4. The cytochrome P_{450} system is located primarily in the kidneys and is responsible for drug elimination.

Answers: 1. true; 2. false; absorption is the movement of the drug from its site of administration to the bloodstream; 3. true; 4. false; the cytochrome P_{450} enzyme system is located primarily in the liver and is responsible for drug metabolism.

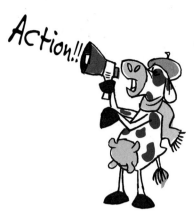

Places everyone!

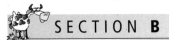

SECTION **B**

PHARMACODYNAMICS

One of the fundamental concepts of *pharmacodynamics*—that is, *what a drug does to the body*—relates to the site of drug action. The site of drug action is the specific cell, tissue, or organ where the drug works; it can be defined at four levels: the molecular level, the cellular level, the tissue level, and the body system level. Most drug molecules bind to cellular receptors, where they initiate a series of biochemical reactions that alter the cell's structure and/or function. To understand pharmacodynamics the nurse needs to also understand the related terminology.

What You NEED TO KNOW

In most cases, the **receptor** is a protein molecule (or perhaps a glycoprotein) present on the cell surface, on an organelle within the cell, or in the cytoplasm, although it can be a cell membrane or an enzyme to which drugs display a chemical or biophysical attraction. Other sites of drug action include ion channels and transport molecules. The term **affinity** is used to describe the strength of the drug's binding to receptors. Some drugs have a stronger affinity for the receptors than other drugs.

One of the following four actions is likely to occur when a drug binds to a receptor: (1) an ion channel is opened or closed; (2) biochemical messengers (e.g., cAMP or cGMP) are activated to initiate a series of chemical reactions within the cell; (3) normal cell function is inhibited; or (4) a cell function is "turned on," or activated.

Drugs, hormones, and neurotransmitters that activate receptors are called **agonists.** In any given dose, some drug molecules find their target receptor while other molecules are being distributed, metabolized, and excreted. Usually, a number of receptors must be occupied by agonists before a measurable change in cell function occurs.

Understanding the difference between drug action and drug effect is important. The interaction between a drug and molecular or cellular components constitutes the **mechanism of action,** or how the drug works. A patient's response to drug action represents the *effect*.

Efficacy refers to the degree to which a drug is able to induce maximal effects. For example, if drug A causes a 50-point drop in total cholesterol levels and drug B produces a 20-point drop, drug A is the more efficacious. The term *efficacious* is used to compare drugs with different mechanisms of action (e.g., nonsteroidal antiinflammatory drugs versus opioids). *Potency* is the amount of drug required to produce 50% of the maximal response possible for that drug. The term *potency* is used to compare drugs within the same chemical class (e.g., morphine versus oxycodone).

Before a new drug can be approved for marketing, its efficacy and safety must be tested in animals and humans. The results of the testing provide us with information regarding the **therapeutic index (TI)** of a drug. The TI is sometimes referred to as the *margin of safety*. The TI is calculated by dividing the dose that would be toxic in 50% of animals (TD_{50}) by the dose that produces the desired therapeutic effect in 50% of animals (ED_{50}). Drugs with a high TI are said to be safe (i.e., to have a wide margin of safety). Drugs with a low therapeutic index have a narrow margin of safety and are unsafe. The closer the ratio is to 1, the greater the possibility for toxicity.

Drug Responses and Effects

In general, when drug use is warranted, the expected benefits should outweigh the potential risks. It should be noted, though, that no drug is totally safe and that all drugs produce a variety of effects. Clinically, an **adverse effect** is any unexpected or unintended response to a therapeutic dose of a drug. An adverse effect usually requires changing dosage, stopping the drug, or administering an antidote to terminate drug action. Adverse effects, sometimes called **side effects,** fall into two groups: predictable effects occur as the result of known, dose-related pharmacologic effects, whereas unpredictable effects are unrelated to the drug's characteristics. Reactions in this second group are often the result of something distinctive to the individual, such as drug allergies, hypersensitivities, or idiosyncratic reactions. Adverse effects can range in severity from those that are merely annoying to those that are life-threatening.

Augmented pharmacologic responses are predictable, dose-related, and known to occur as a result of the pharmacology of the drug. These effects are relatively common and seldom fatal. For example, diphenhydramine (Benadryl) is often used for its side effect of sleepiness in the treatment of insomnia. In another example, hypoglycemia may occur

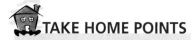

TAKE HOME POINTS

Adverse effects are categorized as those that are predictable and those that are unpredictable. Predictable responses include augmented pharmacologic responses, toxic effects, and cumulative effects. Unpredictable responses include idiosyncratic reactions, pharmacogenetic reactions, allergic reactions, drug tolerance, and dependence.

after an injection of insulin, which is intended to lower blood sugar levels.

Toxic effects are associated with excessive drug levels in a given patient and are predictable. The risk for a toxic response is inversely related to the TI of the drug. For example, toxicity with water-soluble vitamins is rarely seen. However, when drugs, such as digoxin or insulin—each having a narrow TI—are administered, therapy must be closely monitored and carefully managed to avoid toxicity. Many drugs, in and of themselves, are not toxic but may be activated to toxic metabolites through metabolism. The toxic response then depends on the rate at which the toxic metabolite is produced and destroyed.

Cumulative effects result when the effects of one drug have not dissipated before administration of another dose. Cumulative effects occur most often with drugs whose half-lives are measured in days, weeks, or months rather than hours (whose concentrations fall to ineffective levels long before the drug disappears from the body).

Bizarre effects occur unpredictably, and, although uncommon, they have a high rate of morbidity and mortality. These effects include idiosyncratic reactions, pharmacogenetic reactions, allergic reactions, tolerance, and drug dependence. An **idiosyncratic reaction** is a genetically determined unusual or abnormal response to a drug. These reactions affect a small portion of the total population and tend to be unrelated to dose. Idiosyncratic reactions result from (1) extreme sensitivity to a low dose of a drug, (2) extreme insensitivity to a high dose of a drug, indicating abnormal tolerance, or (3) unpredictable and unexplainable symptoms. Sometimes idiosyncratic reactions result in a **paradoxical reaction.** Paradoxical reactions are opposite to that desired. For example, a sedative is given for insomnia but instead keeps the patient awake.

Pharmacogenetic reactions result from genetic differences in drug disposition. Genetic differences are inherited much like inborn errors of metabolism—but with two major differences. Patients with pharmacogenetic disorders lead normal lives and do not have difficulty unless they are challenged with a drug producing an aberrant response. Pharmacogenetic differences result in either increased or decreased intensity of response to a drug and a longer or shorter duration of action.

Allergic reactions such as anaphylaxis, cytotoxicity, and immune complex–mediated reactions are immediate; they are also difficult to predict and to prevent. Contrary to popular belief, these reactions do not occur with the first exposure to a drug but are manifested after a second or subsequent exposure. A review of a physiology or pathophysiology textbook will help to distinguish between these three different allergic reactions.

Delayed reactions are those that occur in the patient sometime after the original treatment or in the children of treated patients. For example, a rash that develops 2 weeks after the start of an antibiotic is a delayed hypersensitivity reaction. Secondary cancers have developed in patients treated with alkylating drugs for Hodgkin's disease. Another example of a delayed effect involves the development of vaginal cancer in the daughters of women who took diethylstilbestrol (DES) during pregnancy.

Tolerance represents a decreased response to a drug; it occurs when the dosage of a drug must be increased to achieve the same effect as that achieved with initial use of the drug. Tolerance can be metabolic, cellular, or behavioral.

Dependence develops when a patient repeatedly needs a drug in order to function normally. This chronic effect is most often seen when the drug is stopped and withdrawal symptoms appear. Dependence may be physical, or it may have a psychological component.

Drug Interactions

The four basic types of drug interactions include additive interactions, synergistic interactions, potentiation, and antagonism. These interactions may be the result of altered absorption, competition for protein binding, or altered metabolism or elimination.

Additive interactions occur when the response elicited by the combined drugs is equal to the combined response of the individual drugs (i.e., 1 + 1 = 2). A *synergistic interaction* is elicited when the effects of the combined drugs are greater than the combined responses of the individual drugs (i.e., 1 + 1 = 3). *Potentiation* occurs when a drug that has no effect itself enhances the effect of a second drug (i.e., 0 + 1 = 2). *Antagonism* occurs when one drug inhibits the action of another drug (i.e., 1 + 1 = 0). Usually, the antagonist drug has no pharmacologic activity of its own, but, by occupying the receptor, the antagonist drug either prevents an agonist drug from binding to the receptor or prevents the agonist from evoking a molecular response when it binds to the receptor.

Anaphylaxis is life-threatening. The signs and symptoms of anaphylaxis include apprehension; itching of the palms, chin, or throat; tearing; laryngeal edema; wheezing; and dyspnea. When severe, the reaction progresses to hypotension, shock, and cardiovascular collapse.

What You DO

Nursing Responsibilities

- Review potential drug interactions prior to drug administration.
- Check for patient's allergies before administering a drug.
- Assess the patient's response to medication.
- Monitor pertinent laboratory results for any abnormalities.
- Observe the patient for adverse effects.

Do You UNDERSTAND?

DIRECTIONS: Fill in the blanks in the following statements.

1. A receptor is a specialized protein molecule present on the _____, on an _____, or in the_____, although it can be a _____ membrane or an _____ to which drugs display a chemical or biophysical attraction.

2. The stronger the _____ for the receptor, the _____ the drug action.

3. _____ is the degree to which a drug is able to induce maximal effects.

4. Antagonism occurs when one drug _____ the action of another drug.

5. An _____ drug reaction is a genetically determined unusual or abnormal response to a drug.

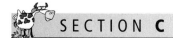

SECTION C

DEVELOPMENTAL CONSIDERATIONS

Prescribing or administering drugs without consideration of the patient's physiologic and psychosocial profile is substandard care. Several physiologic factors influence drug action, interactions, and reactions. These factors include pregnancy, the patient's age, gender, genetics, general state of health, and biologic rhythms. Psychosocial factors influencing a patient's response to drug therapy include the patient's environment and dietary intake, the bioavailability of the drug and its additives, the dosage and number of drugs taken, the route and technique for drug administration, and compliance, noncompliance, and misuse issues.

Pregnancy

Pregnancy and its normal developmental changes during gestation influence pharmacokinetics, pharmacodynamics, and the patient's response to drugs. Although the numerous physiologic changes that occur affect drug action, the pregnant patient is not necessarily at higher risk for adverse effects. Body water and plasma volume increase by as much as 50% during a normal pregnancy, so drug dosages are "diluted" compared with dosages in the nonpregnant patient. Thus dosage requirements may increase for pregnant patients.

Drug treatment of pregnant women (and women who are likely to become pregnant) must take into account the welfare of both the fetus and the mother. Obviously, **teratogenic drugs** (those known to cause fetal harm) must be avoided. However, it is wise to regard all drugs as being potentially harmful.

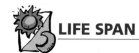

LIFE SPAN

Remember: When you administer a drug to a pregnant patient, the drug will be received by two persons, the mother *and* the fetus. The placenta does not act as a barrier, but rather as a selective filtration system.

Age and Weight

Pharmacokinetic drug actions in infants and older adults are different from actions in other patients. Infants have a greater proportion of total body water than do adults, resulting in expanded distribution and diminished blood levels of water-soluble drugs. Infants and young children also have a low percentage of body fat, thus contributing to increased blood levels of lipid-soluble drugs. A relative lack of gastric acid contributes to an exaggerated absorption of drugs that would normally be inactivated by gastric acid. Furthermore, an infant's body system lacks the enzymes responsible for drug metabolism. However, most of the enzyme systems develop quickly, with levels reaching those of an adult by 1 to 8 weeks after birth. By the first year of life, the enzyme systems are probably as active as they will ever be.

Additionally, rapid dehydration caused by immature temperature regulation mechanisms can elevate serum drug levels. The renal elimination of drugs is also reduced in an infant as a result of decreased blood flow to the kidneys and more widespread drug distribution. The breastfeeding infant can develop adverse reactions to drugs that pass from the mother into breast milk.

On the other end of the age spectrum, the older adult is prone to drug interactions as a result of the normal changes of aging and concomitant disease states. Alterations in drug absorption, distribution, metabolism, and elimination are common in older adults. A high gastric pH decreases the absorption of drugs that are normally nonionized at the low pH of the stomach. Proportional increases in body fat lead to less fat-soluble drug deposition. Reduced body water contributes to higher serum concentrations of water-soluble drugs. Lowered serum albumin levels result in increased amounts of unbound drug, leading to greater drug activity. Furthermore, a reduction in cardiac output and blood flow to the kidneys affects metabolism and elimination of drugs. All of these changes result in higher drug concentration levels and a greater chance for toxicity.

The magnitude of drug response is a function of drug concentration at the site of action. As a general rule, a particular quantity of drug may be less effective in an obese individual compared with another individual of normal weight (assuming normal liver, kidney, and cardiovascular function in both individuals). The average adult dose of a drug is calculated on the basis of the amount that will produce a particular effect in half of the population between the ages of 18 and 65 years who weigh approximately 154 pounds (70 kg). The dosage required to obtain a therapeutic effect is roughly proportional to body size. Any variation in effect is minimized when dosage is calculated using kilograms of body weight. The recommended dosages for many drugs are listed in terms of grams or milligrams per kilogram (g/kg or mg/kg) of body weight. Pediatric dosages should be calculated on the basis of body weight.

Gender

Gender does not play a significant role in drug action. However, women generally require smaller doses of drugs than men to manifest the same magnitude of response, simply because of lower average weight. For women taking drugs with a narrow TI, the differences in drug response may require a reduction in dosage. There can also be gender-related differences in drug response based on different proportions of lean body mass to fat mass.

Genetics

An exaggerated response or lack of response to a drug can be the result of genetically determined susceptibility. Genetically determined drug responses require that the patient be closely assessed and monitored for abnormal susceptibility, especially at the start of therapy.

General State of Health

Almost all pharmacokinetic and pharmacodynamic principles have been formulated using data collected from healthy persons. Drugs, however, are administered to persons in whom a physiologic process is taking place. The presence of disease contributes to variability in drug response, especially when organs responsible for the absorption, distribution, metabolism, and elimination of drugs are affected. For example, drugs tend to accumulate in the presence of liver disease. As the liver ceases to function, the rate of metabolism falls and drug levels rise. As with liver disease, kidney disease interferes with the elimination of water-soluble drugs, causing the drugs to accumulate in the body. A decrease in dosage levels is required so that drug levels remain below toxic range.

Biologic Rhythms

Normal biologic rhythms influence drug action and can, in some cases, lead to adverse drug responses. Circadian rhythms continue to operate even when external factors that influence behaviors, such as clocks and work routines, are removed. For example, cortisol levels normally raise between 8 and 10 a.m., decline toward evening, and then rise again in the morning. Human growth hormone and prolactin secretions peak within the first 2 hours after sleep. Maximum thyroid-stimulating hormone levels are reached the first few hours after sleep begins. Thyroid-stimulating hormone levels fade about 3 hours after awakening. Biologic rhythms must be considered in the interpretation of laboratory results related to drug and hormone levels.

Psychosocial Factors

Even with our present-day knowledge of normal body functioning and the manner in which these functions are affected by disease, it is difficult to separate the pharmacologic effects of drugs from their psychological effects. Certain symptoms of disease, such as headache, nausea, and even

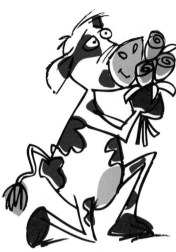

Wanting to please you.

more serious signs, can be brought about by impulses that originate in the cerebral cortex. For example, **placebo effects** are temporally correlated with administration and cannot be attributed to a drug's pharmacodynamic properties. Placebos are usually inert substances (i.e., lactose). The term *placebo* is derived from Latin, meaning "I shall please." An inactive substance is administered specifically for the purpose of satisfying an individual's need for drug dosing.

Physical Environment

Physical environment affects drug response. For example, environmental temperature influences the action and effects of nitrates and antihypertensives. These drugs, when used by a patient exposed to high temperatures, relax peripheral vessels to the extent that excessive vasodilation occurs. Pesticide exposure, smoking, and alcohol use alter the pharmacokinetics of certain drugs, thereby increasing the risk for adverse effects.

Bioavailability and Additives

Numerous brands of the same drug can vary in bioavailability because of differences in manufacturing. Variance in onset, peak concentration levels, and duration of action among the different drugs can lead to adverse effects. Therefore caution must be used when substituting one brand of drug for another or when changing from a brand name to a generic drug and vice versa. Drug additives, such as buffers, stabilizing agents, or dyes can produce adverse responses in susceptible patients. When adverse responses to a specific additive are numerous, the manufacturer may reformulate a drug to remove the offending additive.

Dosage and Number of Drugs Taken

The dosage and number of drugs taken contributes to adverse effects. The probability of an adverse response increases for the patient who is on high doses for extended periods. The risk for adverse effects also increases in direct proportion to the number of drugs the patient takes.

Dietary Intake

The presence of food in the stomach impairs the absorption of certain drugs. For example, excessive intake of foods rich in vitamin K (e.g., green leafy vegetables) decreases the effectiveness of oral anticoagulants (e.g., warfarin). Cabbage, broccoli, charcoal-broiled meats, and products containing caffeine stimulate liver enzymes, thereby increasing the rate of drug metabolism.

Compliance, Noncompliance, and Misuse

Compliance (some prefer the term *adherence*) is defined as the extent to which a prescribed care plan is followed. Drugs are not always taken or administered as prescribed. Doses may be omitted, extra doses may be taken, or the drug may be taken at a wrong time. Patients receiving higher than normal dosages for extended periods are at increased risk for adverse effects. On the other hand, in patients receiving less than the dose prescribed, serum drug levels may remain at or below minimal effective concentrations, and therapeutic drug levels may never be reached.

Misuse (the administration of a drug for the wrong purpose) is often the result of inaccurate self-diagnosis. In addition, the administration of a drug in situations in which contraindications are misunderstood or not recognized contributes to drug misuse. Patients at greatest risk for adverse reactions related to compliance or misuse behaviors are those taking drugs that have a narrow TI, those taking drugs for which the precise timing of the dosage is important, and those in whom underlying medical conditions are likely to be aggravated by a particular drug.

Administration by routes other than those recommended by the manufacturer can cause adverse reactions. Even using the recommended route can cause adverse reactions at times. A parenterally administered drug does not have to be absorbed through the GI tract before entering systemic circulation. For this reason, drugs administered by this route, especially those given intravenously (IV), reach receptor sites quickly and are more likely to cause adverse effects. Administering an IV drug too rapidly may cause an adverse response, because the speed with which a drug is given alters its rate of distribution. Similarly, a drug designed to treat ear problems will cause pain and irritation if administered in the eye.

TAKE HOME POINTS

Noncompliance with (or misuse of) a prescribed drug regimen is viewed as deviant behavior by health care providers. In reality, the patient may not be aware of the proper dose and regimen or may have chosen not to take the drug as prescribed for a variety of reasons.

What You DO

Nursing Responsibilities

- Know that there are many variables that influence drug action, interactions, and reactions.
- Realize that a sound understanding of variables that influence drug action, interactions, and reactions is vital to the safe administration of drug therapy.

- Recognize the physiologic variables that influence drug therapy, including pregnancy, age and weight, gender, genetics, general state of health, and biologic rhythms.
- Know that other variables influencing drug therapy include psychosocial considerations, the physical environment, bioavailability of the drug and its additives, the dosage and number of drugs taken or administered, dietary intake, compliance/noncompliance/misuse issues, and the administration route and technique.
- Realize that no drug should be prescribed or given to a pregnant woman, no matter how innocuous it may seem, unless the drug is considered to be safe for the fetus and there is a clear need for the drug and/or the mother is so ill that the drug is justified even if the fetus may be harmed.
- Recognize that the therapeutic index and margin of safety both refer to the relationship between a drug's therapeutic and adverse effects.
- Recognize that drug interactions refer to a change in the magnitude or duration of a response of one drug because of the presence of another drug.
- Know that placebo effects are temporally related to drug administration rather than to a drug's pharmacodynamic properties.

Do You UNDERSTAND?

DIRECTIONS: Indicate in the space provided whether the statement is *true* or *false*. If the answer is false, correct the statement to make it true (using the margin space).

_____ 1. A fundamental principle of pharmacology states that the intensity of response elicited by a drug is a function of the dose administered.

_____ 2. Drug interactions can be related to the pharmacokinetic or pharmacodynamic characteristics of the interacting drugs.

_____ 3. Adverse drug reactions may be categorized as dose-related or sensitivity-related.

_____ 4. Drugs are considered antagonists when they interact with a receptor to produce an effect of their own.

Answers: 1. true; 2. true; 3. true; 4. false; agonists interact with a receptor to produce an effect of their own; antagonists have no pharmacologic effect of their own.

References

Gutierrez K, Queener S: *Pharmacology for nursing practice*, St Louis, 2003, Mosby.

Hardman J, Limbird L: *Goodman & Gilman's the pharmacologic basis of therapeutics*, ed 10, New York, 2001, McGraw-Hill.

Huether S, McCance K: *Understanding Pathophysiology*, ed 3, St Louis, 2004, Mosby.

Katzung B: *Basic and clinical pharmacology*, ed 9, New York, 2005, Lange Medical Books.

Lehne R: *Pharmacology for nursing care*, ed 5, Philadelphia, 2004, WB Saunders.

Lilley L, Harrington S, Snyder J: *Pharmacology and the nursing process*, ed 4, St Louis, 2005, Mosby.

NCLEX® Review

1. Distribution of drugs to specific tissues:
   1 is independent of blood flow to the organ.
   2 is independent of the solubility of the drug in that tissue.
   3 depends on the unbound drug concentration gradient between blood and the tissues.
   4 has no effect on the half-life of the drug.

2. Regarding termination of drug action:
   1 drugs must be eliminated from the body to terminate their action.
   2 metabolism of drugs always increases their water-solubility.
   3 metabolism of drugs always abolishes their pharmacologic activity.
   4 liver metabolism and renal elimination are the two most important mechanisms involved in termination of drug action.

3. Polar molecules usually:
   1 penetrate cell membranes rapidly if there is a pH gradient.
   2 require specific transport systems to cross membranes.
   3 can move across cell membranes via channels or pores.
   4 are given orally so that they can be absorbed in the stomach.

4. Patients with disorders of peripheral circulation would have problems with which phase of pharmacokinetics?
   1 Absorption
   2 Distribution
   3 Metabolism
   4 Elimination

5. A health care provider would use knowledge of a drug's half-life when determining which of the following?
   1 The dosage and frequency of drug administration
   2 Which brand of a generic drug to mandate
   3 The precise timing of drug elimination
   4 The precise timing of drug distribution

NCLEX® Review Answers

1. **3** The distribution of drug depends on the concentration gradient between bound and unbound drug. Distribution of drugs to specific tissues is *dependent* on the blood flow to the organ, *dependent* on the solubility of the drug in that tissue, and *does* effect the half-life of the drug.

2. **4** Note the "trigger" words *(must, always)* in choices 1, 2, and 3. Liver metabolism and renal elimination are the two most important mechanisms involved in termination of drug action.

3. **3** Polar drug molecules move across cell membranes via channels or pores. All other responses are incorrect.

4. **2** Distribution. Drug distribution is dependent on blood flow to the organ or tissues. Absorption, metabolism, and elimination are not affected by peripheral circulation abnormalities.

5. **1** A drug's half-life is used for determining the dosage and frequency of drug administration. It is not used to determine choice of trade (brand) names. Drug distribution and elimination are influenced by a variety of other factors, including the disease state.

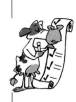

Notes

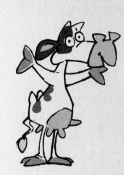

Chapter

2

Drugs Used to Treat Infections

What You WILL LEARN

After reading this chapter, you will know how to do the following:

✔ Contrast the action and uses of penicillin, sulfonamides, aminoglycosides, tetracyclines, macrolides, and fluoroquinolones.
✔ Compare adverse effects of penicillin, sulfonamides, aminoglycosides, tetracyclines, macrolides, and fluoroquinolones.
✔ Identify common adverse effects of antibiotics and antivirals.
✔ Explain common nursing responsibilities of antifungals.

 SECTION **A**

ANTIBIOTICS

This chapter reviews drugs that are used to treat infectious diseases. An antibiotic is a chemical substance that is derived from mold or bacteria and has the ability to destroy or inhibit the growth of one or more causative pathogens in the treatment of infectious conditions. Generally, antibiotic monotherapy (single-drug therapy) is sufficient; however, in some instances, multidrug therapy is necessary to eradicate the infectious process.

β-Lactam Antibiotics

β-Lactam antibiotics have a β-lactam ring in their molecules and exhibit some cross-sensitivity. Penicillins and cephalosporins are β-lactam antibiotics that inhibit enzymes required for the synthesis of bacterial cell walls, which are rigid to protect cytoplasm inside the cells. When β-lactam antibiotics are introduced, bacterial cell walls become weak. Osmotic pressure within weakened cells causes the walls to swell and burst. This process of destroying bacterial cells by osmotic pressure is known as **osmotic lysis.** Human cells are not harmed because they do not use this biochemical process to form cell walls.

What IS a Penicillin Antibiotic?

Penicillin Types	Trade Names	Uses
Natural penicillin penicillin G potassium [pen-ih-SILL-in]	Megacillin	Treatment of moderate-to-severe systemic infections
Penicillinase-resistant penicillin oxacillin [ox-uh-SILL-in]	Prostaphlin	Treatment of staphylococcal infections
Broad-spectrum penicillin (or aminopenicillin) amoxicillin [uh-MOX-ih-sill-in]	Amoxil	Treatment of mild-to-moderate infections
Extended-spectrum penicillin ticarcillin [TIE-car-sill-in]	Ticar	Treatment of septicemia and intraabdominal, skin, soft tissue, and respiratory and GU tract infections

Action

The penicillin classification is separated into four groups: natural, penicillinase-resistant, broad-spectrum, and extended-spectrum penicillins. Natural penicillins inhibit enzymes that are required for bacterial cell wall synthesis; thus they kill bacteria.

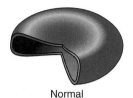

Normal

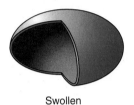

Swollen

LIFE SPAN

Caution should be used when penicillins are given to patients who are pregnant and lactating or those with anemia, thrombocytopenia, granulocytopenia, bone marrow depression, or renal insufficiency.

Overuse of penicillin allows bacteria that were initially sensitive to natural penicillins to develop a protective enzyme (**penicillinase** or **β-lactamase**) and become resistant to therapy. Penicillinase splits open the β-lactam ring of the antibiotic molecule and renders the bacteria resistant to natural penicillins, thereby inactivating natural penicillin antibiotics. Penicillinase-resistant penicillins overcome bacterial resistance because they are stable against penicillinase or β-lactamase enzymes that break down natural penicillins. Other newly developed penicillins include broad-spectrum penicillins (or aminopenicillins), which have an amino group attached to their penicillin nucleus that enhances their activity against gram-negative bacteria. Extended-spectrum penicillins have a wider spectrum of activity than do the other types of penicillin.

Penicillins are bactericidal (i.e., they inhibit the action of enzymes that are necessary for bacterial cell wall formation, thereby killing bacteria). Normally, a microorganism's cell wall lies outside the cytoplasmic membrane and is stiff, penetrable, and meshlike. The high osmotic pressure within the organism's cytoplasmic membrane creates a strong gradient that attracts water; thus the cell swells. Without the stiff cell wall, water would be absorbed to such a degree that the organism would burst. Penicillins suppress substances that are necessary for bacterial cell wall rigidity, making the bacterial cells osmotically unstable, which results in excessive water intake, swelling, and rupture of the bacterial cell, causing bacterial death. Because human cells lack a similar cell wall, the penicillins have virtually no direct effect on host cells.

Uses

Penicillins affect gram-positive and gram-negative aerobes, anaerobes, streptococci, staphylococcus, bacilli, and enterococci. Penicillins are used for the treatment of pharyngitis, tonsillitis, otitis media, pneumonia, endocarditis, soft-tissue infections, meningitis, scarlet fever, rat-bite fever, diphtheria, anthrax, urinary tract infections, syphilis, and gonorrhea. Prophylactically, penicillins may be given before surgery or dental procedures in patients with a history of rheumatic fever.

What You NEED TO KNOW

Contraindications/Precautions

Penicillins are contraindicated for patients with a history of allergic reaction to any penicillin or cephalosporins.

Drug Interactions

Penicillin and penicillinase-resistant groups are less effective when given with tetracyclines. Aminoglycosides are inactivated when given with penicillins. Probenecid slows the excretion of penicillins. Penicillins are believed to decrease the effectiveness of oral contraceptives. The serum level of beta blockers is decreased when given with ampicillin.

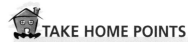

TAKE HOME POINTS

Women who are taking oral contraceptives should be advised to practice an alternate form of birth control throughout penicillin antibiotic therapy.

Adverse Effects

Penicillins are the most common cause of drug allergy. Allergic reactions vary from minor rashes to life-threatening anaphylaxis. The severe reactions are most likely to occur with parenteral use. Immediate penicillin reactions occur within the first 30 minutes after drug administration. Delayed reactions may take days or weeks to develop. Hypersensitivities may appear in the form of rash, pruritus, fever, wheezing, severe dyspnea, stridor, nausea, vomiting, tachycardia, sweating **(diaphoresis),** vertigo, hypotension, loss of consciousness, or death. Because of cross-sensitivity, patients who are allergic to one type of penicillin are generally considered allergic to all penicillins.

TAKE HOME POINTS

Observe for anaphylactic reactions, which are common in penicillin therapy, and immediately treat with epinephrine, antihistamines, and corticosteroid administration.

The adverse effects of penicillins generally involve the gastrointestinal (GI) system with glossitis, mouth sores **(stomatitis),** anorexia, heartburn, gastritis, abdominal pain, nausea, vomiting, and mild-to-severe diarrhea. Taste alterations, sore mouth, and discolored tongue (i.e., black, furry tongue) are primarily a result of the loss of normal flora and the subsequent opportunistic infections called *superinfections.*

Toxicities involve the neurologic, nephrologic, or hematologic systems of the body. Neurologic reactions include lethargy, twitching, confusion, difficulty swallowing **(dysphasia),** agitation, hyperreflexia, depression, hallucinations, psychosis, convulsions, and coma. Hematologic toxicity includes neutropenia, thrombocytopenia, hemolytic anemia, and prolonged bleeding time. Other adverse effects include fever, macular rash, eosinophilia, proteinuria, hematuria, and leukocyturia, which can progress to renal failure.

 Penicillins, when given with anticoagulants, increase bleeding time.

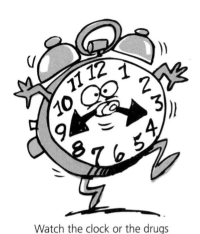

Watch the clock or the drugs
won't rock.

What You DO

Nursing Responsibilities

When administering penicillins, the nurse's prime concern is to be aware of the potential for allergic reactions. Prior to administration, the nurse should ask the patient about allergies.

Some penicillins are well absorbed following oral administration. However, penicillin G is unstable in acid, and most of an oral dose is destroyed in the stomach. Food slows gastric emptying, thus prolonging exposure of the penicillin to gastric acid. Consequently, to produce blood levels comparable in effectiveness to parenteral administration, the oral dose must be four to five times greater, and the drug must be taken on an empty stomach. When administering oral penicillins, the nurse should encourage the patient to take penicillins at the prescribed dose and at evenly spaced intervals. Because of rapid clearance, around-the-clock administration is required for drug efficacy.

All forms of penicillin may be given intramuscularly (IM), but various penicillins (i.e., sodium, potassium, procaine, benzathine) are absorbed at different rates. For example, the sodium and potassium forms of penicillin G are rapidly absorbed, with peak blood levels reached in 15 to 30 minutes after injection. In contrast, procaine and benzathine forms are absorbed at a slower rate. The average peak penicillin drug effect is reached in 4 hours after administration. When administering penicillin, the nurse should:

- Watch the intravenous (IV) sites for phlebitis, and apply warm compresses when they become painful and swollen.
- Discontinue the IV access, and restart another line on discovery of phlebitis.
- Check the patient who is receiving sodium or potassium penicillin drugs for electrolyte imbalance because hyperkalemia can lead to cardiac arrest.
- Examine laboratory results for renal dysfunction, bone marrow depression, and prolonged bleeding time to detect toxicities early.
- Teach patients about the need for additional contraception throughout the duration of penicillin therapy.
- Instruct the patient to report the following to the health care provider: any unusual bleeding or bruising, severe headaches, dizziness, weakness,

sudden fever elevation, chills, sore throat, mouth sores, vaginal itching, hives, rash, severe diarrhea, or difficulty breathing.

- Instruct the patient to take oral doses of penicillin on an empty stomach (1 hour before or 2 hours after meals) with a full glass of water. Fruit juices and soft drinks should be avoided with oral penicillin.
- Inform the patient that antibiotics should be continued for the full course of therapy, usually 10 days, at equally spaced times around the clock for efficacy, even when the infection has subsided.
- Tell the patient to take adequate hydration to replace fluids that are lost from diarrhea. Small frequent meals may help to ensure adequate nutrition.
- Monitor the patient's signs and symptoms of infection for improvement or failure to resolve infection.

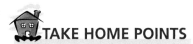

TAKE HOME POINTS

Offer frequent mouth care, ice chips, or sugarless candy to suck, which helps relieve discomfort from stomatitis.

Do You UNDERSTAND?

DIRECTIONS: Provide appropriate responses to the following questions and statement.

1. What is the most unique adverse effect of penicillin therapy?

   _____
   _____

2. What are some examples of hypersensitivity responses to penicillin?

   _____
   _____

3. List four types of penicillins and give one example of each.

   _____
   _____
   _____
   _____

Answers: 1. black, furry tongue; 2. rash, pruritus, fever, wheezing, severe dyspnea, stridor, nausea, vomiting, tachycardia, diaphoresis, vertigo, hypotension, loss of consciousness, and death; 3. natural penicillins (penicillin G), penicillinase-resistant penicillins (oxacillin), aminopenicillins (amoxicillin), extended-spectrum penicillins (ticarcillin).

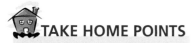

What IS a Cephalosporin?

Cephalosporin	Trade Names	Uses
First generation		
cephalexin	Keflex	Treatment of respiratory, GU, soft tissue, skin, and
[seff-uh-LEX-in]	Biocef	bone infections and otitis media in children
Second generation		
cefoxitin	Mefoxin	Treatment of lower respiratory, GU tract, skin,
[se-FOX-i-tin]		bone, and joint infections
Third generation		
ceftriaxone	Rocephin	Treatment of perioperative prophylaxis and lower
[seff-try-AX-one]		respiratory, meningitis, skin, bone, joint, pelvic,
		and intraabdominal infections
Fourth generation		
cefepime	Maxipime	Treatment of pneumonia and skin and
[SEFF-eh-pim]		GU infections

Action

Cephalosporins are semisynthetic antibiotics that are organized into four generations based on their order of development. Each generation has increasing activity against gram-negative bacteria and anaerobes. Cephalosporins are bactericidal and act on bacteria by interfering with bacterial cell wall synthesis. The bacterial cell walls weaken, swell, and burst from increased osmotic pressure within the cell, causing bacterial cell death.

First-generation cephalosporins are primarily used for gram-positive bacteria and have moderate activity against gram-negative bacteria. Second-generation cephalosporins have enhanced activity against bacteria that are susceptible to the first-generation cephalosporins, as well as gram-negative bacteria. Third-generation cephalosporins have enhanced activity against bacteria that are susceptible to first- and second-generation cephalosporins and unusual strains of enteric bacteria. Fourth-generation cephalosporins have a greater spectrum of antibiotic activity and greater stability against β-lactamase enzymes than third-generations. Fourth generations are also active against both gram-positive and gram-negative bacteria and unusual strains of enteric bacteria.

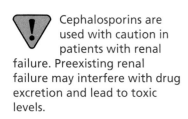

Cephalosporins are used with caution in patients with renal failure. Preexisting renal failure may interfere with drug excretion and lead to toxic levels.

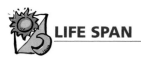

LIFE SPAN

Caution should also be taken in pregnant and lactating women because of the potential risk to the fetus or infant.

Uses

Cephalosporins are effective in treating sinusitis, pharyngitis, laryngitis, tonsillitis, bronchitis, otitis media, skin infections, urinary tract infections, abdominal infections, pelvic inflammatory disease, septicemia, meningitis, and osteomyelitis. They are used prophylactically in patients undergoing surgery involving the GI or genitourinary (GU) tract, bone, or skin.

What You NEED TO KNOW

Contraindications/Precautions

Because of the cross-sensitivity, cephalosporins are contraindicated for patients with known allergies to cephalosporins or penicillins.

Drug Interactions

Consuming alcohol while taking cefmetazole, cefoperazone, or cefotetan will induce a disulfiram-like reaction. A disulfiram reaction involves tremors, nausea, severe vomiting, diarrhea, and either hypotension or hypertension. This reaction may occur up to 72 hours after the drug is discontinued. Drugs that promote anticoagulation may increase bleeding time when used concurrently with cephalosporins. Probenecid delays renal excretion of some cephalosporins and prolongs their effect. Cephalosporins given concurrently with aminoglycosides may lead to an increased risk for nephrotoxicity.

Adverse Effects

Cephalosporins are usually tolerated well and are one of the safest types of antibiotics. Five to ten percent of penicillin-sensitive patients are also sensitive to cephalosporins because of the structural similarity between the two classes of drugs. Common systemic hypersensitivity reactions involve rash, pruritus, fever, chills, urticaria, joint pain or inflammation, edema, erythema, and eosinophilia.

The most common adverse effects of cephalosporins involve the GI effects of anorexia, nausea, flatulence, vomiting, abdominal pain, and diarrhea. Other GI adverse effects that may occur are taste alteration, decreased salivation, dyspepsia, glossitis, and hepatic dysfunction. Additional adverse effects include dizziness, hallucinations, malaise, fatigue, nightmares, headache, bleeding tendencies, paresthesia, menstrual irregularities, vaginitis, genital pruritus, vaginal moniliasis, and nephrotoxicity. An overgrowth of nonsusceptible microorganisms (superinfection) is associated more frequently with third-generation cephalosporins compared with the other generations.

TAKE HOME POINTS

- Cephalosporin antibiotic therapy requires equidistant spacing to maintain an effective blood level.
- Cephalosporins may cause false-positive results for the Coombs' test, and cefotetan can cause falsely elevated serum and urine creatinine concentrations. When cephalosporins are taken concurrently with aminoglycosides, the patient should be monitored frequently for nephrotoxicity (elevated BUN and creatinine levels) to determine any needed dose adjustment.
- Cephalosporin therapy should be continued 48 to 72 hours after the patient reaches an asymptomatic state (usually 10 days) or 24 to 48 hours after surgery when used for perioperative prophylaxis.
- Cefmetazole, cefoperazone, and cefotetan will induce a disulfiram-like reaction when taken with alcohol.
- Monitor prothrombin times when administering cephalosporins because concurrent administration of anticoagulants may increase bleeding time.

What You DO

Nursing Responsibilities

Many cephalosporins can be administered orally, but others must be administered parenterally. Cephalosporin drug therapy is usually continued for 48 to 72 hours after the patient reaches an asymptomatic state. Perioperative prophylaxis is usually discontinued within 24 to 48 hours after surgery. When administering cephalosporins, the nurse should:

- Check the IM site for evidence of local abscess and the IV site for phlebitis. Discontinue the IV site and restart at another location when phlebitis occurs. Warm compresses relieve the pain and edema of a local abscess.
- Schedule cephalosporins at equally spaced times throughout a 24-hour period.
- Monitor renal and hepatic function studies throughout cephalosporin therapy because they have been shown to cause transient alterations in various test results, including blood urea nitrogen (BUN), alanine aminotransferase (ALT), serum glutamic pyruvic transaminase (SGPT), aspartate aminotransferase (AST), alkaline phosphatase, lactate dehydrogenase (LDH), and bilirubin levels.
- Teach the patient who is taking the cephalosporin to continue the full course of treatment.
- Instruct the patient to take the medication with a small meal or snack to decrease GI effects. Small frequent meals can help ensure adequate nutrition.
- Inform the patient to perform adequate hydration to replace fluids that are lost with diarrhea. Frequent oral care and sucking ice chips or sugarless candy may relieve stomatitis discomfort.
- Counsel the patient to avoid consuming alcohol until 72 hours after drug discontinuation to avoid the disulfiram-like reaction.
- Watch prothrombin times for appropriate dose adjustment when oral anticoagulants are administered concurrently with cephalosporins.
- Monitor the patient's signs and symptoms of infection for improvement or failure to resolve infection.
- Instruct the patient to report bleeding gums or bruising, which requires a reduction of the oral anticoagulant dose.
- Advise the patient to report difficulty breathing, severe headache, severe diarrhea, dizziness, weakness, and superinfections to the health care provider.

Do You UNDERSTAND?

DIRECTIONS: Fill in the blanks with appropriate responses to the following question and statements.

1. Which generation cephalosporin is most associated with super-infections? _____

2. List five signs of a disulfiram-like reaction and the three cephalosporins that cause this reaction to alcohol.

   _____

   _____

   _____

   _____

   _____

3. Ceftriaxone (Rocephin) is a _____-generation drug and is used against _____ microorganisms.

4. Cephalexin (Keflex) is a _____-generation drug and is used against _____ microorganisms.

What IS a Sulfonamide?

Sulfonamide	Trade Names	Uses
sulfisoxazole [sull-fih-SOX-uh-zole]	Gantrisin	Treatment of conjunctivitis, otitis media, UTI, and meningococci
trimethoprim-sulfamethoxazole [try-METH-oh-prim–suhl-fuh-meth-OX-uh-zole]	Bactrim Septra	Treatment of UTI, otitis media, and bronchitis
sulfasalazine [SULL-fuh-SAL-uh-zeen]	Azulfidine	Treatment of ulcerative colitis

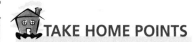

TAKE HOME POINTS

Some bacteria are able to alter their metabolic pathways to use precursors or other forms of folic acid, thereby developing resistance to the antibacterial action of sulfonamides. After resistance to one sulfonamide develops, cross-resistance to other sulfonamides is common.

Action

Sulfonamides (**sulfa drugs**) are synthetic derivatives that are bacteriostatic, which means they have the ability to inhibit the formation of new bacteria but have no effect on bacteria that are already formed. Sulfonamides compete with para-aminobenzoic acid (PABA) and prevent

Answers: 1. third; 2. tremors, nausea, severe vomiting, diarrhea, and hypotension or hypertension; cefmetazole, cefoperazone, and cefotetan; 3. third, gram-positive and negative cocci and unusual strains of enteric microorganisms; 4. first, gram-positive cocci.

PABA from uniting with folic acid to form new bacteria, thereby preventing the growth of bacteria. The sulfonamides, rather than PABA, enter the reaction, competing for the enzyme involved and causing the formation of nonfunctional derivatives of folic acid. Because bacteria require PABA to unite with folic acid—an agent that is required for the synthesis of deoxyribonucleic acid (DNA), ribonucleic acid (RNA), and proteins—bacterial cell replication is halted. Therefore sulfonamides stop growth, development, and multiplication of new bacteria but do not kill mature, fully formed bacteria. Bacteria that can use preformed folic acid are unaffected by sulfonamides. Therefore the growth of human or host cells are unaffected by sulfonamides because they can use preformed folic acid.

Uses

Sulfonamides are bacteriostatic against a wide range of gram-positive and gram-negative bacteria. Sulfonamides are indicated for the treatment of otitis media, bronchitis, urinary tract infections (UTIs), ulcerative colitis, chlamydia, gonorrhea, and other sexually transmitted diseases (STDs), as well as typhoid fever, dermatitis herpetiformis, *Pneumocystis carinii* pneumonia, toxoplasmosis, brucellosis, and shigellosis. Sulfonamides are also used prophylactically in patients with a history of rheumatic fever, penicillin allergies, granulocytopenia, in children who are infected with human immunodeficiency virus (HIV), and in patients with traveler's diarrhea. Because of the emergence of resistant bacteria and the development of newer antibiotics, sulfonamides are no longer widely used. However, sulfonamides remain inexpensive; thus when cost is an issue, they are used for UTIs and chronic contagious conjunctivitis (**trachoma**).

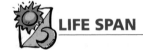

LIFE SPAN

Sulfonamides are contraindicated during pregnancy and lactation.

Sulfonamide antibiotics should be used cautiously in patients with a history of peptic ulcers or renal disorders because these drugs tend to irritate the gastric mucosa and have a potential for nephrotoxicity.

What You NEED TO KNOW

Contraindications/Precautions

Sulfonamides are contraindicated for patients with any known allergy to sulfonamides, sulfonylureas, or thiazide diuretics because of the possibility of cross-sensitivity. Sulfonamides are also contraindicated for patients with blood dyscrasias, porphyria, or those who are within 2 to 3 weeks of an acute gout attack.

Drug Interactions

When sulfonamides are administered concurrently with other drugs, interactions may occur. Alcohol combined with a sulfonamide leads to increased blood urate levels. When taken with a sulfonamide, salicylates decrease uricosuric activity. Concurrent drugs that increase the risk for hypoglycemia include sulfonylurea agents or those that stimulate insulin release. When warfarin is taken with sulfonamides, its effects are increased and bleeding may occur. Other interactions include decreased renal excretion of methotrexate and decreased hepatic clearance of phenytoin, barbiturates, tolbutamide, and uricosurics; increased thrombocytopenia when taken with thiazide diuretics; and increased nephrotoxicity when taken with cyclosporine.

Adverse Effects

Sulfonamide adverse effects have varying degrees of severity and may include hypersensitivity reactions. The most common adverse effects of sulfonamides include rash, headache, fever, anorexia, nausea, vomiting, abdominal pain, and diarrhea. Other adverse effects include urticaria, weakness, flushing, drowsiness, dizziness, stomatitis, glossitis, photosensitivity, ataxia, convulsions, depression, peripheral neuritis, hematuria, oliguria, anuria, uric acid kidney stones, and exacerbations of gout. Older sulfonamides have low solubility and present a high risk for crystalluria, resulting in renal damage. Newer sulfonamides have increased solubility, but the potential for crystalluria remains.

What You DO

Nursing Responsibilities

Sulfonamides are usually administered orally, on an empty stomach, 1 hour before or 2 hours after meals, and with a full glass of water. If GI distress occurs, sulfonamides may be taken with small, frequent meals or snacks. After oral administration, peak plasma levels are generally reached within 4 hours. In severe infections, sulfonamides are given IV for a faster response. The peak action after IV administration occurs in 1 hour. When administering sulfonamides, the nurse should:

- Watch complete blood count (CBC) for early detection of bone marrow depression and the development of blood dyscrasias.

TAKE HOME POINTS

Cross-sensitivity may exist among sulfonamides, sulfonylureas, or thiazide diuretics.

- Life-threatening adverse effects of sulfonamides include anaphylaxis, blood dyscrasias, convulsions, hepatic and renal damage, and Stevens-Johnson syndrome.
- Counsel patients to avoid driving or operating dangerous machinery because of the adverse effects of dizziness, lethargy, and ataxia.

TAKE HOME POINTS

- Antibiotics require appropriate spacing between doses to maintain a certain blood level for effectiveness.
- Teach the patient to increase fluid intake to 2 liters per day to prevent crystalluria and replace fluids.

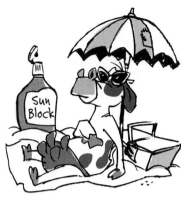

Keep it shady.

- Monitor renal and liver function tests before and throughout administration of sulfonamides to assure adequate functioning of these organs.
- Check glucose levels of patients who are taking sulfonylurea agents or other drugs that stimulate insulin release because dose adjustments of the antidiabetic agents may be required.
- Monitor the patient's signs and symptoms of infection for improvement or failure to resolve infection.
- Teach the patient to increase fluid intake to prevent crystalluria and replace fluids that are lost from diarrhea.
- Tell the patient to store sulfonamides in a tight, light-resistant container at room temperature.
- Inform the patient that frequent oral care and sucking on ice chips or sugarless candy may relieve discomfort of stomatitis.
- Advise the patient to avoid sunlight, use a sunscreen, and wear protective clothing to prevent sunburns.
- Encourage the patient to adhere to the full treatment length for therapeutic effects and to prevent a superinfection.
- Instruct patients to notify their health care provider in the event of hypersensitivity reaction, difficulty breathing, rash, ringing in the ears, fever, sore throat, or blood in the urine.

Do You UNDERSTAND?

DIRECTIONS: **Indicate in the space provided whether the statement is** *true* **or** *false.* **If the answer is false, correct the statement to make it true (using the margin space).**

_____ 1. Sulfonamides may cause increased thrombocytopenia when taken with thiazide diuretics.

_____ 2. Sulfasalazine (Azulfidine) should be taken for 5 days to prevent superinfections.

_____ 3. A unique adverse effect of sulfonamides that is linked to their low solubility is crystalluria.

Answers: 1. true; 2. false; they should be taken for 10 days; 3. true.

What IS an Aminoglycoside?

Aminoglycosides	Trade Names	Uses
gentamicin sulfate [JEN-tuh-MY-sin]	Garamycin	Treatment of serious infections, especially gram-negative
amikacin sulfate [am-ih-KAY-sin]	Amikin	Treatment of serious infections, especially gram-negative
kanamycin sulfate [kan-uh-MY-sin]	Kantrex	Treatment of serious infections, especially gram-negative
tobramycin sulfate [TOE-bruh-MY-sin]	Nebcin	Treatment of serious infections, especially gram-negative

Action

Aminoglycosides are bactericidal; they bind irreversibly to both the 30S and 50S ribosomes to prevent bacterial protein synthesis. When ribosomes stop functioning, protein synthesis is disrupted and the bacterial cell eventually dies.

Uses

Because aminoglycosides are potent, they are usually reserved for more serious, life-threatening infections. These medications kill aerobic gram-positive and gram-negative bacteria, mycobacteria, aerobic gram-negative bacilli, and some protozoa. Aminoglycosides are used to treat serious nosocomial infections (i.e., gram-negative bacteremia, peritonitis, pneumonia).

A synergistic effect may be achieved by administering aminoglycosides in combination therapy with cephalosporins, penicillins, or vancomycin for greater effectiveness. Gentamicin is usually combined with penicillin to treat amebic dysentery. Extended-spectrum penicillins are usually combined with an aminoglycoside to treat serious pseudomonas infections.

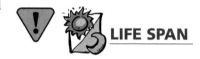

LIFE SPAN

Aminoglycosides should be administered with caution in neonates because of their immature renal systems. Fetal damage may occur when these drugs are given to pregnant or lactating women. Aminoglycosides are contraindicated during lactation.

What You NEED TO KNOW

Contraindications/Precautions

Aminoglycosides are contraindicated for patients with known allergies, renal or hepatic disease, preexisting hearing loss, active herpes, mycobacterial infections, myasthenia gravis, and parkinsonism.

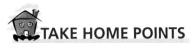

TAKE HOME POINTS

Allergic reactions to aminoglycosides are rare. Evidence of an allergic reaction involves a rash, urticaria, pruritus, generalized burning, and fever.

An IV aminoglycoside should not be mixed in solution with extended-spectrum penicillins because the aminoglycoside will be inactivated.

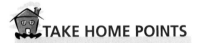

TAKE HOME POINTS

A baseline culture and sensitivity is required before initiating antibiotic therapy.

Drug Interactions

The concurrent administration of dimenhydrinate can mask aminoglycoside toxicity. Co-administrating aminoglycosides and a neuromuscular blocking agent can lead to peripheral nerve toxicity and paralysis. Co-administration with potent diuretics increases the incidence of ototoxicity, nephrotoxicity, and neurotoxicity. Because aminoglycosides decrease intestinal vitamin K synthesis, concurrent use of oral anticoagulants can increase bleeding time.

Adverse Effects

Adverse effects from aminoglycosides include nausea, vomiting, stomatitis, diarrhea, weight loss, headache, paresthesia, neuromuscular blockade, dizziness, vertigo, skin rash, fever, and superinfections. Cardiovascular effects, such as palpitations, hypotension, and hypertension, may also occur.

Aminoglycosides are potent antibiotics and are capable of producing potentially serious toxicities. Common toxicities that may result from aminoglycosides are nephrotoxicity and ototoxicity. Symptoms of ototoxicity or eighth cranial nerve damage include dizziness, tinnitus, vertigo, nystagmus, ataxia, and hearing loss. Gentamicin and streptomycin are the primary culprits that cause toxicity to the vestibular portion of the eighth cranial nerve. Kanamycin, amikacin, and netilmicin primarily are associated with cochlear toxicity, although tobramycin may cause both types of ototoxicity. Nephrotoxicity involves symptoms of urinary casts, proteinuria, and increased BUN and serum creatinine levels. Patients at higher risk for nephrotoxicity are those with preexisting renal impairment and those who are taking other concurrent nephrotoxic drugs. Depressed bone marrow toxicity may result from aminoglycosides, leading to eosinophilia and immune suppression. Toxicity damage is usually associated with high doses, high trough levels, or prolonged therapy.

What You DO

Nursing Responsibilities

Aminoglycosides have negligible GI absorption. When an aminoglycoside is ordered for IV administration, the prepared solution should be refrigerated until use and infused over at least 30 minutes. When administering aminoglycosides, the nurse should:

- Administer an aminoglycoside and a penicillin at least 2 hours apart.
- Draw peak and trough levels periodically throughout aminoglycoside therapy to evaluate effectiveness and for early detection of toxicity. A serum trough level is typically drawn 15 minutes before drug administration, and the peak level is drawn 30 minutes after.
- Monitor renal function tests (creatinine, BUN, and urinalysis) at least every other day in patients with impaired renal function and at least once a week in patients with normal renal function to detect toxicity early.
- Watch the patient's CBC results for evidence of bone marrow suppression.
- Monitor the patient's signs and symptoms of infection for improvement and failure to resolve infection.
- Tell the patient to consume adequate fluids to overcome fluid loss from diarrhea and to decrease nephrotoxicity.
- Encourage the patient to take the full course of treatment.
- Teach the patient safety precautions (i.e., avoidance of driving or operating hazardous machinery).
- Instruct the patient to report any difficulty breathing, severe headache, loss of hearing or tinnitus, or a decreased urine output to the health care provider.
- Instruct the patient to report bleeding to the health care provider immediately because aminoglycosides decrease intestinal vitamin K, and concurrent use of oral anticoagulants can increase bleeding time.

Do You UNDERSTAND?

DIRECTIONS: Provide an accurate response to each of the following statements.

1. List five possible signs of ototoxicity.

   _____

   _____

   _____

   _____

   _____

2. List three possible signs of nephrotoxicity.

   _____

   _____

   _____

3. Identify one nursing measure that can be used to prevent nephrotoxicity during aminoglycoside therapy.

   _____

4. Identify one antibiotic that should not be mixed with an aminoglycoside and should be spaced at least 2 hours apart.

   _____

What IS a Tetracycline?

Because the targeted bacterial protein is similar to a protein found in human cells, tetracyclines in high concentrations can be toxic to humans.

Tetracyclines	Trade Names	Uses
tetracycline [the-truh-SIGH-kleen]	Achromycin	Treatment of gram-positive and gram-negative infections
doxycycline [DOX-ee-SIGH-kleen]	Vibramycin	Treatment of gram-positive and gram-negative infections
demeclocycline [dem-e-klo-SIGH-kleen]	Declomycin	Treatment of gram-positive and gram-negative infections

Action

Tetracyclines are bacteriostatic, semisynthetic antibiotics that enter bacterial cells by passive diffusion and an active transport system.

Answers: 1. dizziness, tinnitus, nystagmus, ataxia, and hearing loss; 2. proteinuria, increased BUN and creatinine levels, and urinary casts; 3. encourage fluids for adequate hydration; 4. extended-spectrum penicillin.

Tetracyclines compete for the binding of the 30S subunit site of the RNA ribosome to decrease bacterial growth, repair, and multiplication, thereby obstructing protein cell wall synthesis in susceptible bacteria. Tetracyclines may be bactericidal in high concentrations or against highly susceptible bacteria.

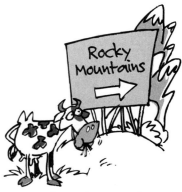

Don't forget the tetracyclines!

Uses

Because broad-spectrum antibiotics are effective against both gram-positive and gram-negative bacteria, tetracyclines are useful in treating several uncommon infections. Tetracyclines are considered the first-line drug defense for Rocky Mountain spotted fever and other rickettsial infections, as well as pneumonia, typhus, trachoma, brucellosis, peptic ulcer disease, lymphogranuloma venereum, urethritis, cervicitis, *Chlamydia*, and cholera. Doxycycline has proven to be effective against malaria.

Additional uses for tetracyclines include treatment of acne, sinusitis, cystitis, tetanus, rat-bite fever, tropical sprue (bacterial infection of the intestine found in tropical regions, characterized by weakness, weight loss, and malabsorption of essential nutrients), tularemia (an acute plague-type infection from an infected tick, other infected insect or animal, or infected food or water), anthrax, yaws (infectious disease that is caused by a spirochete), and plague. When patients are allergic to penicillin, tetracyclines are frequently used to treat certain STDs, urinary and respiratory tract infections, and meningitis.

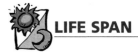

LIFE SPAN

Tetracyclines are contraindicated for women during pregnancy and lactation and for children under 8 years of age because of possible damage of their bones and teeth.

What You NEED TO KNOW

Contraindications/Precautions

Tetracyclines are contraindicated for patients with renal and hepatic dysfunction and bile duct obstruction. Ocular tetracyclines are contraindicated for patients with eye infections that may be exacerbated by the loss of normal bacterial flora.

Tetracyclines should be used cautiously in patients with asthma, myasthenia gravis, or those who are malnourished.

Drug Interactions

With the exception of doxycycline and minocycline, absorption of tetracyclines is compromised when taken with dairy products and concurrent administration of antacids that contain calcium, magnesium, aluminum, or iron. Because these products prevent tetracycline absorption, antibacterial efficacy is decreased.

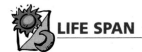

LIFE SPAN

Concurrent use of tetracycline with oral contraceptives leads to breakthrough bleeding, altered GI bacterial flora, decreased contraceptive effectiveness, and increased risk of pregnancy.

Because tetracyclines have a high affinity for calcium, prolonged use during the fourth fetal month through the eighth year of life when tooth development occurs may cause inadequate calcium deposit and discoloration of both deciduous and permanent teeth.

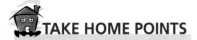

TAKE HOME POINTS

- Instruct patients to avoid tetracyclines during lactation to prevent discoloration of the child's teeth.
- Instruct patients that adequate absorption is prevented when tetracyclines are taken with dairy products, antacids, or iron.
- When tetracyclines are necessary for the woman who is taking oral contraceptives, additional barrier contraceptives must be used.

High-dose IV tetracycline that exceeds 2 g/day has been associated with liver failure and death.

When tetracyclines are taken with penicillin, the bactericidal action of penicillin is decreased. Concurrent use of doxycycline with barbiturates, carbamazepine, and phenytoin increases the metabolism of tetracyclines. Cimetidine, taken concurrently, decreases the absorption of tetracyclines. Nephrotoxicity may occur when tetracyclines are taken with the general anesthetic methoxyflurane. When tetracyclines are given concurrently with digitalis, the risk for digitalis toxicity is increased.

Adverse Effects

The most common adverse effects of tetracyclines are nausea, abdominal cramping and distention, vomiting, diarrhea, and superinfections. A red rash upon exposure to sunlight is more common with demeclocycline and doxycycline compared with other tetracyclines; however, photosensitivity reactions may occur with any tetracycline. Nephrotoxicity may occur following high doses of tetracyclines or when concurrent with other nephrotoxic drugs.

Minocycline may evoke dizziness and vestibular damage resulting in difficulty in maintaining balance. A rash, glossitis, dermatitis, sore throat, dysphagia, hemolytic anemia, eosinophilia, neutropenia, thrombocytopenia, leukopenia, leukocytosis, and hepatotoxicity are other adverse effects of tetracyclines. Rare effects are hemolytic anemia and bone marrow depression. Hypersensitivity reactions include fever, headache, impaired vision, papilledema, intracranial hypertension, and anaphylaxis.

What You DO

Nursing Responsibilities

Absorption can be enhanced when taken on an empty stomach because alterations in gastric pH may decrease the absorption. Ideally, tetracyclines are given 1 hour before meals or 2 hours after meals with a full glass of water. However, when GI upset occurs, a small meal may be consumed with the drug to minimize distress. When administering tetracyclines, the nurse should:

- Space antacid doses at least 3 hours after tetracycline administration when the patient is taking both drugs.

- Provide the patient who is taking tetracyclines with adequate hydration to compensate for fluid loss from diarrhea.
- Check the dose and rate carefully when tetracycline is administered IV.
- Watch CBCs, urinalysis, and liver and kidney function tests. Several laboratory values may be altered from tetracycline therapy. Elevated BUN, creatinine, bilirubin, alkaline phosphatase, ALT and AST, and urinary levels of catecholamines and protein may be present. Additionally, hemoglobin and platelet values may be decreased, and urine glucose results may be falsely positive or falsely negative.
- Monitor the patient's signs and symptoms of infection for improvement and failure to resolve infection.
- Inform the patient that tetracyclines should be avoided during pregnancy and lactation.
- Instruct patients to use protective clothing and sunscreen to protect themselves from sunlight and ultraviolet light exposure because of a possible photosensitivity reaction. The sunscreen should not contain PABA.
- Inform patients that outdated tetracyclines should not be ingested because degraded drugs are highly nephrotoxic.
- Teach the patient to report any difficulty breathing, rash, itching, cramps, severe diarrhea, or a decrease in urine to the health care provider.

Do You UNDERSTAND?

DIRECTIONS: **Indicate in the space provided whether the statement is *true* or *false*. If the answer is false, correct the statement to make it true (using the margin space).**

_____ 1. Iron interacts with tetracyclines and decreases absorption.

_____ 2. A drug interaction of tetracyclines with oral contraceptives may lead to an increased risk for pregnancy.

_____ 3. The maximal IV tetracycline dose is 4 grams per day.

_____ 4. The patient who is taking tetracyclines should use a sunscreen with PABA.

Answers: 1. true; also milk, dairy products, antacids, and cimetidine; 2. true; 3. false; high doses over 2 grams per day have been associated with liver failure and death; 4. false; use sunscreen without PABA.

What IS a Macrolide?

Macrolides	Trade Names	Uses
erythromycin [eh-RITH-row-MY-sin]	E-Mycin	Treatment of ocular infections
azithromycin [UHZ-ith-row-MY-sin]	Zithromax	Treatment of STDs and respiratory tract, pelvic, and skin infections
clarithromycin [kluh-RITH-row-MY-sin]	Biaxin	Treatment of respiratory tract and skin infections
dirithromycin [die-RITH-row-MY-sin]	Dynabac	Treatment of respiratory tract and skin infections

Action

Macrolides are bacteriostatic or bactericidal, depending on their concentration and the offending bacteria. Macrolides bind to the 50S ribosomal subunits and inhibit polypeptide synthesis, thereby inhibiting protein synthesis. By binding to bacterial cell membranes, macrolides change protein function and cause cell death or prevent cell division.

Uses

Macrolides are used in treating mild-to-moderate infections and are effective against gram-positive and gram-negative cocci. Macrolides are also used to treat mild-to-moderate infections of the respiratory tract, sinuses, skin, GI tract, and soft tissue, as well as diphtheria, STDs, and impetigo contagiosa. Macrolides are also the drug of choice in pertussis, diphtheria, Legionnaires' disease, atypical viral pneumonia, syphilis, and Chlamydia. Macrolides are also given prophylactally before dental procedures in patients with valvular heart disease to prevent endocarditis. Erythromycin is also used to treat anthrax infection.

Macrolides should be administered with caution in patients with impaired liver or renal function and in women during pregnancy and lactation.

What You NEED TO KNOW

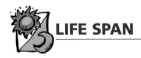

LIFE SPAN

Safety and efficacy of macrolides has not been established for patients under 12 years of age.

Contraindications/Precautions

Macrolides are contraindicated for patients with a known allergy to any macrolide because cross-sensitivity occurs. Ocular macrolides are contraindicated for patients with eye infections that may be exacerbated by the loss of normal bacterial flora.

Drug Interactions

The absorption of macrolides is decreased when they are taken with antacids. Increased effects of anticoagulants, carbamazepine, triazolam, astemizole, corticosteroids, theophylline, valproate, alfentanil, bromocriptine, cyclosporine, terfenadine, tacrolimus, and ergot alkaloids are present when macrolides are given concurrently. Macrolides may decrease the effects of zidovudine. Erythromycin may increase serum levels of digoxin. Aminoglycosides and tetracyclines should not be given together because they have similar actions and compete with each other.

> **!** When macrolides are given concurrently with astemizole, terfenadine, or cisapride, potentially fatal cardiac dysrhythmias may occur.

Adverse Effects

Macrolides are considered to have low toxicity among antibiotics and have relatively few adverse effects. The most common adverse effects of macrolides include dose-related anorexia, abnormal taste, heartburn, nausea, vomiting, abdominal cramping, stomatitis, flatulence, diarrhea, pruritus ani, reversible hearing loss, allergic reactions, and mild acute pancreatitis. These adverse effects usually resolve with continued therapy. Other adverse effects of erythromycin include headache, vertigo, dizziness, confusion, abnormal thinking, uncontrollable emotions, somnolence, tinnitus, palpitations, chest pain, bilateral hearing loss, and superinfections.

Hepatotoxicity with jaundice occurs with estolate and ethylsuccinate forms of erythromycin. Additionally, cholestatic hepatitis (from obstruction of bile flow) has been associated with erythromycin when drug therapy lasts longer than 10 days or when the drug is given repeatedly.

What You DO

Nursing Responsibilities

Macrolides may be inactivated by gastric acid; thus they are enteric-coated or buffered. Ideally, macrolides should be taken 1 hour before or 2 hours after meals for better absorption. However, because of the high incidence of GI distress, macrolides may be taken with a small snack. Erythromycin is not given IM because of painful injections and the potential formation of a sterile abscess. When administering macrolides, the nurse should:

- Teach the patient about safety precautions and using caution when driving vehicles or operating machinery.

> **!** Erythromycin stearate should not be administered with food. Macrolides should not be mixed for IV use with incompatible drugs (e.g., vitamin B complex, vitamin C, cephalothin, tetracycline, heparin, colistimethate sodium, furosemide, metaraminol bitartrate, metoclopramide hydrochloride).

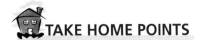

TAKE HOME POINTS

A baseline culture and sensitivity is required before initiating antibiotic therapy. IV solutions should be administered within 4 hours after reconstitution.

- Monitor liver and renal function tests to ensure adequate functioning.
- Ascertain that culture and sensitivity tests are performed before macrolide therapy to ensure that the most effective drug is given.
- Watch the patient for phlebitis during IV infusion.
- Check digoxin levels because increased levels occur when the drug is taken concurrently with macrolides. The digoxin dose may need to be adjusted throughout macrolide therapy.
- Monitor the patient's signs and symptoms of infection for improvement and failure to resolve infection.
- Inform patients that frequent mouth care and sucking on ice chips or sugarless candy may relieve discomfort.
- Tell the patient to drink an adequate amount of fluids and maintain nutrition to compensate for any nausea, vomiting, and diarrhea.
- Instruct patients to report changes in hearing, signs of cholestatic hepatitis (i.e., nausea, vomiting, abdominal pain, jaundice, rash), and allergic reactions to the health care provider.

Do You UNDERSTAND?

DIRECTIONS: Provide accurate responses to the following statements and question.

1. List three of the most common adverse effects of macrolides.

   _____

   _____

2. Macrolides are contraindicated for patients with what condition?

   _____

3. List two preferred routes of macrolide administration.

   _____

   _____

Answers: 1. GI distress, anorexia, abnormal taste; 2. preexisting liver disease; 3. orally, IV.

What IS a Fluoroquinolone?

Fluoroquinolones	Trade Names	Uses
ciprofloxacin [sip-ROW-FLOX-ah-sin]	Cipro	Treatment of STDs and lower respiratory, GU, bone, skin, and joint infections
levofloxacin [lee-voe-FLOX-ah-sin]	Levaquin	Treatment of respiratory, GU, and skin infections

Action

Fluoroquinolones are bactericidal against a broad spectrum of bacteria. Fluoroquinolones interfere with DNA gyrase, which is an enzyme that is required to synthesize bacterial DNA and for growth and reproduction.

Uses

Fluoroquinolones are active against a wide range of gram-positive and gram-negative bacteria and are used to treat infections involving the respiratory, urinary, and GI tracts, infections of the sinus, skin, soft tissue, bones, joints, and prostate, as well as anthrax infection, infectious diarrhea, and STDs. Newer fluoroquinolones—gatifloxacin and moxifloxacin—are available for once-a-day treatment of community-acquired pneumonia, acute bacterial exacerbations of chronic bronchitis, and acute sinusitis.

What You NEED TO KNOW

Contraindications/Precautions

Fluoroquinolones are contraindicated for women during pregnancy and lactation and for children under 18 years of age.

Drug Interactions

Fluoroquinolones increase xanthine effects of theophylline and caffeine, both of which predispose a patient to seizures. When given concurrently with fluoroquinolones, the effects of anticoagulants are increased. Probenecid interferes with renal tubular secretion. Sucralfate and antacids that contain magnesium or aluminum hydroxide decrease the effect of fluoroquinolones. The risk for nephrotoxicity may be increased

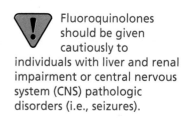 Fluoroquinolones should be given cautiously to individuals with liver and renal impairment or central nervous system (CNS) pathologic disorders (i.e., seizures).

when fluoroquinolones are taken concurrently with cyclosporine. Nitrofurantoin may interfere with the antibacterial effects of norfloxacin. The elimination of fluoroquinolones may be decreased by cimetidine. When fluoroquinolone administration is combined with nonsteroidal antiinflammatory drugs (NSAIDs), an increased risk for CNS stimulation occurs. Additionally, dairy products and other food reduce the absorption of ciprofloxacin. Food also delays the absorption of lomefloxacin.

Adverse Effects

Instruct patients to avoid using machinery or activities that require alertness because of potential dizziness and confusion.

Fluoroquinolones may cause mild-to-moderate adverse effects, which usually disappear after the drug is discontinued. Common adverse effects include nausea, vomiting, abdominal discomfort, headache, dizziness, insomnia, confusion, restlessness, and depression. Other adverse effects include fever, skin rash, photosensitivity, photophobia, flushing, dry mouth, unpleasant taste, anorexia, pruritus, urticaria, visual difficulty, superinfections, and renal impairment. Crystalluria may occur with large doses of fluoroquinolone. The most serious adverse effects are seizures and tendon injury. Rare adverse effects include tendonitis, vasculitis, palpitations, syncope, atrial flutter, myocardial infarction (MI), respiratory difficulty, leukopenia, eosinophilia, anaphylaxis, and heart attack. Cross-sensitivity among fluoroquinolones may occur. Serious adverse effects may occur after a single dose.

What You DO

Nursing Responsibilities

Ciprofloxacin is the most widely used fluoroquinolone and can be administered in oral, injectable, and topical forms. When administering ciprofloxacin IV, the nurse should infuse the drug over 60 minutes. When administration is too rapid, seizures may occur. When giving fluoroquinolones, the nurse should:

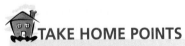

TAKE HOME POINTS

Frequent mouth care and sucking on ice chips or sugarless candy may relieve discomfort.

- Instruct the patient to complete the full course of treatment to prevent the development of resistant strains of bacteria.
- Watch theophylline, carbamazepine, and warfarin levels because these drugs may require dose adjustment.
- Check renal and liver function tests for impairment and possible dose reduction.

- Instruct patients to maintain an adequate fluid intake to compensate for diarrhea and to prevent crystalluria.
- Teach the patient to avoid milk products, antacids, iron, or sucralfate because these agents decrease the fluoroquinolone effect.
- Tell patients to use protective clothing and sunscreen to protect themselves from exposure to sunlight and ultraviolet light.
- Instruct patients to report difficulty breathing, severe headache, severe diarrhea, fainting, and heart palpitations to the health care provider.
- Monitor the patient's cardiac rhythm because taking fluoroquinolones concurrently with drugs that prolong the Q-T interval or cause torsades de pointes (i.e., quinidine, procainamide, amiodarone, sotalol, bepridil, erythromycin, terfenadine, astemizole, cisapride, pentamidine, tricyclics, phenothiazines) may lead to fatal cardiac dysrhythmias.
- Watch the patients who are taking fluoroquinolones and NSAIDs for seizures.
- Monitor the patient's signs and symptoms of infection for improvement or failure to resolve infection.

Do You UNDERSTAND?

DIRECTIONS: Match the statements from Column A to the corresponding responses in Column B.

Column A	Column B
_____ 1. Peak fluoroquinolone serum level	a. 60 minutes
_____ 2. Concurrent fluoroquinolones and NSAIDs can lead to these	b. Crystalluria
_____ 3. IV Cipro should be infused over	c. 1 to 3 hours
_____ 4. Adverse effect of large doses of fluoroquinolones	d. Seizures

Answers: 1. c; 2. d; 3. a; 4. b.

What IS a Miscellaneous Antibiotic?

Miscellaneous Antibiotics	Trade Names	Uses
aztreonam [azz-TREE-oh-nam]	Azactam	Treatment of urinary, lower respiratory, skin, and intraabdominal infections
clindamycin [KLIN-duh-MY-sin]	Cleocin	Treatment of serious abdominal and pelvic infections
imipenem-cilastatin [ih-mih-PEN-em–SIGH-luh-STAT-in]	Primaxin	Treatment of serious urinary, lower respiratory, skin, bone, joint, and intraabdominal infections
vancomycin [van-koe-MY-sin]	Vancocin	Treatment of serious infections
telithromycin [teh-lih-throw-MY-sin]	Ketek	Treatment of chronic bronchitis, acute bacterial sinusitis, and mild-to-moderate community-acquired pneumonia

Action

Several other antibiotics that do not fit into the previous classifications are discussed in this section. Aztreonam disrupts cell wall synthesis of bacteria that causes a leakage of intracellular contents and cell death. This drug is the only antibiotic in the monobactam classification and is bactericidal against gram-negative aerobic bacteria; thus it has a narrow spectrum of activity. Clindamycin is an example of the lincosamide antibiotic classification, which binds to the 50S subunit of the bacterial ribosomes and inhibits protein synthesis.

Imipenem/cilastatin is composed of imipenem (a β-lactam antibiotic) and cilastatin (an inhibitor of dipeptidase inactivation of imipenem). Imipenem is bacteriocidal because mucopeptide synthesis in bacterial cell walls is inhibited, which leads to cell death. This drug has the greatest spectrum of any β-lactam antibiotic. Vancomycin inhibits bacterial cell wall synthesis and promotes bacterial lysis and death. Vancomycin also binds to the molecules that serve as precursors for cell wall biosynthesis, thereby disrupting the bacterial cell wall.

Telithromycin is the first drug in a new classification called *ketolide*. The action is similar to macrolides, but ketolides have two binding sites on the bacterial ribosomes.

Uses

Aztreonam is indicated in the treatment of septicemia and for skin, intraabdominal, urinary tract, and gynecologic infections. Because aztreonam differs greatly in structure from β-lactam antibiotics, little cross-allergenicity exists between aztreonam with penicillins and cephalosporins. Therefore aztreonam appears to be a safe alternative for patients with β-lactam allergies.

Clindamycin is used in severe anaerobic infections outside the CNS. Clindamycin is a preferred drug for abdominal and pelvic infections and is also used for acne vulgaris and bacterial vaginosis.

Imipenem/cilastatin is used to treat serious infections in the respiratory tract, urinary tract, bones, joints, skin, intraabdominal area, gynecologic system, endocarditis, and bacterial septicemia.

Vancomycin is used to treat life-threatening infections and is the treatment of choice for antibiotic-associated pseudomembranous colitis (AAPC).

Telithromycin is effective for mild-to-moderate respiratory tract infections, such as acute exacerbation of chronic bronchitis, acute bacterial sinusitis, and community-acquired pneumonia.

What You NEED TO KNOW

Contraindications/Precautions

Clindamycin is contraindicated for patients with lincosamide hypersensitivity, regional enteritis, and ulcerative colitis. Imipenem/cilastatin is contraindicated for patients with hypersensitivity. Vancomycin is contraindicated for patients with hypersensitivity, previous hearing loss, and concurrent ototoxic or nephrotoxic drugs.

Telithromycin is contraindicated in patients with a hypersensitivity to a ketolide or any macrolide antibiotic. This new drug is also contraindicated in patients who are taking cisapride or pimozide and those who have myasthenia gravis, hypokalemia, or hypomagnesemia.

Drug Interactions

The renal elimination of aztreonam is slowed when it is given concurrently with probenecid. When clindamycin is given with neuromuscular blocking agents, the neuromuscular blocking action is enhanced. Clindamycin, erythromycin, and chloramphenicol may antagonize the effects of one another when given together because the ribosomal sites (at which the lincosamides bind) overlap. The antibiotic effect of imipenem/cilastatin may be antagonized by aztreonam, penicillin, or cephalosporins. Vancomycin leads to the risk for otic and renal toxicities when given

 Aztreonam should be used with caution in patients with hypersensitivity to penicillin or cephalosporins and patients with renal or hepatic dysfunction.

Aztreonam is contraindicated for women during pregnancy and lactation and for children. Clindamycin is contraindicated for women during pregnancy and lactation and for infants under 1 month of age. Imipenem/cilastatin is contraindicated for women during pregnancy and for children under 12 years of age. Vancomycin is contraindicated during pregnancy.

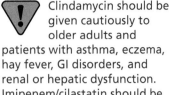

Clindamycin should be given cautiously to older adults and patients with asthma, eczema, hay fever, GI disorders, and renal or hepatic dysfunction. Imipenem/cilastatin should be used with caution in lactating women, as well as in patients with seizures, head injuries or other CNS disorders, renal impairment, and penicillin hypersensitivity. Vancomycin should be given cautiously to neonates and patients with renal dysfunction.

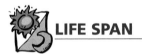

LIFE SPAN

The most severe toxicity of clindamycin is pseudomembranous colitis which is a superinfection with profuse, watery diarrhea of up to 10 to 20 stools per day. The condition may be fatal without treatment. Rapid IV administration may cause hypotension, dysrhythmias, and cardiac arrest.

concurrently with aminoglycosides, amphotericin B, colistin, polymyxin B, and other ototoxic or nephrotoxic drugs.

Adverse Effects

Because aztreonam is well tolerated, adverse effects are few. The most common adverse effects are pain and thrombophlebitis at the injection site. Other adverse effects include headache, dizziness, confusion, tinnitus, nasal congestion, sneezing, diplopia, nausea, vomiting, diarrhea, paresthesia, insomnia, seizures, urticaria, rash, superinfections, elevation of liver function tests, and eosinophilia.

Adverse effects of clindamycin include hypersensitivity, rash, skin dryness, loss of taste, nausea, vomiting, abdominal pain, flatulence, diarrhea, abnormal liver function tests, and blood dyscrasias.

Imipenem/cilastatin is well tolerated. Adverse effects include hypersensitivity, rash, pruritus, fever, nausea, vomiting, and diarrhea. Rare adverse effects from imipenem/cilastatin include superinfections and seizures.

Vancomycin can cause highly toxic adverse effects. Adverse effects that are associated with vancomycin include superinfections, ototoxicity, and renal failure. "Red man syndrome" or "red neck syndrome" can also occur as a result of an increase in histamine release following an infusion that is too rapid. Fever, rash, chills, paresthesia, tachycardia, sudden and severe hypotension, and flushing or redness on the neck and back are characteristics of "red man syndrome."

What You DO

Nursing Responsibilities

When administered IM, aztreonam should be injected deeply into large muscle mass. (Refer to *Saunders Nursing Survival Guide: Drug Calculations and Drug Administration*, edition 2, for injection sites.) Clindamycin is unaffected by food and may be given orally, IM, or IV. When given orally, clindamycin should be followed by a full glass of water. Pseudomembranous colitis usually begins in the first week of treatment but may develop 4 to 6 weeks after treatment. Pseudomembranous colitis is treated with oral vancomycin or metronidazole, with the diarrhea subsiding in 3 to 5 days. Vancomycin can be administered orally or IV. Infusions should be administered slowly for 60 minutes or more. The vancomycin IV site should be monitored for thrombophlebitis. When administering antibiotics, the nurse should:

- Ascertain that culture and sensitivity tests are performed before administering an antibiotic to ensure that the most effective drug is given.
- Draw peak and trough levels periodically throughout vancomycin therapy to evaluate effectiveness and detect toxicity. A serum trough level is typically drawn 15 minutes before administering the drug, and the peak level is drawn 30 minutes after administration.
- Monitor hepatic and renal function tests throughout the course of treatment for early detection of dysfunction and necessary dose alteration.
- Prevent thrombophlebitis from IV antibiotic infusions by diluting the drug appropriately and frequently changing the infusion site.
- Instruct the patient to report more than five watery stools per day for the early detection of pseudomembranous colitis.

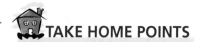

TAKE HOME POINTS

Baseline culture and sensitivity testing is required before initiating antibiotic therapy.

Do You UNDERSTAND?

DIRECTIONS: Answer the following questions with the appropriate responses.

1. Which miscellaneous antibiotic is likely to cause pseudomembranous colitis?

   _____

2. Which miscellaneous antibiotic causes "red neck syndrome"?

   _____

3. Which miscellaneous antibiotic causes severe ototoxicity?

   _____

Answers: 1. clindamycin; 2. vancomycin; 3. vancomycin.

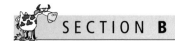

SECTION **B**

ANTIVIRALS

Viruses are intracellular parasites with no metabolic machinery of their own; they lack both a cell wall and a cell membrane and do not carry out metabolic processes. To replicate, viruses must attach to and enter a living host cell—animal, plant, or bacterium—and use its metabolic processes. Viral replication requires DNA or RNA synthesis and synthesis of viral proteins and glycosylation.

All viruses require cells to replicate. Most antiviral drugs must penetrate cells that are already infected to produce a therapeutic antiviral response. Few drugs are sufficiently selective to prevent viral replication without injury to the host. Some drugs discriminate sufficiently between cellular and viral reactions to be effective and yet relatively nontoxic. Unfortunately, only a few viral groups respond to these drugs. Many antiviral agents inhibit single steps in the viral replication cycle. These agents are considered virustatic and do not destroy a given virus but temporarily halt replication. Optimal antiviral effectiveness requires a competent host immune system that can eliminate or effectively halt virus replication. This section reviews selected antivirals, including protease inhibitors, nucleoside reverse transcriptase inhibitors, nonnucleoside reverse transcriptase inhibitors, and nucleoside analogs.

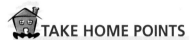

TAKE HOME POINTS

Retrovirus is a common name for the family of RNA-containing tumor viruses. These viruses induce tumors such as sarcomas, leukemias, and lymphomas. These viruses contain reverse transcriptase, which is essential for the production of a DNA molecule from RNA.

What IS a Protease Inhibitor Antiretroviral?

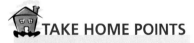

TAKE HOME POINTS

Protease inhibitors are not curative.

Protease Inhibitors	Trade Names	Uses
saquinavir [sack-KWIN-uh-vihr]	Invirase	Treatment of advanced HIV infection
nelfinavir [nell-FIN-ah-veer]	Viracept	Treatment of HIV infection

Action

Protease inhibitors block protease activity of the human immunodeficiency virus (HIV). Aspartate proteinase is essential for the final step of viral proliferation and is encoded with the HIV genome; thus it is absent in uninfected CD4 cells. Protease inhibitors interfere with HIV protease enzyme, thereby impeding the viral replication of retroviruses, including HIV type I (HIV-1) and type II (HIV-2). The active enzyme generates proteins, which are necessary to the virus. The HIV protease inhibitors interfere in this process and lead to the assembly of nonfunctional virions. In summary, protease inhibitors interfere with the multiplication of the virus and slow the progression of the disease, which may prolong survival.

LIFE SPAN

Protease inhibitors should be administered with caution in older adults and patients with diabetes mellitus and renal or hepatic dysfunction.

Uses

Protease inhibitors are used to treat HIV infection in adults.

What You NEED TO KNOW

Contraindications/Precautions

Protease inhibitors are contraindicated for patients with hypersensitivity or hemophilia.

Drug Interactions

Because the hepatic cytochrome P-450 family of enzymes metabolizes protease inhibitors, they interact with other drugs, leading to further interactions. When more than one protease inhibitor is given together, liver metabolism may be inhibited, or a synergistic or antagonistic action may occur. Rifampin markedly reduces the plasma concentration and action of protease inhibitors. Ketoconazole, clarithromycin, and quinidine sulfate increase indinavir levels when given concurrently. Indinavir increases isoniazid levels when given together. Anticonvulsants decrease nelfinavir levels.

Adverse Effects

Although protease inhibitors are usually well tolerated, headache, alopecia, dizziness, rash, dry skin, fatigue, cough, taste alteration, nausea, vomiting, diarrhea, back pain, hyperglycemia, and paresthesias around the mouth may occur. More serious adverse effects include nephrolithiasis, anaphylaxis, hepatic failure, and Stevens-Johnson syndrome. Elevated hepatic aminotransferase, serum glutamicoxaloacetic transaminase, SGPT, and triglyceride levels have been reported.

What You DO

Nursing Responsibilities

When administering protease inhibitors, the nurse should:

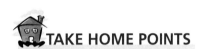
TAKE HOME POINTS

Advise patients that when they are unable to swallow tablets, the tablets may be dissolved in water and mixed with milk or chocolate milk.

- Instruct the patient to take protease inhibitors with water or milk 1 hour before meals or 2 hours after meals. If the patient develops GI distress, the medication may be taken with a light snack, such as dry toast with jelly.
- Tell the patient to avoid mixing nelfinavir with an acidic juice or food because of the bitter taste.
- Watch renal and hepatic function, as well as blood glucose.
- Monitor nutritional status. Ensure adequate intake if GI distress is severe.
- Encourage the patient to drink at least 1.5 liters of fluids within a 24-hour period when taking protease inhibitors to prevent nephrolithiasis.
- Teach the patient to take protease inhibitors at least 1 hour apart from didanosine.
- Instruct the patient to take the full dose of medication as ordered. These drugs must be given in doses sufficiently high to completely suppress viral replication; otherwise, resistant viruses can emerge. Cessation of treatment results in reemergence of the virus.
- Inform the patient that if a dose of protease inhibitors is missed, that dose should be disregarded and the next dose should be taken at the usual time.

Do You UNDERSTAND?

DIRECTIONS: **Indicate in the space provided whether the statement is *true* or *false*. If the answer is false, correct the statement to make it true (using the margin space).**

_____ 1. Protease inhibitors interfere with the first step of viral proliferation.

_____ 2. Protease inhibitors eliminate aspartate proteinase.

_____ 3. Protease inhibitors are curative.

_____ 4. Protease inhibitors should be given at the lowest possible dose to prevent adverse effects.

_____ 5. Protease inhibitors are safe to use, with rare drug interactions.

What IS a Nucleoside Reverse Transcriptase Inhibitor Antiretroviral?

Nucleoside Reverse Transcriptase Inhibitors	Trade Names	Uses
zidovudine (AZT) [sid-OH-vue-deen]	Retrovir	Treatment of HIV infection
didanosine [die-DAN-oh-SEEN]	Videx	Treatment of HIV infection

Action

Nucleoside reverse transcriptase inhibitors (NRTIs) interfere with viral RNA-directed DNA polymerase (reverse transcriptase), thereby impeding the replication of retroviruses, including HIV. NRTIs exert a virustatic effect against retroviruses.

Zidovudine, also known as azidothymidine (AZT), is an analog of thymidine, which is a nucleoside present in DNA. In retroviruses (i.e., HIV), zidovudine is an active inhibitor of reverse transcriptase. This drug is combined with triphosphate by cellular enzymes. The triphosphate

Answers: **1.** false; protease inhibitors interfere with multiplication of the virus; **2.** true; **3.** false; protease inhibitors slow progression of the disease; **4.** false; protease inhibitors need to be given in high enough doses to suppress viral replication; **5.** false; hepatic cytochrome P-450 enzymes metabolize protease inhibitors, leading to interactions with other drugs.

form competes with equivalent cellular triphosphates, which are the essential basis for the formation of proviral DNA by viral reverse transcriptase (viral RNA-dependent DNA polymerase). The incorporation of this substance into growing viral DNA strands results in chain termination. Mammalian alpha DNA polymerase is relatively resistant to the effect. However, gamma DNA polymerase in the host cell mitochondria is fairly sensitive to the compound, which may be the basis of unwanted effects.

Because of rapid mutation, the HIV virus is a constantly moving target; thus the therapeutic response decreases with long-term usage, particularly in the later stage of the disease. Resistant strains can be transferred between individuals. Another factor that contributes to the loss of drug efficacy includes increased viral load, resulting from a reduction in immune mechanisms.

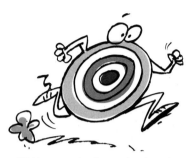

HIV is a constantly moving target.

Uses

NRTIs are used in the treatment of HIV infection in adults or children over 3 months of age. Retroviral therapy should be started before immunodeficiency becomes evident. The aim is to reduce plasma viral concentration as much as possible and for as long as possible. NRTIs have greater effectiveness in the treatment of HIV-acquired immunodeficiency syndrome (AIDS) when used in combination of at least three drugs (i.e., two reverse transcriptase inhibitors and one protease inhibitor). When plasma viral concentration increases, the health care provider can change to a new regimen.

What You NEED TO KNOW

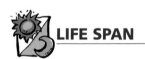

LIFE SPAN

NRTIs are contraindicated for women during pregnancy and lactation.

Contraindications/Precautions

NRTIs are contraindicated for patients with hypersensitivity. NRTIs should be used with caution in patients with peripheral vascular disease, neuropathy, chronic pancreatitis, renal or liver dysfunction, and compromised bone marrow function.

Drug Interactions

When didanosine is taken with aluminum and magnesium antacids, the adverse effects are increased. When they are taken with zalcitabine, an additive neuropathy may develop. NRTIs decrease the effectiveness of dapsone. When zidovudine is taken with acetaminophen, bone marrow suppression may occur. The risk for AZT toxicity is increased when taken with amphotericin B, aspirin, dapsone, indomethacin, interferon, and vincristine.

Adverse Effects

Common adverse effects associated with NRTIs include anemia and neutropenia, particularly with long-term administration. Other adverse effects include dizziness, headache, fever, insomnia, confusion, nervousness, anxiety, depression, dry mouth, cough, dyspnea, weakness, poor coordination, seizures, abdominal pain, nausea, vomiting, diarrhea, constipation, paresthesias, myopathy, and liver dysfunction. Influenza-like syndrome, hypocalcemia, hypokalemia, hypomagnesemia, elevated hemoglobin and white blood count, severe bone marrow suppression, visual disturbance, palpitations, and dysrhythmias have also been reported. The short-term prophylactic use in relatively healthy adults who have specific exposure to the virus is associated with only minor reversible adverse effects.

What You DO

Nursing Responsibilities

NRTIs are administered orally or IV. When administering NRTIs, the nurse should:

- Administer oral NRTIs on an empty stomach, either well before or well after meals.
- Monitor nutritional status. Ensure adequate intake if GI distress is severe.
- Instruct the patient to take oral NRTIs with water, not with fruit juice or other acidic liquid. Tablets should be chewed thoroughly or crushed to disperse in 30 mL of water and swallowed immediately.
- Watch the patient's plasma viral load, CD4 count, CBC, and renal and liver function studies throughout NRTI therapy. When the plasma viral count increases in a patient who is taking NRTIs, a new treatment regimen is indicated.
- Tell the patient to avoid doubling doses. When a dose is missed, the patient should take the missed dose only if it is more than 4 hours before the next dose. Otherwise, the missed dose should be disregarded and the next dose should be taken at its normal time.
- Tell the patient to report a rash, particularly when blisters and fever are present.

Do You UNDERSTAND?

DIRECTIONS: **Select the word(s) from the italicized list below to complete the following statements.**

1. When a patient is taking an NRTI, the nurse should monitor _____.

2. The most common adverse effect of NRTIs is _____.

   polycythemia   *liver function tests*   *cough*
   anemia   *potassium level*

What IS a Nonnucleoside Reverse Transcriptase Inhibitor Antiretroviral?

Nonnucleoside Reverse Transcriptase Inhibitors	Trade Names	Uses
nevirapine [nuh-VEER-uh-peen]	Viramune	Treatment of HIV infection
delavirdine [dell-ah-VIR-deen]	Rescriptor	Treatment of HIV-1 infection

Action

A nonnucleoside reverse transcriptase inhibitor (NNRTI) antiviral is different from an NRTI in structure and action. NNRTIs bind to the active center of reverse transcriptase to block RNA and DNA polymerase activities. This action causes a disruption of the enzyme's catalytic site and prevents replication of HIV-1 virus.

Uses

NNRTIs are used in the treatment of HIV infection. Usually, treatment with NNRTIs is in combination with other antiviral agents.

What You NEED TO KNOW

Contraindications/Precautions

NNRTIs are contraindicated for patients with hypersensitivity.

Drug Interactions

Antacids and didanosine decrease absorption of delavirdine. When given concurrently, delavirdine increases serum levels of indinavir, saquinavir, alprazolam, midazolam, dapsone, quinidine, clarithromycin, warfarin, ergot alkaloids, calcium channel blockers, and antidysrhythmics. Nevirapine decreases concentrations of protease inhibitors and oral contraceptives when given together. Rifampin and rifabutin decrease the action of nevirapine.

Adverse Effects

The most common adverse effect of NNRTIs is a rash, which can be benign or life-threatening. The rash may be associated with fever, conjunctivitis, blistering, oral lesions, muscle or joint pain, erythema multiforme, and Stevens-Johnson syndrome. Other common adverse effects include headache, fatigue, nausea, vomiting, and diarrhea. Anemia and neutropenia may also develop.

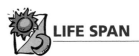

LIFE SPAN

NNRTIs are contraindicated for women during lactation.

NNRTIs should be used with caution in children, in patients with hepatic dysfunction and CNS disorders, and in women during pregnancy.

What You DO

Nursing Responsibilities

NNRTIs may be given with or without food. Delavirdine should be mixed with at least 3 ounces of water before administration. Antacids and didanosine should not be administered within 1 hour of delavirdine. Because acidity enhances absorption, these agents may be given with an acidic beverage, such as orange or cranberry juice. When administering NNRTIs, the nurse should:

- Check the liver and renal function studies for early detection of dysfunction.
- Watch the CBC reports for early detection of blood dyscrasias.
- Monitor nutritional status. Ensure adequate intake if GI distress is severe.

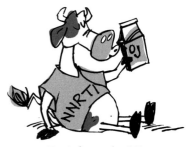

Don't forget the OJ!

- Warn the patient that drowsiness and fatigue may occur when taking NNRTIs and that safety must be considered when operating hazardous equipment.
- Instruct patients who are taking NNRTIs to withhold the drug and notify the prescribing health care provider immediately if a severe rash occurs. A severe rash may indicate erythema multiforme or Stevens-Johnson syndrome.

Do You UNDERSTAND?

DIRECTIONS: **Indicate in the space provided whether the statement is *true* or *false*. If the answer is false, correct the statement to make it true (using the margin space).**

_____ 1. NNRTIs are used primarily in the treatment of herpes simplex.

_____ 2. Delavirdine decreases serum levels of warfarin.

_____ 3. The most common adverse effect of NNRTIs is a headache.

What IS a Nucleoside Analog Antiviral?

Nucleoside Analogs	Trade Names	Uses
acyclovir [A-SIGH-klo-vihr]	Zovirax	Treatment of herpes simplex viruses, varicella zoster, and genital herpes
famciclovir [fam-SIGH-klo-vihr]	Famvir	Treatment of herpes simplex, herpes zoster, and genital herpes

Action

Acyclovir acts by being converted by the viral cell into its active form of triphosphate and inhibits viral DNA polymerase. Acyclovir preferentially interferes with DNA synthesis of herpes simplex types 1 and 2 and varicella-zoster virus.

Answers: 1. false; NNRTIs prevent replication of the HIV-1 virus; 2. false; delavirdine increases serum levels; 3. false; rash.

Uses

Nucleoside analog antivirals are used to inhibit viral replication of herpes, types 1 and 2 herpes simplex, and varicella (chickenpox) viruses. These agents also exert antiviral activity against Epstein-Barr virus (infectious mononucleosis) and cytomegalovirus.

What You NEED TO KNOW

Contraindications/Precautions

Nucleoside analog antivirals are contraindicated for patients with hypersensitivity and blood dyscrasias.

Drug Interactions

Nucleoside analog antivirals have some drug interactions with other drugs. When probenecid is given with acyclovir, the action of acyclovir is prolonged. Zidovudine causes increased acyclovir levels, increasing the risk for toxicity.

Adverse Effects

The adverse effects of acyclovir include hypotension, headache, dizziness, confusion, insomnia, tremors, rash, malaise, nausea, vomiting, and diarrhea. Other more serious adverse effects include hallucinations, depression, hematuria, seizures, and coma.

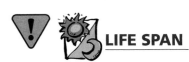

LIFE SPAN

Nucleoside analog antivirals should be used with caution in patients with neurologic, renal, or hepatic dysfunction, dehydration, in older adults, and in patients who are taking nephrotoxic drugs.

What You DO

Nursing Responsibilities

Nucleoside analog antivirals are given orally or via IV infusion but not subcutaneously (Sub-Q), IM, IV bolus, or ophthalmically. The absorption of nucleoside analog antivirals is unaffected by food. Oral acyclovir may be taken with food to decrease GI distress. When administering the nucleoside analog antivirals, the nurse should:
- Check the IV site carefully during administration and for several days after drug completion. An infusion pump and a microdrip infusion

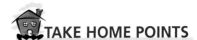

TAKE HOME POINTS

- Administer an IV dose of nucleoside analog antivirals over 1 hour to prevent renal damage. Be certain that the patient who is taking nucleoside analog antivirals is well hydrated.
- Other precautions must be taken to prevent spreading viruses. Teach the patient that after herpes simplex virus is controlled, latent viruses can be activated by exposure to sunlight, fever, stress, menstruation, sexual intercourse, and trauma.

set are preferred to avoid inflammation, phlebitis, extravasation, or sloughing of tissues at the injection site.

- Ascertain that the patient is well hydrated during and for 2 hours after drug infusion to prevent renal damage.
- Monitor the patient's creatinine and BUN levels because these values may elevate after drug infusion.
- Inform the patient that these drugs can only manage the disease; they cannot cure it or keep it from spreading to others.
- Instruct the patient to avoid sexual intercourse when either partner has evidence of a herpes infection.
- Instruct the patient to report any unexplained redness or pain in the eye. An untreated eye infection can lead to corneal keratitis and blindness.
- Tell the patient to take the full course of treatment.

Do You UNDERSTAND?

DIRECTIONS: **Indicate in the space provided whether the statement is** *true* **or** *false.* **If the answer is false, correct the statement to make it true (using the margin space).**

_____ 1. Nucleoside analog antivirals are used in the treatment of chickenpox.

_____ 2. Probenecid decreases the action of acyclovir.

_____ 3. Keep the patient NPO prior to and during the drug infusion of a nucleoside analog antiviral.

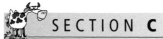 SECTION C

ANTIFUNGALS

Fungal infections may be superficial or systemic. Systemic infections occur mostly in the immunocompromised, such as patients with AIDS or those who are taking corticosteroids or anticancer drugs.

Two main groups of fungi can cause disease in humans:

1. Molds (**filamentous fungi**) grow as long filaments that intertwine to form a mycelium. Examples of molds are the dermatophytes and *Aspergillus fumigatus.* Dermatophytes (given their name because of their ability to digest keratin) cause infections of the skin, nails, and hair. *Aspergillus fumigatus* may cause pulmonary or disseminated aspergillosis.

2. True yeast is either a unicellular round or oval fungus. An example of a type of yeast is *Cryptococcus neoformans,* which may cause cryptococcal meningitis or pulmonary infections, usually in immunocompromised patients.

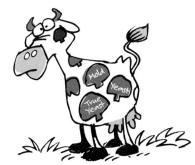

There's a fungus among us.

Currently, few effective antifungal drugs exist, and the first-line drug that is used in severe and potentially fatal systemic mycoses is highly toxic. Flucytosine is much less toxic than is amphotericin, but its use is limited because of its narrow spectrum, and resistance can develop rapidly during therapy. Flucytosine is converted in fungal cells into fluorouracil, which inhibits DNA synthesis. Flucytosine fails to undergo this conversion in human cells. The imidazoles, which are widely used topically, are broad-spectrum antifungal drugs that inhibit ergosterol synthesis. The triazoles are newer drugs, structurally similar to the imidazoles, but with a wider range of antifungal activity. These agents have a lower incidence of adverse effects because they are much more specific inhibitors of lanosterol x-demethylase action that results in inhibition of ergosterol synthesis. The antifungals discussed in this section include polyenes and azoles.

What IS a Polyene Antifungal?

Polyene Antifungals	Trade Names	Uses
amphotericin B [am-foe-TER-ih-sin B]	Amphotec Fungizone	Treatment of systemic fungal infections
nystatin [nye-STAT-in]	Mycostatin	Treatment of candidal infections

Action

Amphotericin B is an amphoteric polyene macrolide antibiotic that exerts its antifungal action primarily by binding to sterols, such as ergosterol, in the fungal cell membrane. The fungal cell membrane is then no longer able to function as a selective barrier. As a result, cell membrane permeability is changed, allowing leakage of intracellular components and causing cell death. The drug is selectively toxic because, in human cells, the major sterol is cholesterol rather than ergosterol. The binding to sterols in cells (i.e., kidney cells, erythrocytes) may account for some of the toxicities. Nystatin (another polyene) is too toxic for parenteral use.

Uses

The first-line antifungal drug is amphotericin B. This agent is used for most pathogenic fungi, including yeasts and protozoa. Amphotericin B is a wide-spectrum antifungal drug that is used to treat potentially fatal systemic infections from *Aspergillus, Candida*, or *Cryptococcus*. Nystatin is used primarily for *Candida albicans* infections of the skin and mucous membranes and has little systemic effect.

Polyene antifungals are contraindicated for women during pregnancy and lactation.

What You NEED TO KNOW

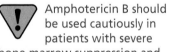 Amphotericin B should be used cautiously in patients with severe bone marrow suppression and renal impairment.

Contraindications/Precautions

Polyene antifungals are contraindicated for patients with hypersensitivity.

Drug Interactions

Amphotericin B interacts with corticosteroids and digitalis to increase the risk for hypokalemia. Concurrent use of amphotericin B with furosemide, vancomycin, aminoglycosides, capreomycin, carboplatin, and cisplatin increase the risk for nephrotoxicity.

Adverse Effects

The adverse effects of amphotericin B are common; most patients develop paresthesia, flushing, fever, chills, anorexia, nausea, vomiting, dyspepsia, and abdominal cramping. Long-term therapy inevitably causes renal damage, especially when given in high doses. Nephrotoxicity is reversible only when detected early. Amphotericin B may cause headache, hypotension, weight loss, hypokalemia, hypomagnesemia, malaise, arthralgia, ototoxicity, anemia, pseudomembranous colitis, and thrombocytopenia. Local irritation, burning, and thrombophlebitis at the IV site may also occur.

> **!** Febrile reactions of fever, chills, headache, and nausea occur in up to 90% of patients who receive amphotericin B and generally begin 1 to 2 hours after initiation of infusion, subsiding within 4 hours after the drug is discontinued.

What You DO

Nursing Responsibilities

Amphotericin B is poorly absorbed orally and is given by IV infusion or intrathecally when the CNS is involved. Heparin and saline should not be used to flush the amphotericin B IV line. Long-term therapy with amphotericin B usually requires placement of a central line. When administering the polyene antifungals, the nurse should:

- Protect amphotericin B IV solutions from light exposure, particularly when given over 8 hours. This drug is usually infused slowly over a minimum of 6 hours.
- Administer nystatin oral suspension by rinsing the mouth or by using a "swish and swallow" technique. The solution should then be kept in the mouth as long as possible (at least 2 minutes).
- Instruct the patient to avoid food or drink for 30 minutes after oral administration of nystatin.
- Instruct the patient to remove dentures before oral administration and at night because superinfections, such as oral candidiasis, are more likely to occur in patients who wear dentures 24 hours per day.
- Insert vaginal suppositories and creams high into the vagina.
- Instruct the patient to lie recumbent for 10 to 15 minutes after vaginal insertion.
- Instruct patients to continue suppository-cream therapy during menses.
- Inform the patient that topical or vaginal administration should be discontinued when sensitivity or rash occurs; otherwise, the treatment should be continued for the full course to eradicate the fungus and to prevent reoccurrence.

TAKE HOME POINTS

- When a test dose of amphotericin B is given (usually 1 mg over 20 to 30 minutes), the vital signs should be monitored every 30 minutes for at least 4 hours.
- Potassium supplements are usually given concurrently with amphotericin B to prevent hypokalemia.

- Watch intake and output and daily weight (checking for weight loss or gain).
- Monitor electrolytes, hepatic and renal function, and hematological studies frequently. Compare these with baseline studies for early detection of dysfunction.
- Withhold amphotericin B and report to the health care provider when the BUN exceeds 40 mg/dL or when the serum creatinine is elevated above 3 mg/dL.
- Check vital signs frequently during the beginning phase of therapy.
- Inspect skin for rash daily and report to health care provider promptly.
- Instruct the patient to report tinnitus, vertigo, unsteady gait, or hearing loss because ototoxicity is common with amphotericin B administration.

Some prescribing health care providers take prophylactic measures by ordering aspirin or acetaminophen, antiemetics, antihistamines, and corticosteroids 1 hour before amphotericin B infusion to reduce intensity of adverse reactions.

Do You UNDERSTAND?

DIRECTIONS: Provide appropriate responses to the following statement and question.

1. Identify two drugs or drug groups that increase the risk for hypokalemia when given concurrently with amphotericin B.

   _____

2. Amphotericin B should be administered IV over a minimum of how many hours?

   _____

Answers: 1. corticosteroids, digitalis; 2. 6.

What IS an Azole Antifungal?

Azole Antifungals	Trade Names	Uses
fluconazole *[flew-KOE-nuh-zole]*	Diflucan	Treatment of candidal infections and cryptococcal meningitis
ketoconazole *[KEY-toe-KOE-nuh-zole]*	Nizoral	Treatment of systemic and cutaneous fungal infections
itraconazole *[eye-tra-CON-ah-zoll]*	Sporanox	Treatment of tinea pedis and blastomycosis, histoplasmosis, aspergillosis, onychomycosis, and dermatophyte skin infections
clotrimazole *[kloe-TRIM-a-zole]*	Lotrimin	Treatment of skin, oropharyngeal, and vulvovaginal candidiasis
oxiconazole *[ox-I-CON-a-zole]*	Oxistat	Treatment of tinea pedis, tinea cruris, and tinea corporis

Action

Azoles are wide-spectrum antifungal drugs to which resistance rarely develops. These agents bind to sterols in the fungal cell membrane, which changes cell membrane permeability. Azoles can be fungistatic or fungicidal, depending on the drug concentration and the organism. Ketoconazole is classified as an imidazole antifungal, while fluconazole is classified as triazole antifungal.

Uses

Fluconazole is used for cryptococcal meningitis, pneumonia, peritonitis, urinary tract infections, oropharyngeal and vaginal candidiasis, systemic fungal infections, and prophylactically to decrease the incidence of candidiasis in bone marrow transplant recipients. Triazoles have been used successfully in a wide range of superficial and systemic mycoses (not *Aspergillus*). Ketoconazole has been used in the treatment of local and systemic mycoses. Itraconazole is used in the treatment of blastomycosis, histoplasmosis, aspergillosis, onychomycosis, dermatophyte skin infections, and tinea pedis. Clotrimazole is widely used topically in the treatment of dermatophyte and *Candida albicans* infections. Oxiconazole is used to treat cutaneous candidiasis, tinea pedis, tinea cruris, and tinea corporis. Tinea is a fungal skin infection occurring on various body parts (i.e., pedis affects the foot and is commonly called "athlete's foot"; cruris affects scrotal, anal, or genital areas and is commonly called "jock itch"; corporis affects the body and is commonly called "ringworm").

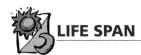

LIFE SPAN

Azole antifungals are contraindicated for women during pregnancy or lactation.

 Ketoconazole should be used with caution in patients with achlorhydria and hepatic dysfunction.

Co-administration of itraconazole with pimozide, triazolam, oral midazolam, and quinidine may cause life-threatening dysrhythmias.

What You NEED TO KNOW

Contraindications/Precautions

Azole antifungals are contraindicated for patients with hypersensitivity. Ketoconazole is contraindicated for patients with chronic alcoholism and fungal meningitis.

Drug Interactions

When fluconazole is given concurrently with cimetidine and rifampin, fluconazole levels are reduced. An increase in fluconazole level occurs when given concurrently with hydrochlorothiazide. Fluconazole increases the level of cyclosporine, phenytoin, warfarin, oral hypoglycemics, and theophylline when it is given together with any of these drugs.

Ketoconazole and itraconazole decrease the efficacy of oral contraceptives and increase the effects of warfarin, buspirone, cyclosporine, corticosteroids, benzodiazepines, zolpidem, tacrolimus, protease inhibitors, and vinca alkaloids. Itraconazole increases the effects of digoxin, simvastatin, lovastatin, alfentanil, ritonavir, losartan, and felodipine. Ketoconazole may also increase the effects of tricyclic antidepressants, carbamazepine, quinidine, sulfonylureas, donepezil, and nisoldipine. The effects of theophylline may be reduced when given together with ketoconazole. Antacids, anticholinergics, H_2 blockers, didanosine, and sucralfate decrease the absorption and action of ketoconazole. There are no drug interactions with clotrimazole and oxiconazole.

Adverse Effects

Most adverse effects of azole antifungals are mild-to-moderate. Common adverse effects include hypersensitivity, headache, drowsiness, dizziness, confusion, depression, nausea, vomiting, abdominal pain, and diarrhea. Other adverse effects include photophobia, taste perversion, tinnitus, hypertension, fainting, orthostatic hypotension, insomnia, myalgia, menstrual disorders, impotence, gynecomastia, suicidal tendencies, thrombocytopenia, leukopenia, hemolytic anemia, angioedema, decreased secretion of adrenal corticosteroids, and hepatic dysfunction. Anaphylactic reactions rarely occur.

What You DO

Nursing Responsibilities

Itraconazole capsules and oral solution cannot be used interchangeably. When fluconazole is given as an IV infusion, the maximal rate is 200 mg/hr. IV admixtures of other drugs are not recommended. When administering azole antifungals, the nurse should:

- Administer itraconazole capsules after a full meal (oral solutions should be taken without food).
- Instruct the patient to report evidence of liver dysfunction (i.e., unusual fatigue, anorexia, nausea, vomiting, dark urine, pale stools, jaundice).
- Apply topical administration sparingly and protect hands with latex gloves when applying the drug. Occlusive dressings should be avoided, unless otherwise directed. Before topical use, cleanse the skin according to the prescribing health care provider's orders and dry the skin thoroughly. Avoid contact with eyes.
- Monitor hepatic function studies, BUN, and serum creatinine periodically for 1 month or when suggestive symptoms occur for early detection of dysfunction.
- Obtain fungal culture specimens before initiating drug therapy.
- Avoid administering ketoconazole concurrently with antacids, anticholinergics, or H_2 blockers.
- Allow clotrimazole oral lozenge to dissolve slowly in the mouth over 15 to 30 minutes for maximal effectiveness.
- Instruct the patient that when a dose is missed, the next dose should not be doubled. Rather, take the missed dose only if the next scheduled dose is more than 4 hours away.

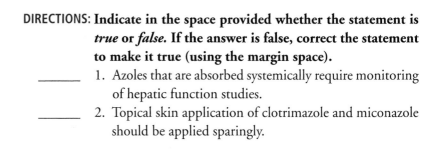

Do You UNDERSTAND?

DIRECTIONS: Indicate in the space provided whether the statement is *true* or *false*. If the answer is false, correct the statement to make it true (using the margin space).

_____ 1. Azoles that are absorbed systemically require monitoring of hepatic function studies.

_____ 2. Topical skin application of clotrimazole and miconazole should be applied sparingly.

References

Abramowicz M: Gatifloxacin and moxifloxacin: two new fluoroquinolones, *Med Let Drugs Ther* 42(1072):315, 2000.

Abrams AC, Lammon CB, Pennington SS: *Clinical drug therapy: rationales for nursing practice*, ed 8, Philadelphia, 2007, Lippincott.

Gutierrez K, Queener SF: *Pharmacology for nursing practice*, St Louis, 2003, Mosby.

Hardman JG, Limbird LE: *Goodman & Gilman's the pharmacological basis of therapeutics*, ed 10, New York, 2001, McGraw-Hill.

Ignatavicius DD, Workman ML: *Medical-surgical nursing: critical thinking for collaborative care*, ed 5, St Louis, 2006, Elsevier.

Karch AM: *Focus on nursing pharmacology*, ed 3, Philadelphia, 2006, Lippincott.

Kee JL, Hayes ER, McCuistion LE: *Pharmacology: a nursing process approach*, ed 5, Philadelphia, 2006, Elsevier.

Lehne RA: *Pharmacology for nursing care*, ed 5, Philadelphia, 2004, WB Saunders.

McKenry, LM, Salerno, E: *Mosby's pharmacology in nursing*, ed 21, St Louis, 2003, Mosby.

Smeltzer SC, Bare BG: *Brunner and Suddarth's textbook of medical-surgical nursing*, ed 10, Philadelphia, 2004, Lippincott.

Wilson BA, Shannon MT, Stang CL: *Nurses drug guide*, Upper Saddle River, New Jersey, 2006, Pearson.

Answers: 1. true; 2. true.

NCLEX® Review

Section A

1. A patient asks the nurse how penicillin G potassium (Megacillin) can help her otitis media. The nurse knows that:
   1 this drug has a spectrum of action wider than that of any other penicillin.
   2 natural penicillins have a structure that was developed to resist splitting of the β-lactam ring.
   3 bacteria may develop a protective mechanism and become resistant to natural penicillins.
   4 natural penicillins have an amino group attached to the nucleus that increases the action against gram-negative bacteria.

2. A patient who is taking cefoxitin (Mefoxin) states she heard that it was bacteriocidal and asks the nurse what *bacteriocidal* means. How should the nurse respond?
   1 A narrow spectrum of action against bacteria
   2 A wide spectrum of action against bacteria
   3 Inhibits the formation and growth of new bacteria
   4 Inhibits enzymes that are necessary for bacterial cell wall maintenance and life

3. A patient is taking trimethoprim-sulfamethoxazole (Bactrim). Which should the nurse teach the patient?
   1 Limit fluid intake.
   2 Drink 2 liters of fluid per day.
   3 Take the drug with orange juice.
   4 Lie down for 30 minutes after the initial dose of the drug.

4. A patient who is taking tobramycin (Nebcin) should be monitored for which of the following?
   1 Seizures
   2 Ototoxicity
   3 Photosensitivity
   4 Teeth discoloration

5. A 24-year-old pregnant female who has a serious respiratory tract infection is prescribed an antibiotic. Which drug is contraindicated during pregnancy?
   1 Amoxicillin (Amoxil)
   2 Azithromycin (Zithromax)
   3 Gentamicin (Garamycin)
   4 Levofloxacin (Levaquin)

Section B

6. A patient asks the nurse how zidovudine (AZT; Retrovir) can help his HIV infection. Which response by the nurse about AZT is incorrect?
   1 AZT must be converted to the nucleotide form to express antiviral activity.
   2 AZT is incorporated into growing viral but not mammalian nuclear DNA.
   3 AZT is currently used to treat severe herpesvirus and respiratory syncytial viral infections, as well as AIDS.
   4 AZT is toxic to bone marrow and causes adverse hematologic effects.

7. A patient who is told that his leukemia is due to a retrovirus asks for more information. The nurse knows that retroviruses contain which of the following?
   1 Fungi
   2 DNA only
   3 RNA only
   4 Reverse transcriptase

8. A patient who is taking nelfinavir (Viracept) should be instructed to take the medication with which food or drink?
   1 Wine
   2 Meals
   3 Acidic juice
   4 Chocolate milk

9. Identify one of the principles of retroviral therapy.
   1 Use monotherapy regimen.
   2 Initiate treatment before immunodeficiency becomes evident.
   3 Discontinue one drug when plasma viral loads decrease.
   4 Antiviral agents do not affect the viral replication cycle.

10. A patient is taking acyclovir (Zovirax) for genital herpes. Which nursing responsibility should the nurse perform?
    1 Restrict the patient's fluids.
    2 Monitor for Stevens-Johnson syndrome.
    3 Administer the medication 1 hour before meals.
    4 Monitor the patient's BUN and creatinine for renal damage.

Section C

11. A patient has a serious systemic infection. Which antifungal medication does the nurse expect to be used as a first-line drug of defense?
    1 Nystatin
    2 Clotrimazole
    3 Oxiconazole
    4 Amphotericin B

12. A patient is taking nystatin (Mycostatin) to treat an oral candidal infection. Which nursing responsibility should the nurse perform?
    1 Monitor the patient for hypertension.
    2 Tell the patient to eat a meal or snack immediately after the medication.
    3 Have the patient keep the dentures in during administration and especially at bedtime.
    4 Tell the patient to keep the solution in the mouth for 2 minutes after a "swish and swallow" technique.

13. A patient is taking amphotericin B (Amphotec). Which is not a corresponding nursing responsibility?
    1 Administer deep intramuscularly.
    2 Infuse IV amphotericin B slowly over 6 hours.
    3 Protect IV amphotericin B solution from light exposure.
    4 Expect an antihistamine or corticosteroid to be given prior to amphotericin B administration.

14. A patient is prescribed fluconazole (Diflucan) for a vaginal candidal infection. For which adverse effect should the nurse expect to monitor?
    1 Diarrhea
    2 Convulsions
    3 Renal dysfunction
    4 Stevens-Johnson syndrome

15. A patient is taking delavirdine (Rescriptor). Which nursing responsibility is not necessary for the nurse to perform?
    1 Monitor liver enzymes.
    2 Monitor BUN and creatinine.
    3 Warn the patient about drowsiness and safety precautions.
    4 Instruct the patient to avoid orange juice when taking delavirdine.

NCLEX® Review Answers

Section A

1. 3 Bacteria may develop a protective mechanism and become resistant to natural penicillins. The spectrum of action is wider with extended-spectrum penicillins compared with any other penicillin. Penicillinase-resistant penicillins have a structure that was developed to resist splitting of the β-lactam ring. Aminopenicillins have an amino group that is attached to the penicillin nucleus, which increases the action against gram-negative bacteria.

2. 4 *Bacteriocidal* indicates that the antibiotic inhibits enzymes that are required for bacterial cell wall maintenance; thus they kill bacteria. *Narrow-spectrum* or *wide-spectrum action* refers to the antibiotic's effectiveness against a variety of microorganisms. *Bacteriostatic* means that these antibiotics inhibit the formation and growth of new bacteria, thus keeping bacteria in check but not killing them.

3. 2 When taking sulfonamides, the patient should drink 2 L of fluid per day to prevent crystalluria and resultant renal damage. Therefore limiting fluid intake is incorrect. Taking the drug with orange juice is incorrect because sulfonamides should preferably be taken on an empty stomach.

The patient need not lie down after the initial dose.

4. 2 Aminoglycosides, such as tobramycin, are known to cause ototoxicity as an adverse effect; the nurse should monitor for this effect. Penicillins, sulfonamides, aztreonam, and imipenem-cilastatin—but not aminoglycosides—may lead to seizures. Sulfonamides, tetracyclines, and fluoroquinolones—but not aminoglycosides—may lead to photosensitivity. Tetracyclines, not aminoglycosides, may lead to teeth discoloration.

5. 4 Fluoroquinolones, such as levofloxacin, are contraindicated during pregnancy, as are tetracyclines, sulfonamides, aztreonam, clindamycin, vancomycin, and imipenem-cilastatin. Penicillins, macrolides, and aminoglycosides should be used cautiously during pregnancy.

Section B

6. 3 AZT is currently used only in the treatment of HIV infections. AZT must be converted to the nucleotide form to express antiviral activity. It is incorporated into growing viral DNA but not mammalian nuclear DNA. AZT is toxic to bone marrow and causes adverse hematologic effects.

7. 4 Retroviruses contain reverse transcriptase and tumor viruses, which induce tumors (i.e., sarcomas, leukemias, lymphomas). Reverse transcriptase is essential for the production of a DNA molecule from RNA. Retroviruses do not contain fungi; they contain DNA only or RNA only.

8. 4 Protease inhibitors should be taken with water, milk, or chocolate milk. Protease inhibitors should not be mixed with acidic juices or wine or taken with meals.

9. 2 A principle of retroviral therapy is to initiate treatment before immunodeficiency is evident. NRTIs have greater effectiveness in HIV and AIDS treatment when used in combination with at least three drugs. A drug should not be discontinued when plasma viral loads decrease. Antivirals inhibit single steps in the viral replication cycle.

10. 4 BUN and creatinine should be monitored because levels may elevate, indicating renal damage. The patient should be well hydrated during and for 2 hours after drug administration to prevent renal damage. When the drug is administered orally, it should be taken with food to decrease GI distress. Acyclovir does not have an adverse effect of Stevens-Johnson syndrome.

Section C

11. 4 The first-line antifungal drug for systemic use is amphotericin B. Nystatin has little systemic effect. Clotrimazole is used topically for skin and *Candida albicans* infections. Oxiconazole is used for cutaneous candidiasis.

12. 4 Nystatin should be kept in the mouth as long as possible (at least 2 minutes) after a "swish and swallow" technique. Hypertension does not commonly occur as an adverse effect of nystatin. The patient should avoid food or drink for 30 minutes after nystatin administration. Dentures should be removed before oral administration and at night because oral infections are more likely to occur when dentures are in.

13. 1 Amphotericin B is not given intramuscularly but by IV. Amphotericin B solution should be protected from light and infused slowly over 6 hours, and the nurse should expect an antihistamine or corticosteroid to be given prior to administration.

14. 1 Diarrhea is a common adverse effect of fluconazole. Convulsions, renal dysfunction, and Stevens-Johnson syndrome are not associated with fluconazole.

15. 4 Delavirdine absorption is enhanced by acidic beverages, such as orange juice or cranberry juice. Monitoring liver enzymes, BUN, and creatinine, as well as warning the patient about safety are necessary nursing responsibilities for the patient receiving delavirdine.

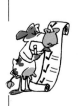

Notes

Drugs Used to Alter Immune Function

What You WILL LEARN

After reading this chapter, you will know how to do the following:

✔ Contrast the action of an immunosuppressant, interferon, interleukin, and a colony-stimulating factor.
✔ Discuss common adverse effects of cytotoxic antineoplastics.
✔ Explain common nursing responsibilities when administering biologic response modifiers, antineoplastics, and targeted therapies.

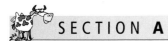 SECTION **A**

BIOLOGIC RESPONSE MODIFIERS

Biologic response modifiers augment and use the body's immune system to counteract the side effects of various treatments, particularly cancer chemotherapy. The selected pharmacologic agents that are discussed in this section include immunosuppressants and immunomodulators, such as interferons, interleukins, colony-stimulating factors, and monoclonal antibodies.

What IS an Immunosuppressant?

Immunosuppressants	Trade Names	Uses
azathioprine [AZE-uh-THIGH-oh-preen]	Imuran	Prevents rejection of kidney transplantation
cyclosporine [SIGH-kloe-spore-EEN]	Sandimmune	Prolongs survival of transplants involving skin, heart, kidneys, pancreas, bone marrow, small intestine, liver, and lungs
tacrolimus [ta-kroe-LEE-mus]	Prograf, Protopic	Treats rejection of heart, renal, and liver transplantation

Action

An immunosuppressant acts to suppress the body's natural immune response to an antigen. Azathioprine, cyclosporine, and tacrolimus inhibit T-helper cells and T-suppressor cells, thereby suppressing humoral immunity and cell-mediated immune reactions (e.g., delayed hypersensitivity, T-cell effects, allograft rejection, collagen-induced arthritis). Immunosuppressants help block an inflammatory response and thereby decrease cell damage. Azathioprine also alters antibody production. Tacrolimus blocks antibody production by B cells, inhibits T cells, and modifies release of interleukins. In contrast, immunomodulating agents augment and promote the host's own defense mechanisms.

Uses

Immunosuppressants are given primarily to prevent rejection of transplanted organs, such as heart, kidney, and liver. Azathioprine and cyclosporine are also used in the treatment of rheumatoid arthritis.

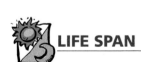

TAKE HOME POINTS

T and B cells are the two major types of lymphocytes, forming approximately 20% of white blood cells. Several different types of T cells exist, including T-helper cells and T-suppressor cells. T-helper cells carry out different immune functions, such as assisting in the reproduction of memory cells that provide long-lasting immunity against specific antigens. T-suppressor cells have immunosuppressive and regulatory functions. B cells produce antibodies against an antigen and have antibody-type receptors on their cell surface, which assists in immunity.

LIFE SPAN

Most immunosuppressants are contraindicated for children and for women during pregnancy and lactation.

What You NEED TO KNOW

Contraindications/Precautions

Immunosuppressants are contraindicated for patients with hypersensitivity. Cyclosporine is contraindicated for patients with renal dysfunction, uncontrolled hypertension or malignancies, and psoriasis.

Drug Interactions

Azathioprine decreases the action of anticoagulants, decreases cyclosporine levels, reverses neuromuscular blockers, induces severe leukopenia when given with angiotensin-converting enzyme (ACE) inhibitors, increases action and toxic effects of allopurinol, and increases 6-MP metabolite levels when given together.

When cyclosporine is given with other nephrotoxic drugs (e.g., anti-inflammatories, antibiotics, antifungals, GI agents), the risk for renal dysfunction is increased. When it is given with lovastatin, increased digoxin levels, severe myopathy, or rhabdomyolysis may occur. Androgens, amiodarone, azole antifungals, calcium channel blockers, macrolide antibiotics, metoclopramide, and oral contraceptives increase cyclosporine and tacrolimus levels. Anticonvulsants decrease cyclosporine and tacrolimus levels. Colchicine and corticosteroids increase the adverse effects and toxicities of cyclosporine.

Adverse Effects

Immunosuppressants commonly cause nausea, vomiting, diarrhea, rash, fever, malaise, and pulmonary edema. They may also cause malignancies if given over a prolonged period. Azathioprine may also cause joint and muscle pain, hypotension, temporary infertility, and fetal damage. This drug may lead to dose-related severe leukopenia, thrombocytopenia, macrocytic anemia, and severe bone marrow depression.

Additional adverse effects of cyclosporines include photosensitivity, anxiety, confusion, depression, increased LDLs, diabetes mellitus, nephrotoxicity, hepatotoxicity, CNS toxicity, convulsions, tremors, hirsutism, hypertension, gum hyperplasia, chest pain, and myocardial infarction (MI). Other adverse effects of tacrolimus are headache, insomnia, nightmares, hair loss (alopecia), hyperglycemia, hyperkalemia, hypomagnesemia, hypertension, anorexia, diarrhea, and leg cramping.

What You DO

Nursing Responsibilities

Azathioprine is usually administered with food or in divided doses to decrease gastric distress. This medication is usually initiated 1 to 3 days before and repeated within 24 hours after transplantation. When giving immunosuppressants, the nurse should:

- Monitor the patient's CBC weekly during the first month of therapy, every 2 weeks during the second and third months, and monthly thereafter.

- Cyclosporine should be given with caution to patients with renal or hepatic dysfunction, diabetes mellitus, elevated low-density lipoproteins (LDLs), and cancer.
- Immunosuppressed patients with an infection require immediate treatment with the appropriate antibiotic or antifungal agent. Delays in treatment may be life-threatening for the individual.

TAKE HOME POINTS

- Azathioprine should be discontinued or the dose reduced at the first indication of a significant decrease or a continued decrease in leukocytes or platelets to avoid irreversible bone marrow depression.
- Instruct the patient who is taking azathioprine to report the following symptoms immediately: fever of 100.5° F or more, sore throat, unusual bruising, bleeding, pale stools, or darkened urine.
- Patients who are receiving immunosuppressant drugs may not show the classic symptoms of infection. Look for slight to moderate rises in temperature, changes in behavior, changes in breath sounds, and complaints of painful urination or defecation.

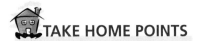

TAKE HOME POINTS

Monitor patients for 48 hours after first dose for early signs of first-dose reaction (e.g., high fever, chills, malaise, dyspnea).

- Teach the patient who is taking an immunosuppressant to report any abnormal bleeding or signs of infection immediately.
- Instruct patients to avoid contact with people who have known infections, thereby protecting themselves and preventing infections.
- Ascertain that cyclosporine is given as a single dose, initially 4 to 12 hours before transplantation. Cyclosporine may be given IV when the patient is unable to tolerate the drug orally.
- Mix oral solutions of cyclosporine with milk, chocolate milk, or orange or apple juice in a glass container (never plastic) at room temperature. Grapefruit juice should be avoided because it affects the metabolism of cyclosporine.
- Inform patient to thoroughly stir oral cyclosporine solutions, take immediately, and follow with more diluent in the same glass to ensure that the entire dose is consumed. The outside of the glass should be dried, but the glass should not be rinsed with water.
- Instruct patients to take cyclosporine on a consistent schedule every day.
- Encourage patients who are taking cyclosporine to practice thorough oral hygiene and to inspect the mouth daily for swollen gums, sores, and white patches.
- Monitor the patient who is receiving IV cyclosporine for at least 30 minutes after initiating drug administration and frequently thereafter for hypersensitivity and other adverse effects.
- Watch the patient who is receiving IV cyclosporine for infection, nephrotoxicity, and neurotoxicity.
- Monitor baseline renal and liver function tests and potassium before therapy, then periodically thereafter for comparison and early detection of toxicity.
- Instruct the patient who is taking cyclosporine to wear sunscreen and protective clothing, thus limiting exposure to sunlight.
- Inform patients who are taking cyclosporine that hirsutism is reversible after drug therapy is discontinued.
- Warn women to use effective contraception before immunosuppressant therapy, during therapy, and up to 6 weeks after this drug has been discontinued.
- Instruct patients who are taking immunosuppressants to report evidence of infection, hematuria, and peripheral edema.
- Monitor the patient for early signs of acute pulmonary edema and have resuscitation equipment available (i.e., intubation, oxygen, corticosteroids). First-dose reaction usually occurs 45 to 60 minutes after the first and second doses.

- Assess the patient for fever. If the patient has a fever of 37.8° C (100° F) or pulmonary edema, or both, the health care provider should be consulted before treatment to prevent acute pulmonary edema and possible death.

Do You UNDERSTAND?

DIRECTIONS: **Indicate in the space provided whether the statement is** *true* **or** *false*. **If the answer is false, correct the statement to make it true (using the margin space).**

_____ 1. Immunosuppressants are given primarily to prevent rejection of transplanted organs.

_____ 2. Immunosuppressants are contraindicated for women during pregnancy.

_____ 3. Immunosuppressants predispose patients to infection.

Immunomodulators

Immunomodulators have the ability to improve or promote immune responses by the host. The selected immunomodulators that are discussed in this section include interferons, interleukins, and colony-stimulating factors.

What IS an Interferon?

Interferons	Trade Names	Uses
interferon α-2a [IN-ter-FEAR-ahn]	Roferon-A	Treatment of hairy cell and chronic myelogenous leukemia, AIDS-related Kaposi's sarcoma, and chronic hepatitis C
interferon α-2b [IN-ter-FEAR-ahn]	Intron A	Treatment of hairy cell leukemia, malignant melanoma, follicular lymphoma, condylomata acuminata, Kaposi's sarcoma, and chronic hepatitis B and C

Answers: 1. true; 2. true; 3. true.

Action

An interferon acts on the body by exerting antitumor activity. The mechanism is not clearly understood. The belief is that interferons modulate the host's immune response, preventing tumor cells and viral particles from reproducing.

Uses

Interferon α-2a is indicated in the treatment of hairy cell leukemia, AIDS-related Kaposi's sarcoma, and chronic myelogenous leukemia. Interferon α-2b is used in the treatment of hairy cell leukemia, malignant melanoma, condylomata acuminata (genital and perianal warts), AIDS-related Kaposi's sarcoma, and chronic hepatitis B and C.

Interferon α-2a should be given with caution to patients with cardiac disease, severe renal or hepatic impairment, seizure disorders, myelosuppression, and compromised CNS function. Serious adverse effects include suicidal ideation, GI hemorrhage, life-threatening anemia, renal or hepatic impairment, and cardiac dysrhythmias.

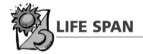

LIFE SPAN

Caution is to be used in women during pregnancy and lactation and in children.

What You NEED TO KNOW

Contraindications/Precautions

Interferon α-2b is contraindicated for any patient with a hypersensitivity, thyroid abnormality, or preexisting psychiatric condition or history of a severe psychiatric disorder. Caution should be used when giving interferon α-2b to patients with thrombocytopenia, influenza symptoms, pneumonia, cardiovascular disease, retinal damage, hepatic impairment, autoimmune diseases, hyperglycemia, and infertility.

Drug Interactions

The effects of theophylline and aminophylline are exacerbated when interferon α-2a and interferon α-2b are given concurrently. When interferon α-2a is given concurrently with interleukin-2, a potential risk for renal failure exists. When interferon α-2b is given with zidovudine, the patient may have an increased risk for neutropenia.

Adverse Effects

Adverse effects of interferon α-2a and interferon α-2b include fever, fatigue, headache, chills, weight loss, photosensitivity, dizziness, rash, diaphoresis, anxiety, lethargy, alopecia, and itching. Other adverse effects include depression, suicidal ideation, paresthesia, sleep disturbance, decreased mental status, anorexia, nausea, vomiting, diarrhea, bone and joint pain, coughing, dyspnea, and bone marrow depression. Adverse effects may be severe to the extent that these drugs must be discontinued.

What You DO

Nursing Responsibilities

Interferon α-2a is given Sub-Q or IM. After the initial dose, maintenance doses are usually given three times weekly. Interferon α-2b is given IV, Sub-Q, or IM but should not be given IM to patients with thrombocytopenia and platelet counts less than 60,000/mm. This population may receive interferon α-2b Sub-Q as a substitute. When administering interferons, the nurse should:

- Monitor frequent CBCs, platelet counts, blood chemistries, electrolytes, thyroid-stimulating hormone (TSH) levels, liver function tests, chest x-ray studies, and electrocardiogram (ECG) data in patients who are receiving interferon for early detection of toxicities.
- Instruct the patient who is taking interferon to report any hives, itching, cough, difficulty breathing, wheezing, tightness in the chest, dizziness, or suspected pregnancy to the health care provider.
- Recommend contraceptive measures during interferon therapy.
- Warn patients who are taking interferon α-2a to avoid changing brands of interferon because changes in the dose may result.
- Advise patients who are taking interferon α-2a to maintain adequate hydration.
- Instruct the patient that photosensitivity may occur and to take precautions in sunlight.
- Warn the patient to use caution when driving or operating hazardous machines that require alertness and coordination because interferon may cause drowsiness or dizziness.

When administering interleukins, the nurse should:

- Teach the patient to use mild soap and rinse well.
- Instruct the patient to avoid lotions or skin products containing alcohol or perfumes.
- Advise the patient to avoid sunlight.

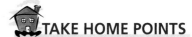

TAKE HOME POINTS

Instruct the patient who is taking interferon to use sunscreens and protective clothing and to decrease ultraviolet exposure until tolerance is determined.

Do You UNDERSTAND?

DIRECTIONS: **Indicate in the space provided whether the statement is**
true or _false_. If the answer is false, correct the statement
to make it true (using the margin space).

_____ 1. Patients who are taking interferon should take precautions regarding ultraviolet light exposure.

_____ 2. Patients should not receive interferon when the platelet count is less than 100,000/mm.

What IS an Interleukin?

Interleukins	Trade Names	Uses
interleukin-11 or oprelvekin [oh-prel-vee-kin]	Neumega	Prevents severe thrombocytopenia in myelosuppression
interleukin-2 or aldesleukin [IN-ter-LU-kin]	Proleukin	Treatment of metastatic melanoma or renal cell carcinoma

Action

Oprelvekin is a thrombopoietic growth factor that stimulates platelet production. Aldesleukin is a recombinant protein that enhances lymphocyte mitogenesis, stimulates long-term growth of human interleukin-2-dependent cell lines, enhances lymphocyte cytotoxicity, and induces interferon-gamma production. Interleukins inhibit tumor growth and activate cellular immunity with profound lymphocytosis, eosinophilia, thrombocytopenia, and the production of cytokines (including tumor necrosis factor, interleukin-1, and gamma interferon).

Uses

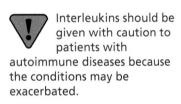

Interleukins should be given with caution to patients with autoimmune diseases because the conditions may be exacerbated.

Oprelvekin is indicated in the prevention of severe thrombocytopenia; it can also be used to reduce the need for platelet transfusions following myelosuppressive chemotherapy. Oprelvekin and aldesleukin are used in the treatment of metastatic renal-cell carcinoma.

Answers: 1. true; 2. false; less than 60,000/mm.

What You NEED TO KNOW

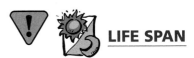

LIFE SPAN

Contraindications/Precautions

Interleukins are contraindicated for patients with hypersensitivity, abnormal thallium stress test, pulmonary function tests, uncontrolled dysrhythmias, pericardial tamponade, angina, or MI.

Drug Interactions

Interleukins may cause leakage of plasma proteins and fluid into the extravascular space and loss of vascular tone, leading to hypovolemia, significant hypotension, tachycardia, and hypoprofusion. These agents may also cause mental changes, renal and hepatic toxicity, infertility, allograft rejection in transplant patients, and thyroid impairment. When aldesleukin is given with other nephrotoxic or hepatoxic drugs, the risk for toxicity in increased. Antihypertensives increase the hypotension caused by aldesleukin.

Adverse Effects

Most adverse effects following oprelvekin administration are mild or moderate in severity and reversible after the drug is discontinued. These adverse effects include blurred vision, chills, fever, nervousness, alopecia, anorexia, dyspepsia, constipation, abdominal pain, ecchymosis, weakness, muscle and bone pain, and infection. Other adverse effects include nausea, vomiting, dyspnea, cough, rhinitis, edema, headache, rash, eye hemorrhage, amblyopia, paresthesia, skin discoloration, and exfoliative dermatitis.

Aldesleukin may cause many cardiovascular adverse effects, including dysrhythmias, MI, congestive heart failure (CHF), cardiac arrest, stroke, pericardial effusion, and thrombosis. Aldesleukin may also cause pulmonary congestion, wheezing, apnea, pneumothorax, respiratory failure, GI bleeding, intestinal perforation, coma, seizures, coagulation disorders, thrombocytopenia, and electrolyte disturbances.

Oprelvekin should be used with caution in children, in women during pregnancy, and in patients with papilledema or congestive heart, renal, or liver failure. Aldesleukin should not be given to children under 18 years of age.

Additional adverse effects of aldesleukin are often fatal, including capillary leak syndrome (CLS). This condition is a result of plasma proteins and fluid escaping into extracellular spaces, with a loss of vascular tone. This process leads to a drop in mean arterial blood pressure (BP), edema, reduced organ perfusion, and may cause death.

What You DO

Nursing Responsibilities

Oprelvekin is administered by an IV infusion over 15 minutes every 8 hours and is administered Sub-Q as a single dose in the abdomen, thigh, hip, or upper arm. Drug administration may begin at least 6 hours after the completion of chemotherapy. When giving interleukins, the nurse should:

- Monitor platelet counts periodically to ensure effectiveness of therapy. Interleukin therapy should continue until the platelet count postnadir is greater than 50,000 cells/microliter. A treatment course of more than 21 days is not recommended.
- Teach the patient who is self-administering interleukin at home about proper reconstitution and administration techniques, necessary caution, and disposal of materials. Reconstituted solution may be stored at 36° to 46° F until used but do not freeze the solution. The reconstituted interleukin solution should be used within 3 hours. Do not use solution that is discolored or contains particles.

TAKE HOME POINTS

When reconstituting oprelvekin solution, gently swirl vial, but do not shake the solution. Do not administer this agent with an in-line filter, or mix with normal saline or bacteriostatic water. This drug should not be mixed with other medications.

Do You UNDERSTAND?

DIRECTIONS: Fill in the blanks to complete the following statements.

1. Oprelvekin is given to stimulate _____ cell production.
2. Oprelvekin therapy is usually initiated at least _____ hours after chemotherapy is completed.
3. Aldesleukin therapy may lead to an often fatal condition known as _____.

Answers: 1. platelet; 2. 6; 3. capillary leak syndrome.

What IS a Colony-Stimulating Factor?

Colony-Stimulating Factor	Trade Names	Uses
erythropoietin [e-RITH-roe-po-E-tin]	Epogen	Treatment of low hematocrit levels in anemia
filgrastim [fil-GRASS-tim]	Neupogen	Treatment of neutropenia
sargramostim [sar-GRA-mos-tim]	Leukine	Restores red bone marrow after transplantation

Action

Erythropoietin is a serum protein that promotes monocyte differentiation. A colony-stimulating factor called **erythropoietin** is a glycoprotein (a compound of carbohydrate and protein) that stimulates red blood cell production. Normally, erythropoietin is produced primarily in the kidneys in response to hypoxia; however, in chronic renal failure (CRF), erythropoietin production is impaired. The impaired erythropoietin production is the main cause of anemia in CRF. Erythropoietin stimulates erythropoiesis and is indicated in patients with anemia. After administration, the reticulocyte count is usually increased within 10 days. The red cell count, hemoglobin, and hematocrit are usually increased within 2 to 6 weeks. Filgrastim (G-CSF) is a glycoprotein that regulates the production of neutrophils. Sargramostim (GM-CSF) is a hematopoietic growth factor that stimulates neutrophils, monocytes, and macrophages.

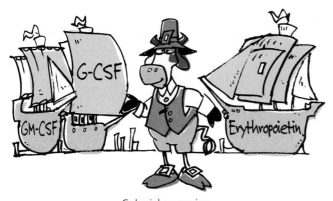

Colonial expansion.

Uses

Erythropoietin is indicated in patients with anemia and zidovudine-treated HIV-infected patients with cancer who are taking chemotherapy, as well as those on postsurgical status. Erythropoietin is also used in patients with CRF, whether they require dialysis or not. This agent decreases the number of transfusions that are usually required in patients with CRF, and it improves cardiovascular status, cognitive function, exercise tolerance, and quality of life. G-CSF is used to promote a regeneration of neutrophils, thereby decreasing the incidence of infection in patients who are receiving myelosuppressive anticancer drugs. GM-CSF is effective in the treatment of bone marrow deficiency from cancer chemotherapy or bone marrow transplantation. Sargramostim is used to restore red bone marrow following bone marrow transplantation.

Colony-stimulating factors should be given with caution to patients with hematologic malignancies because of the potential risk for increased growth of cancer cells in patients who are taking this drug.

LIFE SPAN

Caution should be taken when administering erythropoietin to children and women who are pregnant or lactating. G-CSF should be given with caution to patients with hypothyroidism, pregnant or lactating women, and children. This agent should be given with caution to patients with cardiovascular or respiratory disease, renal or hepatic impairment, and those with fluid retention.

What You NEED TO KNOW

Contraindications/Precautions

Erythropoietin is contraindicated for patients with uncontrolled hypertension and known hypersensitivity. GM-CSF is contraindicated for patients with excessive leukemic myeloid blasts in the bone marrow.

Drug Interactions

When corticosteroids and lithium are given with GM-CSF, myeloproliferative effects may be increased. Myeloproliferative effects are a rapid reproduction of bone marrow elements. When erythropoietin is given concurrently with heparin, anticoagulation effects may decrease.

Adverse Effects

Elevated BP is an adverse effect of erythropoietin, which may require antihypertensive medication. Seizures and hypertensive encephalopathy have occurred in patients who are taking erythropoietin and those with CRF. Other adverse effects of erythropoietin include headache, dizziness, anxiety, fatigue, sweating, hypertension, insomnia, fever, nausea, vomiting, diarrhea, constipation, joint pain, clotting of arteriovenous (AV) fistula, and seizures.

Adverse effects from G-CSF include bone pain, transient decrease in BP, nausea, vomiting, diarrhea, and fatigue. First-dose syndrome from G-CSF is an adverse effect that includes respiratory distress, hypoxia, flushing, syncope, tachycardia, hypotension, neutrophils above 20,000/mm or a platelet count greater than 500,000/mm. Other adverse effects include peripheral edema, nausea, vomiting, diarrhea, abdominal pain, GI hemorrhage, blood dyscrasia, hyperglycemia, fever, chills, malaise, weight loss, asthenia, muscle and bone pain, and hypertension.

Cardiovascular adverse effects from GM-CSF include hypertension, hypotension, edema, tachycardia, and MI. Other adverse effects include dyspnea, paresthesia, insomnia, anxiety, fever, rash, itching, alopecia, anorexia, nausea, vomiting, diarrhea, abdominal pain, stomatitis, GI bleeding, bilirubinemia, blood dyscrasias, and hyperglycemia.

 Because lithium may cause the release of neutrophils, G-CSF should be given with caution to patients who require both drugs. Because lithium and corticosteroids may cause myeloproliferative effects, caution should be used with GM-CSF. G-CSF and GM-CSF are never given concurrently with cytotoxic cancer therapy.

What You DO

Nursing Responsibilities

Erythropoietin can be given Sub-Q or IV three times a week. Dose adjustment should not be made more than once a month. When administering colony-stimulating factors, the nurse should:

- Monitor the BP before erythropoietin therapy. Hypertension may occur as an adverse effect, particularly when the hematocrit is rising quickly.
- Discard any unused portion of the vial, because erythropoietin contains no preservatives.
- Watch the hematocrit, fluid and electrolyte balance, and renal function. After reaching target hematocrit or when the hematocrit rises more than four points in a 2-week period, notify the health care provider for dose reduction. When the hematocrit fails to rise five to six points or is still below target range after 8 weeks of therapy, notify the health care provider for dose increase.
- Monitor patients who are taking erythropoietin and those undergoing hemodialysis treatment carefully because they may require heparin anticoagulation to prevent arteriovenous shunt clotting.
- Instruct the patient to avoid driving or engaging in hazardous activity when the possibility of seizures is present.
- Do not give G-CSF within 24 hours of cytotoxic chemotherapy. G-CSF is usually given daily for 2 weeks until the neutrophil count reaches 10,000/mm.

TAKE HOME POINTS

- Do not shake the solution because this may denature the glycoprotein, making it biologically inactive. Erythropoietin doses should be decreased if the hematocrit elevates more than four points in a 2-week period. The BP should be closely monitored and controlled in patients who are receiving erythropoietin.
- When necessary, G-CSF may be diluted in 5% dextrose solution but never in saline because the medication may precipitate.
- Monitor the hematocrit twice weekly after beginning erythropoietin therapy (until the dose is stabilized) and throughout therapy; the risk for seizures is greater when the hematocrit increases rapidly.
- Premature discontinuation of G-CSF is not recommended before recovery from the expected neutrophil nadir.

The nurse must use extreme caution when administering chemotherapy drugs, many of which have potentially serious, even lethal, adverse effects and toxicities.

- Monitor a baseline CBC and platelet count drawn before G-CSF therapy. Following initiation of therapy, these tests should be monitored two times a week during therapy. G-CSF should be discontinued after neutrophil counts remain at normal levels for at least 3 days.
- Administer GM-CSF over a 2-hour IV infusion for a 21-day treatment at least 24 hours after the last chemotherapy dose and 12 hours after the last radiation dose.
- Check the CBC with differential two times a week during therapy. When the neutrophils increase 20,000/mm or the platelet count is greater than 500,000/mm, GM-CSF therapy should be interrupted or the dose reduced by one half.

Do You UNDERSTAND?

DIRECTIONS: Fill in the blanks with the appropriate responses.

1. The first-dose syndrome of GM-CSF involves the following symptoms:

   _____

   _____

   _____

   _____

   _____

2. GM-CSF should be discontinued or the dose reduced by one half when the neutrophil reaches _____ or the platelet count is _____.

Answers: 1. respiratory distress, hypoxia, flushing, syncope, tachycardia, hypotension; 2. a level less than 20,000/mm, less than 500,000/mm.

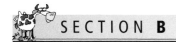

SECTION **B**

ANTINEOPLASTIC AGENTS

Antineoplastic agents are used to treat a wide variety of diseases and disorders, including many different types of cancers and autoimmune disorders. Cytotoxic agents tend to interfere with growth and replication of rapidly dividing cells. Normal tissue that is characterized by rapid growth and replication includes the hair follicles, the bone marrow, and the lining of the GI tract that extends from the mouth to the anus. Cancer therapy affects these parts of the body in varying degrees. Nearly all chemotherapeutic agents have potential organ-specific toxicities that the nurse should identify before administration; thus appropriate evaluation and monitoring may be implemented before, during, and after the drugs are given. Because of the high toxicity profile, the dosing schedule of these drugs is calculated according to the patient's body surface area, which is calculated based on height and weight.

Cytoxic antineoplastic drugs are not tumor-specific; therefore they can exert damaging effects on normal healthy cells in addition to cancer cells. Within the last decade, newer targeted therapies have been developed that are highly specific against certain components of the tumor cell or its environment, which results in less toxic effects against normal tissue. Examples of these therapies include monoclonal antibodies, cell signal transduction inhibitors, and angiogenesis inhibitors. Antineoplastic drugs are prescribed with one of three goals in mind: to cure, control, or obtain palliation of malignant disease. Newer treatment regimens combining cytotoxic agents with targeted therapies offer improved treatment outcomes and in some cases cures for many cancer patients.

Cytotoxic agents are classified according to their mechanism of action, the point at which they act within the cell's life cycle, and their chemical structure. To maximize therapeutic outcomes, combination regimens consist of two or more drugs. Most cancer treatment protocols use drugs that act at different points within the cell cycle, maximizing tumor cell kill and decreasing the severity of adverse effects. The term *cell cycle* refers to the reproductive process that occurs in both normal and malignant cells. The cell cycle or replication of body cells is a predetermined sequence of events that occurs in the interval between the origination of the cell and its division into two new cells.

The cell cycle involves several phases:

1. G_0 is the resting phase, during which the cell performs all functions except replication.
2. G_1 is the first active phase, during which RNA and enzymes required for the creation of DNA are developed.
3. S is the phase during which DNA is synthesized for chromosomes.
4. G_2 is the phase during which RNA is synthesized and the mitotic spindle is formed.
5. M is the last phase, during which mitosis occurs, allowing the cell to split into two cells.

There exists a broad range of potentially dangerous complications and safety issues associated with antineoplastic therapy treatment. Only a registered nurse with special educational preparation may assume responsibility for preparing and administering antineoplastic drugs.

Because antineoplastic agents are also classified as biohazardous substances, special precautions must be taken when preparing, handling, and administering these drugs. In the event of an accidental spill, special cleaning procedures must be observed. These safety procedures are beyond the scope of this book but are available online at the Oncology Nursing Society's website.

Because these drugs are potentially lethal, the nurse must always ensure that the patient has given informed consent before therapy can begin. Also, special precautions should be taken to verify that the dosage and drug has been appropriately calculated and prepared.

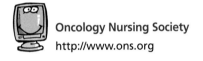

Oncology Nursing Society
http://www.ons.org

What IS an Antimetabolite Agent?

Antimetabolite Agents	Trade Names	Uses
cytarabine [sye-TARE-a-been]	ARA-C	Treatment of leukemias, Hodgkin's disease, and non-Hodgkin's lymphoma
5-fluorouracil [flure-oh-YOUR-a-sil]	5FU	Treatment of carcinoma of the breast, colon, rectum, liver, pancreas, stomach, and esophagus and head and neck cancers
floxuridine [flox-YOUR-i-deen]	FUDR	Treatment of carcinoma of the GI tract with metastasis to the liver, gallbladder, or common bile duct

Antimetabolite Agents	Trade Names	Uses
methotrexate [meth-oh-TREX-ate]	MTX	Treatment of leukemia, lymphoma, and lung, breast, and head and neck cancers; in lower doses, also useful in the treatment of rheumatoid arthritis
capecitabine [cap-e-SI-ta-been]	Xeloda	Treatment of breast cancer and metastatic colon cancer

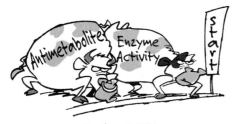

Ready, set, GO!

Action

Antimetabolites are similar in structure to normal metabolites. These agents compete for enzyme activity within the cell and prevent the synthesis of DNA. Cellular division is stopped, which results in cell death. These drugs act within the S phase of the cell's life cycle.

Uses

Because of the limited time in the cell's life cycle during which these drugs are effective, antimetabolites are typically prescribed for rapidly growing tumors, such as leukemias and lymphomas. Antimetabolites are useful in the treatment of many different types of tumors, including acute and chronic leukemias and some solid tumors.

What You NEED TO KNOW

Contraindications/Precautions

Antimetabolite agents are contraindicated for patients with hypersensitivity. Floxuridine is contraindicated for patients with a current or recent viral infection. 5-Fluorouracil is contraindicated for patients with malnutrition and myelosuppression. Patients with impaired liver function may require reduced dosages of floxuridine and fluorouracil.

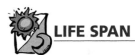 **LIFE SPAN**

5-Fluorouracil is contraindicated for women during pregnancy and lactation. Floxuridine is contraindicated during pregnancy.

5-Fluorouracil should be used cautiously in patients who have had major surgery within 1 month. Floxuridine should be used with caution in patients who are malnourished or have bone marrow depression. Capecitabine should be used with caution in patients with infections. Caution should also be used for antimetabolite drugs in patients with renal or hepatic dysfunction.

Drug Interactions

Patients who use over-the-counter medications, herbal and vitamin preparations, and other alternative therapies may encounter drug interactions when taking antimetabolite therapy (e.g., folic acid decreases the effect of methotrexate). When cytarabine is given together with digoxin, decreased serum levels of digoxin may occur. Serum levels of fluorouracil are increased, which then leads to fluorouracil toxicity when fluorouracil is given with cimetidine or α-interferon. Increased methotrexate toxicity may occur when methotrexate is given with aspirin, NSAIDs, or sulfonamides. When thioguanine is given concurrently with myelosuppressants, an increased risk for toxicity, bleeding, and liver damage may occur.

Adverse Effects

Antimetabolite drugs tend to exert their main toxicities in the bone marrow, the lining of the GI tract, and hair follicles. High doses of these drugs may also cause renal and neurologic damage.

Similar to most chemotherapy agents, these drugs tend to reach their lowest point (**nadir**) 10 to 14 days after administration. When renal and hepatic functions are normal, the body gradually resumes normal function approximately 21 days after these drugs are last administered.

Cellular debris is thought to cause increased inflammation and hypermotility of the GI tract, which causes abdominal pain, cramping, and diarrhea. Mucosal surfaces of the GI tract tend to develop ulcers because the body is unable to replace cells that are worn away by the normal processes of eating and digestion. When the patient has visible mouth ulcers, the intestines are likely to be similarly affected.

Temporary suppression of bone marrow function may occur. The degree and duration of suppression is a function of the dose and the patient's overall health status. White blood cells are most likely to show a decrease in number, placing the patient at risk for a variety of infections. A decrease in white blood cells leaves the patient unable to mount a normal immunologic or inflammatory response to tissue injury or infection.

Patients may experience delayed wound healing, tissue repair, and life-threatening infections. Early signs and symptoms of infection in these patients include mild-to-moderate fever, chills, malaise, weakness, fatigue, and inadequate oxygenation. In patients with neutropenia, these symptoms may be subtle and easily overlooked.

What You DO

Nursing Responsibilities

When administering antimetabolites, the nurse should:

- Provide the patient with written and verbal explanation about possible toxic effects, precautions, and measures to manage and minimize adverse effects.
- Confirm that the patient has given informed consent before therapy begins.
- Evaluate CBC, BUN, creatinine clearance, and liver function studies before initiating therapy. The patient with preexisting organ damage or bone marrow suppression may not be a candidate for this category of drugs or may require a dose reduction.
- Establish reliable IV access before therapy begins.
- Monitor all chemotherapy infusions carefully for patency of the IV site because these drugs may cause pain and tissue damage during infiltration.
- Assess patients who have already received treatment for evidence of chemotherapy-related mouth ulcers (**stomatitis**), GI distress (particularly vomiting and diarrhea), and symptoms of infection.
- Evaluate patients carefully for evidence of infection.
- Teach the patient the proper way to avoid potential sources of infection. Reinforce the need for ongoing medical follow-up visits.
- Assess the patient for GI distress and changes in bowel habits.
- Monitor intake and output of patients with diarrhea because they may require fluid replacement and treatment with antidiarrheal agents.
- Teach patients about the importance of maintaining good oral care and of avoiding potential sources of infection.
- Adjust the patient's diet as necessary to maximize oral intake. Small portions of soft, bland, room-temperature foods are generally tolerated.

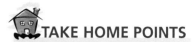

TAKE HOME POINTS

Assess oral cavity daily for ulceration. Patients experiencing diarrhea should be placed on intake and output and will require additional monitoring for electrolyte imbalances.

Do You UNDERSTAND?

DIRECTIONS: **Indicate in the space provided whether the statement is *true* or *false*. If the answer is false, correct the statement to make it true (using the margin space).**

_____ 1. Antimetabolites compete for enzymatic activity within the cell and prevent DNA synthesis.

_____ 2. Antimetabolites particularly cause toxicity of the cardiovascular system.

What IS a Mitotic Inhibitor?

Mitotic Inhibitors	Trade Names	Uses
vincristine [vin-KRIS-teen]	Oncovin	Treatment of carcinoma, Hodgkin's disease, acute lymphoblastic leukemia, and Wilms' tumor
paclitaxel [pac-li-TAX-el]	Taxol	Treatment of breast cancer or ovarian cancer, non-small-cell lung cancer, and head and neck cancer
topotecan [toe-po-TEE-can]	Hycamtin	Treatment of metastatic ovarian, lung, and colorectal cancers; AIDS-related Kaposi's sarcoma
etoposide [e-toe-PO-side]	Toposar	Treatment of testicular and small-cell lung carcinoma, acute lymphocytic leukemia, multiple myeloma

Action

Mitotic inhibitors are all plant derivatives that are grouped into four classes: vinca alkaloids, taxines, camptothecins, and podophyllotoxins. Most of the drugs in this category are cell-cycle–specific and act either within the G or S phase of cellular reproduction.

The vinca alkaloids (e.g., vincristine, vinblastine, vinorelbine, vindesine) are cell-cycle–specific and inhibit the formation of the mitotic spindle and the replication of DNA and RNA, thereby stopping cell mitosis. Taxines (e.g., docetaxel, paclitaxel) inhibit the division of tumor cells in the M and G phases of the cell cycle. Camptothecins (**topoisomerase I inhibitors**), such as irinotecan and topotecan, produce irreparable breaks in the cell's DNA, causing cell death. These agents inhibit the enzyme

Answers: **1. true; 2. false; antimetabolites cause renal, neurologic, GI, and bone marrow damage.**

that is needed for DNA replication. Podophyllotoxins (**topoisomerase II inhibitors**), such as etoposide and teniposide, act in the G_2 phase of the cell cycle to prevent mitosis, thereby stopping cellular replication.

Uses

Mitotic inhibitors are used to treat tumors of various body parts, such as the lung, breast, testes, and ovaries. Vincristine is used to treat Hodgkin's disease, acute lymphoblastic leukemia, oat cell carcinoma of the lung, and Wilms' tumor. Paclitaxel is used for the treatment of advanced breast and ovarian cancers. Topotecan is used for lung, ovarian, and colorectal cancer. Etoposide is used for small cell lung and testicular cancer.

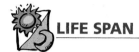
LIFE SPAN

Mitotic inhibitors are contraindicated for women during pregnancy and lactation and for children.

What You NEED TO KNOW

Contraindications/Precautions

Mitotic inhibitors are contraindicated for patients with hypersensitivity. Paclitaxel is also contraindicated for patients with a neutrophil count of less than 1500 cells/mm^3. Topotecan is further contraindicated for patients with acute infection. Etoposide is contraindicated for patients with severe bone marrow depression, current or recent infection, and severe renal and hepatic dysfunction.

Drug Interactions

Vinca alkaloids may cause severe bone marrow suppression. Vinblastine reaches a nadir 4 to 10 days after administration. When vinblastine is given concurrently with mitomycin, bronchospasms may occur. When paclitaxel and ketoconazole are given together, serious toxicities may occur.

Topoisomerase I inhibitors and vincristine are all capable of causing severe peripheral neuropathy and autonomic neuropathy, which may be permanent if dose reductions are not implemented when the symptoms first appear. When irinotecan is taken with laxatives, severe, prolonged diarrhea may occur, leading to volume depletion and electrolyte imbalances. When irinotecan is taken with Decadron, an increased risk for hyperglycemia and decreased lymphocyte count occurs. When prochlorperazine is taken within 24 hours of irinotecan, an increased risk of akathisia may occur. Topoisomerase II inhibitors may cause dose-limiting bone marrow suppression and stomatitis. Topotecan may cause stomatitis,

 Vincristine should be used cautiously in patients with infection, leukopenia, bone marrow suppression, chickenpox, current neurologic or neuromuscular disorders, and hepatic dysfunction. Paclitaxel should be used with caution in patients with cardiac dysrhythmias. Topotecan should be used cautiously in patients with a history of bleeding disorders, previous radiation therapy, and myelosuppression. Etoposide should be used with caution in patients with gout.

nausea, vomiting, and headache. Myelosuppression is the major dose-limiting toxicity for the taxines.

Adverse Effects

Mitotic inhibitors are all plant derivatives; thus they have a relatively high incidence of allergic reactions. All of the vinca alkaloids are vesicants, which means that these drugs are capable of causing permanent tissue damage and necrosis when allowed to extravasate into tissues.

TAKE HOME POINTS

- Obtain reliable IV access with an intact vein to decrease the risk for tissue damage from extravasation of vesicant agents. Remember "V" for vesicant and take precautions!
  * Vincristine
  * Vinblastine
  * Velban
  * Vindesine
- Patients who will require prolonged treatment with vesicant agents should have a central venous line placed in order to decrease their risk for tissue damage from these drugs.
- Always check laboratory studies and diagnostic test results before starting antineoplastic therapy, even if the patient has never received previous treatment.

Failure to address peripheral neuropathy may result in irreversible neurologic damage.

What You DO

Nursing Responsibilities

When vesicant drugs are administered via a peripheral IV route, extreme caution must be taken to establish reliable IV access in an area that has not been subjected to recent venipuncture. Leakage of drug from a recent venipuncture site or unsuccessful attempt to establish an IV allows the drugs to infiltrate into soft tissues around the venipuncture site (**extravasation**). When administering mitotic inhibitors, the nurse should:

- Follow established protocol for administration of antidotes and application of heat or cold before administrating a vesicant drug; thus treatment may be provided immediately in the event of an extravasation. Research indicates that heat or cold applications, or both (depending on the drug), may minimize tissue damage.
- Administer an antidote to minimize the damage caused by extravasation. Some, but not all, vesicant drugs have antidotes.
- Verify that informed consent has been given before beginning treatment.
- Check the patient's laboratory and diagnostic studies before beginning therapy, with special attention being given to the CBC, platelet count, and liver function studies. Counts that are unacceptably low or reflective of organ dysfunction may indicate the need to delay treatment or decrease the dose, particularly when the patient has recently received previous treatment with cytotoxic agents.
- Monitor the patient for evidence of treatment-related toxicities, particularly bone marrow depression and peripheral neuropathy.
- Teach the patient about signs and symptoms of peripheral neuropathy, including paresthesias in the hands or feet, difficulty with fine-motor skills, and numbness. Other signs and symptoms include constipation, paralytic ileus, urinary retention, and jaw pain.

- Instruct the patient to report any of these complaints immediately to the health care provider, who will generally choose either to delay treatment or to decrease the dose.
- Teach the patient about measures to prevent constipation and decrease the risk for infection.
- Teach the patient the proper way to manage adverse effects and the point at which to seek medical assistance.

Do You UNDERSTAND?

DIRECTIONS: Fill in the blanks to complete the following statements.

1. Mitotic inhibitors are used to treat tumors in the _____, _____, _____, and _____.

2. The nurse should carefully monitor the patient for evidence of adverse effects that include _____ and _____.

What IS an Alkylating Agent?

Alkylating Agents	Trade Names	Uses
cyclophosphamide [sye-kloe-FLOSS-fa-mide]	Cytoxan	Treatment of neoplasms
busulfan [byoo-SUL-fan]	Myleran	Treatment of chronic myelogenous leukemia
cisplatin [sis-PLAT-in]	Platinol	Treatment of ovarian, testicular, bladder, cervical, breast, prostate, lung, and head and neck cancers

Action

Alkylating agents cause single- and double-strand breaks in DNA, thereby preventing cellular replication. Although these drugs are cell-cycle–nonspecific, they tend to be most effective against rapidly dividing cells.

Answers: 1. lung, breast, testes, ovaries; 2. bone marrow suppression, neuropathy.

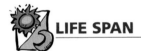

Alkylating drugs should be used with caution in patients with gout, urate renal stones, or patients who have undergone recent radiation or cytotoxic drug therapy. Cyclophosphamide should be used with caution in patients with renal or hepatic dysfunction, leukopenia, and thrombocytopenia or in those who are undergoing steroid drug therapy. Adequate renal function must be ascertained prior to the administration of cisplatin. Patients receiving this drug should have aggressive hydration in order to maintain adequate renal function. The drug should not be given if the patient's serum creatinine is above 1.5 mg/dl.

LIFE SPAN

Alkylating drugs are contraindicated for patients of childbearing age and women during pregnancy and lactation.
  Birth defects in the children of patients who have been treated with alkylating drugs are not uncommon.

Uses

This group of agents has demonstrated activity against lymphoma, Hodgkin's disease, breast cancer, cervical, bladder and lung cancer, and multiple myeloma.

What You NEED TO KNOW

Contraindications/Precautions

Alkylating drugs are contraindicated for patients with serious infections and myelosuppression.

Drug Interactions

When cyclophosphamide is given with succinylcholine, prolonged neuro-muscular blocking activity may occur. Doxorubicin may increase cardiac toxicity when given together with cyclophosphamide. When busulfan is given concurrently with probenecid and sulfinpyrazone, uric acid levels may increase.

Adverse Effects

Alkylating agents are highly effective against a wide variety of cancers. However, when given in high doses, these agents appear to increase the patient's risk for developing a second primary cancer. After repeated doses, these drugs may produce cumulative myelosuppression, with a prolonged recovery period.

  Cisplatin is considered one of the most emetogenic (i.e., capable of causing nausea and vomiting) drugs. Gonadal atrophy may occur in varying degrees, according to the age of the patient at the time that the agents are administered. Decreased sperm production is frequently observed in men and may be permanent, depending on the age of the individual at the time of treatment and the size of the dose that is administered. Chemotherapy-related alopecia is frequently severe with this class of drugs, although the hair growth typically returns to normal soon after the drugs are discontinued. The byproduct of cyclophosphamide may cause sterile hemorrhagic cystitis that can be severe enough that surgical removal of the bladder is required.

What You DO

Nursing Responsibilities

Melphalan is a vesicant and should be administered with extreme care when a peripheral IV is used. Carmustine and lomustine deserve special mention because they are associated with an extremely long nadir of 5 to 6 weeks after the drugs are administered; the nadir may continue for several weeks afterward. When administering an alkylating agent, the nurse should:

- Validate that laboratory and diagnostic studies are within acceptable limits before initiating chemotherapy.
- Monitor the therapy tolerance of patients who are receiving highly emetogenic therapy (e.g., cisplatin) and report adverse effects to the health care provider immediately.
- Provide treatment with antiemetic drugs prior to administering emetogenic drugs before nausea and vomiting become severe.
- Direct nursing care toward preventing damage that is associated with antineoplastic therapy and maximizing the patient's comfort.
- Prepare patients for their eventual hair loss; encourage them to shop for attractive head coverings and wigs before the hair loss is noticeable. Hair loss from antineoplastic therapy may be particularly devastating for some patients because it is a visible reminder of a life-threatening illness.
- Provide vigorous hydration before, during, and after cyclophosphamide administration.
- Instruct the patient who is taking the oral form to do so early in the day and to empty the bladder at least every 2 hours to avoid damaging the bladder mucosal lining.

TAKE HOME POINTS

- Lomustine and carmustine are noted for prolonged nadirs of 5 to 6 weeks; thus comprehensive education regarding self-care measures, adequate medical care, and follow-up after discharge is essential.
- Adverse effects of alkylating agents include severe nausea, vomiting, hair loss, and sterile hemorrhagic cystitis.

Do You UNDERSTAND?

DIRECTIONS: Fill in the blanks to complete the following statements.

1. One of the most emetogenic drugs is _____.
2. Melphalan is a vesicant that should be administered by the _____ _____ route.

Answers: 1. cisplatin; 2. peripheral IV.

What IS an Antitumor Antibiotic?

Antitumor Antibiotic	Trade Names	Uses
doxorubicin [dox-oh-ROO-bi-sin]	Adriamycin	Treatment of neoplasms of the breast, ovary, prostate, stomach, lung, and liver
dactinomycin [dak-ti-know-MY-sin]	Actinomycin-D	Treatment of Ewing's sarcoma, Wilms' tumor, testicular cancer, and rhabdomyosarcoma
idarubicin [ida-RUB-icin]	Idamycin	Acute nonlymphocytic leukemia

Antitumor antibiotics should be used with caution in patients with renal or hepatic dysfunction and those with antineoplastic or radiation therapy within 3 to 6 weeks. Dactinomycin should be used with caution in patients who are obese or those with gout.

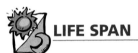

LIFE SPAN

Antitumor antibiotics are contraindicated for pregnant or lactating women and for infants under 6 months of age.

Action

Antitumor antibiotics were derived originally from fungi in soil and are cell-cycle–nonspecific drugs. These agents exert their mechanism of action by combining with cell DNA to form complexes that inhibit DNA activity.

Uses

Antitumor antibiotics are highly effective in the treatment of a wide variety of tumors, including malignancies of the breast, lymphatics, and ovaries.

What You NEED TO KNOW

Contraindications/Precautions

Doxorubicin is contraindicated for patients with myelosuppression, jaundice, and cardiac or pulmonary dysfunction. Additionally, dactinomycin is contraindicated for patients with viral infections.

Drug Interactions

When doxorubicin is given with barbiturates, body metabolism may be increased, which may necessitate an increased dose of doxorubicin. Conversely, streptozocin may prolong doxorubicin, necessitating a dose reduction. Because dactinomycin may elevate uric acid level, dose adjustments may be required when given together with antigout drugs. Effects of dactinomycin may be increased when given concurrently with other myelosuppressants or radiation. Dactinomycin decreases the effects of vitamin K, leading to an increased risk for hemorrhage.

Adverse Effects

Because antitumor antibiotics are derived from a naturally occurring substance, they have the potential to cause anaphylaxis. Alopecia, stomatitis, nausea, and vomiting are the most commonly occurring nonorgan-specific adverse effects. Daunorubicin and doxorubicin may cause dose-limiting myelosuppression. The anthracyclines may cause severe irreversible cardiac and pulmonary toxicity. Bleomycin and mitomycin-C may cause severe pulmonary toxicity. When reconstituted, daunorubicin and doxorubicin have a bright reddish-orange color, which causes the patient's urine to turn a similar color. Dactinomycin is a radiation sensitizer and may cause a phenomenon called *radiation recall*. This condition means that tissue that was damaged by radiation may become reddened and inflamed in response to antineoplastic therapy.

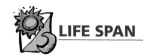

LIFE SPAN

Risk factors for cardiac toxicity include certain dosing schedules, children, adults over the age of 50, and patients with previous cardiac damage or previous radiation therapy to the chest wall.

What You DO

Nursing Responsibilities

Because cardiac toxicity is well documented for doxorubicin, recommendations are that patients should not exceed a cumulative lifetime dose of 550 mg/m^2 or 450 mg/m^2 when previous radiation therapy to the chest has been administered.

The cardiac health of all patients should be carefully evaluated before initiating treatment. Currently, a radiologic examination of the heart (known as a *gated blood pool scan*) is used to measure the left ventricular ejection fraction. This test provides information on the pumping ability of the heart and correlates well with cardiac damage. In most cases, by the time the patient manifests cardiac symptoms, irreversible damage has occurred. Patients in high-risk groups may require a decrease in the dose. When administering antitumor antibiotics, the nurse should:

- Evaluate the patient's cardiopulmonary status thoroughly before initiating antitumor antibiotic therapy and before each treatment. Patients who need a prolonged treatment regimen or those who require large doses of doxorubicin may benefit from the concurrent administration of a cardioprotective agent called *dexrazoxane.*
- Obtain a baseline evaluation of cardiac and pulmonary function before beginning therapy.

TAKE HOME POINTS

- Most antitumor antibiotics are toxic to the heart and lungs.
- Monitor the patient's CBC and chemistry laboratories because a low white blood cell count or inadequate renal function may indicate the need to delay or stop therapy.
- Provide comprehensive patient education regarding management of symptoms and the point at which to seek medical care. Many antitumor antibiotics are vesicants and must be administered with the appropriate precautions.

- Monitor the patient for early signs and symptoms of CHF and progressive cardiomyopathy (e.g., dry cough, tachycardia, dyspnea at rest) and report all abnormal findings to the health care provider immediately.
- Evaluate the patient's CBC, platelet count, and serum chemistry studies before starting treatment.
- Administer antitumor antibiotics with the appropriate precautions to avoid tissue damage because these drugs are vesicants.
- Administer an antiemetic before starting antitumor antibiotic therapy to prevent nausea and vomiting.
- Provide the patient with antiemetics that are suitable for home use before discharge.
- Provide the patient a detailed verbal and written explanation of the proper way to manage adverse symptoms (e.g., fatigue, food aversion, appetite changes, nausea, vomiting) before discharge.
- Provide the patient with a written list of symptoms that require immediate medical intervention.

Do You UNDERSTAND?

DIRECTIONS: **Indicate in the space provided whether the statement is** *true* **or** *false***. If the answer is false, correct the statement to make it true (using the margin space).**

_____ 1. Antitumor antibiotics are toxic to the GI tract and kidneys.

_____ 2. A low red blood cell count or inadequate renal function may indicate the need to delay or stop therapy.

Answers: 1. false; toxic to the heart and lungs; 2. false; low white blood cell count.

What IS a Miscellaneous Antineoplastic Drug?

Miscellaneous Antineoplastics	Trade Names	Uses
hydroxyurea [hye-DROX-ee-yoo-ree-ah]	Hydrea	Palliative treatment of CML or metastasis
asparaginase [a-SPAR-a-gi-nase]	l-Asparaginase	Treatment of acute lymphocytic leukemia
procarbazine [pro-CAR-ba-zeen]	Matulane	Palliative treatment of Hodgkin's disease

Action

Not all antineoplastic agents can be neatly classified. The exact mechanism of action in some drugs is unknown or the chemical structure is not well understood. Hydroxyurea is a cell-cycle–specific drug that inhibits DNA synthesis. In some patients, hydroxyurea appears to act as a radiation sensitizer, although this effect does not consistently occur and is poorly understood. Asparaginase exerts its mechanism of action by depriving cells of an essential nutrient **(asparagines).** Procarbazine disrupts chromatin arrangement in the cell and interferes with mitosis.

Uses

Hydroxyurea is used in palliative treatment of chronic myelocytic leukemias (CML). Asparaginase is helpful in the treatment of myeloproliferative disorders. This drug is commonly used in conjunction with vincristine and prednisone as induction therapy for acute lymphocytic leukemia. Procarbazine is used for palliation of Hodgkin's disease and advanced carcinoma of the adrenal cortex.

These antineoplastics should be given with caution to patients with renal or hepatic dysfunction, diabetes mellitus, and those who have undergone radiation or antineoplastic therapy within 1 month. Hydroxyurea should be given with caution to patients with asthma, epilepsy, migraines, cardiac dysfunction, or mental depression. Asparaginase should be given with caution to patients with gout. Procarbazine should be given with caution to patients who are undergoing concurrent CNS depressant therapy.

What You NEED TO KNOW

Contraindications/Precautions

Miscellaneous antineoplastics are contraindicated for patients with myelosuppression. Asparaginase is also contraindicated for patients with herpes infections and pancreatitis.

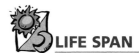

LIFE SPAN

Miscellaneous antineoplastics are contraindicated for women during pregnancy and lactation.

Drug Interactions

Asparaginase decreases the hypoglycemic effects of sulfonylureas and insulin. When asparaginase is given concurrently with corticosteroids or vincristine, the risk for toxicity is increased. When asparaginase is given concurrently with methotrexate, the antitumor effect is counteracted. Procarbazine is a monoamine oxidase inhibitor (MAOI) and may precipitate a hypertensive crisis when the patient consumes foods that contain tyramine. CNS depression is increased when given with alcohol, phenothiazines, or other CNS depressants.

Adverse Effects

Adverse effects of hydroxyurea include headache, malaise, fever, chills, dizziness, anorexia, nausea, vomiting, diarrhea, constipation, seizures, hallucinations, and bone marrow suppression. Asparaginase is a naturally occurring compound that has the potential to cause hypersensitivity reactions, ranging in severity from itching to anaphylaxis. Asparaginase is different from most antineoplastic agents in that it does not usually cause myelosuppression or hair loss (**alopecia**). Asparaginase may cause prolonged bleeding times, pancreatitis, hepatic dysfunction, and acute renal insufficiency. Adverse affects of procarbazine include bone marrow suppression, nausea, vomiting, and neuropathy.

What You DO

Nursing Responsibilities

When administering asparaginase, the nurse should:
- Obtain baseline clotting, as well as renal and hepatic function tests before asparaginase therapy begins.
- Have resuscitation equipment and emergency drugs readily available.
- Monitor the patient carefully, particularly when the drug is infused IV.
- Instruct the patient to report any unusual symptoms immediately, particularly those suggestive of hypersensitivity (e.g., itching, respiratory distress, rash).
- Check glucose levels daily and anticipate orders for subcutaneous doses of vitamin K to restore normal clotting function.
- Monitor the CBC and platelet count routinely for the patient who is undergoing procarbazine therapy.

- Assess the patient carefully for evidence of neuropathy or poor oral intake.
- Report any abnormal findings or laboratory values to the health care provider before beginning treatment.
- Be aware that MAOIs should be discontinued 14 days before initiating procarbazine therapy. Some foods that must be avoided when given concurrently with procarbazine include aged cheeses, chocolates, and red wine.

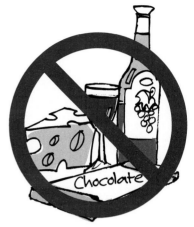

Not with MAOIs.

Do You UNDERSTAND?

DIRECTIONS: Fill in the blanks to complete the following statements.

1. _____ does not usually cause myelosuppression or alopecia.

2. _____ is a drug that disrupts chromatin arrangement in the cell and interferes with mitosis. This agent is used for palliation of Hodgkin's disease and advanced carcinoma of the adrenal cortex.

What IS Targeted Therapy?

The term *targeted therapy* refers to the administration of biologic agents that have a specific molecular target within the malignant cell. These agents exploit the basic molecular differences between cancerous and normal cells, such as how the cells grow and multiply. These drugs have varying different mechanisms of action. In general, they act by interfering with proteins that stimulate the transformation of normal cells into cancer cells and the progression and growth of cancer cells. These agents offer an advantage in that they usually impose minimal damage on normal healthy cells.

Answers: 1. Asparaginase; 2. Procarbazine.

Targeted Therapies	Trade Name	Uses
imatinib mesylate [I-MAT-in-ib MES-i-late]	Gleevec	Treatment of CML in adults in chronic or acute blast crisis phase
cetuximab [Ce-TUX-i-mab]	Erbitux	Treatment of patients with metastatic colorectal cancer who no longer are responding to other chemotherapeutic agents
bevacizumab [Bev-a-CIZ-u-mab]	Avastin	Treatment of patients with previously untreated metastatic colorectal cancer

Action

Imatinib mesylate acts by interfering with cellular growth signals that ordinarily move from the outside of the cell to the nucleus. Cetuximab is a monoclonal that also interferes with cellular activation and signaling and blocks the ability of endothelial growth factor (EGF) to activate cell growth. This agent also inhibits the progression of tumor cells through the cell cycle and causes cellular apoptosis (cell death). Bevacizumab is a recombinant antibody that blocks the ability of vascular endothelial growth factor to bind with cell receptors, thereby preventing the tumor cell from stimulating the growth of blood vessels, which is needed to receive nutrients.

What You NEED TO KNOW

Contraindications/Precautions

Imatinib is contraindicated for any patient who is severely neutropenic or thrombocytopenic. Prior to administration, the patient's liver function studies, hepatic transaminases, and serum bilirubin levels should be reviewed. Elevated levels may be a contraindication for receiving this drug. As of this time, special laboratory effects of cetuximab are unknown. The drug does have a high risk for anaphylaxis, particularly with the initial infusion. Patients should be directly observed during the first 15 minutes of an infusion of cetuximab and monitored frequently thereafter. Bevacizumab should not be given to patients with a low platelet count, white cell count, or proteinuria. Because this drug inhibits the growth of blood vessels, it should not be given for at least 1 month after major surgery because it may impair wound healing. Patients receiving this therapy are also at risk for gastrointestinal perforation and should be monitored accordingly.

Drug Interactions

Imatinib should not be given concurrently with CYP3A4 inhibitors such as itraconazole or ketoconazole because they may increase plasma concentrations. Imatinib may also decrease metabolism of simvastin, causing serum levels to increase as much as 300%. Dexamethasone, phenytoin, rifampicin, phenobarbital and St. John's wort may increase metabolism of imatinimib, causing a decrease in serum plasma concentration with the possibility of a less than optimal therapeutic outcome. Cetuximab tends to act synergistically with most cytotoxic forms of chemotherapy.

Adverse Effects

Imatinib has been reported to cause severe skin reactions, including Stevens-Johnson syndrome and erythema multiforme. Other complications of this drug include serious fluid retention and edema, including pleural effusions, cerebral edema, and pericardial tamponade. Hematologic effects associated with this drug include anemia, neutropenia, and thrombocytopenia.

Cetuximab has been reported to cause severe infusion reactions, characterized by bronchospasm, stridor, hoarseness, coughing, itching, and a sudden precipitate fall in blood pressure. Malaise, vomiting, diarrhea, and abdominal pain may also occur following cetuximab administration.

Bevacizumab may cause hypertension, mouth sores, diarrhea, anorexia, weakness, intestinal bleeding, low white blood cell count, and heart failure. On rare occasions, bevacizumab has been known to cause perforation of the gastrointestinal tract and dehiscence of surgical wounds. Other complications of this drug include hemoptysis (especially in patients with small cell lung cancer) and arterial thromboembolism.

> ⚠ Patients receiving antibodies should be premedicated prior to the infusion in order to decrease the risk for infusion reactions. Resuscitation equipment should also be readily available.

What You DO

Nursing Responsibilities

When administering targeted therapy, the nurse should:
- Take special care to store and reconstitute these products correctly. Many targeted therapies are protein-based and require refrigeration. If the product is lyophilized, it should not be shaken, nor should the diluent be injected directly into the powder.

- Verify adequate organ function and informed consent prior to beginning therapy according to the preference of the health care provider and the policies of the institution.
- Teach the patient receiving targeted therapies regarding the signs and symptoms of bleeding, anemia, and infection because these drugs either may cause these complications in and of themselves or may potentiate the effect of concurrently administered cytotoxic agents.
- Report unusual bruising or bleeding, painful urination or defecation, cough, shortness of breath, or fever greater than or equal to 100.5° F promptly to the health care provider.
- Instruct patients receiving bevacizumab to inform their health care provider immediately if they have abdominal pain or refractory nausea and vomiting because this may signal a gastrointestinal perforation.
- Warn the patient to avoid exposure to the sun or the use of harsh soaps or topical agents containing alcohol or perfumes because many of these products adversely affect the skin.
- Instruct patients receiving antibodies regarding the signs and symptoms of anaphylaxis and infusion reactions so that they can seek assistance before the reactions become severe.

Do You UNDERSTAND?

DIRECTIONS: **Match the following drugs to the characteristics that apply. (Note: Characteristics may apply to more than one drug. Some drugs may match more than one characteristic.)**

Drug	Characteristic
1. imatinib mesylate	a. Acts by causing cellular apoptosis
2. cetuximab	b. Is not given when neutropenia is present
3. bevacizumab	c. May cause Stevens-Johnson syndrome
	d. May cause heart failure

Answers: 1. b, c; 2. a; 3. b, d.

References

Abrams AC, Lammon CB, Pennington SS: *Clinical drug therapy: rationales for nursing practice*, ed 8, Philadelphia, 2007, Lippincott.

Gutierrez K, Queener SF: *Pharmacology for nursing practice*, St Louis, 2003, Mosby.

Hardman JG, Limbird LE: *Goodman & Gilman's the pharmacological basis of therapeutics*, ed 10, New York, 2001, McGraw-Hill.

Ignatavicius DD, Workman ML: *Medical-surgical nursing: critical thinking for collaborative care*, ed 5, St Louis, 2006, Elsevier.

Karch AM: *Focus on nursing pharmacology*, ed 3, Philadelphia, 2006, Lippincott.

Kee JL, Hayes ER, McCuistion LE: *Pharmacology: a nursing process approach*, ed 5, Philadelphia, 2006, Elsevier.

Lehne RA: *Pharmacology for nursing care*, ed 5, Philadelphia, 2004, WB Saunders.

Lilley LL, Harrington S, Snyder JS: *Pharmacology and the nursing process*, ed 4, St Louis, 2005, Mosby.

McKenry, LM, Salerno, E: *Mosby's pharmacology in nursing*, ed 21, St Louis, 2003, Mosby.

Polovich M, White JM, Kelleher LO: *Chemotherapy and biotherapy guidelines and recommendations for practice*, ed 2, Pittsburgh, 2005, Oncology Nursing Society.

Smeltzer SC, Bare BG: *Brunner and Suddarth's textbook of medical-surgical nursing*, ed 10, Philadelphia, 2004, Lippincott.

Wilson BA, Shannon MT, Stang CL: *Nurses drug guide*, Upper Saddle River, New Jersey, 2006, Pearson.

NCLEX® Review

Section A

1. A patient is prescribed oprelvekin (Neumega). Which action does the nurse expect from this drug?
   1 Stimulates platelet production
   2 Stimulates red blood cell production
   3 Increases the body's ability to produce antibodies
   4 Regulates the production of neutrophils

2. Interleukin therapy should continue until the postnadir platelet count is greater than what value?
   1 0.005 to 0.015 micromole/mL
   2 15 to 35 micromole/mL
   3 50,000 cells/microliter
   4 500,000 cells/mm

3. Which drug exerts antitumor activity?
   1 Cyclosporine
   2 Interleukin-11
   3 Interferon α-2a
   4 Sargramostim

4. Which drug action prevents rejection of organ transplantation?
   1 Erythropoietin
   2 Interferon α-2a
   3 Cyclosporine or Imuran
   4 Interleukin-1 or interleukin-2

5. By what method should cyclosporine be administered?
   1 IM
   2 In a plastic container
   3 Mixed with grapefruit juice
   4 Mixed with chocolate milk or orange juice

Section B

6. Doses for chemotherapy are based on which factor?
   1 The patient's ideal body weight
   2 Milligrams per kilogram
   3 Body surface area
   4 The patient's actual weight

7. When chemotherapy drugs are prepared, special precautions must be taken because the drugs have which characteristic?
   1 Irritating to the GI tract
   2 Ability to cause vomiting
   3 Acidic
   4 Biohazardous substances

8. Cytotoxic agents tend to exert their effect on which type of cells?
   1 Rapidly growing cells
   2 Cells that are poorly supplied with oxygen
   3 Cells with a long doubling time
   4 Cells with a poor blood supply

9. Patients with a low white blood cell count may experience which problem?
   1 Acidosis
   2 Delayed wound healing
   3 Hyperviscosity of the blood
   4 Prolonged bleeding times

10. Which of the following drugs is not a vesicant?
    1 Vincristine
    2 Methotrexate
    3 Vinblastine
    4 Melphalan

11. DNA is synthesized for chromosomes during the
    _____ phase.
    1 G_1
    2 G_2
    3 S
    4 M

12. Bevacuzamib acts by:
    1 Interfering with the formation of DNA.
    2 Inhibiting the formation of microtubules.
    3 Blocking apoptosis.
    4 Blocking the binding of growth factors to cell
      receptors.

NCLEX® Review Answers

Section A

1. 1 Oprelvekin is a thrombopoietic growth factor that
   stimulates platelet production. Erythropoietin
   stimulates red blood cell production. An
   immunosuppressant suppresses the body's natural
   response to an antigen. Filgrastim (Neupogen) is a
   colony-stimulating factor that regulates the
   production of neutrophils.

2. 3 Interleukin therapy should continue until
   the postnadir platelet count is greater than
   50,000 cells/microliter. The desirable dATP
   trough level is 0.005 to 0.015 micromole/mL.
   The desirable ADA trough level is 15 to
   35 micromole/mL. Interleukin therapy should
   not continue if the postnadir count is at
   500,000 cells/mm.

3. 3 Interferon α-2a is an immunomodulator that
   exerts antitumor activity. Cyclosporine is an
   immunosuppressant that prevents rejection of
   transplanted organs. Interleukin-11 is a
   thrombopoietic growth factor that stimulates
   platelet production. Sargramostim is a colony-
   stimulating factor that restores red bone marrow
   after transplantation.

4. 3 Immunosuppressants, cyclosporine, and Imuran
   prevent rejection of organ transplantation.
   Erythropoietin is a colony-stimulating factor
   that stimulates red blood count production.
   Interferon α-2a is an immunomodulator that
   treats leukemia and Kaposi's sarcoma.

Interleukin-1 or interleukin-2 treats melanoma or
renal cell cancer.

5. 4 Cyclosporine should be mixed with milk,
   chocolate milk, or apple or orange juice for
   oral administration. Cyclosporine is given orally
   or, when not tolerated, IV, but it is never given
   IM. Cyclosporine must be given in a glass
   container. Cyclosporine may adhere to a
   plastic container, which reduces the dose.
   Styrofoam is also porous and may absorb
   the drug. Grapefruit juice affects cyclosporine
   metabolism.

Section B

6. 3 Chemotherapy doses are based on body surface
   area, which is calculated based on height and
   weight. Chemotherapy doses should not be based
   on ideal body weight, mg/kg of body weight, or
   actual weight.

7. 4 Special precautions must be taken when
   preparing chemotherapy drugs because these
   agents are irritating to the skin, are liable to cause
   hypersensitivity reactions, and are biohazardous.
   Chemotherapy drugs may cause GI tract
   irritability and vomiting, but this reaction is not
   the reason for which these agents are administered
   with special precautions. Chemotherapy drugs are
   not acidic.

8. 1 Cytotoxic drugs tend to exert their effect on
   rapidly growing cells. These drugs do not exert
   their effect on cells that have poor oxygen or
   blood supply or on cells with a long doubling
   time.

9. 2 Patients with a low white blood cell count
   experience delayed wound healing because white
   blood cells (leukocytes) are involved in the
   inflammatory response to injury and aid in tissue
   repair. Acidosis is associated with a low red blood
   cell count. Viscosity of blood is related more to a
   high red blood cell count. Bleeding times are
   associated more with platelets, which affect blood
   coagulation and hemostasis.

10. 2 Methotrexate is not a vesicant. Vincristine,
    vinblastine, and melphalan are vesicants.

11. 3 DNA synthesis takes place within the S phase of the cell cycle.

12. 4 Bevacuzamib is an antibody that acts by blocking the ability of vascular endothelial growth factor to bind with cell receptors, thereby preventing the tumor cell from stimulating the growth of blood vessels that it needs to receive nutrients.

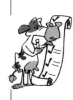

Notes

Drugs Used to Treat Nervous System Disorders

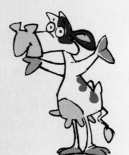

What You WILL LEARN

After reading this chapter, you will know how to do the following:

✔ Compare the action of an adrenergic agonist with an α-adrenergic antagonist and a β-adrenergic antagonist.

✔ Identify three direct-acting cholinergic agonists and their uses.

✔ Explain common nursing responsibilities for patients taking anticonvulsants.

✔ Discuss common adverse effects of intravenous nonbarbiturate anesthetic agents.

 SECTION **A**

SYMPATHETIC NERVOUS SYSTEM DRUGS

Hormones (norepinephrine and epinephrine) activate the sympathetic nervous system. Sympathetic nerves release both of these hormones, whereas the adrenal gland also releases epinephrine. Norepinephrine and epinephrine stimulate four types of receptor sites found in autonomic nerve pathways: α_1-adrenergic, α_2-adrenergic, β_1-adrenergic, and β_2-adrenergic receptors. Several physiologic responses result when each type of receptor is activated. The nurse must be aware of the different receptor sites and the associated responses; thus the effects of the agents can be predicted. These responses include:

α_1-*Receptors affect:*

- Pupil dilation (facilitates eye examinations and ocular surgery)
- Gastrointestinal (GI) tract motility (decreases secretions and peristalsis)
- Vasoconstriction of arterioles (increases blood pressure, decreases bleeding and nasal congestion)
- Bladder contraction (promotes urethral sphincter closure for treating urinary incontinence)
- Prostate contraction (improves symptoms of benign prostatic hypertrophy)

α_2-*Receptors affect:*

- GI tract motility (decreases secretions and peristalsis)
- Vasoconstriction of arterioles (increases blood pressure, decreases bleeding and nasal congestion)

β_1-*Receptors affect:*

- Heart rate, contractility, automaticity, and conduction (increases heart rate and contractility)

β_2-*Receptors affect:*

- Bronchodilation (improves breathing)
- Heart rate and contractility (increases heart rate and contractility)
- Conversion of glycogen to glucose (causes hyperglycemia)
- Uterus (relaxes uterus)
- GI tract motility (decreases secretions and peristalsis)

Sympathetic nervous system agents either stimulate or inhibit α- or β-receptors or both. Most agents either stimulate or inhibit more than one receptor but usually activate one more strongly than the other. Sympathetic nervous system agents are classified as adrenergic agonists (stimulators) and adrenergic antagonists (inhibitors).

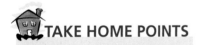

TAKE HOME POINTS

Most adrenergic agonists frequently stimulate more than one adrenergic receptor site, producing a variety of effects.

Adrenergic Agonists

What IS an Adrenergic Agonist?

Adrenergic Agonists	Trade Names	Receptor Site	Primary Use
phenylephrine [fen-ill-EH-frin]	Neo-synephrine	α_1, α_2	Treat shock and nasal congestion
pseudoephedrine [soo-doe-e-FED-rin]	Sudafed	α_1, β_1	Relieve nasal, sinus, and eustachian tube congestion
ephedrine [eh-FED-rin]	Ephedsol Ectasule Vatronol	α_1, β_1, β_2	Temporary relief of nasal and sinus congestion; treat hypotension
dobutamine [doe-BYOOT-uh-meen]	Dobutrex	α_1	Inotropic support in congestive heart failure and cardiogenic shock
ritodrine [RI-toe-dreen]	Yutopar	β_1, β_2	Reduces and/or stops uterine contractions
albuterol [al-BYOO-ter-ahl]	Proventil Ventolin	β_2	Bronchospasm associated with asthma or bronchitis

Action

Adrenergic agonists (adrenergics or sympathomimetic agents) can stimulate any one or any combination of α- or β-receptors. Adrenergic agonists that stimulate only one type of receptor can be further classified as either an α-agonist or β-agonist. α-Agonists constrict arterioles, thereby elevating blood pressure (BP).

Adrenergic agonists that stimulate β-receptors are called *β-adrenergic agonists*. The type of β-receptor they primarily stimulate further classifies them as selective or nonselective agents. β_1-Agonists speed conduction and automaticity and increase myocardial contractility, which restores cardiac rhythm. β_2-Agonists cause bronchodilation, vasodilation, hyperglycemia, and decreased peristalsis.

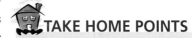

TAKE HOME POINTS

- Many of the adrenergic agents are emergency agents that are used to treat cardiovascular collapse or arrest.
- Be familiar with which drug stimulates receptor site to predict the effects of various adrenergic agonists.

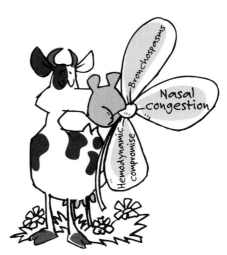

Use an adrenergic agent.

Uses

Adrenergic agonists are used primarily for three reasons: hemodynamic compromise (e.g., hypotension resulting from any type of shock, acute congestive heart failure, or depressed cardiac rhythm), bronchospasm, and nasal or sinus congestion.

The adrenergic agonist agents that are commonly used for hypotension include dopamine, norepinephrine, ephedrine, and phenylephrine. α-Agonists are used to treat shock. β_1-Agonists are used to restore cardiac rhythm in profound bradycardia, second-degree type II heart block, or complete heart block until the insertion of a pacemaker, as well as acute congestive heart failure and cardiogenic shock. β_2-Agonists are used primarily for pulmonary disorders and to treat or prevent bronchospasm by causing bronchodilation.

Dopamine is a unique drug that is different from the other adrenergic agonists because its actions depend on the dose. Doses of 5 to 10 mcg/kg/min stimulate β_1-receptors, and doses greater than 10 mcg/kg/min stimulate α-receptors. Doses of 2 to 3 mcg/kg/min stimulate dopaminergic receptors, causing dilation of the mesenteric and renal arteries. Dopamine is frequently used to increase blood flow to the kidneys when renal insufficiency is present or to prevent renal failure from shock.

Phenylephrine is used to promote drainage of sinus secretions, as well as treating severe hypotension and shock. Ritodrine is used to prevent or delay preterm labor by reducing intensity and frequency of uterine contractions.

What You NEED TO KNOW

Contraindications/Precautions

Phenylephrine is contraindicated in patients with pheochromocytoma. α-Agonists are contraindicated in patients who have tachycardia and severe hypertension because stimulation of α-receptors causes vasoconstriction further potentiating hypertension. Because α-agonists cause pupil dilation **(mydriasis)**, they are contraindicated for patients with narrow-angle glaucoma. Ritodrine should be used with caution in patients concurrently receiving potassium-depleting diuretics.

Drug Interactions

Agents that increase the effects of adrenergic agonists on the cardiovascular and central nervous system (CNS) include monoamine oxidase inhibitors (MAOIs), theophylline, and tricyclic antidepressants. Antihistamines and atropine increase the risk for tachycardia. Digoxin, when taken with adrenergic agonists, increases the risk for ventricular dysrhythmias.

Adverse Effects

The most common adverse effects of all adrenergic agonists involve the cardiovascular and CNS. Cardiovascular effects include palpitations, tachycardia, ectopic beats, tachydysrhythmias, hypertension, myocardial ischemia, chest pain, and pulmonary edema. CNS effects include nervousness, weakness, tremors, and anxiety. Adrenergic agonists also cause blurred vision, pupil dilation, drowsiness, and hyperglycemia. Additive adverse effects may occur when more than one adrenergic agent is administered together.

Adrenergic agonists should be avoided in patients with cardiac disease because these agents may precipitate angina or myocardial infarction (MI).

Giving an adrenergic agonist by direct IV push when it is intended for continuous infusion can be lethal to the patient.

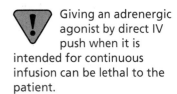

TAKE HOME POINTS

- Be aware of which adrenergic agents may be given by direct IV push and which should be diluted and given only by continuous infusion.
- Titrate continuous infusions slowly until the desired effect (i.e., increased BP or myocardial contractility) or dose is achieved to promote hemodynamic stability.

⚠ Agents such as norepinephrine and dopamine can cause a serious local reaction when they infiltrate into the surrounding tissues. Infiltration of these agents can cause extravasation and sloughing of local tissues. When an IV infiltrates with any of these agents, a local antidote must be given to prevent tissue necrosis. The antidote is 5 to 10 mg of phentolamine in 10 mL of normal saline injected into the infiltrated tissue through multiple injections with a tuberculin needle. This procedure should be performed within 12 hours after an infiltration is suggested, preferably immediately.

What You DO

Nursing Responsibilities

Gastric acid inactivates many adrenergic agonists; thus most are given intravenously (IV) or through inhalation or both. When given IV, the effects are usually immediate or within minutes. After the agents enter the bloodstream, they are rapidly metabolized. The rapid metabolism results in a short duration of action for these agents.

All the adrenergic agonists that are used for hemodynamic compromise are given IV, but some may be given intramuscularly (IM) or subcutaneously (Sub-Q). The IV route may be given by direct IV or diluted and given only as a continuous infusion.

When an adrenergic drug is given as a continuous infusion, it should be titrated until the desired effect is achieved. The prescribing health care provider will order the desired effect or dose range. Titration of these agents should be done slowly (i.e., 2 to 3 mL every 3 to 5 minutes). Continuous infusions should not be discontinued abruptly, but rather, titrated down slowly.

Sudden discontinuation may cause extreme fluctuations in BP and heart rate. All continuous infusions should be infused through microdrip tubing via an infusion pump. Macro-drip tubing and manual rate control does not ensure accurate titration.

Most adrenergic agonists that are used to treat bronchospasm are given by inhalation therapy. Inhalation therapy includes use of a nebulizer, intermittent positive-pressure breathing (IPPB), and metered-dose inhaler (MDI). Albuterol may be given orally. These agents are commonly found as over-the-counter (OTC) oral preparations or nasal sprays. Many of these agents are absorbed into the systemic circulation from the respiratory tract; thus cardiovascular and CNS effects may be observed during or after an inhalation treatment.

When administering adrenergic agonists to treat hemodynamic compromise or bronchospasm, the nurse should:

• Avoid giving α-agonists to patients with narrow-angle glaucoma because they increase intraocular pressure.
• Calculate the dose of adrenergic agonists carefully because small errors may lead to severe adverse effects.

- Monitor for cardiovascular and CNS effects during and after inhalation treatments because these are the most common adverse effects of adrenergic agonists.
- Check blood glucose levels closely, particularly in patients with diabetes.
- Monitor the patient for signs and symptoms of pulmonary edema.
- Teach patients with ischemic heart disease that they should check with the health care provider before taking any OTC adrenergic agonists.
- Place the patient receiving ritodrine IV in the left lateral recumbent position throughout the entire IV dose to reduce possible hypotension.
- Discard ritodrine IV solution if it is cloudy or a precipitate is seen.
- Monitor IV site for extravasation. Phentolamine should be available for antidote-injections in the affected site.
- Instruct the patient not to abruptly discontinue self-administration of adrenergic agonists because sudden withdrawal may result in the development of dysrhythmias, rebound hypertension, encephalopathy, and death.

Most adrenergic agents that are used to treat nasal and sinus congestion are given intranasally or orally. These agents consist of common OTC "cold medicines." Similar to other adrenergic agonists, these agents may also cause cardiovascular and CNS effects; thus they should be avoided in the presence of ischemic heart disease.

Do You UNDERSTAND?

DIRECTIONS: Fill in the blanks with the name of the receptor that produces the effect listed.

1. Stimulating _____-receptors results in bronchodilation.
2. Stimulating _____-receptors increases myocardial contractility.
3. Stimulating _____-receptors increases BP.
4. Stimulating _____-receptors decreases GI motility.

Answers: 1. β_2; 2. β_1; and β_2; 3. α_1; and α_2; 4. α and β_2.

Adrenergic Antagonists

Adrenergic antagonists inhibit or block the effects of the sympathetic nervous system neurotransmitters and are antagonists to the adrenergic agonists. Adrenergic antagonists are also called *adrenergic blockers* or *sympatholytic agents* because they block sympathetic effects throughout the body **(lyse).** Agents that block sympathetic receptors produce responses similar to those occurring when parasympathetic receptors are activated. Adrenergic antagonists do not occur naturally in the body. Dissimilar to adrenergic agonists, which can stimulate more than one receptor type, most adrenergic antagonists block only one type of receptor, either the α- or β-receptors. These adrenergic antagonist agents can be further classified as either α-antagonists or β-antagonists.

What IS an α-Adrenergic Antagonist?

α-Adrenergic Antagonists	Trade Names	Uses
doxazosin mesylate [dox-A-zo-sin]	Cardura	Treatment of hypertension
terazosin [tear-ah-ZOE-sin]	Hytrin	Treatment of hypertension and benign prostatic hypertrophy (BPH)
tamsulosin hydrochloride [TAM-su-lo-sin]	Flomax	Treatment of benign prostatic hypertrophy

Action

α-Adrenergic antagonists (also called α-*adrenergic blockers*) block receptors throughout the body. The following responses result when these sites are blocked:

- Pupil constriction **(miosis)**
- Increased GI tract motility
- Vasodilation of arterioles (decreases BP)
- Bladder neck relaxation (increases urinary flow)
- Prostate relaxation (reduces signs and symptoms of BPH)

The primary effects of α-adrenergic antagonists involve the cardiovascular system. Because the α-receptors are blocked, the arterioles dilate, which decreases BP and peripheral vascular resistance.

Uses

α-Adrenergic antagonists are used primarily to treat five conditions: hypertension, migraine headaches, Alzheimer's disease, benign prostatic hypertrophy, and vasoactive disorders. Most agents are used for only one condition.

α-Adrenergic antagonists can be used to treat benign prostatic hypertrophy because they dilate blood vessels along the urinary tract and enhance urine outflow. Terazosin is used to treat hypertension and improve signs and symptoms of BPH.

What You NEED TO KNOW

Contraindications/Precautions

α-Adrenergic antagonists, except doxazosin, prazosin, and terazosin, should be avoided in patients with bradycardia, hypotension, heart blocks, acute coronary syndrome, heart failure, and shock.

Drug Interactions

The only specific drug interactions with α-antagonists involve the use of agents that are classified as α-agonists because they counteract the desired effects.

> ⚠ When other antihypertensive agents are used, α-antagonists should be used cautiously to prevent hypotension. Avoid α-adrenergic antagonists, except doxazosin, prazosin, and terazosin, in patients with ischemic heart disease.

Adverse Effects

The major adverse effect of α-adrenergic antagonists is orthostatic hypotension. The sympathetic nervous system is stimulated when a person stands up quickly, causing vasoconstriction to prevent blood from pooling in the legs. When a person is taking α-adrenergic antagonists, the vessels are unable to constrict because α-receptors are blocked. As a result, BP rapidly falls, and blood flow to the brain decreases, causing the person to become dizzy and develop syncope. The decrease in BP from most α-adrenergic antagonists also tends to cause reflexogenic cardiac stimulation. This reflex causes tachycardia and an increase in the force of myocardial contractions. Therefore the cardiac stimulation may increase the workload of the heart and result in myocardial ischemia or infarction.

Doxazosin and terazosin are α-adrenergic antagonists that cause minimal cardiac stimulation. These agents usually do not cause reflex tachycardia because they block only one type of α-receptor (α_1)—and not the type (α_2) that causes cardiac stimulation.

Other adverse effects are also related to blocking of α-receptor sites, including insomnia, headache, miosis, increase in lacrimation, blurred vision, drowsiness, nasal congestion, pharyngitis, an increase in GI motility, nausea, vomiting, peripheral edema, and impotence.

What You DO

Nursing Responsibilities

When administering α-adrenergic antagonists, the nurse should:

- Monitor for orthostatic hypotension, particularly after the initial dose. Instruct patients to rise to a standing position slowly and to sit immediately when dizziness or lightheadedness occurs to prevent falling.
- Monitor patients who are taking α-adrenergic antagonists for tachycardia.
- Advise patients to avoid participating in any activity that may be dangerous (e.g., driving) until the drug response is determined (at least 12 hours after the first dose).
- Instruct patients to report any weakness or dizziness immediately to the health care provider.
- Administer an α-adrenergic antagonist given for hypertension at the same time every day and spaced equally throughout a 24-hour period to optimize its effect on BP. For example, administering the drug every 8 hours is preferable to three times during the day (tid).
- Encourage the patient to check with the health care provider prior to taking OTC medications, especially adrenergic drugs.
- Instruct the patient to report a 1- to 2-pound weight gain, especially when accompanied by peripheral edema.

Phentolamine is the drug of choice to prevent tissue extravasation in the event of either a dopamine or a norepinephrine IV infiltration. Usually, 5 to 10 mg is diluted in 10 mL of normal saline. A tuberculin-size needle is used to make multiple injections into the infiltrated tissue. This procedure must be performed within 12 hours of the infiltration; otherwise tissue extravasation and sloughing may occur. Phentolamine is most effective when given immediately after the infiltration.

Do You UNDERSTAND?

DIRECTIONS: Fill in the blanks with appropriate responses.

1. _____ should be closely monitored after the initial dose of an α-adrenergic antagonist.
2. _____ is the drug of choice for a norepinephrine IV infiltration.
3. _____ is an α-adrenergic antagonist that is used to treat Alzheimer's disease.

What IS a β-Adrenergic Antagonist?

Refer to Chapter 7 for a discussion of β-adrenergic antagonists.

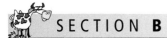 **SECTION B**

PARASYMPATHETIC NERVOUS SYSTEM DRUGS

The parasympathetic nervous system is concerned primarily with conserving energy and promoting digestion. Several responses occur when the parasympathetic nervous system is stimulated:

- Pupil constriction (**miosis**)
- Lacrimation
- Salivation
- Bronchoconstriction
- Decrease in heart rate, conduction, and automaticity
- Stimulation of gastric secretions and increase in GI motility
- Contraction of bladder and relaxation of the sphincter

Several groups of agents that affect parasympathetic activity are discussed in this section. Most of these agents either enhance or inhibit the parasympathetic nervous system receptors. Direct-acting cholinergic agonists and cholinesterase inhibitors enhance parasympathetic activity. Agents that reduce or inhibit parasympathetic activity are classified as anticholinergics.

Agents that are used to treat Parkinson's disease are reviewed in this section. These agents are generally classified as antiparkinsonism agents. Selective anticholinergic agents and dopaminergics are used to relieve some of the major symptoms that are associated with Parkinson's disease.

What IS a Direct-Acting Cholinergic Agonist?

Direct-Acting Cholinergic Agonists	Trade Names	Uses
bethanechol chloride [beth-AN-ih-kole KLOR-ide]	Urecholine	Treatment of urinary retention
dexpanthenol [dex-PAN-the-nole]	Ilopan	Prevention or treatment of postoperative abdominal distention, intestinal atony, and paralytic ileus
metoclopramide [MET-oh-KLOE-pra-mide]	Reglan	Treatment of gastroparesis, nausea, and vomiting associated with antineoplastics and gastroesophageal reflux

Action

Acetylcholine (ACh) is the primary neurotransmitter involved in the parasympathetic nervous system. ACh stimulates cholinergic receptors that are classified as either muscarinic or nicotinic. Muscarinic receptors are located in the CNS, heart, glands, and smooth muscle of organs. The response of muscarinic receptors is generally inhibitory, except for stimulation of glandular secretions (i.e., stimulation of gastric secretions, salivation). Nicotinic receptors are located in skeletal muscle cells and autonomic ganglia. The nicotinic response is an excitatory effect (i.e., increase in GI motility). Direct-acting cholinergic agonists affect primarily the muscarinic receptors. These agents act similarly to ACh in stimulating muscarinic receptors and producing parasympathetic responses or cholinergic effects. Direct-acting cholinergic agonists are also called *parasympathomimetic agents* and *cholinergic agonists*.

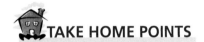

TAKE HOME POINTS

- Be familiar with the parasympathetic responses that are produced by direct-acting cholinergic agonists to ensure safe administration.
- Be aware that alcohol and CNS depressants can enhance sedation.

Uses

Bethanechol is used for urinary retention because it contracts the bladder, allowing the bladder to empty. Several of the direct-acting cholinergic agonists are used to treat GI disturbances because they increase GI motility. Dexpanthenol is used to prevent or treat postoperative abdominal distention, intestinal atony, and paralytic ileus. Metoclopramide is effective in relieving gastroparesis, nausea, and vomiting that are associated with antineoplastic agents and gastroesophageal reflux.

What You NEED TO KNOW

Contraindications/Precautions

Direct-acting cholinergics are contraindicated for patients with asthma because they can precipitate bronchospasm. These agents are also contraindicated for patients with mechanical obstruction in either the GI or the urinary tract because stimulation may cause tearing of body tissues.

Drug Interactions

Several agents can alter the effects of direct-acting cholinergic agonists. Cholinesterase inhibitors can augment the cholinergic effects. Procainamide, quinidine, atropine, and epinephrine antagonize the effects of cholinergic agents. Alcohol and CNS depressants enhance sedation. Metoclopramide can cause extrapyramidal symptoms (e.g., acute dystonia), and phenothiazines may increase the potential of these symptoms.

Adverse Effects

Most of the adverse effects that are associated with direct-acting cholinergic agonists are related to the parasympathetic responses that they produce. These effects include dry mouth, sedation or drowsiness, excessive lacrimation, miosis, decreased BP with reflex tachycardia, excessive salivation, diarrhea, cramping, and abdominal pain.

What You DO

Nursing Responsibilities

When direct-acting cholinergics are used for GI tract symptoms, they should be given before meals and at bedtime for optimal effect. Metoclopramide should be given 30 minutes before meals.

When administering direct-acting cholinergics, the nurse should:

- Monitor the patient for signs and symptoms of cholinergic overdose, including salivation, sweating, flushing, abdominal cramps, and nausea.
- Administer the antidote or antagonist for cholinergic overdose (atropine sulfate), which is administered IM, slow IV, or Sub-Q and repeated every 2 hours as needed.
- Monitor respiratory status of patients who are taking direct-acting cholinergic agonist therapy and immediately report dyspnea to the health care provider.
- Give direct-acting cholinergics that are used for GI disorders before each meal and at bedtime.

TAKE HOME POINTS

Atropine sulfate is the antidote for cholinergic overdose.

Do You UNDERSTAND?

DIRECTIONS: Place a check mark next to the responses that occur with direct-acting cholinergic agonists.

_____ 1. Decreased salivation
_____ 2. Decreased heart rate
_____ 3. Increased gastric motility
_____ 4. Increased cardiac conduction

Answers: 2. Decreased heart rate; 3. Increased gastric motility.

What IS a Cholinesterase Inhibitor?

Cholinesterase Inhibitors	Trade Names	Uses
neostigmine bromide *[nee-oh-STIG-meen]*	Prostigmin	Diagnoses myasthenia gravis; differentiates between myasthenic and cholinergic crisis
edrophonium chloride *[eh-droe-FOE-nee-uhm]*	Tensilon	Diagnoses myasthenia gravis; differentiates between myasthenic and cholinergic crisis
pyridostigmine bromide *[pier-id-oh-STIG-meen]*	Mestinin, Regonal	Improves muscle strength in myasthenia gravis; reverses nondepolarizing skeletal muscle relaxants
donepezil hydrochloride *[dawn-EPP-uh-zill]*	Aricept	Treatment of Alzheimer's disease
rivastigmine tartrate *[riv-ah-STIG-meen]*	Exelon	Treatment of Alzheimer's disease

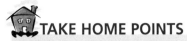

TAKE HOME POINTS

- Cholinesterase inhibitors inhibit AChE, thereby improving skeletal muscle function.
- Cholinesterase inhibitors are used primarily to restore skeletal muscle function, particularly in patients with myasthenia gravis.

Action

Cholinesterase inhibitors are also referred to as *acetylcholinesterase inhibitors*. ACh is released in the peripheral nerves, as well as the central nerves. When released in the peripheral nerves, ACh reacts with target cells to stimulate the skeletal muscles. Immediately after ACh interacts with target cells, the enzyme acetylcholinesterase (AChE) stops its action on the target cells. Cholinesterase inhibitors are agents that inhibit AChE. Inhibiting this enzyme allows the actions of ACh to be prolonged and more intense (i.e., excess vasodilation can lead to shock).

Uses

Because cholinesterase inhibitors prolong the effect of ACh, most of these agents are used to restore skeletal muscle function from either myasthenia gravis or from nonpolarizing skeletal muscle relaxants. Some of these agents are used to improve memory in patients with Alzheimer's disease. Edrophonium chloride and neostigmine have a short duration of action; thus they are not used for maintenance therapy in treating myasthenia gravis, but rather, to diagnose myasthenia gravis and to differentiate between a myasthenic and cholinergic crisis.

A myasthenic crisis occurs when the dose of a cholinesterase inhibitor is subtherapeutic; therefore skeletal muscle function declines. When a cholinesterase inhibitor becomes toxic, a cholinergic crisis results, leading to cholinergic effects. Donepezil hydrochloride and rivastigmine are used to improve memory in patients with Alzheimer's disease.

Edrophonium and neostigmine should be used cautiously in patients with bronchial asthma and hyperthyroidism and in those with a history of ulcers and GI bleeding.

The nurse should know the difference between a cholinergic and myasthenic crisis. Cholinesterase inhibitor underdosing may lead to a myasthenic crisis. Overdosing may lead to a cholinergic crisis.

Edrophonium and neostigmine are used to reverse the neuromuscular blockade effects produced by nonpolarizing skeletal muscle relaxants that are commonly used to produce paralysis during surgery.

What You NEED TO KNOW

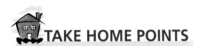

TAKE HOME POINTS

The nurse should know which agents enhance or antagonize the effects of cholinesterase inhibitors.

Life-threatening cholinergic effects include excessive pulmonary secretions, bronchospasm, respiratory depression, and respiratory paralysis.

Contraindications/Precautions

Donepezil and neostigmine are contraindicated for patients with bradycardia or hypotension. Donepezil, edrophonium, and neostigmine are contraindicated for patients with urinary tract and intestinal obstruction.

Drug Interactions

Several drug interactions may occur with cholinesterase inhibitors. Depolarizing muscle relaxants, such as succinylcholine and decamethonium, have prolonged action when administered with cholinesterase inhibitors. Tubocurarine, atracurium, vecuronium, pancuronium, procainamide, quinidine, and atropine, as well as any drug with anticholinergic properties (i.e., antihistamines, antidepressants, phenothiazines, disopyramide), inhibit the effects of cholinesterase inhibitors. Procainamide, quinidine, mecamylamine, and succinylcholine can intensify the toxicity of ambenonium. The metabolism of donepezil is inhibited by ketoconazole and quinidine, and its elimination is increased by carbamazepine, dexamethasone, phenobarbital, phenytoin, and rifampin.

Adverse Effects

Common adverse effects that are associated with cholinesterase inhibitors are related to excessive cholinergic stimulation. These effects include salivation, sweating, flushing, headache, and abdominal cramps. Individuals who take pyridostigmine may develop bronchoconstriction, hypotension, bradycardia, and muscle weakness. Rivastigmine has few adverse effects, which include dizziness, anorexia, nausea, vomiting, and diarrhea. Food may affect the absorption of cholinesterase inhibitors.

What You DO

Nursing Responsibilities

Two problems can develop in patients with myasthenia gravis who are receiving cholinesterase inhibitor therapy. Either a myasthenic crisis from underdosing or a cholinergic crisis from overdosing of a cholinesterase inhibitor can develop. Both conditions are difficult to differentiate because they have similar symptoms of skeletal muscle weakness and respiratory depression. An edrophonium test (**Tensilon test**) is performed (usually by the health care provider) to differentiate between a myasthenic crisis and a cholinergic crisis. Edrophonium is administered IV, and improvement is observed within 1 minute when the patient is experiencing a myasthenic crisis. When the condition worsens, the problem is a cholinergic crisis. No response indicates an optimal treatment regimen.

When administering cholinesterase inhibitors, the nurse should:

- Place atropine sulfate at the bedside for immediate administration to reverse the cholinergic effects when a cholinergic crisis is present before the Tensilon test is performed.
- Place intubation equipment nearby for potential respiratory depression or arrest. Atropine is an anticholinergic drug that antagonizes the cholinergic stimulation that is produced by cholinesterase inhibitors.
- Report any respiratory distress or depression immediately.
- Teach the patient to recognize adverse effects because dose adjustments may be necessary.
- Warn patients that they may become resistant when undergoing long-term treatment. However, when the drug is withdrawn for several days or the dose is reduced, individuals usually become responsive again.
- Give pyridostigmine with food to minimize cholinergic effects.
- Assess muscle strength for effectiveness prior to administration of pyridostigmine.
- Protect the patient who is taking donepezil or rivastigmine because dizziness and fainting episodes may occur.
- Teach patients to report any signs of GI ulceration or bleeding immediately.

Do You UNDERSTAND?

DIRECTIONS: **Indicate in the space provided whether each statement is** *true* **or** *false*. **If the answer is false, correct the statement to make it true (using the margin space).**

_____ 1. AChE inhibits the actions of ACh.

_____ 2. Inhibiting AChE causes less stimulation of skeletal muscles.

_____ 3. ACh stimulates skeletal muscles.

_____ 4. Cholinesterase inhibitors intensify and prolong the action of ACh.

What IS an Anticholinergic?

Anticholinergics	Trade Names	Uses
atropine sulfate [A-troe-peen]	Isopto atropine	Treatment of GI hyperacidity, hypermotility, and spasms; preoperative drug to dry secretions
glycopyrrolate [glye-koe-PYE-roe-late]	Robinul	Treatment of GI hyperacidity, hypermotility, and spasms; preoperative drug to dry secretions
propantheline bromide [proe-PAN-the-leen]	Pro-Banthine	Treatment of GI hyperacidity, hypermotility, and spasms; preoperative drug to dry secretions
oxybutynin chloride [ox-I-BYOO-ti-nin]	Ditropan, Oxytrol	Treatment of neurogenic bladder; relieves bladder spasms
tolterodine [toll-TEAR-oh-deen]	Detrol	Treatment of overactive bladder, urinary frequency, urgency, and incontinence
scopolamine [skoe-POL-a-meen]	Hyoscine	Controls spasticity; preoperative drug to dry secretions; relieves motion sickness

Action

Anticholinergics block muscarinic receptors, thereby antagonizing the effects of ACh and inhibiting parasympathetic actions. Anticholinergics are also called *parasympatholytic* and *antimuscarinic agents*. Because these agents block the actions of the parasympathetic nervous system, the

Answers: 1. true; 2. false; inhibiting AChE allows the action of ACh to be prolonged and restores skeletal muscle function; 3. true; 4. true.

effects produced mimic many of the sympathetic effects. Anticholinergic agents produce the following responses:

- Pupil dilation (**mydriasis**)
- Decreased lacrimation
- Increased heart rate, automaticity, conduction, and contractility
- Decreased GI motility and gastric acid secretion
- Decreased salivary gland secretion
- Decreased sweat gland activity
- Bladder muscle contraction and relaxation of sphincter

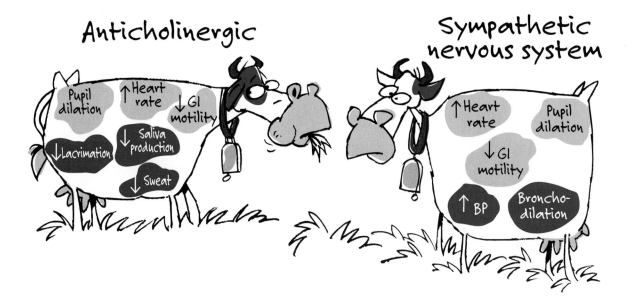

Uses

Anticholinergics are used for three primary reasons: to dry salivation and pulmonary secretions; to relieve symptoms that are associated with Parkinson's disease; and to relieve spasms of the GI tract, genitourinary (GU) tract, and those associated with menstrual cramps. Some agents may be used for one or more of the three primary uses.

Agents that dry secretions are used as preoperative medications to dry salivation, perspiration, and respiratory secretions during surgery. In addition to use as a "drying" agent, scopolamine is used for a sedative effect in obstetric patients and to relieve motion sickness.

Atropine is used as an agent to dry secretions and as an antidote to treat cholinergic overdose produced by other medications (e.g., cholinesterase inhibitors, direct-acting cholinergic agonists), as well as to treat cholinergic crisis in patients with myasthenia gravis. Another important use for atropine is its use in emergency cardiovascular situations. Atropine increases the heart rate in patients who have sinus bradycardia, second-degree type II atrioventricular block, complete heart block, or asystole. Atropine is also an antidote for organophosphate poisoning from insecticides, and it dries excessive pulmonary secretions that organophosphates produce.

Anticholinergic agents, used as antispasmodics, help relieve symptoms that are associated with GI disorders that produce hyperacidity, hypermotility, and spasms (e.g., peptic ulcer, irritable bowel syndrome, neurogenic bowel disorder, pylorospasms, and spasms of the biliary tract). Some anticholinergics, used as antispasmodics, are also used to relieve symptoms that are associated with dysmenorrhea or various GU disorders (e.g., bladder spasms, nocturnal enuresis, and neurogenic bladder). Oxybutynin and tolterodine are used to relieve urgency, frequency, nocturia, and incontinence in patients with neurogenic bladder.

What You NEED TO KNOW

Contraindications/Precautions

Anticholinergics should be used cautiously in patients with coronary artery disease and renal or liver dysfunction.

Anticholinergics are contraindicated for patients with narrow-angle glaucoma because they cause pupil dilation, for male patients who have an enlarged prostate, and for patients with myasthenia gravis because they inhibit the effects of ACh. Anticholinergics are also contraindicated in individuals with ulcerative colitis and GI or GU obstruction.

Drug Interactions

Several agents affect or can be affected by anticholinergics. Antihistamines, tricyclic antidepressants, quinidine, procainamide, disopyramide, and amantadine may increase the anticholinergic effects. Anticholinergics decrease the antipsychotic effects of phenothiazines. Methotrimeprazine may precipitate extrapyramidal symptoms when taken with an anticholinergic. Alcohol enhances the sedative effects of anticholinergics, particularly in anticholinergics that are used to treat Parkinson's disease (e.g., benztropine, biperiden, procyclidine, scopolamine, trihexyphenidyl). Antacids decrease the absorption of anticholinergics.

Adverse Effects

Several adverse effects are associated with anticholinergics, most of which are related to antimuscarinic properties. Common adverse effects include dry mouth, tachydysrhythmias, hypertension, decreased sweating, drowsiness, nervousness, insomnia, confusion, hallucinations, flushing, blurred vision, mydriasis, and constipation. Because anticholinergics increase the heart rate, conduction, contractility, and automaticity, an increase in myocardial oxygen demand may occur, resulting in myocardial ischemia. Anticholinergics may cause acute urinary retention in patients with an enlarged prostate or benign prostatic hypertrophy.

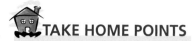

TAKE HOME POINTS

- Antacids decrease the absorption of anticholinergics; thus 1 hour should be spaced between administering an antacid and an anticholinergic. Alcohol enhances the sedative effects in anticholinergics.
- Atropine should be used to treat symptomatic and not asymptomatic bradycardia.

What You DO

Nursing Responsibilities

When administering anticholinergics, the nurse should:

- Space 1 hour between administering an antacid and an anticholinergic.
- Decrease doses in patients with hepatic or renal dysfunction because most anticholinergics are metabolized by the liver and eliminated through the kidneys.
- Monitor intake and output.
- Palpate bladder to assess urinary retention.
- Advise patients who are taking an anticholinergic to avoid high temperatures because their ability to perspire is inhibited, making them susceptible to heat stroke.
- Warn the patient to avoid driving or engaging in any activity that requires alertness until the sedative effects of the anticholinergic are determined.
- Instruct the patient to avoid concurrent use of alcohol and other depressants.
- Instruct the patient to check with the health care provider before taking any OTC agents, particularly any antihistamines because they increase anticholinergic effects.
- Instruct the patient to perform frequent mouth care to relieve dry mouth.
- Instruct the patient to report any anticholinergic adverse effects (e.g., urinary retention, constipation, drowsiness, confusion) to the health care provider.

When administering atropine, the nurse should:

- Use atropine only when the patient with ischemic heart disease is symptomatic. Atropine increases the myocardial oxygen demand and should be used to treat symptomatic bradycardia (not asymptomatic bradycardia), particularly in patients with coronary artery disease. When atropine is used for treatment of bradycardia, a minimum IV dose of 0.5 mg should be given to the adult patient because a dose less than 0.5 mg may cause paradoxical bradycardia.
- Inform the health care provider about any patient who complains of chest pain and who is receiving atropine or an anticholinergic immediately.
- Realize that atropine is the drug of choice for treatment of bradydys-rhythmias and heart blocks.
- Recognize that atropine is used to treat an overdose of cholinesterase inhibitors (**cholinergic crisis**) and direct-acting cholinergic agonists, as well as to treat organophosphate poisoning. Be aware of the doses for atropine when used as an antidote for these conditions.

Do You UNDERSTAND?

DIRECTIONS: Match each item listed in Column A with the appropriate response in Column B.

Column A	Column B
_____ 1. antacids	a. May precipitate extrapyramidal effects when taken with an anticholinergic.
_____ 2. methotrimeprazine	b. May increase the anticholinergic effects of anticholinergics.
_____ 3. alcohol	c. Decrease(s) the absorption of anticholinergics.
_____ 4. antihistamines	d. Increase(s) the sedative effects in anticholinergics.

Answers: 1. b; 2. d; 3. a; 4. c.

What IS a Dopaminergic?

Dopaminergics	Trade Names	Uses
levodopa [LEE-voe-DOE-puh]	Dopar, Larodopa	Treatment of Parkinson's disease
carbidopa-levodopa [CAR-bih-doe-puh]	Sinemet Sinemet-CR Lodosyn	Treatment of Parkinson's disease
amantadine hydrochloride [a-MAN-ta-deen]	Symmetrel	Treatment of Parkinson's disease and drug-induced extrapyramidal symptoms
bromocriptine mesylate [BROE-moe-KRIP-teen MEH-sih-LATE]	Parlodel	Treatment of Parkinson's disease
ropinirole [row-PIN-ih-role]	Requip	Treatment of Parkinson's disease and restless leg syndrome
pramipexole [pram-ih-PECKS-all]	Mirapex	Treatment of Parkinson's disease

Action

A variety of pharmacologic actions exist among the dopaminergic agents, but all optimize the availability of dopamine in the brain. Levodopa is a metabolic precursor of dopamine. Amantidine releases dopamine from dopaminergic neurons. Amantidine also has antiviral properties and is used to treat symptoms that are associated with influenza A. Bromocriptine, pramipexole, and ropinirole are dopamine agonists.

Uses

Dopaminergics are used to treat Parkinson's disease. This disease is progressive and chronic, involving the areas of the brain that control balance, posture, and coordination. Three primary symptoms observed in Parkinson's disease are rigidity, tremors, and slow movements (**bradykinesia**). These symptoms result because of a deficiency of dopamine in the brain's extrapyramidal system and basal ganglia. Dopaminergic nerves are either degenerated or a depletion of the neurotransmitter stores occurs.

Levodopa is a common, primary dopaminergic used to treat Parkinson's disease because it is identical to the chemical in the body called *dihydroxyphenylalanine (DOPA)*. The enzyme DOPA decarboxylase converts to dopamine. One way to enhance the effects of levodopa without increasing the dose is to administer the drug in a preparation combined with carbidopa, which inhibits DOPA decarboxylase in the GI tract.

⚠️ Dopaminergics should be used cautiously in patients with a history of arrhythmias, MI, hypertension, peptic ulcers, and renal or hepatic impairment.

This inhibition prevents the conversion of levodopa to dopamine before the latter reaches the brain; thus more dopamine becomes available in the brain. Some of the dopaminergics are ineffective alone; thus they are used only as adjuncts to levodopa. These adjunctive agents include bromocriptine.

What You NEED TO KNOW

Contraindications/Precautions

Administration of dopaminergics is contraindicated for individuals who have glaucoma and within 2 weeks of administering MAOIs. Amantidine should be avoided in patients with a history of seizures because it may precipitate seizure activity.

Drug Interactions

Several agents interact with dopaminergics. Anticholinergics may increase the anticholinergic effects of amantidine. Alcohol may increase CNS depression caused by dopaminergics.

MAOIs may precipitate a hypertensive crisis, particularly with levodopa and levodopa-carbidopa. Pyridoxine, MAOIs, benzodiazepines, phenytoin, and phenothiazines antagonize the effects of levodopa. Butyrophenones, metoclopramide, and phenothiazines antagonize the effects of the dopaminergic agents, bromocriptine, pramipexole, and ropinirole. Selegiline with opioids may result in possible life-threatening reactions, including excitation, sweating, rigidity, hypertension, hypotension, and coma.

🏠 **TAKE HOME POINTS**

- Consumption of alcohol or other depressants with a dopaminergic drug increases CNS depression; thus these drug combinations should be avoided.
- Life-threatening reactions may result when selegiline is taken with opioids.

Adverse Effects

A variety of adverse effects may occur with dopaminergics. Dopaminergics frequently cause dry mouth, weakness, headache, dizziness, nausea, vomiting, insomnia, and sudden sleep attacks. Dopaminergics may also produce cardiovascular effects, including orthostatic hypotension, rhythm disturbances, and palpitations. Levodopa or carbidopa-levodopa may cause blurred vision, mydriasis, leukopenia, and hemolytic anemia. Amantidine may precipitate seizure activity in patients with a history of seizures. All of the dopaminergics may become toxic and produce

🏠 **TAKE HOME POINTS**

- Monitor for postural hypotension when administering dopaminergics.
- Levodopa or carbidopa-levodopa may cause leukopenia or hemolytic anemia; thus complete blood counts should be monitored.

CNS effects, such as involuntary movements, ataxia, twitching, agitation, confusion, delusions, depression, hallucinations, and hepatic dysfunction.

What You DO

Nursing Responsibilities

The doses of dopaminergics that are metabolized by the liver and eliminated by the kidneys should be decreased in patients with either hepatic or renal failure. When administering dopaminergics, the nurse should:

- Assess possible extrapyramidal and parkinsonian symptoms before initiating dopaminergics and throughout therapy. Symptoms include akinesia, tremors, rigidity, shuffling gait, twisting motions, and drooling. Worsening of symptoms may indicate drug toxicity.
- Monitor the patient's BP for hypotension, particularly when the patient rises to a standing position.
- Warn patients to make postural changes slowly.
- Monitor complete blood counts, including white blood cell counts, hemoglobin, and hematocrit, in patients who are taking either levodopa or carbidopa-levodopa because these agents may cause leukopenia and hemolytic anemia.
- Check renal and hepatic function tests to determine early dysfunction.
- Teach the patient to take medication with meals to avoid GI irritation.
- Encourage patient to void prior to drug administration.
- Instruct patients to avoid driving or any activity that requires alertness until the sedative response is determined.
- Advise patients who are taking dopaminergics to avoid alcohol and other depressants.
- Inform patients to avoid abrupt discontinuation of dopaminergics because sudden parkinsonian symptoms may occur.
- Instruct patients to report any symptoms of mental changes or dizziness so that doses may be decreased.

Do You UNDERSTAND?

DIRECTIONS: **Indicate in the space provided whether each statement is *true* or *false*. If the answer is false, correct the statement to make it true (using the margin space).**

_____ 1. Dopaminergics optimize the availability of dopamine in the brain.

_____ 2. Phenothiazines antagonize the therapeutic effect of pramipexole.

_____ 3. Bromocriptine is used as a single agent to treat Parkinson's disease.

_____ 4. Amantidine is a metabolic precursor of dopamine.

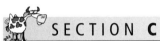

SECTION C

CENTRAL NERVOUS SYSTEM DRUGS

This section reviews pharmacologic agents that stimulate the CNS and relax skeletal muscles. Some CNS stimulants can produce severe psychologic dependence. The Controlled Substances Act of 1970 classifies these drugs as schedule II drugs. Continuous use of CNS stimulants may lead to drug tolerance and dependence.

CNS stimulants are used in the treatment of narcolepsy and obesity, as well as attention-deficit/hyperactivity disorder (ADHD), attention-deficit disorder (ADD), or hyperkinetic syndrome. The medications discussed in this section include psychomotor stimulants, anorexiants, analeptics, centrally acting muscle relaxants, and peripherally acting muscle relaxants. Xanthines (e.g., theophylline) are also CNS stimulants. However, prescription use of xanthines as CNS stimulants is rare; thus xanthines will be discussed in Chapter 8 (Section C) as a treatment of respiratory disorders.

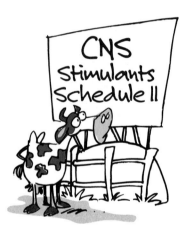

Don't depend on us!

Answers: 1. true; 2. true; 3. false; bromocriptine is an adjunctive agent to levodopa; 4. false; levodopa is a metabolic precursor of dopamine, and amantidine releases dopamine from dopaminergic neurons.

What IS a Psychomotor Stimulant?

Psychomotor Stimulants	Trade Names	Uses
amphetamine sulfate [am-FET-uh-meen]	Adderall	Treatment of narcolepsy and ADHD
dextroamphetamine sulfate [DEX-troe-am-FET-uh-meen]	Dexedrine	Treatment of narcolepsy, ADHD, and exogenous obesity
pemoline [PEM-oh-leen]	Cylert	Treatment of ADHD
methylphenidate [meth-ill-FEN-ih-date]	Ritalin	Treatment of narcolepsy and ADHD

Action

Psychomotor stimulants affect the CNS. These drugs cause a release of brain neurotransmitters involving serotonin, dopamine, and norepinephrine. Small doses of amphetamines tend to act selectively to elevate mood, decrease perception of fatigue, reduce appetite, stimulate the respiratory and cardiovascular systems, and increase alertness, concentration, metabolism, and motor performance. Large doses of amphetamines tend to stimulate the entire CNS and produce restlessness, insomnia, tremors, and motor performance deterioration. By exerting a direct blocking action on central receptors for serotonin, psychomotor stimulants affect the individual psychologically by increasing initiative and self-confidence. Physiologic effects include systolic and diastolic BP elevation, bronchial relaxation, increased sphincter tone in urinary bladder, increased peristalsis, and suppressed rapid-eye-movement (REM) sleep.

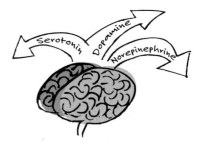

Uses

The therapeutic uses of amphetamines include treatment of narcolepsy, exogenous obesity, and ADHD.

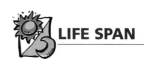

LIFE SPAN

Methylphenidate is used in treating ADHD in children and narcolepsy in adults. Pemoline is a schedule IV controlled drug and is used only in treating ADHD in children. Psychomotor stimulants are contraindicated for women during pregnancy and lactation. Psychomotor stimulants are not recommended for children under 6 years of age for ADHD or in children under 12 years of age for appetite suppression.

What You NEED TO KNOW

Contraindications/Precautions

Psychomotor stimulants are contraindicated for patients with hypertension, cardiovascular disease, anxiety, agitation, glaucoma, psychopathologic disorders, hyperthyroidism, and Gilles de la Tourette's syndrome.

! Caution must be taken when administering amphetamines to older patients with malnutrition, insomnia, renal dysfunction, diabetes mellitus, seizures, or a history of drug abuse.

! When drug administration is initiated or in subsequent titrations, extended-release or resin preparations should not be used.

These agents are contraindicated for patients with suicidal tendencies or those who are homicidal. Psychomotor stimulants are also contraindicated during or within 14 days of MAOI therapy. Pemoline is contraindicated in individuals who have hepatic dysfunction.

Drug Interactions

When amphetamines are taken concurrently with adrenergic or tricyclic antidepressants, the adrenergic effects are intensified. Taking MAOIs and phenothiazines together with amphetamines can lead to a hypertensive crisis. The effects of antihypertensives may be antagonized when they are given with amphetamines. Phenothiazines decrease the effect of amphetamines. When amphetamines are taken with anticonvulsants, the anticonvulsant effects are delayed. Psychomotor stimulants cause an alteration in insulin requirements. Acid urine promotes drug elimination, and when the urine is alkaline (e.g., due to cranberry juice consumption), reabsorption is promoted and the drug action is prolonged.

Adverse Effects

Adverse effects of amphetamines include irritability, restlessness, nervousness, anxiety, headache, perceptual disturbances, hallucinations, depression, euphoria, insomnia, tremors, and hyperactive reflexes. GI adverse effects include dry mouth, metallic taste, anorexia, nausea, vomiting, abdominal cramps, diarrhea, and constipation. More serious adverse effects include cardiac stimulation, angina, palpitations, tachycardia, hypertension, dysrhythmias, seizures, psychosis, and hepatic failure.

What You DO

Nursing Responsibilities

After the dose of psychomotor stimulant is stabilized, the extended-release preparations are safe and convenient. The first dose of the day should be administered early in the day and the last dose given no later than 6 hours before bedtime to avoid insomnia. When administering psychomotor stimulants, the nurse should:
- Instruct the patient to rinse the mouth frequently with clear water and increase fluid intake to prevent dryness.
- Instruct patients to avoid using psychomotor stimulants to overcome fatigue and sleep deficit (e.g., students studying for tests, athletes, or

TAKE HOME POINTS

- Instruct the patient that meticulous oral hygiene with gentle brushing of the tongue is required because decreased saliva may lead to demineralization of tooth surfaces and oral mucosal erosion.
- Psychomotor stimulants should be gradually withdrawn after prolonged use to avoid profound depression or other psychopathologic conditions that may last several weeks.

long-distance drivers). The stimulating drug effect masks fatigue. After the exhilaration has disappeared, fatigue and depression are usually greater than previously experienced, requiring a longer rest period.

- Inform patients that use of these drugs may impair the ability to engage in hazardous activities, such as operating an automobile or machinery.
- Warn patients to anticipate that height and weight suppression occurs as a result of appetite suppression.
- Monitor liver function for early detection of hepatic failure.
- Check vital signs and cardiac monitor for early detection of cardiovascular adverse effects.
- Monitor the glucose level in the patient with diabetes who is taking psychomotor stimulants for potential dose adjustments of insulin.
- Instruct patients to avoid concurrent intake of caffeine and psychomotor stimulants to prevent intensified effects.
- Encourage the patient to relieve dry mouth with sugarless gum.
- Interrupt therapy periodically to evaluate the patient's need for continued drug use and to allow for normal growth and development. Prolonged therapy is inappropriate because of a potential risk for drug tolerance with long-term usage.

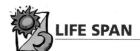

LIFE SPAN

- Children should be given psychomotor stimulants after meals to minimize appetite suppression and interference with nutrition and growth.
- Closely monitor children who are taking psychomotor stimulants because long-term effects are unknown. Older patients are likely to experience mental confusion, anxiety, nervousness, and insomnia from psychomotor stimulants.

Do You UNDERSTAND?

DIRECTIONS: Place a check mark next to each of the following descriptions that demonstrate the adverse effects of psychomotor stimulants.

_____ 1. Shaking (tremors)
_____ 2. Coughing
_____ 3. Opening door to bathroom
_____ 4. Drinking large glass of water
_____ 5. Sleeping soundly

What IS an Anorexiant?

Anorexiants	Trade Names	Uses
diethylpropion [die-ETH-uhl-PRO-pee-ahn]	Tepanil, Dospan, Teniate	Treatment of exogenous obesity
benzphetamine [benz-FET-uh-meen]	Didrex	Treatment of exogenous obesity
phentermine [fen-TER-meen]	Fastin, Zantryl, adipex-P, Ionamin, Obe-Nix-30	Treatment of exogenous obesity
phenmetrazine [fen-MET-ra-zeen]	Preludin	Treatment of exogenous obesity

Action

The action of anorexiants is unknown, but they are thought to stimulate the satiety center in the hypothalamus. Appetite receptors in the satiety center respond specifically to hunger messages and trigger a feeling of fullness, reducing the need to consume food.

Uses

Anorexiants are used for short-term treatment in the adjunctive management of exogenous obesity. Adjunctive treatment modalities include exercise, diet, and behavior modification.

What You NEED TO KNOW

Contraindications/Precautions

Anorexiants are contraindicated for patients with hypersensitivity, glaucoma, severe cardiovascular disease, hyperthyroidism, and agitation.

Drug Interactions

Drug interaction between anorexiants and insulin leads to a reduction of insulin requirements. When anorexiants are given concurrently with guanethidine, the hypotensive effect of guanethidine is decreased. When they are given concurrently with, or within 14 days of, MAOIs, a hypertensive crisis may be triggered. Other CNS depressants (e.g., alcohol, general anesthetics) create an intensified effect to anorexiants.

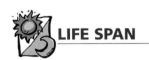

LIFE SPAN

Anorexiants are contraindicated for children less than 12 years of age.

Adverse Effects

Adverse effects of anorexiants include dyspnea, blurred vision, restlessness, dry mouth, altered taste, vomiting, diarrhea, abdominal pain, constipation, sweating, rash, menstrual irregularities, and bone marrow suppression. Cardiovascular related adverse effects include dizziness, fatigue, palpitations, tachycardia, hypertension, and dysrhythmias. Psychologically related adverse effects include euphoria, insomnia, confusion, depression, and psychosis.

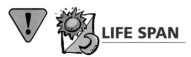 **LIFE SPAN**

Caution should be taken in older adults who require anorexiant therapy. Caution should be taken in patients who have diabetes mellitus or psychosis and require anorexiant therapy.

What You DO

Nursing Responsibilities

A single anorexiant dose is usually taken midmorning or midafternoon, depending on the patient's eating habits. Anorexiants should be given on an empty stomach, approximately 30 to 60 minutes before meals. To avoid insomnia, the daily dose should be administered no later than 6 hours before bedtime.

When administering anorexiants, the nurse should:

- Teach the patient who is taking anorexiants about safety from potential dizziness.
- Monitor the patient with diabetes who is taking both insulin and an anorexiant because dose adjustments may be necessary.
- Monitor CBC results for early detection of bone marrow suppression.
- Encourage the patient to weigh three times a week at the same time of day with the same amount of clothing.
- Inform the patient that the anorexiant effect is temporary and seldom lasts more than a few weeks. Because this tolerance may occur, short-term use is appropriate.
- Tell the patient that a potential exists for dependence on these drugs.
- Teach the patient that abrupt withdrawal of the drug following prolonged high doses may result in GI distress, abdominal cramping, tremors, extreme fatigue, and mental depression.

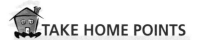**TAKE HOME POINTS**

Warn patients to avoid driving any vehicle or operating hazardous machinery until the reaction to the drug is determined. Anorexiant therapy should not exceed 12 weeks.

 Advise patient to avoid abrupt discontinuation of anorexiants.

Do You UNDERSTAND?

DIRECTIONS: **Match each statement in Column A with the appropriate term in Column B.**

Column A	Column B
_____ 1. When given concurrently or within 14 days, this drug can trigger hypertensive crisis.	a. Alcohol
	b. MAOIs
	c. Bradycardia
_____ 2. Anorexiants typically cause this alteration in the heart rate.	d. Tachycardia
	e. Bedtime
_____ 3. This is the best time of day to take an anorexiant	f. Mid morning

What IS an Analeptic?

Analeptics	Trade Names	Uses
caffeine [kaf-EEN]	Caffedrine Vivarin	Promotes mental alertness and wakefulness
doxapram [DOX-a-pram]	Dopram	Treatment of postanesthesia and drug-induced respiratory depression

Action

Analeptics release epinephrine and norepinephrine from the adrenal medulla, producing CNS stimulation. These agents (e.g., caffeine, doxapram) inhibit the phosphodiesterase enzyme, which results in higher concentrations of cyclic adenosine monophosphate (cAMP). In small doses, caffeine stimulates the cerebral cortex, reducing drowsiness and fatigue while increasing awareness. Higher doses stimulate respiratory, medullary, vasomotor, and vagal centers. The peak time of caffeine effects is 15 to 45 minutes.

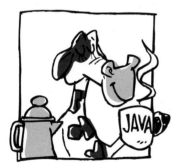

Caffeine is an analeptic.

Uses

Analeptics are used as mild CNS stimulants to restore mental alertness and aid in remaining awake. Doxapram stimulates the CNS at all levels, but clinical use is generally for stimulating respirations. Doxapram promotes arousal and the return of pharyngeal and laryngeal reflexes and is generally used for short-term adjunctive therapy of respiratory depression from drugs or anesthesia. Caffeine is found in many beverages and foods, such as coffee, tea, cola, and chocolate. Caffeine is also an ingredient in many OTC headache medications (e.g., Anacin, Excedrin).

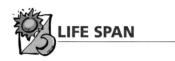

LIFE SPAN

Caffeine is contraindicated for women during lactation.

What You NEED TO KNOW

Contraindications/Precautions

Caffeine is contraindicated for patients with depression, duodenal ulcers, and diabetes mellitus. Doxapram is contraindicated for patients with seizures, flail chest, pneumothorax, acute chronic obstructive pulmonary disease (COPD), severe hypertension, coronary artery disease, head injury, and cerebral vascular accident (CVA).

Drug Interactions

Caffeine increases CNS effects when taken concurrently with cimetidine, ciprofloxacin, enoxacin, phenylpropanolamine, disulfiram, and oral contraceptives. Doxapram produces increased effects when given with anesthetics (e.g., halothane, cyclopropane, and enflurane). When doxapram is given concurrently with MAOIs or sympathomimetics, hypertensive effects are increased. The effects of caffeine are reduced when taken while the patient is smoking. When caffeine is taken together with iron, it decreases the absorption of iron.

Adverse Effects

The adverse effects of analeptics include headache, dizziness, tachycardia, nausea, vomiting, and diarrhea. Additional adverse effects following caffeine use include restlessness, nervousness, insomnia, abdominal pain, and diuresis. Adverse effects of doxapram include flushing, disorientation, sweating, hyperactivity, increased reflexes, elevated BP, seizures, laryngospasm, and bronchospasm.

Doxapram should be used with caution during pregnancy and lactation.

Doxapram should also be given cautiously to patients who have dysrhythmias, hyperthyroidism, pheochromocytoma, cerebral edema, increased intracranial pressure, peptic ulcers, and acute agitation.

↑ caffeine consumption = ↓ iron absorption

What You DO

Nursing Responsibilities

When administering analeptics, the nurse should:

- Delay doxapram treatment at least 10 minutes after discontinuation of anesthetics.
- Instruct patients to take iron at least 2 hours before or after caffeine in the form of coffee, tea, cola, and chocolate.
- Instruct patients that caffeine withdrawal effects include headache, anxiety, and increased muscle tension.

Do You UNDERSTAND?

DIRECTIONS: **Provide appropriate responses to the following statements.**

1. List three beverages that contain caffeine.

   _____

   _____

   _____

2. List an OTC medication that contains caffeine.

   _____

3. State the peak time for caffeine effects.

   _____

4. List at least three adverse effects of analeptics or caffeine.

   _____

   _____

   _____

Answers: 1. coffee, tea, cola; 2. Anacin or Excedrin; 3. 15 to 45 minutes; 4. headache, dizziness, tachycardia, nausea, vomiting, diarrhea, restlessness, nervousness, insomnia, abdominal pain, diuresis, flushing, disorientation, sweating, hyperactivity, increased reflexes and BP, seizures, laryngospasm, and bronchospasm.

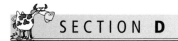

SECTION D

ANTICONVULSANTS

This section reviews drugs that manage seizure disorders. The primary aim of treatment is seizure control. The two types of seizure disorders include isolated events as observed in a febrile illness and recurrent events, such as in epilepsy.

Seizures are classified internationally for uniformity. Common generalized seizures include tonic-clonic (formerly known as *grand mal*) and absence (formerly known as *petit mal*). Tonic-clonic seizures are the most prevalent form, involving skeletal muscle contraction for 3 to 5 seconds in the tonic phase and a jerkiness of the body for 2 to 4 minutes in the clonic phase. Absence seizures involve a momentary loss of consciousness lasting approximately 10 seconds. Partial seizures may be either focal (which do not involve a loss of consciousness) or complex (involving loss of consciousness). Focal seizures (also known as *simple* or *jacksonian*) involve spontaneous movement that may spread. Complex seizures usually include repetitive behavior.

Anticonvulsant drugs decrease the excess firing, inhibit the spread of nerve impulses, and elevate the seizure threshold, thereby promoting the stabilization of abnormal brain cells. No single drug is available that controls all types of seizures; drug choice is individualized for each patient. This section explains the various anticonvulsant medications, which include hydantoins, barbiturates, benzodiazepines, succinimides, valproic acid, carbamazepine, and gabapentins.

What IS a Hydantoin?

Hydantoins	Trade Names	Uses
phenytoin [FEN-ih-toyn]	Dilantin	Controls tonic-clonic mal and psychomotor seizures
mephenytoin [me-FEN-ih-toyn]	Mesantoin	Controls tonic-clonic, psychomotor, focal, and jacksonian seizures
fosphenytoin [fos-FEN-ih-toyn]	Cerebyx	Controls generalized status epilepticus

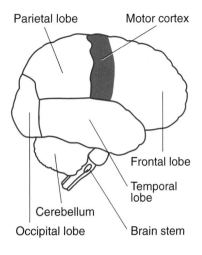

Parietal lobe   Motor cortex

Frontal lobe

Temporal lobe

Cerebellum

Occipital lobe   Brain stem

Action

The mechanism of action in anticonvulsants is not completely known. Theories suggest that anticonvulsants stabilize neuronal membranes and limit the spread of irritability or seizure activity. Hydantoins appear to act on the motor cortex. Anticonvulsants inhibit seizure activity by promoting sodium outward flow (**efflux**) from neurons and inhibiting the production of repetitive action potentials at synapses. Because hyper-excitability is a result of excessive stimulation or environmental changes, which reduces the membrane sodium gradient, hydantoins tend to stabilize the hyperexcitability threshold. Hydantoins lower the activity of brain stem centers, which controls the tonic phase of tonic-clonic seizures.

Uses

Hydantoins are used primarily to control tonic-clonic and psychomotor seizures. Phenytoin is the oldest and most well known of the hydantoins. Phenytoin remains one of the most effective and commonly used anticonvulsants. Phenytoin is also used in the prevention and treatment of seizures in patients who are undergoing neurosurgery and has been effective in controlling status epilepticus. Because of their efficacy, hydantoins are used in all age groups. In addition to controlling tonic-clonic and psychomotor seizures, mephenytoin is used to control focal or jacksonian seizures.

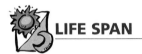

LIFE SPAN

Hydantoins are contraindicated for pregnant and nursing women.

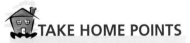

TAKE HOME POINTS

Carefully monitor patients with cardiac function impairment, such as Stokes-Adams syndrome, second- and third-degree atrioventricular block, sinoatrial node block, and sinus bradycardia because of the antiarrhythmic effect of phenytoin.

What You NEED TO KNOW

Contraindications/Precautions

Hydantoins are contraindicated for patients with hypersensitivity. Intravenous phenytoin is contraindicated for patients with sinus bradycardia, sinoatrial node block, second- and third-degree atrioventricular block, and Stokes-Adams syndrome.

Drug Interactions

Several drugs interact adversely with hydantoins, particularly phenytoin. Prolonged use of acetaminophen together with hydantoins may increase the risk for hepatotoxicity. Because hydantoin anticonvulsants may cause hyperglycemia, persons with diabetes may require medication adjustments. Hydantoins increase the action of anticoagulants and aspirin.

Antacids and calcium preparations decrease the absorption and efficacy of hydantoins, whereas cimetidine and sulfonamides increase the action of hydantoins.

Adverse Effects

The most frequent adverse effects include constipation, headache, dizziness, drowsiness, blurred vision, gingival hyperplasia, nausea, vomiting, diarrhea, and enlargement of facial features. Other adverse effects occurring at high plasma levels include CNS toxicity, including ataxia, confusion, nystagmus, slurred speech, stuttering, trembling of hands, excitement, nervousness, irritability, and hyperglycemia. Peripheral neuropathies, blood dyscrasias (e.g., agranulocytosis), and Stevens-Johnson syndrome are rare adverse effects.

What You DO

Nursing Responsibilities

Anticonvulsants are usually administered orally; however, some of the hydantoins may be given IM or IV in emergency situations. When administering hydantoins, the nurse should:

- Monitor periodic blood studies to ensure therapeutic plasma levels, particularly in the initial stages of therapy. The therapeutic serum concentration is 10 to 20 mcg/mL.
- Observe the patient closely for possible adverse reactions to anticonvulsants, particularly at the initiation of therapy.
- Monitor periodic hepatic and hematologic laboratory studies to identify potential adverse reactions.
- Provide clear and accurate information for the proper use of hydantoins so that patients can self-administer their medication successfully and achieve seizure control. The proper dose, compliance with therapy, and taking medications as prescribed are three important aspects of therapy.
- Teach the patient the proper way to address missed doses of medication. The patient should be advised to contact the health care provider when doses are missed for 2 or more days in a row.
- Advise the patient on precautions (e.g., older patients tend to metabolize hydantoins slowly). Other medications should not be taken

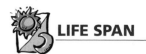

LIFE SPAN

Adverse effects are more likely to occur in the geriatric population compared with the younger populations.

TAKE HOME POINTS

- Although rare, the occurrence of blood dyscrasias may be a significant adverse effect of treatment.
- Monitor laboratory tests for therapeutic hydantoin levels, hepatic function, and hematologic status. Instruct patients that if a dose is omitted, the next dose should not be doubled. Impress on the patient the importance of avoiding abrupt discontinuation of the medication.

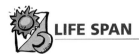

LIFE SPAN

Older patients tend to metabolize hydantoins slowly, increasing the potential for toxic serum levels. Older patients frequently require decreased doses and subsequent dose adjustment.

concurrently, nor should the brand or dose forms of phenytoin be changed without contacting the health care provider.

- Instruct patients to avoid alcoholic beverages and other CNS depressants when taking hydantoins.
- Advise the patient to avoid abrupt discontinuation of the medication. A gradual dose reduction is required to maintain seizure control and should be designed by the health care provider.
- Instruct patients to take oral hydantoin with meals to lessen gastric irritation.
- Report skin rash, unusual depression, or personality change to the health care provider because the drug may need to be discontinued.
- Inform the patient that phenytoin may change the color of urine to pink or reddish-brown.
- Provide the patient with information on obtaining MedicAlert information.

Do You UNDERSTAND?

DIRECTIONS: **Indicate in the space provided whether the statement is *true* or *false*. If the answer is false, correct the statement to make it true (using the margin space).**

_____ 1. Hydantoins are used to control absence and psychomotor seizures.

_____ 2. Adverse effects are more likely to occur in the geriatric population.

_____ 3. Older patients frequently require higher doses of hydantoins because of this population's metabolism.

_____ 4. Hydantoins should not be discontinued abruptly.

Answers: 1. false; hydantoins are used to control tonic clonic and psychomotor seizures; 2. true; 3. false; older patients tend to metabolize hydantoins slowly and require decreased doses and subsequent dose adjustment; 4. true.

What IS a Barbiturate?

Barbiturates	Trade Names	Uses
phenobarbital [fee-noe-BAR-bi-tal]	Luminal	Long-term treatment of tonic-clonic and partial seizures; controls status epilepticus, eclampsia, and febrile convulsions in children
mephobarbital [me-foe-BAR-bi-tal]	Mebaral	Controls tonic-clonic and absence seizures
metharbital [Meth-ARE-bi-tal]	Gemonil	Controls tonic-clonic and absence seizures
primidone [PRIH-mih-doan]	Mysoline	Controls tonic-clonic and partial seizures

Action

Phenobarbital was the first widely effective, long-acting antiepileptic drug. The primary anticonvulsant mechanism is the decrease of nerve transmission and excitability of the nerve cell. Barbiturates also increase the threshold for electrical stimulation of the motor cortex.

Uses

Barbiturates are indicated in long-term anticonvulsant therapy for the treatment of generalized tonic-clonic seizures and focal-partial seizures. Mephobarbital and metharbital are indicated as alternatives to phenobarbital. Although other more effective, selective, and less sedating anticonvulsants are available, barbiturates may still be used because of their efficacy in seizure reduction. Primidone is used for partial seizures and generalized tonic-clonic seizures.

Cautious use should be taken in older adults or patients who are debilitated. Caution should also be used in the presence of fever, severe anemia, hyperthyroidism, renal and liver dysfunction, and diabetes mellitus.

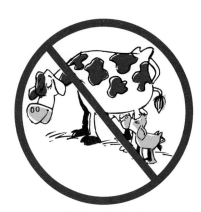

Not now junior!

What You NEED TO KNOW

Contraindications/Precautions

Barbiturates are contraindicated for patients with hypersensitivity, severe respiratory dysfunction, renal impairment, or those with a history of porphyria.

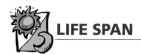

LIFE SPAN

Barbiturates are contraindicated for women who are pregnant and lactating. Barbiturates cross the placenta and are present in breast milk.

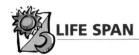

LIFE SPAN

Older patients may react to typical doses of barbiturates with excitement, confusion, or depression. Older patients are more likely than younger patients to have age-related hepatic or renal impairment that requires dose reduction. Be aware of the need for reduced barbiturate doses in the older patient.

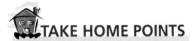

TAKE HOME POINTS

Female patients who are taking estrogen-containing oral contraceptives should be advised to use an additional alternative method of birth control for the duration of barbiturate treatment.

Drug Interactions

Several drugs interact with barbiturates. The effects of anticoagulants may be decreased when used concurrently with barbiturates. Bleeding may result when the barbiturate is discontinued; thus periodic monitoring of prothrombin time may be indicated. The concurrent use of another hydantoin anticonvulsant may result in its unpredictable metabolism. Barbiturates may also reduce the contraceptive reliability of estrogen-containing oral contraceptives. Alcohol or other CNS depressants may increase the depressant effect of either of the previously mentioned substances.

Adverse Effects

Barbiturates are depressants of both respiratory and GI motility, although the degree of depression is dose-dependent. Common adverse effects include drowsiness, respiratory depression, lethargy, hypothermia, vertigo, headache, bradycardia, insomnia, nightmares, paradoxical excitement, liver dysfunction, blood dyscrasias, and CNS depression. Allergic reactions, exfoliative dermatitis, hallucinations, hypotension, and blood dyscrasias (e.g., agranulocytosis, thrombocytopenia) may occur in rare instances. Withdrawal symptoms may occur after as little as 2 weeks of uninterrupted barbiturate therapy.

What You DO

Nursing Responsibilities

Barbiturates are administered orally, rectally, or parenterally. Emergency treatment of status epilepticus may require IV administration. When administering barbiturates, the nurse should:

- Monitor seizure activity for changes with regard to character, frequency, and duration.
- Warn the patient about concurrent use of other CNS depressants (e.g., analgesics, antihistamines, alcohol).
- Advise the patient to seek medical approval before taking OTC cold or allergy medications.
- Teach the patient about safety measures while taking barbiturates.
- Instruct the patient to avoid abrupt discontinuation of barbiturate therapy because seizures may be precipitated.

- Monitor the patient for respiratory and liver function, CNS depression, and bone marrow suppression.
- Monitor the patient's serum for drug concentration to detect toxic levels early.
- Warn the patient about the potentially addictive nature of long-term barbiturate use.
- Instruct the patient to avoid alcohol while taking barbiturates.

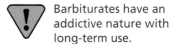 Barbiturates have an addictive nature with long-term use.

Do You UNDERSTAND?

DIRECTIONS: Indicate in the space provided whether the statement is *true* or *false*. If the answer is false, correct the statement to make it true (using the margin space).

_____ 1. Mephobarbital was the first widely effective antiepileptic drug.

_____ 2. Phenobarbital is a long-acting barbiturate that is indicated for long-term anticonvulsant therapy.

_____ 3. Older patients may react to barbiturate therapy with depression.

_____ 4. Medical approval is unnecessary for OTC cold or allergy medications.

What IS a Benzodiazepine?

Benzodiazepine	Trade Names	Uses
lorazepam [lore-AZE-uh-pam]	Ativan	Treatment of status epilepticus
diazepam [DIE-aze-uh-pam]	Valium	Treatment of status epilepticus
clorazepate [klor-AZE-uh-PATE]	Tranxene	Treatment of partial seizures
clonazepam [kloe-NAY-ze-pam]	Klonopin	Treatment of absence, myoclonic, and akinetic seizures

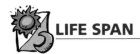

LIFE SPAN

Benzodiazepines are contraindicated for pregnant and nursing women and for children under 12 years of age. Benzodiazepines should be used cautiously in older or debilitated patients.

Benzodiazepines should also be used cautiously in patients with suicidal tendencies and those with renal or hepatic dysfunction, myasthenia gravis, and GI disorders.

Action

Benzodiazepines act as CNS depressants that produce all levels of CNS depression, ranging from mild sedation to coma, depending on the dose. All benzodiazepines have both antiepileptic and anxiolytic properties that reduce seizures and anxiety.

Uses

Several of the benzodiazepines (e.g., diazepam, clonazepam, clorazepate, parenteral lorazepam) are used as anticonvulsants. Clorazepate and clonazepam are particularly useful in treating seizures that are difficult to control. Parenteral diazepam is the drug of choice in treating status epilepticus.

What You NEED TO KNOW

Contraindications/Precautions

Benzodiazepines are contraindicated for patients with acute narrow-angle glaucoma, coma, shock, and acute alcohol intoxication.

Drug Interactions

Concurrent use of antacids may delay the absorption of some benzodiazepines. Alcohol and other CNS depressants exacerbate benzodiazepines. Lorazepam and diazepam may increase the antiparkinsonism effects of levodopa. Benzodiazepines may increase phenytoin levels. Smoking decreases the antianxiety and sedative effects of lorazepam.

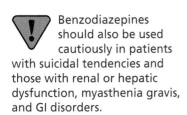

LIFE SPAN

Use of benzodiazepines in children may result in drug-induced personality changes and learning disabilities. The older population is sensitive to the development of CNS adverse effects of benzodiazepines.
   In the older population, lower-than-normal doses of benzodiazepines are required because of the development of CNS effects.

Adverse Effects

The most common adverse effects include drowsiness, reduced mental and physical alertness, dizziness, visual disturbances, and cardiovascular irregularities. Constipation, nausea, and vomiting have also been noted. Prolonged use of benzodiazepines can cause physical dependency and result in withdrawal syndrome when they are discontinued. Symptoms of toxicity range from problems with short-term memory, confusion, and vertigo to bradycardia, ataxia, severe weakness, shortness of breath, and depression.

What You DO

Nursing Responsibilities

Diazepam and lorazepam may be given orally or parenterally. When giving diazepam by direct IV push, inject the drug slowly over at least 1 minute for every 5 milligrams. Because diazepam adheres to plastic infusion tubing, care must be taken during parenteral administration. Clorazepate and clonazepam are given orally. When administering benzodiazepines, the nurse should:

- Teach the patient the correct dose and administration schedule and the importance of taking the medication exactly as prescribed.
- Inform the patient of the potential for physical and psychologic dependence on benzodiazepines and the risk for withdrawal when these drugs are abruptly discontinued.
- Teach the patient to recognize signs and symptoms of benzodiazepine dependence and when to report them.
- Monitor renal and hepatic function periodically to assess adequate drug metabolism and excretion.

TAKE HOME POINTS

- Administer IV diazepam as close as possible to the IV insertion site
- Advise the patient to take antacids (when needed) at least 1 hour before or after the scheduled dose of benzodiazepines to ensure maximal drug absorption and effectiveness. Use of benzodiazepines results in reduced tolerance for alcohol, narcotics, antihistamines, MAOIs, analgesics, and other sedatives.
- All benzodiazepines have CNS depressant effects. Significant changes in BP and heart rate may indicate impending toxicity.

Do You UNDERSTAND?

DIRECTIONS: Indicate in the space provided whether the statement is *true* or *false*. If the answer is false, correct the statement to make it true (using the margin space).

_____ 1. All benzodiazepines have either an antiepileptic or an anxiolytic property.

_____ 2. Parenteral diazepam is used for the treatment of status epilepticus.

_____ 3. The level of CNS depression with benzodiazepines is dose-dependent.

Answers: 1. true; 2. true; 3. true.

What IS a Succinimide?

Succinimides	Trade Names	Uses
ethosuximide *[ETH-oh-SUX-ih-mide]*	Zarontin	Treatment of absence seizures
methsuximide *[meth-SUX-ih-mide]*	Celontin	Treatment of absence seizures
phensuximide *[fen-SUX-ih-mide]*	Milontin	Treatment of absence seizures

Action

Succinimides diminish nerve transmission in the motor cortex, thereby decreasing the frequency of absence seizures in children and adults. Succinimides also reduce the focal activity that produce spike and wave patterns on electroencephalograms (EEGs) more effectively than does phenytoin. This action increases the seizure threshold and decreases seizure activity by blocking calcium channels and delaying the entrance of calcium into neurons.

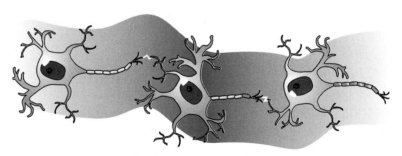

Controlling synaptic activity.

Uses

Phensuximide should be used with caution in patients with acute intermittent porphyria.

Succinimides are used in the treatment of absence seizures. Ethosuximide is the first drug of choice of the three succinimides. Methsuximide has a high risk for toxicity, and phensuximide is less effective than are the other succinimides.

What You NEED TO KNOW

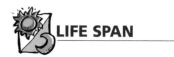

LIFE SPAN

Contraindications/Precautions

Succinimides are contraindicated for patients with hypersensitivity, blood dyscrasias, and severe renal or hepatic disease.

Succinimides are contraindicated for women during pregnancy.

Drug Interactions

Only a few drug interactions are associated with the succinimides. When given concurrently with hydantoins, succinimides may increase hydantoin levels. Isoniazid may significantly increase ethosuximide levels when these drugs are given together. Carbamazepine may decrease the concentration of a succinimide when given concurrently. When ethosuximide and phenobarbital are given together, the drug levels of both may be altered and may lead to increased seizure frequency. Valproic acid may increase or decrease succinimide levels when these drugs are given together.

Adverse Effects

Adverse effects following succinimide administration include GI effects of anorexia, nausea, vomiting, swollen tongue, weight loss, abdominal pain, constipation, and diarrhea. Neurologic adverse effects include flushing, headache, inability to concentrate, drowsiness, dizziness, euphoria, restlessness, irritability, sleep disturbances, depression, night terrors, hyperactivity, aggressiveness, lethargy, confusion, and ataxia. Psychosis and suicidal ideation are rare adverse effects. GU adverse effects include vaginal bleeding, urinary frequency, hematuria, and albuminuria. Hematologic adverse effects involve leukopenia, thrombocytopenia, eosinophilia, agranulocytosis, aplastic anemia, and pancytopenia. Hypersensitivity reactions following succinimides include pruritic skin eruptions, exfoliative dermatitis, systemic lupus erythematosus (SLE), and Stevens-Johnson syndrome. Additional adverse effects from methsuximide therapy include renal and hepatic damage as well as alopecia.

What You DO

TAKE HOME POINTS

Instruct the patient to take succinimides with meals to reduce GI adverse effects.

Impress on the patient the importance of avoiding abrupt discontinuation of the medication.

Nursing Responsibilities

Liquid forms of succinimides should be stored at 59° to 86° F (15° to 30° C) in light-resistant containers. Capsules should be stored in airtight containers. Suspensions should be shaken before administration. Adjustments in the succinimides dose must be made carefully and slowly. Succinimides are administered orally. Ethosuximide may be taken with food when GI distress occurs. When administering succinimides, the nurse should:

• Monitor the patient's serum succinimide drug level for a therapeutic effect. A normal serum level in adults ranges from 40 to 100 micrograms/mL.

• Monitor complete blood counts and signs of infection in patients who are taking succinimides to detect blood dyscrasias early.

• Instruct the patient to report any evidence of infection (e.g., sore throat) for early treatment of infection and detection of blood dyscrasias.

• Watch the patient who is taking succinimides for behavioral changes and report these changes to the health care provider. Succinimides should be withdrawn at the first signs of depression or aggression to prevent further psychosis.

• Instruct the patient to avoid abrupt discontinuation of the medication because abrupt withdrawal may precipitate seizures. A gradual dose-reduction schedule, designed by the health care provider, is required to maintain seizure control.

• Inform the patient that phensuximide may color the urine pink, red, or reddish-brown.

• Instruct the patient to avoid operating potentially hazardous machinery while undergoing succinimide therapy.

• Protect the patient who is taking succinimides when the mental status is altered through the use of safety precautions (e.g., side rails, low bed position, assistance with ambulation).

Do You UNDERSTAND?

DIRECTIONS: **Indicate in the space provided whether the statement is** *true* **or** *false*. **If the answer is false, correct the statement to make it true (using the margin space).**

_____ 1. Mental depression is a common side effect of succinimide anticonvulsants.

_____ 2. When given together, succinimides increase the metabolism of hydantoin anticonvulsants.

_____ 3. Severe adverse effects following succinimides include Stevens-Johnson syndrome, SLE, and renal and hepatic damage.

What IS a Miscellaneous Anticonvulsant?

Miscellaneous Anticonvulsants	Trade Names	Uses
valproic acid [val-PROE-ic]	Depakote	Treatment of absence seizures
carbamazepine [kar-ba-MAZ-e-peen]	Tegretol	Treatment of tonic-clonic or psychomotor seizures
gabapentin [GAB-uh-PEN-tin]	Neurontin	Adjunctive therapy in treatment of partial seizures

Action

A group of miscellaneous drugs, including valproic acid, carbamazepine, and gabapentin, are effective anticonvulsants and have different actions. Valproic acid inhibits the enzyme breakdown of gamma-aminobutyric acid (GABA) to a simpler form, thereby selectively increasing the concentration of GABA in the synapses, which reduces seizure activity. The increase of GABA decreases impulse transmission. Carbamazepine blocks sodium and calcium channels, which prevents the formation of repetitive action potentials in the abnormal focus, thereby reducing polysynaptic responses and blocking posttetanic potentiation. Gabapentin affects the

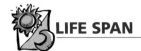

LIFE SPAN

Valproic acid is contraindicated for women during pregnancy and lactation. Valproic acid should be used with extreme caution in children under 2 years of age, particularly when they are undergoing multiple-combination anticonvulsant therapy. Additionally, caution should be used when administering valproic acid to patients who have congenital metabolic disorders, a history of severe seizures with accompanying mental retardation, or organic brain disease. This drug is strongly related to fatal hepatotoxicity, particularly in children under 2 years of age.

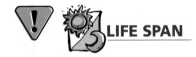

LIFE SPAN

- Gabapentin should be used cautiously in women during pregnancy and lactation and in children under 12 years of age.
- Carbamazepine and gabapentin should be given with caution to older patients.

transport of amino acids across neuronal membranes, which reduces seizure activity.

Uses

Valproic acid is approved for the treatment of simple and complex absence seizures. Effectiveness has also been demonstrated in mixed seizures, such as myoclonic and tonic-clonic seizures. Carbamazepine is one of the drugs of choice used in the control of tonic-clonic or focal seizures and trigeminal neuralgia. Carbamazepine is also effective in managing partial and mixed seizures. Gabapentin is used as adjunctive therapy for focal seizures.

What You NEED TO KNOW

Contraindications/Precautions

Valproic acid is contraindicated for patients with bleeding disorders and hepatic disease. Carbamazepine is contraindicated for patients with increased intraocular pressure, systemic lupus erythematosus (SLE), and hepatic or renal disease. These drugs are contraindicated for patients with hypersensitivity.

Drug Interactions

CNS depressants and alcohol increase the depressant effects when given concurrently with anticonvulsants. When these agents are administered with other anticonvulsants and barbiturates, anticonvulsant and barbiturate levels and the risk for toxicity are increased. Salicylates, chlorpromazine, erythromycin, felbamate, and cimetidine may increase valproic acid levels and toxicity when given with valproic acid. In addition to the anticonvulsant action, valproic acid inhibits the secondary phase of platelet aggregation. Therefore when valproic acid is administered concurrently with aspirin, dipyridamole, or warfarin, the risk for decreased clotting and spontaneous bleeding increases. When valproic acid is given with clonazepam, absence seizures may be exacerbated. Cholestyramine, rifampin, carbamazepine, topiramate, lamotrigine, and charcoal may decrease the absorption of valproic acid when given together.

When taken concurrently with oral contraceptives, carbamazepine increases the metabolism of estrogen, which decreases contraceptive effectiveness. Other anticonvulsant serum concentrations may decrease when these miscellaneous anticonvulsants are taken because of increased metabolism. Carbamazepine decreases the hypoprothrombinemia effects of concurrent oral anticoagulants. Increased carbamazepine levels may result when this agent is taken with verapamil, erythromycin, ketoconazole, or nefazodone.

Gabapentin may cause an increase in phenytoin levels when given concurrently. Antacids reduce the absorption of gabapentin. Lamotrigine levels may be decreased when given with carbamazepine, phenytoin, phenobarbital, and primidone. Tiagabine levels may be decreased when given with carbamazepine, phenytoin, and phenobarbital. Increased CNS depression occurs when topiramate is taken together with alcohol and other CNS depressants. When given concurrently, carbamazepine, phenytoin, and valproic acid may decrease topiramate levels.

Adverse Effects

Common adverse effects of these agents include drowsiness, dizziness, weakness **(asthenia),** and incoordination **(ataxia).** Valproic acid appears to have a low incidence of adverse effects. Other adverse effects that may occur after valproic acid therapy include emotional upset, hallucinations, aggression, and prolonged bleeding. GI adverse effects from valproic acid include hypersalivation, anorexia or increased appetite, nausea, indigestion, vomiting, weight loss or gain, abdominal cramps, diarrhea, and constipation. Valproic acid may also cause skin rash, transient hair loss, curliness or waviness of hair, breakthrough seizures, tremors, amenorrhea, irregular menses, photosensitivity, hyperammonemia, and hepatic failure. Bone marrow depression may occur in the form of anemia, leukopenia, and thrombocytopenia.

When carbamazepine anticonvulsant drug therapy begins slowly and with gradually increasing dose increments, adverse effects are minor and tolerable. Adverse effects of carbamazepine include diplopia, nystagmus, increased intraocular pressure, headache, dry mouth, hives, tremors, urine retention, and constipation. Severe adverse effects include syncope, increased or decreased BP, dysrhythmias, MI, and congestive heart failure (CHF). Rare adverse effects involve hematologic toxicity with aplastic anemia, agranulocytosis, thrombocytopenia, leukopenia, Stevens-Johnson syndrome, hepatotoxicity, latent psychosis, and mental depression. In most patients, the adverse effects of carbamazepine usually disappear within 2 to 3 weeks after initiating therapy. Other adverse effects of gabapentin include blurred vision, slurred speech, headache, impaired concentration, weight gain, nystagmus, nausea, and vomiting.

- Valproic acid should be administered with caution to patients with renal disease or to those who are undergoing other anticonvulsant adjunctive therapy.
- Carbamazepine should be administered with caution to patients with a history of cardiac disease.
- Gabapentin should be given with caution to patients who are taking digoxin, other CNS depressants, or neuromuscular blocking agents, as well as to patients with impaired hepatic or renal function.

TAKE HOME POINTS

- Instruct the patient to avoid alcohol and OTC medications, particularly aspirin, sedatives, or allergy medications, to prevent exacerbating CNS depressant effects.
- Instruct women who are taking oral contraceptives to use an alternate form of birth control for the duration of their treatment with carbamazepine.

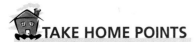

TAKE HOME POINTS

- The patient may take anticonvulsants with food to decrease GI distress.
- Emphasize the importance of avoiding abrupt discontinuation of the medication.

What You DO

Nursing Responsibilities

These anticonvulsants are initially administered in small doses and gradually increased. Administration with meals enhances the absorption and decreases GI distress. Carbamazepine should be protected from heat and stored at 59° to 86° F (15° to 30° C). When administering miscellaneous anticonvulsants, the nurse should:

- Initiate valproic acid therapy gradually to minimize GI adverse effects. The therapeutic range for valproic acid is 50 to 100 mcg/mL.
- Instruct the patient who is taking valproic acid to swallow capsules whole and to avoid chewing medication or taking the drug with carbonated drinks to avoid mouth and throat irritation.
- Monitor the patient for early detection of neurologic toxicity.
- Evaluate platelet counts, bleeding time, serum ammonia, and liver function tests at least every 2 months during the first 6 months of valproic acid therapy for the early detection of blood dyscrasias or hepatic dysfunction.
- Instruct the patient to report any fever, sore mouth or throat, unusual fatigue, spontaneous bleeding, bruising, nosebleeds, bleeding gums, rash, visual disturbances, jaundice, light-colored stools, vomiting, and diarrhea to the health care provider.
- Warn the patient to avoid hazardous activities (e.g., driving) that require alertness until the drug response is known.
- Monitor laboratory test results for the patient taking carbamazepine for early detection of myelosuppression. The following results should be reported to the health care provider: hematocrit below 32%, hemoglobin below 11 g/dL, red blood cell count below 4 million/mm, reticulocyte count below 20,000/mm, white blood cell count below 4000/mm, platelet count below 100,000/mm, and serum iron above 150 mcg/dL.
- Protect the patient when the mental status is altered through the use of safety precautions (e.g., side rails, low bed position, assistance with ambulation).
- Encourage the patient to avoid abrupt discontinuation of these drugs because this action may precipitate seizures, possibly status epilepticus. A gradual dose-reduction schedule designed by the health care provider is required to maintain seizure control.

- Tell the patient to report signs of fluid retention, oliguria, and changes in BP or pulse patterns.
- Instruct the patient who is taking carbamazepine suspension to avoid taking the drug with any other liquid medication to prevent a precipitate forming in the stomach.
- Warn the patient to avoid excessive sunlight or to use sunscreen with sun protection factor (SPF) of 12 or above because photosensitivity reactions may occur.

Do You UNDERSTAND?

DIRECTIONS: Complete the following statements.

1. A _____ laboratory test should be initially monitored at least every 2 months when taking valproic acid.
2. Extra contraceptive precautions should be used to prevent pregnancy when taking _____.
3. Anticonvulsants should be discontinued _____.

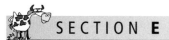

SECTION **E**

ANESTHETICS

This section reviews the pharmacologic agents used to produce anesthesia. Legally, only nurse anesthetists are permitted to administer anesthetic agents; however, other nurses should be aware of these agents and their effects on patients, primarily because these nurses will be providing nursing care in the perioperative period. Anesthetics are classified as local and general. Local anesthetics (**regional anesthesia**) block pain sensation in a limited region of the body but do not reduce consciousness. Local anesthetics are administered topically or by local infiltration into the tissues. A nerve block is a blockage of pain in a specific nerve of the body with local anesthetic agents. Blocking nerve transmission in the spinal cord is called *epidural* or *spinal anesthesia.*

Answers: 1. platelet count; 2. carbamazepine; 3. gradually.

General anesthetics block the body's response to painful stimuli. These blocked responses produce unconsciousness, muscle relaxation, and amnesia. General anesthetics can be administered IV, rectally, or by inhalation. This section includes local and IV anesthetic agents.

What IS a Local Anesthetic?

Local Anesthetics	Trade Names	Type	Uses
procaine HCl [PROE-kane]	Novocaine	Ester	Infiltration anesthesia, spinal anesthesia, epidural, peripheral nerve block
lidocaine [LYE-doe-kane]	Xylocaine	Amide	Nerve block or dental procedures
bupivacaine [byoo-PIV-a-kane]	Marcaine	Amide	Local infiltration and sympathetic block; lumbar epidural; caudal block; peripheral nerve block; dental block

Action

Local anesthetics block pain at the injection site while allowing the continuation of consciousness. Local anesthetics inhibit ionic flux into nerve cells, slow nerve impulse production, and reduce the rate of electrical action potential of a nerve fiber, thereby preventing the conduction of nerve impulses. The order of nerve function loss proceeds in the following manner: pain, temperature, touch, proprioception, and skeletal muscle tone. When vasoconstrictors (e.g., epinephrine) are added to local anesthetics, they decrease systemic absorption, promote local hemostasis, and prolong the duration of action. The rate of absorption of local anesthetics depends on the dose and concentration of the drug, vascular supply, and the presence of vasoconstrictors.

To some extent, local anesthetics are distributed to all body tissues. Local anesthetics are classified into two types: esters and amides. Esters are derivatives of PABA and are metabolized by hydrolysis of the ester linkage by plasma cholinesterase. Hypersensitivities are more common with the ester type. Amides are derivatives of aniline and are metabolized in the liver and excreted in urine.

- Caution should be taken when administering local anesthetics to children, older adults, and pregnant or lactating women.
- Caution should be taken when administering local anesthetics to patients with dysrhythmias, shock, and renal or hepatic dysfunction.

Uses

Local anesthetics are used in infiltration anesthesia and are used in spinal, epidural, caudal, brachial plexus, and peripheral nerve blocks.

What You NEED TO KNOW

Contraindications/Precautions

These local anesthetic agents are contraindicated for patients with hypersensitivity. Procaine is contraindicated for patients with cerebrospinal diseases, hypotension, hypertension, and heart block.

Drug Interactions

When different local anesthetic agents are mixed, the drug interaction produces an increased risk for toxicity. When sedatives are given concurrently, the drug interaction produces intensified CNS effects. Local anesthetics inhibit the action of sulfonamides when given together.

Adverse Effects

Adverse effects of local anesthetics are generally dose-related. Most adverse effects involve CNS or cardiovascular depression. Adverse effects of local anesthetic agents include dizziness, fainting, blurred vision, double vision, tinnitus, euphoria, anxiety, restlessness, chills, nausea, vomiting, hypotension, bradycardia, convulsions, respiratory impairment, and ventricular dysrhythmias. Additionally, sensation of heat, cold or numbness, redness, itching, sneezing, excessive sweating, postspinal headache, and paralysis may occur. Some rare adverse effects include fecal or urinary incontinence, urinary retention, weakness, and loss of perineal sensation and sexual function.

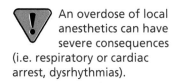 An overdose of local anesthetics can have severe consequences (i.e. respiratory or cardiac arrest, dysrhythmias).

What You DO

Nursing Responsibilities

Acute emergencies from local anesthetics are usually a result of high concentrations in the plasma. Prevention of emergency situations is of major importance. The nursing responsibilities for caring for a patient who has received local anesthetic are to:

- Observe for evidence of an overdose (e.g., hypotension, bradycardia, convulsions, apnea, hypoxia, acidosis). Be prepared to provide respiratory support to patients who have experienced an overdose.
- Monitor the patient closely in the postoperative period.

- Inform patients who are receiving caudal or epidurals that they may experience temporary loss of sensation and motor activity, usually in the lower portion of the body.
- Caution patients who are having dental procedures to avoid eating food or hot liquids until sensation returns.

Do You UNDERSTAND?

DIRECTIONS: Indicate in the space provided whether each statement is *true* or *false*. If the answer is false, correct the statement to make it true (using the margin space).

_____ 1. Local anesthetics are not systemically absorbed into the body.

_____ 2. The nurse should be prepared to provide respiratory support after local anesthetic use.

What IS an IV Nonbarbiturate Anesthetic Agent?

Nonbarbiturate Anesthetics	Trade Names	Uses
midazolam [MID-ah-ZOE-lam]	Versed	Anesthesia induction; conscious sedation
ketamine [KET-uh-MEEN]	Ketalar	Used in young children for minor procedures that are surgical and diagnostic but do not require skeletal muscle relaxation; ideal for burn cases because it causes immobility
propofol [PRO-puh-fole]	Diprivan	Induction and maintenance of anesthesia; conscious sedation
fentanyl [FEN-tuh-nill]	Sublimaze	Short-acting neuroleptic analgesia and tranquilizer during operative and perioperative period of surgical or diagnostic procedures
droperidol [droe-PER-I-dahl]	Inapsine	Reduces nausea and vomiting; produces tranquilizing effect; adjunct drug during induction and maintenance of anesthesia

Answers: 1. false; local anesthetics are distributed to all body tissues to some extent; 2. true.

Action

Midazolam is a short-acting benzodiazepine that interferes with the reuptake of GABA and promotes its accumulation at nerve cell synapses, thereby intensifying GABA activity. Ketamine is a rapid-acting general anesthetic that selectively interrupts association pathways of the brain, producing somatesthetic sensory blockade. This action blocks consciousness of body sensations and is called *dissociative anesthesia.* Propofol acts as a sedative-hypnotic. Fentanyl is a short-acting neuroleptic analgesic and tranquilizer that blocks receptors for dopamine, which causes analgesia. Droperidol is a short-acting neuroleptic analgesic and tranquilizer that antagonizes emetic effects of drugs that act on the chemoreceptor trigger zone (CTZ). This agent acts primarily at the subcortical level to produce sedative effects, reduce anxiety, and decrease motor activity.

Uses

IV nonbarbiturate anesthetics are CNS depressants that serve as supplements to anesthesia. These agents are used throughout the perioperative period for their desired effects. IV nonbarbiturate anesthetics are also used for the induction and maintenance of anesthesia, conscious sedation, reduction of nausea and vomiting, short-acting neuroleptic analgesia, and production of a tranquilizing effect.

What You NEED TO KNOW

Contraindications/Precautions

Nonbarbiturate anesthetics are contraindicated for patients with hypersensitivity. Midazolam is contraindicated for acute narrow-angle glaucoma, acute alcohol intoxication, coma, and shock. Ketamine is contraindicated for patients with significant hypertension and a history of psychiatric illness. Propofol is contraindicated for patients with increased intracranial pressure and impaired cerebral circulation. Fentanyl is contraindicated for patients with severe renal or hepatic dysfunction, increased intracranial pressure, and severe respiratory depression.

Drug Interactions

Drug interactions that may occur with droperidol include peripheral vasodilation and hypotension when given concurrently with other anesthetics. CNS depressants have an additive or intensifying effect when

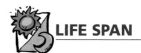

LIFE SPAN

Midazolam, propofol, and fentanyl are contraindicated for women during pregnancy and lactation.

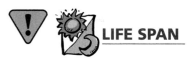

LIFE SPAN

Midazolam should be used with caution in older adults and in patients with heart failure, COPD, and renal failure. Fentanyl is contraindicated for children, patients with myasthenia gravis, or those who have received an MAOI within 14 days. Droperidol should be used with caution in older adults, pregnant and lactating women, children, and patients with renal or hepatic dysfunction.

! Ketamine should be used with caution in chronic alcoholics and those with acute alcohol intoxication. Propofol should be used with caution in patients with severe cardiac or respiratory dysfunction and in those with a history of seizures. Fentanyl should be used with caution in older adults, debilitated patients, and individuals with COPD, head injuries, and bradydysrhythmias.

given together with IV nonbarbiturate anesthetics. When ketamine is given together with muscle relaxants, prolonged respiratory depression may develop. Administration of thyroid hormones and ketamine together may lead to hypertension and tachycardia. When halothane and ketamine are given concurrently, decreased cardiac output, BP, and heart rate may occur. The hypnotic effect of thiopental may be antagonized when given with ketamine.

Adverse Effects

Nonbarbiturates may cause respiratory depression. Midazolam may cause cardiac arrest. The adverse effects of ketamine include emergence delirium, hallucinations, confusion, excitement, irrational behavior, diplopia, nystagmus, elevated intraocular pressure, hypotension, hypertension, tachycardia, bradycardia, dysrhythmia, anorexia, nausea, vomiting, and laryngospasm. Adverse effects of propofol include cough, hiccups, headache, dizziness, hypotension, twitching, vomiting, abdominal cramping, jerking, decreased intraocular pressure, and ventricular asystole. Fentanyl may cause hypotension. Adverse effects of droperidol include drowsiness, tachycardia, hypotension, hypertension, muscular rigidity, chills, dizziness, shivering, laryngospasm, bronchospasm, hallucinations, restlessness, anxiety, hyperactivity, and extrapyramidal symptoms (e.g., dystonia, akathisia, oculogyric crisis).

What You DO

Nursing Responsibilities

Administering slowly over 2 or more minutes and allowing 2 or more minutes between injections can reduce the adverse effects of midazolam. Fentanyl and droperidol are available premixed as Innovar. When administering IV nonbarbiturate anesthetics, the nurse should:

- Monitor the cardiac and respiratory status of a patient who is receiving IV nonbarbiturate anesthetics.
- Evaluate the patient for drug-induced excitation (e.g., twitching, tremors, spasmodic muscular contractions between antagonistic muscle groups).
- Advise the patient to avoid driving, operating hazardous machinery, or engaging in hazardous activity for 24 hours after anesthesia with ketamine.

Do You UNDERSTAND?

DIRECTIONS: Fill in the blanks with the appropriate responses.

1. The dissociative anesthetic agent is _____.
2. _____ is an IV nonbarbiturate anesthetic that is contraindicated when a patient has received an MAOI 1 week earlier.

References

Abrams AC, Lammon CB, Pennington SS: *Clinical drug therapy: rationales for nursing practice,* ed 8, Philadelphia, 2007, Lippincott.

Gutierrez K, Queener SF: *Pharmacology for nursing practice,* St Louis, 2003, Mosby.

Hardman JG, Limbird LE: *Goodman & Gilman's the pharmacological basis of therapeutics,* ed 10, New York, 2001, McGraw-Hill.

Hodgson B, Kizior R: *Saunders nursing drug handbook 2005,* St. Louis, 2005, Elsevier.

Hodgson B, Kizior R: *Mosby's 2006 drug consult for nurses,* 2006, St Louis, 2005, Elsevier.

Ignatavicius DD, Workman ML: *Medical-surgical nursing: critical thinking for collaborative care,* ed 5, St Louis, 2006, Elsevier.

Karch AM: *Focus on nursing pharmacology,* ed 3, Philadelphia, 2006, Lippincott.

Kee JL, Hayes ER, McCuistion LE: *Pharmacology: a nursing process approach,* ed 5, Philadelphia, 2006, Elsevier.

Lehne RA: *Pharmacology for nursing care,* ed 5, Philadelphia, 2004, WB Saunders.

McKenry, LM, Salerno, E: *Mosby's pharmacology in nursing,* ed 21, St Louis, 2003, Mosby.

Smeltzer SC, Bare BG: *Brunner and Suddarth's textbook of medical-surgical nursing,* ed 10, Philadelphia, 2004, Lippincott.

Spratto G, Woods A: *PDR nurse's drug handbook,* Montvale, NJ, 2001, Delmar Publishers and Medical Economics.

Wilson BA, Shannon MT, Stang CL: *Nurses drug guide,* Upper Saddle River, New Jersey, 2006, Pearson.

Answers: 1. ketamine; 2. fentanyl.

NCLEX® Review

Section A

1. A patient who is diagnosed with emphysema is receiving albuterol treatments via a nebulizer. The most important responsibility is for the nurse to assess the _____ and _____ during and after each treatment.
   1 Pupils, breath sounds
   2 Capillary refill, heart sounds
   3 Pulse rate, blood pressure
   4 Bowel sounds, skin color

2. A patient is receiving doxazosin mesylate (Cardura). Which adverse effects should the nurse expect?
   1 Mydriasis and decreased gastric motility
   2 Miosis and increased gastric motility
   3 Hypertension
   4 Hemorrhage

3. A patient is taking pseudoephedrine (Sudafed) for sinus congestion. Which drug(s) might interact to increase cardiovascular effects and should be avoided?
   1 Alcohol
   2 Metoclopramide
   3 Muscle relaxants
   4 Tricyclic antidepressant

4. A patient is taking tamsulosin (Flomax) for BPH. Which is the related nursing intervention for this patient?
   1 Monitor for weight loss
   2 Monitor for bronchoconstriction
   3 Warn the patient of possible constipation
   4 Instruct the patient to rise slowly to a standing position

5. A patient is receiving albuterol (Proventil) for bronchospasm attacks. Which is the related nursing responsibility?
   1 Administer quickly by metered-dose inhaler
   2 Administer albuterol intramuscularly in emergencies
   3 Use IV direct push method of controlling bronchospasm
   4 Use micro-drip IV tubing for tight control of administration

Section B

6. A patient is taking bethanechol (Urecholine) for urinary retention. Which drug is the antidote for an overdose of a direct-acting cholinergic agonist?
   1 Procainamide
   2 Lidocaine
   3 Artane
   4 Atropine

7. A patient who takes pyridostigmine for myasthenia gravis is given an edrophonium (Tensilon) test, and the patient's skeletal muscle weakness improves. The nurse then knows that the dose of pyridostigmine is:
   1 Not enough.
   2 Too much.
   3 Therapeutic.
   4 Overdose level.

8. Which drug(s) may precipitate a hypertensive crisis when taken with a dopaminergic?
   1 Methyldopa
   2 Tricyclic antidepressants
   3 Alcohol
   4 MAOIs

9. Opioids may cause possible life-threatening reactions when taken with which of the following drugs?
   1 Selegiline
   2 Bromocriptine
   3 Amantadine
   4 Ropinirole

10. Which of the following agents are used as maintenance therapy for myasthenia gravis?
   1 Ambenonium and pyridostigmine
   2 Edrophonium and neostigmine
   3 Donepezil and rivastigmine
   4 Neostigmine and pyridostigmine

Section C

11. A 10-year-old child is taking methylphenidate (Ritalin). For which use is this drug typically prescribed in children?
   1 To overcome obesity
   2 As a sleeping aid at bedtime
   3 Found to be safe for long-term use
   4 Primarily for ADHD therapy

12. A patient is taking phentermine (Zantrly). Which time of day should the nurse instruct the patient to take this drug?
   1 Before breakfast
   2 Midmorning
   3 With the evening meal
   4 At bedtime

13. Which substance does not contain caffeine?
   1 Cola
   2 Ritalin
   3 Excedrin
   4 Chocolate

14. A patient is taking an amphetamine (Adderall). Which adverse effect is common with this drug?
   1 Hypotension
   2 Bradycardia
   3 Somnolence
   4 Nervousness

15. A patient is taking diethylpropion (Tenuate). Which nursing responsibility is correct?
   1 Instruct the patient to take diethylpropion after meals
   2 Teach the patient about safety from potential dizziness
   3 Inform the patient that long-term therapy is most effective
   4 Warn the patient that the insulin dose may need to be increased

Section D

16. A patient who is taking an anticonvulsant has slurred speech, enlargement of facial features, nystagmus, or gingival hyperplasia. Which drug does the nurse expect to lead to these adverse effects?
   1 Phenytoin
   2 Phenobarbital
   3 Lorazepam
   4 Carbamazepine

17. When taking barbiturates, elderly patients usually develop which of the following adverse effects?
   1 Lethargy, drowsiness, and faintness
   2 Excitement, confusion, or depression
   3 Hypertension and diuresis
   4 Bleeding or gingival hyperplasia

18. What can be assumed about patients who are taking benzodiazepines?
   1 Patients should take benzodiazepines with antacids.
   2 Patients develop an increased tolerance for alcohol.
   3 Patients may develop toxicity of short-term memory.
   4 Patients are generally affected by CNS-stimulating properties of benzodiazepines.

19. SLE and Stevens-Johnson syndrome may develop as adverse effects of which drug?
   1 Ethosuximide
   2 Lorazepam
   3 Phenytoin
   4 Valproic acid

20. Which is the drug of choice in treating status epilepticus?
    1 Phenytoin
    2 Diazepam
    3 Phenobarbital
    4 Valproic acid

Section E

21. In which condition would procaine be contraindicated?
    1 Heart block
    2 Spinal block
    3 Elderly adult
    4 Peripheral nerve block

22. Which anesthetic agent would be *least* likely to cause laryngospasm?
    1 Regional
    2 Inhalation
    3 IV barbiturate
    4 IV nonbarbiturate

23. Which condition might indicate a local anesthetic overdose?
    1 Hypertension
    2 Bradycardia
    3 Tachycardia
    4 Alkalosis

24. Which anesthetic agent would require cautious use or be contraindicated in patients with acute alcohol intoxication?
    1 Fentanyl
    2 Enflurane
    3 Midazolam
    4 Thiopental sodium

25. Which agent is known as the dissociative anesthetic?
    1 Propofol
    2 Droperidol
    3 Fentanyl
    4 Ketamine

NCLEX® Review Answers

Section A

1. **3** Albuterol, an adrenergic that stimulates β-receptors (primarily β_2-receptors), has adverse effects of tachycardia and hypertension. α-Agonists, not β-agonists, cause pupil dilation. Capillary refill, heart sounds, bowel sounds, and skin color are unrelated to β_2-adrenergic agonists.

2. **2** α-Adrenergic antagonists, such as doxazosin, cause pupil constriction (miosis) and increased GI motility. Mydriasis and decrease gastric motility are opposite effects. α-Adrenergic antagonists cause vasodilation and decreased blood pressure. Hemorrhage is unrelated to α-adrenergic antagonists.

3. **4** Tricyclic antidepressants are prone to drug interactions with β-adrenergic antagonists, such as pseudoephedrine. Alcohol, metoclopramide, and muscle relaxants are not known to cause drug interactions with pseudoephedrine.

4. **4** The patient should be taught to rise to a standing position slowly to avoid orthostatic hypotension, which is a common adverse effect of tamsulosin. Weight loss, constipation, and bronchoconstriction are not commonly associated with tamsulosin.

5. **1** Albuterol is administered orally or by inhalation, not IV or intramuscularly.

Section B

6. **4** A direct-acting cholinergic agonist (which stimulates muscarinic glandular secretions; stimulates receptors in the heart, CNS, and smooth muscles of organs; and excites nicotinic responses) requires a drug that produces the opposite for an antidote. Atropine is the antidote for cholinergic overdose because it blocks muscarinic responses with an antisecretory action and blocks vagal impulses to the heart. Procainamide and lidocaine are incorrect because these drugs are antiarrhythmics. Artane is used as a treatment for Parkinson's disease and extrapyramidal disorders. Procainamide, lidocaine, and Artane do not block muscarinic responses.

7. 1 When the edrophonium test is performed and the patient's skeletal muscle weakness improves, the patient is experiencing a myasthenic crisis from underdosing of a cholinesterase inhibitor. When the patient's condition worsens, the patient is experiencing a cholinergic crisis from overdosing or receiving excessive pyridostigmine.

8. 4 MAOIs may precipitate a hypertensive crisis when taken with a dopaminergic. When a dopaminergic is given with methyldopa, the risk for toxic effects in the CNS is increased. When combined with tricyclic antidepressants, postural hypotension may occur. Alcohol exacerbates CNS depression, not a hypertensive crisis, when given with a dopaminergic.

9. 1 Opioids may cause life-threatening reactions when taken with selegiline. Bromocriptine, amantadine, and ropinirole have no drug interaction with opioids.

10. 1 Ambenonium and pyridostigmine are used as maintenance therapy for myasthenia gravis. Edrophonium and neostigmine are used for diagnosing myasthenia gravis and for differentiating between myasthenic and cholinergic crisis. Donepezil and rivastigmine are used to improve memory in patients with Alzheimer's disease.

Section C

11. 4 Ritalin is primarily used in children for ADHD therapy. Anorexiants are used to treat obesity. Ritalin should be given early in the day, no later than 6 hours before bedtime, not at bedtime. The long-term effects of Ritalin are unknown.

12. 2 Anorexiants should be administered midmorning or midafternoon, depending on the patient's eating habits. Anorexiants should be given on an empty stomach, approximately 30 to 60 minutes before meals and no later than 6 hours before bedtime.

13. 2 Ritalin contains no caffeine. Caffeine is found in many beverages, such as coffee, tea, cola, and chocolate. Caffeine is also an ingredient in many OTC headache medications (e.g., Anacin, Excedrin).

14. 4 Nervousness, hypertension, insomnia, and tachycardia are common adverse effects of amphetamine. Hypotension, somnolence, and bradycardia are not associated with this drug.

15. 2 The nurse should teach the patient about safety precautions because of the potential for dizziness from anorexiants, such as diethylpropion. Anorexiants should be taken 30 to 60 minutes before meals. The anorexiant effect is temporary and seldom lasts more than a few weeks. Therefore short-term use is more effective. The insulin dose may need to be decreased.

Section D

16. 1 Hydantoins are associated with the peculiar adverse effects of nystagmus and gingival hyperplasia. Phenobarbital and lorazepam do not cause these adverse effects. Carbamazepine may cause nystagmus but not slurred speech, enlargement of facial features, or gingival hyperplasia.

17. 2 Elderly patients commonly develop the adverse effects of depression, confusion, and the paradoxic effect of excitement when taking barbiturates. Barbiturates lead to hypotension (but not hypertension) and excitement (but not lethargy). Although barbiturates can cause thrombocytopenia, gingival hyperplasia is not an adverse effect.

18. 3 Benzodiazepines are associated with toxicity, ranging from loss of short-term memory, confusion, and vertigo to bradycardia, ataxia, severe weakness, shortness of breath, and depression. Antacids delay absorption of benzodiazepines. A reduced, not increased, tolerance for alcohol occurs when taking benzodiazepines. Benzodiazepines lead to CNS-depressing effects.

19. 1 Ethosuximide is associated with causing the adverse effect of SLE. Lorazepam, phenytoin, and valproic acid are not associated with this effect.

20. 2 Diazepam is the drug of choice in treating status epilepticus. Phenytoin and valproic acid are not used for the treatment of status epilepticus. Phenobarbital may be used to control status epilepticus, but it is not the drug of choice.

Section E

21. **1** Procaine is contraindicated for the patient who has heart block. Common uses of procaine include infiltration anesthesia in spinal and peripheral nerve block. Procaine may be given to older adults when caution is taken.

22. **1** Regional anesthetic agents are least likely to cause laryngospasm. Inhalation, IV barbiturate, and IV nonbarbiturate anesthetics are all likely to cause laryngospasm as an adverse effect.

23. **2** Bradycardia is an indication of local anesthetic overdose, not tachycardia. Other indications of local anesthetic overdose include hypotension (not hypertension) and acidosis (not alkalosis).

24. **3** Midazolam is contraindicated in patients with acute alcohol intoxication. Fentanyl, enflurane, and thiopental sodium do not require cautious use, nor are they contraindicated in patients with acute alcohol intoxication.

25. **4** Ketamine is known as the dissociative anesthetic by blocking consciousness of body sensation. Propofol, droperidol, and fentanyl are not known as dissociative anesthetics.

Notes

Drugs Used to Treat Neuropsychiatric Disorders

What You WILL LEARN

After reading this chapter, you will know how to do the following:

- ✔ Contrast the action of a benzodiazepine and nonbenzodiazepine anxiolytic agent.
- ✔ Explain drug interactions of sedative-hypnotics.
- ✔ Explain the adverse effects of various antidepressants.
- ✔ Contrast the action of psychotherapeutic agents.
- ✔ Discuss the nursing responsibilities for lithium.

Antianxiety (**anxiolytic**) medications are nonspecific CNS depressants that alleviate symptoms of distress but do not affect underlying factors that cause the anxiety. Antianxiety medications are dose-dependent, with increasing dose resulting in sedation and hypnosis. The actions of the antianxiety medications are not well known. Antianxiety agents may act to exacerbate the effects of the inhibitory neurotransmitter GABA, reduce serotonin turnover in cortical tissues, and depress the CNS at the limbic and subcortical levels of the brain. The medications discussed in this section are benzodiazepines, nonbenzodiazepines, and sedative-hypnotics.

Thoughts, feelings, and actions are transmitted in the CNS as electro-chemical impulses. When an impulse reaches the end of one neuron **(presynaptic neuron),** chemicals **(neurotransmitters)** are released that cross the synaptic cleft and bind to specific receptor sites on the next neuron **(postsynaptic neuron).** This binding action triggers electrical changes that either inhibit or continue the conduction of the impulse. After the neurotransmitter's function has been completed, the chemicals are either inactivated by enzymes or stored for future use **(reuptake).** The reuptake process is important in understanding the actions of certain psychotropic drugs. The availability or concentration of neurotransmit-ters at the postsynaptic receptors is significant. Any alteration or decrease is associated with some form of neuropathologic condition.

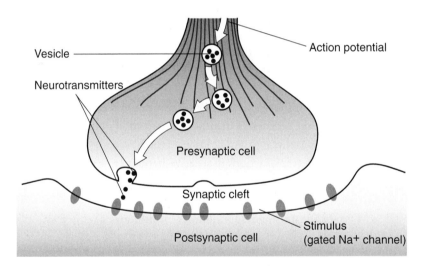

The major categories of neurotransmitters are cholinergics, mono-amines, and neuropeptides. Each type of neurotransmitter is associated with the conduction of impulses in different areas of the CNS. For exam-ple, serotonin is a monoamine transmitter that innervates receptors in the pons, medulla, thalamus, and limbic system. A decrease in serotonin level is associated with clinical depression. Another important example is the amino acid inhibitory transmitter, which is a type of GABA. GABA innervates receptors in the hypothalamus, cortex, cerebellum, basal ganglia, and hippocampus. A decrease in GABA availability is associated with anxiety disorders and schizophrenia. The psychotherapeutic medications discussed in this chapter are antidepressants, antipsychotics, and mood stabilizers.

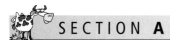

SECTION A

ANXIOLYTICS/SEDATIVE-HYPNOTICS

What IS a Benzodiazepine?

Benzodiazepine	Trade Names	Uses
diazepam [dye-AZ-eh-pam]	Valium	Treatment of anxiety disorders and seizures
alprazolam [al-PRAY-zoe-lam]	Xanax	Treatment of anxiety and panic disorders
temazepam [tem-AZ-eh-pam]	Restoril	Short-term treatment of insomnia
lorazepam [low-RAZ-pam]	Ativan	Treatment of anxiety disorders, status epilepticus, preoperative sedation, amnesia

Action

Benzodiazepines (BZDs) are composed of a large group of chemically similar drugs that are believed to act on neural BZD receptors in the CNS. Stimulation of these receptors leads to stronger impulse inhibition at postsynaptic neurons by the neurotransmitter GABA. As a result, depression of the CNS is observed at the limbic and subcortical levels of the brain. In initial metabolism, many of the BZDs are converted into metabolites that are active CNS depressants. Chronic administration of BZDs that have long-lasting, active metabolites can cause an accumulation of both the medication and the metabolite, resulting in oversedation and CNS depression.

The BZDs work quickly to reduce anxiety symptoms, with the most improvement occurring within the first week of treatment. The efficacy of BZD therapy decreases after 3 to 4 months of continuous use.

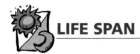

LIFE SPAN

Short-acting BZDs (i.e., those with a short-acting plasma half-life), such as temazepam and lorazepam, are preferred for older adults or patients who are debilitated, because these agents are less likely to accumulate in the body.

Because of altered metabolism that may allow BZDs or their metabolites to accumulate in the plasma and lead to excessive sedation and ataxia, caution must be used when BZDs are administered to older or debilitated patients.

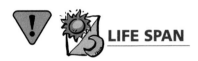

LIFE SPAN

BZDs are believed to cause fetal anomalies when taken during the early stages of pregnancy. BZDs may cause fetal dependence with resulting withdrawal symptoms in the neonate when taken at the end of the third trimester of pregnancy. BZDs taken at the time of labor will cause CNS depression in the neonate. Therefore BZDs are contraindicated for women during pregnancy and lactation, unless no other alternatives are available.

Uses

BZDs are used for treatment of mild-to-severe anxiety (including panic disorder), seizure control in acute alcohol withdrawal, sleep induction, muscle relaxation, and as preoperative medication. The BZDs are ineffective in treating severe psychotic disorders or severe clinical depression, although they may be used in conjunction with other medications when depression is accompanied by severe anxiety. Medications, such as alprazolam and diazepam, are approved for treatment of anxiety and panic disorder. Other BZDs, such as estazolam, flurazepam, quazepam, and triazolam, are used primarily for their hypnotic effect and are approved for the treatment of insomnia.

What You NEED TO KNOW

Contraindications/Precautions

BZDs are contraindicated for patients with renal or hepatic dysfunction, unless no other options are available. Certain BZDs (e.g., alprazolam, lorazepam, midazolam) may aggravate acute angle-closure glaucoma and are contraindicated for these patients.

Drug Interactions

Administering cimetidine with BZDs, other than oxazepam or lorazepam, results in increased serum levels of the BZD. This action results in prolonged sedation, drug hangover, and an increased likelihood of adverse effects. Concurrent use of BZDs and digoxin increases serum digoxin levels, decreases digoxin elimination, and increases the risk for digoxin toxicity.

The use of BZDs in combination with other CNS depressants (e.g., barbiturates, opioids, alcohol, antihistamines) results in additive effects. Additive effects include deepened and prolonged sedative effect, motor impairment, enhanced CNS and respiratory depression, and death.

Adverse Effects

Adverse effects from BZDs include headache, dry mouth, blurred vision, dizziness, hypotension, GI disturbances (e.g., nausea, constipation), jaundice, incontinence, urinary retention, rash, and leukopenia. Additional infrequent adverse effects include anterograde amnesia and paradoxical effects. Anterograde amnesia is an inability to remember events that occur after BZD administration. Paradoxical effects are opposite of that expected; they are rare but can be serious. The paradoxical effects most likely to be observed include increased excitation, euphoria, palpitations, insomnia, and hallucinations.

What You DO

Nursing Responsibilities

Chronic use of BZDs can produce physiologic dependence and cross-tolerance to other members of the benzodiazepine group. BZD use should be closely monitored and time-limited. Therefore BZDs should be used at the lowest effective dose for the shortest time possible. BZDs are administered either orally or parenterally, with the oral route preferred. Absorption rates for IM administration are slower and vary according to the injection site used. For example, when diazepam is given IM, the preferred injection site is the deltoid because the rate of absorption from that area is more constant when compared with other areas. The nurse's primary responsibility in administering BZDs is patient safety. To maintain patient safety:

- Review the patient's medical, medication, and substance abuse history. Excessive CNS depression may occur when the patient has history of hepatic or renal impairment and a likelihood of medication or active metabolite accumulation in the body.
- Assess the patient for suicidal behaviors or suicidal ideation because BZDs (frequently in combination with other CNS depressants) have been used in attempted suicides.
- Instruct the patient to urinate prior to drug administration to prevent sleep disruption.
- Counsel patients who have taken BZDs for a long time to avoid abrupt discontinuation of the therapy. The abrupt discontinuation, particularly of the short-acting BZDs, may cause rebound CNS excitation (including seizures) or withdrawal symptoms.
- Monitor renal and hepatic function periodically to assess adequate drug metabolism and excretion.

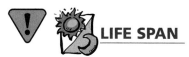

LIFE SPAN

- Although overdose of BZDs is rarely fatal, combined use of BZDs and other CNS depressants is dangerous.
- The outcome of these common effects is an increased risk for falls and subsequent injuries.
- Sedation and ataxia are the most common adverse effects of BZDs, with older adults being the most susceptible.

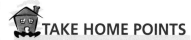

TAKE HOME POINTS

Assess the patient for history of substance abuse and current use of CNS depressants (e.g., opioids, alcohol, or OTC sleep aids). BZDs should be given in the smallest dose possible for the shortest period possible. Severe respiratory depression may occur when drugs are combined.

Do You UNDERSTAND?

DIRECTIONS: **Indicate in the space provided whether each statement is** *true* **or** *false.* **If the answer is false, correct the statement to make it true (using the margin space).**

_____ 1. Because of their sedative, antispasmodic, and antiseizure effects, BZDs are appropriate medications for the treatment of acute alcohol withdrawal symptoms.

_____ 2. Chronic use of BZDs can produce physiologic dependence and cross-tolerance to other classifications of CNS depressants.

_____ 3. Caution must be used in administering BZDs to a patient who is concurrently taking digoxin because the interaction of the drugs can prolong the half-life of the BZD, allowing oversedation and CNS depression.

_____ 4. Concurrent administration of cimetidine with a BZD is contraindicated.

What IS a Nonbenzodiazepine?

Nonbenzodiazepine	Trade Names	Uses
buspirone [byoo-SPEAR-rone]	BuSpar	Short-term treatment of anxiety disorders

Action

Nonbenzodiazepine agents produce CNS depression and a reduction in anxiety symptoms. Buspirone is a member of the azapirone classification of drugs. The exact action of buspirone is unknown, but it is believed to inhibit neuronal firing and to reduce serotonin turnover in certain CNS structures. Buspirone appears to stimulate the serotonin receptors of the CNS.

Answers: 1. true; **2.** false; chronic use of BZDs can produce physiologic dependence and cross-tolerance to other members of the BZD group; **3.** false; concurrent BZD and digoxin leads to increased digoxin levels and predisposes the patient to digitalis toxicity; **4.** true, because it raises BZD levels.

Uses

Buspirone is considered to be as efficient as the BZD group in treating chronic or generalized anxiety. This medication has a gradual onset of approximately 1 to 4 weeks. Therefore buspirone is inappropriate for acute anxiety or panic attacks.

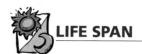

LIFE SPAN

Nonbenzodiazepine anxiolytic agents are contraindicated for lactating and pregnant women. Buspirone is contraindicated for children under 18 years of age.

What You NEED TO KNOW

Contraindications/Precautions

Nonbenzodiazepine anxiolytic agents are contraindicated for patients with hypersensitivity.

Drug Interactions

Although buspirone does not usually cause sedation, administration of this medication with other CNS depressants can increase the effects of the depressant and cause oversedation. Buspirone should not be given to anyone who has received a monoamine oxidase inhibitor (MAOI) within the preceding 14 days. Concurrent use of these medications can cause a dangerous and possibly lethal elevation in BP.

Oversedation, CNS depression, and respiratory depression occur when hydroxyzine or meprobamate is administered in conjunction with other CNS depressants, such as alcohol, opioids, or barbiturates.

TAKE HOME POINTS

Buspirone should not be administered when the patient has taken an MAOI within the previous 14 days to avoid a lethal elevation of BP.

Adverse Effects

Adverse effects that may occur with nonbenzodiazepines include dizziness, drowsiness, headache, nervousness, insomnia, nausea, dry mouth, and blurred vision. Buspirone may cause tremors, decreased concentration, mood changes, tachycardia, and palpitations.

What You DO

Nursing Responsibilities

Nonbenzodiazepines are administered orally. The onset of action from buspirone is gradual, and optimal results may not appear for 3 to 4 weeks.

The nursing responsibilities with regard to patients who are taking nonbenzodiazepines include the following:

- Monitor the patient who is taking nonbenzodiazepines for CNS and respiratory depression, particularly when the patient has a history of taking barbiturates, opioids, or BZDs.
- Assess the patient a history of suicidal behaviors or ideation. Any patient who has a history of these behaviors must be monitored closely because the medication has a history of being used in attempted suicides.
- Instruct the patient to take buspirone with food for increased drug effectiveness.
- Warn the patient to avoid abrupt discontinuation of the BZD when buspirone is to be given to a patient who is already taking a benzodiazepine.
- Teach the patient to taper buspirone when on other combination BZD therapy to prevent withdrawal symptoms and possible seizure activity.

Do You UNDERSTAND?

DIRECTIONS: **Match Column A with Column B.**

Column A	Column B
_____ 1. Does not increase the effects of alcohol and is not associated with withdrawal	a. 14 days
_____ 2. Is comparable to benzodiazepine anxiolytics but does not produce sedation or impair motor function.	b. Buspirone
_____ 3. After receiving an MAOI, wait this time period before giving buspirone.	c. 7 days

What IS a Sedative-Hypnotic Agent?

Sedative-Hypnotics	Trade Names	Uses
butabarbital [byoo-ta-BAR-bi-tal]	Butisol	Treatment of insomnia and anxiety
secobarbital [see-koe-BAR-bi-tal]	Seconal	Treatment of insomnia and acute agitation
zolpidem [ZOL-pi-dem]	Ambien	Treatment of insomnia

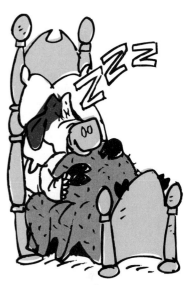

Sweet dreams!

Action

The groups of medications that comprise the sedative-hypnotic classification include barbiturates, selected BZDs, and other miscellaneous CNS depressants. Sedative-hypnotic agents are nonspecific CNS depressants that act in a dose-dependent fashion. These agents produce drowsiness, a calming effect, activity reduction, and sleep induction. These drugs also alleviate symptoms of insomnia but do not affect underlying causative factors.

The precise action of barbiturates (butabarbital and secobarbital) has not been established, but they appear to decrease the excitability of the presynaptic and postsynaptic neurons in the cerebral cortex and the reticular formation of the CNS. Zolpidem is a general depressant that acts on the GABA receptor sites of the CNS. Dissimilar to barbiturates, zolpidem preserves all stages of sleep, including REM and deep sleep. This action is the result of its preference for the omega receptors in the GABA receptor complex.

Uses

Sedative-hypnotic agents should be used as aids to minimize distress that interrupts rest and sleep. Short-acting sedative-hypnotics help the patient to achieve sleep while intermediate-acting agents help to sustain sleep. These medications cannot take the place of natural sleep cycles, and long-term use can adversely affect or diminish necessary sleep and dreaming. Relatively low doses of barbiturates will depress the sensory cortex, depress motor activity, and produce sedation. Most barbiturates suppress REM sleep and decrease stages III and IV of normal sleep. After discontinuing barbiturates, it is not unusual for a patient to experience sleep disturbances from REM rebound.

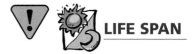

LIFE SPAN

Barbiturates have been associated with fetal abnormalities and are contraindicated for pregnant and lactating women. Zolpidem should be used with caution in children under 18 years of age.

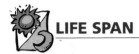 **LIFE SPAN**

Butabarbital and secobarbital are contraindicated for patients with porphyria, a history of addiction, and uncontrolled pain.

 Zolpidem should be used with caution in patients with renal or hepatic dysfunction.

Sedative-hypnotics should be used with caution in patients with renal or hepatic impairment, as well as patients with depression, suicidal tendencies, and a history of drug dependence.

What You NEED TO KNOW

Contraindications/Precautions

Sedative-hypnotics are contraindicated for patients with severe respiratory disorders.

Drug Interactions

The concurrent use of barbiturates may increase the metabolism and decrease drug effectiveness of corticosteroids, digoxin, estrogen, oral contraceptives, theophylline, verapamil, beta blockers, quinidine, tricyclic antidepressants, griseofulvin, and doxycycline. Administration of zolpidem with other CNS depressants can cause oversedation and respiratory depression.

Adverse Effects

Short-term agents usually do not have lingering side effects in the morning, whereas intermediate-acting agents typically have residual drowsiness or hangover effects. When taken for a prolonged period, sedative-hypnotic agents may produce psychologic and physiologic dependence and drug tolerance. The most common adverse effects of zolpidem include headache, dizziness, drowsiness, diarrhea, vomiting, amnesia, ataxia, myalgia, and bradycardia.

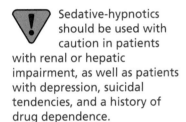 **LIFE SPAN**

Older patients are more likely than are younger patients to experience oversedation and CNS depression because of aging changes, such as slowed metabolic rate and decreased renal function. Therefore when a barbituate is being administered to an older patient, the initial dose should be reduced.

What You DO

Nursing Responsibilities

Barbiturates can be administered orally, rectally, IM, or IV. Zolpidem is administered orally. Short-term treatment (7 to 14 days) of insomnia is appropriate; long-term use is not recommended. When zolpidem has been used long-term, discontinuation of the therapy must be gradual over the period of at least 2 weeks. Rapid termination of can result in severe seizure activity and withdrawal symptoms. Because of the respiratory depression from zolpidem, closely monitor any patient with a history of respiratory insufficiency. This medication should be administered in the lowest possible effective dose. The presence of food significantly reduces the absorption of zolpidem; therefore administer zolpidem at bedtime. When administering sedative-hypnotics, the nurse should:

- Instruct patient to take zolpidem immediately before bedtime.
- Monitor the patient who is taking sedative hypnotics to prevent medication hoarding and self-administration of larger than prescribed doses.
- Instruct the patient that abrupt discontinuation of sedative-hypnotics may lead to withdrawal symptoms.
- Provide safety to prevent falls.

TAKE HOME POINTS

- Patients who are taking sedative-hypnotics and have a history of suicidal ideation or behaviors must be closely monitored because these drugs have a history of use in suicide attempts.
- Sedative-hypnotics that are taken in conjunction with other CNS depressants can cause oversedation and respiratory depression.

Do You UNDERSTAND?

DIRECTIONS: Indicate in the space provided whether each statement is *true* or *false*. If the answer is false, correct the statement to make it true (using the margin space).

_____ 1. Barbiturates that are given in conjunction with oral contraceptives will result in a lower serum barbiturate level and a decreased effectiveness of the sedative-hypnotic.

_____ 2. The best use of sedative-hypnotic medications is as a short-term therapy for insomnia.

_____ 3. Zolpidem is known to cause fetal abnormalities and must not be given during the first trimester of a pregnancy.

_____ 4. Patients with hepatic, renal, or respiratory insufficiency have an increased risk for oversedation and CNS depression when given sedative-hypnotics.

SECTION B

ANTIDEPRESSANTS

Depressive symptoms are related to the sensitivity of catecholamine receptors in the presence of low serotonin levels. This alteration of chemicals allows changes in affective states that are governed by the

Answers: 1. false; barbiturates result in increased metabolism and decreased drug effectiveness of oral contraceptives, corticosteroids, digoxin, estrogen, theophylline, verapamil, tricyclic antidepressants, griseofulvin, and doxycycline; 2. true; 3. false; barbiturates; 4. true.

neurotransmitter norepinephrine. Lowered norepinephrine levels cause depression. Increased norepinephrine levels cause mania. Antidepressants alter levels of serotonin and norepinephrine, which moderate the patient's depression.

Four categories of antidepressants have been identified: tricyclic antidepressants (TCAs), selective serotonin reuptake inhibitors (SSRIs), MAOIs, and miscellaneous antidepressants. Lithium is an antidepressant with only one specific use.

What IS a Tricyclic Antidepressant?

Tricyclic Antidepressants	Trade Names	Uses
amitriptyline [am-eh-TRIP-tih-leen]	Elavil	Treatment of depression
doxepin [DOX-uh-pin]	Sinequan	Treatment of depression and anxiety
imipramine [im-IPP-ruh-meen]	Tofranil	Treatment of depression

Action

TCAs block the uptake of neurotransmitters to decrease the reabsorption of norepinephrine and serotonin in the brain. The decreased rate of reabsorption at the nerve terminals allows more of the neurotransmitters to be available to the postsynaptic receptors. This onset of therapeutic action occurs after 2 to 4 weeks.

Uses

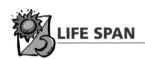

LIFE SPAN

Pregnancy complicates TCA use.

TCAs are most useful for treating major depressive episodes that reflect disturbances in sleep, hunger, appetite, sexual activity, and physical activity. Other indications for administration of a tricyclic medication include panic disorder, obsessive-compulsive disorders, enuresis, and idiopathic chronic pain.

TCAs were, at one time, the drug of choice for treating depression. Because of the possibility of multiple adverse effects and the strong potential for overdose, TCAs are no longer the preferred initial choice for treatment. TCAs are more likely to be reserved for patients who fail to respond well to other antidepressant medications.

What You NEED TO KNOW

Contraindications/Precautions

TCAs are contraindicated for patients during the acute recovery phase following an MI or for those with severe coronary artery disease. Because of possible cardiotoxic effects, TCAs are contraindicated for patients with hyperthyroidism or those who are undergoing thyroid hormone therapy. Other medical conditions that complicate TCA use are benign prostatic hypertrophy, seizure disorders, narrow-angle glaucoma, diabetes, and cardiovascular instability. When antithyroid agents are taken with amitriptyline, the risk for dysrhythmias is increased.

> ⚠️ Precautions must be taken when TCAs are prescribed for a patient with a history of either suicidal behaviors or ideation.

Drug Interactions

The use of other CNS depressants (e.g., barbiturates, opioids, alcohol) can increase CNS depression. Concurrent use of these medications with TCAs should be avoided. Smoking may lower the plasma concentration of the prescribed medication. When cimetidine, SSRIs, and oral contraceptives are given together with TCAs, TCA blood levels and the risk for adverse effects are increased. Concurrent administration of TCAs with clonidine, epinephrine, and norepinephrine leads to an increased risk for hypertensive effects or hypertensive crisis. Concurrent use of TCAs and MAOIs may cause extreme excitation, hyperpyrexia, and seizures.

Older or debilitated patients who are taking TCAs are particularly susceptible to morning orthostatic hypotension.

Adverse Effects

Amitriptyline and doxepin have a slow onset of therapeutic antidepressant effects but strong anticholinergic effects that rapidly appear. These two drugs are the most sedating of the TCAs. Cholinergic effects include dry mouth and mucus membranes, urinary difficulty, blurred vision, and constipation. Other adverse effects include drowsiness, dizziness, headache, migraine headache, tremor, weight gain, amenorrhea, impotence, insomnia, photosensitivity, and orthostatic hypotension.

TCAs are highly dangerous when taken in overdose amounts, causing cardiovascular effects (e.g., tachycardia, life-threatening dysrhythmias, CHF, CVA). TCA overdose can also produce respiratory depression, apnea, seizures, confusion, delirium, hallucinations, hyperpyrexia, bowel and bladder paralysis, blood dyscrasias, and coma. Even at nontoxic levels, TCAs frequently cause orthostatic hypotension. TCAs may also cause extrapyramidal symptoms (EPS), which includes mask-like facies, tremors, rigidity, and shuffling gait.

What You DO

Nursing Responsibilities

When TCA therapy is initiated, a prolonged period of 2 to 4 weeks may elapse before the therapeutic effects are noted. TCAs are administered either orally or IM. TCAs are easily absorbed through the GI tract and the presence of food does not adversely affect the rate of absorption.

TCAs are extremely dangerous in overdose amounts. Any patient who is prone to overdose should be issued only a small number of pills, or another responsible person in the family should control the patient's access to the medication.

When administering TCAs, the nurse should:
- Administer these medications at bedtime, which helps alleviate daytime sedation.
- Check hematologic laboratory studies for early onset of blood dyscrasias.
- Monitor the patient for EPS and cardiac dysrhythmias.
- Monitor patients with a history of suicidal behaviors or suicidal ideation for attempted drug overdose.
- Warn patients of the possibility of morning orthostatic hypotension.
- Teach patient smoking cessation methods when needed.
- Monitor the patient with heart disease for cardiotoxic symptoms.

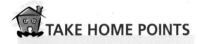

TAKE HOME POINTS

Advise patients who are taking TCAs against smoking.

Do You UNDERSTAND?

DIRECTIONS: **Indicate in the space provided whether each statement is *true* or *false*. If the answer is false, correct the statement to make it true (using the margin space).**

_____ 1. Neurotoxicity or seizure activity is not associated with TCA overdose.

_____ 2. Because of the multiple side effects of the TCAs and the risk for overdose, these medications are no longer the initial drug of choice in dealing with depression.

_____ 3. Orthostatic hypertension is an early indicator of TCA toxicity in older or debilitated patients.

_____ 4. Because of the propensity for cardiac arrhythmias, TCA therapy is contraindicated for anyone who is recovering from a recent heart attack.

_____ 5. The interaction of thyroid hormone and TCAs can increase the danger of cardiotoxicity.

What IS a Selective Serotonin Reuptake Inhibitor?

Selective Serotonin Reuptake Inhibitors	Trade Names	Uses
fluoxetine [flew-OX-uh-teen]	Prozac	Treatment of depression and obsessive-compulsive disorders
paroxetine [puh-ROCKS-uh-teen]	Paxil	Treatment of depression and panic disorders
sertraline [SIR-truh-leen]	Zoloft	Treatment of depression and panic disorders
escitalopram [es-sih-TAIL-oh-pram]	Lexapro	Treatment of major depressive disorder
citalopram [sigh-TAIL-oh-pram]	Celexa	Treatment of depression

Answers: 1. false; 2. true; 3. false; orthostatic hypertension occurs at nontoxic levels; 4. true; 5. true.

Action

SSRIs are a potent and widely prescribed class of antidepressants that block the reuptake of serotonin at selected nerve terminals in the CNS. These agents also have weak effects on the reuptake of norepinephrine and dopamine. The increased availability of serotonin enhances transmission and prolongs the stimulatory potential of the receptors, resulting in mood elevation and reduced anxiety. The elevated mood follows a similar time course as do TCAs.

Uses

Because SSRIs are well tolerated, they are usually considered as a first line of therapy for treating major depression. Fluoxetine is appropriate for the treatment of obsessive-compulsive disorder. Paroxetine and sertraline are used in the treatment of panic disorder. Phobias and post-traumatic stress disorders are also managed by SSRIs.

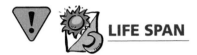

Fluoxetine should be used cautiously in patients with diabetes mellitus, renal and hepatic dysfunction, suicidal ideations, and hyponatremia. Paroxetine should be used with caution in patients with renal or hepatic dysfunction.

LIFE SPAN

Fluoxetine and escitalopram should not be used in patients who are pregnant and lactating. Paroxetine should be used with caution in patients who are pregnant and lactating. SSRI use in children has not been established and should be used cautiously in older adults.

What You NEED TO KNOW

Contraindications/Precautions

SSRIs are contraindicated for patients with a hypersensitivity to these agents. Paroxetine, citalopram, and escitalopram are contraindicated for patients with concurrent use of MAOIs.

Drug Interactions

Fluoxetine and paroxetine cause inhibition of certain hepatic enzymes. This action can lead to increased plasma levels of medications, such as phenothiazines, BZD, and antidysrhythmics. Concurrent administration of cimetidine can decrease the rate of SSRI metabolism, allowing accumulation of the SSRI and an increased risk for adverse effects. Use of warfarin during SSRI therapy can result in an increased prothrombin time and possible bleeding.

Concurrent administration of lithium, TCAs, barbiturates (e.g., phenobarbital), or alcohol may increase the CNS effects of SSRIs. Concurrent use of SSRIs and phenytoin can increase the serum levels of phenytoin.

Adverse Effects

Because of selectivity, SSRIs are as efficient as the TCAs and produce fewer anticholinergic effects. The common adverse effects of SSRIs are usually mild and dissipate within 4 to 6 weeks. Agitation, nervousness, overstimulation, blurred vision, insomnia, and jitteriness are usually found in the beginning phase of SSRI therapy. Patients with a history of panic disorder are more likely to experience these adverse effects. Both male and female patients may experience some sexual dysfunction (usually occurring late in the course of therapy). Other adverse effects include dry mouth, headache, anorexia, nausea, diarrhea, seizures, and suicidal ideation.

SSRIs can stimulate manic activity with patients who have a history of mania. For patients who demonstrate anxiety as part of their disease process, overstimulation can exacerbate the patient's feelings of anxiety.

> Administration of an SSRI with an MAOI may lead to potentially lethal effects. When given concurrently, these drugs can cause serotonergic syndrome, including hyperthermia, hyperactivity, rigidity, rapid fluctuations in vital signs, mental status changes, delirium, coma, and death.

What You DO

Nursing Responsibilities

SSRIs are administered orally and are slowly absorbed into the system. Elimination of the medication from the body is slow, taking as long as 5 weeks for the medication to clear the system completely.

Before beginning SSRI therapy, an in-depth history of past suicidal tendencies, depressive episodes, and previous antidepressant drug use should be obtained. When the patient has used an MAOI, a minimum of a 2-week washout period is required to clear the patient's system to prevent any drug interaction with the initiation of an SSRI. Conversely, when the patient is changing from SSRI therapy to the administration of an MAOI, the washout period must be 5 weeks.

When administering SSRIs, the nurse should:

- Monitor the patient's liver function studies before administering SSRIs and throughout therapy.
- Observe the patient with a history of seizures for potential of a lowered seizure threshold.
- Advise the patient to take SSRIs at bedtime to reduce the danger of sedation (e.g., falls).
- Inform the patient that the therapeutic effect may be delayed for 2 to 4 weeks after initiation of the drug.

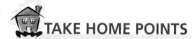**TAKE HOME POINTS**

Limit the suicidal patient's access to SSRIs to prevent a suicide attempt. *SSRIs should never be given together with an MAOI.* When the MAOI is being discontinued, 14 days should elapse before starting the SSRI. Caution the patient against self-medication with OTC drugs.

- Teach the patient the importance of compliance with the prescribed regimen.
- Caution the patient against using other prescriptions, OTC medications, or herbal remedies to control depression (e.g., TCAs, MAOIs, or St. John's wort) that might interfere with the action or metabolism of SSRIs or lead to toxicity.
- Advise the patient who is taking SSRIs to avoid alcohol and other CNS depressants.

Do You UNDERSTAND?

DIRECTIONS: **Indicate in the space provided whether each statement is *true* or *false*. If the answer is false, correct the statement to make it true (using the margin space).**

_____ 1. Patients who have been prescribed an SSRI should be concerned when they experience insomnia because this is an early symptom of neurotoxicity.

_____ 2. A thorough knowledge of a patient's history of suicidal behavior or suicidal ideation is essential to prevent self-administered SSRI overdose.

_____ 3. When an SSRI is administered in conjunction with an MAOI, the patient may experience rapid fluctuations in vital signs that are difficult to control and potentially lethal.

What IS a Monoamine Oxidase Inhibitor?

Monoamine Oxidase Inhibitors	Trade Names	Uses
phenelzine [FEN-el-zeen]	Nardil	Treatment of depression
tranylcypromine [tran-ill-SIP-roe-meen]	Parnate	Treatment of severe depression

Answers: 1. false; insomnia is an adverse effect usually found in the beginning of SSRI therapy; 2. true; 3. true.

Action

MAOIs block the action of monoamine oxidase in the presynaptic nerves. Monoamine oxidase is an enzyme that is found in cells of the brain, liver, spleen, kidneys, and in blood cells. The primary action of monoamine oxidase is to metabolize amines that are found in the body, such as epinephrine, norepinephrine, tyramine, and serotonin. These enzymes then accumulate in the liver, brain, and sympathetic nerves. Inhibiting the metabolism of the neurotransmitters increases their availability for impulse conduction in the CNS. Current studies indicate that depression is partly a reflection of decreased levels of norepinephrine and dopamine. With the increase in transmitters, depressive effects are reduced.

Uses

MAOIs alleviate symptoms of clinical depression. Phenelzine is also used in the treatment of manic-depressive psychosis. Tranylcypromine is usually reserved for severe depression in patients who have failed to respond to other treatment.

What You NEED TO KNOW

Contraindications/Precautions

MAOIs are contraindicated for patients with impaired renal or hepatic function, coronary artery disease, CHF, hypertension, and cerebrovascular defects.

Drug Interactions

Most of the drug interactions affect the cardiovascular and hepatic systems and the CNS. These interactions can be severe. For example, MAOIs should not be administered concurrently with opioids, barbiturates, or alcohol, because marked exacerbating effects occur. Hypertensive crisis, convulsions, coma, and respiratory depression can result when MAOIs are given concurrently with meperidine and sympathomimetics (e.g., vasoconstrictors). Drugs that interact with MAOIs to produce increased BP include diuretics, antihistamines, antihypertensives, and ephedrine (frequently found in OTC cold medications). General anesthetics also interact adversely with MAOIs.

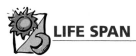

LIFE SPAN

MAOIs cross the placental barrier, causing fetal damage and are excreted in breast milk. MAOI therapy is contraindicated for pregnant or lactating women.

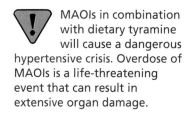

MAOIs in combination with dietary tyramine will cause a dangerous hypertensive crisis. Overdose of MAOIs is a life-threatening event that can result in extensive organ damage.

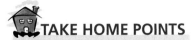

TAKE HOME POINTS

Closely monitor patients because MAOIs have the potential to cause severe and unpredictable adverse effects. Monitor liver function and a blood test to determine monoamine oxidase activity before initiating MAOIs. Repeat this procedure on a regular basis during the course of therapy. MAOI therapy should be discontinued at least 10 days before elective surgery.

Adverse Effects

MAOIs have the potential for severe and unpredictable adverse effects. Primary adverse effects of the MAOIs include orthostatic hypotension, weight gain, sexual dysfunction, and edema. These effects are usually transitory and diminish as the patient adjusts to the medications. An interaction of MAOIs and foods that are high in tyramine and caffeine-containing beverages can lead to hypertensive crisis.

What You DO

Nursing Responsibilities

At the beginning of MAOI therapy, a blood test to assess the monoamine oxidase activity of platelets is recommended. The patient should have this test repeated on a regular basis throughout the course of treatment to monitor toxicity levels. Before initiating MAOI therapy, obtain a thorough history from the patient, including information regarding cardiovascular, hepatic, and neurologic status. After a stable serum drug level is obtained, the dose is then decreased to a maintenance level.

After discontinuing MAOIs, resumption of normal monoamine oxidase metabolism is slow. Inactivation of monoamine oxidase by phenelzine is irreversible, and the enzymes must be redeveloped. A period of up to 2 weeks is needed to reestablish normal metabolism. The return to normal metabolism, after administration of tranylcypromine, is only slightly faster.

When administering MAOIs, the nurse should:

- Instruct the patient who is taking MAOIs to avoid foods that are high in tyramine and to limit caffeine intake as well. These foods and beverages include coffee, red wines, beer, cheese, sour cream, yogurt, nuts, raisins, bananas, yeast extracts, liver, sausage, smoked meats, and soy sauce. The dietary limitations can be one of the most difficult problems for the patient who is undergoing MAOI therapy. The patient may need considerable support and assistance to maintain compliance.
- Administer MAOIs at bedtime to reduce the danger of sedation.
- Instruct the patient to take MAOIs with food if GI distress occurs.
- Monitor the patient who is receiving MAOI therapy for signs of suicidal activity or ideation.
- Limit the patient's access to MAOIs to prevent overdose.

Do You UNDERSTAND?

DIRECTIONS: Indicate in the space provided whether each statement is *true* or *false*. If the answer is false, correct the statement to make it true (using the margin space).

_____ 1. Current literature associates depression with low levels of the neurotransmitters norepinephrine and dopamine.

_____ 2. Because of their unpredictable nature, MAOIs are usually prescribed only when the patient fails to respond to other less dangerous antidepressants.

_____ 3. Therapeutic effects of MAOIs appear between 1 and 4 weeks after initiating therapy.

_____ 4. MAOIs are contraindicated for patients with renal impairment.

_____ 5. MAOIs must be discontinued 1 month before elective surgery to prevent complications during recovery.

_____ 6. Patients who are taking MAOIs need not decrease their coffee intake during the course of the therapy.

What IS a Miscellaneous Antidepressant?

Miscellaneous Antidepressants	Trade Names	Uses
bupropion [byoo-PRO-pee-ahn]	Wellbutrin	Treatment of depression
venlafaxine [VEN-luh-fax-een]	Effexor	Treatment of depression

Action

Miscellaneous antidepressants are also known as *second-generation antidepressants*. These antidepressants include medications that have different chemical properties but share the same mood-elevating effects.

Bupropion is an aminoketone that inhibits the reuptake of dopamine and blocks serotonin and norepinephrine reuptake. Venlafaxine is a phenylamine and a strong inhibitor of both norepinephrine and serotonin reuptake. Venlafaxine is also a weak blocker of dopamine reuptake.

Uses

These miscellaneous antidepressants are appropriate for the treatment of mild-to-moderate depression. These agents are also frequently used as alternative therapy when patients are unable to tolerate or respond to other antidepressants, such as SSRIs.

What You NEED TO KNOW

Contraindications/Precautions

Bupropion is contraindicated for patients with a history of head trauma, CNS tumor, seizure disorders, or with concurrent administration of drugs that lower seizure threshold. Bupropion is not recommended in patients with a history of a recent heart attack, unstable angina, and hepatic or renal insufficiency.

Drug Interactions

Concurrent administration of bupropion with levodopa, phenothiazines, or TCAs is contraindicated because these drugs increase the risk for seizure activity. Administering bupropion concurrently with a rapid withdrawal of BZD is associated with an increased risk for seizure activity. Smoking cessation medications (e.g., Zyban) contain bupropion; thus concurrent administration of bupropion and smoking cessation medication can cause an overdose, leading to seizures. Concurrent administration of venlafaxine and MAOIs can lead to symptoms that are similar to those of neuroleptic malignant syndrome, including myoclonus, seizures, and hyperthermia; death may also occur.

Adverse Effects

Bupropion has a rapid onset that is frequently associated with nausea, agitation, and CNS stimulation. Bupropion is associated with dose-dependent seizure activity. Common adverse effects of bupropion include headache, anxiety, sedation, tremor, insomnia, decreased appetite, dry mouth, and weight loss.

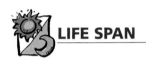
LIFE SPAN

Miscellaneous antidepressants (with the exception of bupropion) are contraindicated for women during pregnancy because they present a risk for adverse fetal development.

Common adverse effects of venlafaxine include nausea, sleepiness, dizziness, dry mouth, sweating, and headaches. Venlafaxine is associated with a dose-dependent, sustained elevation in BP.

What You DO

Nursing Responsibilities

All miscellaneous antidepressants are administered orally. When giving miscellaneous antidepressants, the nurse should:

- Observe the patient who is taking any of the miscellaneous antidepressants for suicidal activity or ideation. The smallest possible amount of medication should be given, or a reliable family member should be given responsibility for administering the medication.
- Monitor the patient who is taking venlafaxine with a history of hypertensive disease because venlafaxine is associated with sustained (dose-dependent) elevations in BP.
- Monitor the patient who is taking bupropion for seizure activity.
- Caution the female patient who is taking one of the miscellaneous antidepressants to notify her health care provider if she becomes pregnant.

TAKE HOME POINTS

- Teach patients that a 14-day hiatus must occur between the last dose of an MAOI and the initiation of venlafaxine.
- Monitor patients for overdose of these antidepressants because these agents may cause severe and possibly lethal effects.

Do You UNDERSTAND?

DIRECTIONS: **Indicate in the space provided whether each statement is *true* or *false*. If the answer is false, correct the statement to make it true (using the margin space).**

_____ 1. Concurrent administration of an MAOI and venlafaxine can result in effects that are similar to those of neuroleptic malignant syndrome.

_____ 2. Among the miscellaneous antidepressants, bupropion is the least likely to cause seizure activity.

Answers: 1. true; 2. false; bupropion is associated with dose-dependent seizure activity.

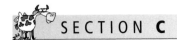

SECTION C

ANTIPSYCHOTICS

Antipsychotic agents are also referred to as neuroleptics. Usually, antipsychotic agents manage psychotic behavior by blocking dopamine transmission. Antipsychotic agents are classified as either typical or atypical. Typical antipsychotics are further categorized as phenothiazines and nonphenothiazines. Atypical antipsychotics are newer and are less likely to have the harsh adverse effects as the older typical antipsychotics.

What IS a Typical Antipsychotic Agent?

Typical Antipsychotic Agents	Trade Names	Uses
Aliphatic phenothiazine chlorpromazine [klor-PROE-ma-zeen]	Thorazine	Management of psychosis and schizophrenia; behavioral problems in children
Piperazine phenothiazine fluphenazine [flew-PHEN-ah-zeen]	Prolixin	Management of psychosis and schizophrenia
Butyrophenone nonphenothiazine haloperidol [hal-oh-PEAR-ih-dawl]	Haldol	Management of psychosis, agitated/delirious patients, and severe behavioral problems in children
Dibenzoxazepine nonphenothiazine loxapine [LOX-ah-peen]	Loxitane	Management of psychosis and schizophrenia

Action

Antipsychotic drugs interfere with the transmission of dopamine in lower brain structures (i.e., midbrain, hypothalamus, limbic system, brain stem, basal ganglia). These drugs inhibit neuronal uptake of norepinephrine and serotonin, as well as suppress the release of ACh. These medications also improve mood and thought disorders, as well as cause hallucinations, delusions, and agitation. Prolonged use of these drugs is not associated with habituation or addiction.

Typical antipsychotics can be further divided into two groups: phenothiazines and nonphenothiazines. The phenothiazine group contains the majority of the neuroleptic medications. This group is divided into three subcategories: the aliphatic, piperidine, and piperazine phenothiazines. Each of these subcategories has special properties and differs from the others in the type and strength of its adverse effects. Selection of a specific phenothiazine neuroleptic may be based in part on the type and strength of the anticipated adverse effects. Piperazine phenothiazines have mild anticholinergic, hypotensive, and antiemetic effects.

Piperidine phenothiazines are effective for organic brain disease (in older adults) and severe behavioral problems in children. Nonphenothiazines are divided into the following groups: butyrophenones, dibenzoxazepines, dihydroindolones, and thioxanthenes. Phenothiazines and thioxanthenes block norepinephrine as well as dopamine transmission, leading to more sedation and hypotensive adverse effects.

Uses

These drugs are effective in relieving the symptoms of acute and chronic psychoses. Although antipsychotic medications are not curative, they are able to suppress symptoms and improve quality of life. The aliphatic group contains chlorpromazine and promazine, which are particularly effective in controlling hallucinations and delusions. Piperidine phenothiazines include thioridazine and mesoridazine, useful for short-term treatment of major depression and sleep disturbances. Piperazine phenothiazines include trifluoperazine, which is particularly useful in patients who are withdrawn or apathetic.

Nonphenothiazine antipsychotics may be selected when the patient is unable to tolerate phenothiazines. Thiothixene is frequently used in treating chronic schizophrenia when other medications have been ineffective. Loxapine is useful in treating patients with both psychosis and symptoms of a mood disorder.

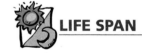

LIFE SPAN

Phenothiazines are not recommended in women during pregnancy and lactation.

What You NEED TO KNOW

Contraindications/Precautions

Because of the likelihood of orthostatic hypotension and tachycardia, phenothiazines are contraindicated for patients with known cardiovascular disease or a recent MI. These drugs are contraindicated for patients with a history of bone marrow depression because the effects can mask or exacerbate agranulocytosis. Phenothiazines are contraindicated for patients with renal or hepatic dysfunction, hypothyroidism, and Parkinson's disease. Because of the anticholinergic effects, phenothiazines are contraindicated for patients with glaucoma or those with a history of peptic ulcer disease, prostatic hypertrophy, and urinary retention. Haloperidol, a nonphenothiazine, is contraindicated for patients with Parkinson's disease or those who display symptoms similar to those of Parkinson's.

Drug Interactions

Concurrent administration of antacids with the antipsychotics can block the absorption of the antipsychotic from the GI tract. Concurrent administration of CNS depressants with antipsychotics can increase the depressive effects of both drugs and may produce severe respiratory depression. Concurrent administration of the antipsychotics and anticonvulsants may require an increased dose of the anticonvulsant because many phenothiazines and nonphenothiazines lower the seizure threshold.

Administering antihypertensives, diuretics, and epinephrine in conjunction with neuroleptics can exacerbate the potential for orthostatic hypotension. When phenothiazines are given with antiarrhythmics, this combination may produce problems for patients with known cardiovascular disease symptoms.

Older patients (generally over age 60) experience an increased occurrence of adverse side effects.

Some individuals (particularly older patients) may experience difficulty in regulating body temperature (**poikilothermia**), and changes in room temperature may produce hypothermia or hyperthermia.

Adverse Effects

Aliphatic phenothiazines produce strong sedative effects, pronounced hypotension, and moderate-to-strong extrapyramidal symptoms (EPS). Piperazine phenothiazines cause EPS but very little sedation and hypotension. Piperidine phenothiazines typically lead to strong sedative effects, moderate hypotension, and very few EPS.

The most prominent of the adverse effects of the phenothiazine neuroleptics are the extrapyramidal symptoms (EPS). Six reactions have been identified: acute dystonia, parkinsonism, akathisia, neuroleptic malignant syndrome, periorbital tremor, and tardive dyskinesia. Among the six reactions, the first four are usually present early in therapy (within the first 60 days). The remaining two (periorbital tremor and tardive dyskinesia) generally occur after prolonged therapy, which may be a result of delayed clearance of medication via the renal system or of an increased sensitivity to the drug's anticholinergic effects.

Other adverse effects of phenothiazines include photosensitivity, tachycardia, impaired thermoregulation, constipation, breast engorgement (in both men and women), abnormal lactation, blood dyscrasias, and neuroleptic malignant syndrome (NMS). The rare but potentially fatal condition of NMS involves altered mental status, high fever, tachycardia, dysrhythmias, muscle rigidity, seizures, rhabdomyolysis, respiratory and renal failure, and coma.

Nonphenothiazine antipsychotics also have the ability to cause significant EPS, including malignant neuroleptic syndrome and tardive dyskinesia. Among all nonphenothiazines, haloperidol has the strongest EPS effects. Thiothixene causes strong EPS but weak anticholinergic, hypotensive, and sedative effects.

What You DO

Nursing Responsibilities

Antipsychotic medications are available for administration either orally or IM. The antipsychotic medications (particularly phenothiazines) tend to have erratic absorption patterns, particularly when administered orally. When administering antipsychotics, the nurse should:

- Administer antipsychotic medications IM to provide a more stable rate of absorption and up to ten times more active medication in the system. Most of these drugs are stored in the fatty tissues and may take weeks to be totally cleared from the body.
- Monitor the patient's vital signs for orthostatic hypotension.
- Monitor WBC for early detection of blood dyscrasia. (e.g., leucopenia, agranulocytosis).

- Observe the patient for EPS and NMS.
- Encourage the patient to discontinue smoking because smoking increases the metabolism of some antipsychotics.
- Warn the patient that sexual dysfunction, menstrual irregularities, and breast enlargement may occur.
- Remain while the patient takes the medication because some patients may hide drugs.
- Teach the patient that antipsychotics should be discontinued gradually to avoid a reoccurrence of psychotic symptoms.
- Inform the patient that taking the medication with food or milk will decrease gastric distress.
- Instruct the patient to use sunscreen and protective clothing when in the sun.

Do You UNDERSTAND?

DIRECTIONS: Indicate in the space provided whether each statement is *true* or *false*. If the answer is false, correct the statement to make it true (using the margin space).

_____ 1. Phenothiazine neuroleptics may cause a patient (particularly a patient over age 60) to experience difficulty in maintaining normal body temperature.

_____ 2. Concurrent administration of CNS depressants with neuroleptics can result in exacerbation of depressant effects and may cause respiratory depression.

_____ 3. The normal slowing of hepatic and renal function as a result of age may be one of the factors that cause older patients to experience increased adverse effects from antipsychotic medications.

_____ 4. Among the EPS that can occur with the neuroleptic medications, only tardive dyskinesia may be anticipated to appear within the first 60 days of therapy.

_____ 5. Administering an antipsychotic to a patient with a known history of seizure may require a decrease of the patient's anticonvulsant dose because of the potential of anticonvulsants by neuroleptics.

Answers: 1. true; 2. true; 3. true; 4. false: acute dystonia, parkinsonism, akathisia, neuroleptic malignant syndrome usually occur within the first 60 days of treatment; other EPS (e.g., periorbital tremors, tardive dyskinesia) occur after prolonged therapy; 5. false: antipsychotics require an increase in dose.

What IS an Atypical Antipsychotic Agent?

Atypical Antipsychotics	Trade Names	Uses
risperidone [ris-PEAR-ih-doan]	Risperdol	Management of schizophrenia
olanzapine [oh-LAN-sah-peen]	Zyprexa	Management of schizophrenia
ziprasidone [zip-RAH-zih-doan]	Geodon	Management of schizophrenia
aripiprazole [air-ee-PIP-rah-zole]	Abilify	Management of schizophrenia

Action

Atypical antipsychotics interfere with the transmission of dopamine and serotonin. These drugs inhibit neuronal uptake of dopamine and serotonin, as well as suppress the release of ACh. These medications produce CNS depression and anticholinergic effects.

Uses

Atypical antipsychotics are effective in managing psychoses and schizophrenia. Atypical antipsychotic medications treat both positive and negative symptoms of schizophrenia.

What You NEED TO KNOW

Contraindications/Precautions

Atypical antipsychotics are contraindicated for patients with hypersensitivity, dysrhythmias, hepatic dysfunction, and blood dyscrasias. Because of the anticholinergic effects, these agents are contraindicated for patients with glaucoma or those with a history of peptic ulcer disease, prostatic hypertrophy, or urinary retention.

Drug Interactions

Concurrent administration of cisapride with atypical antipsychotics may cause dysrhythmias. Risperidone levels may be decreased when given concurrently with carbamazepine. Alcohol and other CNS depressants potentiate depression. Administering antihypertensives in conjunction with neuroleptics can exacerbate the potential for orthostatic hypotension. Paroxetine may increase the risk for EPS when given with risperidone.

Adverse Effects

Atypical antipsychotics may cause weight gain, headache, blurred vision, photosensitivity, insomnia, nervousness, dizziness, GI distress, malaise, dry skin, and orthostatic hypotension. The occurrence of EPS and NMS is low with atypical antipsychotics.

What You DO

Nursing Responsibilities

Atypical antipsychotic medications are available for administration either orally or IM. When administering antipsychotics, the nurse should:

- Monitor the patient for orthostatic hypotension and other adverse effects, such as EPS and NMS.
- Reassess the patient periodically for drug effectiveness to allow the lowest effective dose.
- Check liver function test for early detection of dysfunction.
- Teach the patient that antipsychotics should be discontinued gradually to avoid a reoccurrence of psychotic symptoms.
- Inform the patient that taking the medication with food or milk will decrease gastric distress.
- Instruct the patient to use sunscreen and protective clothing when in the sun.

Do You UNDERSTAND?

DIRECTIONS: Fill in the blank with the appropriate answer.

1. Atypical antipsychotics treat _____.
2. Atypical antipsychotics are contraindicated for patients with _____.
3. The occurrence of EPS and NMS is _____ with atypical antipsychotics.
4. Atypical antipsychotic medications are available for administration either _____.

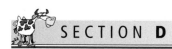

SECTION D

MOOD STABILIZERS

What IS a Mood Stabilizer?

Mood Stabilizer	Trade Name	Uses
lithium carbonate [LITH-ee-um]	Eskalith, Lithobid	Prophylaxis and treatment of acute mania
lithium citrate [LITH-ee-um]	Cibalith-S	Prophylaxis and treatment of acute mania

Action

Lithium, the most commonly used mood stabilizer, is available as lithium carbonate and lithium citrate. Both drugs are alkali metals that change biochemical, electrolyte, and endocrine function in the body. The actions of lithium are thought to inhibit the release of both norepinephrine and dopamine, as well as increase the reuptake of catecholamines in the CNS. This action may be a result of lithium's ability to compete with or replace sodium ions in brain cells. Lithium provides the patient with a feeling of calmness and controls other manic symptoms, such as motor hyperactivity, elation, flight of ideas, restlessness, aggressiveness, hostility, insomnia, and poor judgment. When lithium is given in maintenance therapy, recurrent manic episodes are prevented or diminished in frequency and intensity.

Uses

Lithium is used for the stabilization of bipolar affective disorder. This drug is the medication of choice for individuals who are experiencing acute manic and hypomanic episodes.

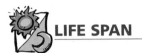

LIFE SPAN

Lithium is contraindicated for patients who are pregnant and those who are lactating.

Lithium should be used with extreme caution in any patient who is on a sodium-restricted diet or receiving concurrent diuretics. Caution should also be used in patients with diabetes or a thyroid disorder. Serum concentrations of lithium in excess of 3.5 mEq/L can cause coma, cardiovascular collapse, and death.

What You NEED TO KNOW

Contraindications/Precautions

Lithium is contraindicated for patients with renal dysfunction, leukemia, CHF, organic brain disease, dehydration, and sodium depletion.

Drug Interactions

Concurrent administration of aminophylline and sodium bicarbonate can cause an increased excretion rate of lithium and lower serum levels. Administering carbamazepine, fluoxetine, methyldopa, probenecid, spironolactone, thiazide diuretics, or nonsteroidal antiinflammatory drugs (NSAIDs) can increase the effects of lithium and toxicity. Concomitant use of neuroleptics (usually chlorpromazine and haloperidol) may cause encephalopathy and may result in acute extrapyramidal effects. Finally, when neuromuscular blockers are given in conjunction with lithium, prolonged paralysis or weakness may occur.

Adverse Effects

Most patients experience some adverse effects from the administration of lithium, but toxicity usually depends on the dose given and the length of therapy. Adverse effects include dizziness, headache, confusion, recent memory loss, dry mouth, metallic taste, drying and thinning hair, weight gain or loss, edema of hands and ankles, reversible leukocytosis (14,000 to 18,000/mm^3), cardiac dysrhythmias, and nephrotoxicity. The margin between therapeutic and toxic lithium levels is extremely narrow. The development of toxic symptoms is gradual and includes anorexia, nausea, vomiting, diarrhea, fine tremors (particularly of the upper extremities),

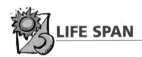

LIFE SPAN

Monitor older patients who are taking lithium more frequently than younger patients.

Warn the female patient to use contraceptive measures during lithium therapy because of the risk to the fetus.

and urinary frequency. Without treatment, the tremors become coarse, the gastric distress intensifies, and the CNS effects increase.

What You DO

Nursing Responsibilities

Lithium is administered orally and is available in both liquid and tablet form. When initiating treatment, the therapeutic effect may not occur for 5 to 6 days. This agent is also available in a sustained-release formula. When administering lithium, the nurse should:

- Monitor regular lithium levels for patients who are receiving lithium therapy to determine serum levels of the medication biweekly after initiation until therapeutic level is achieved, then monthly. Therapeutic serum lithium levels are 0.5 to 1.5 mEq/L.
- Report lithium levels over 1.5 mEq/L to the physician.
- Evaluate sodium levels because sodium levels may be depleted while taking lithium.
- Monitor renal and liver function tests and CBC for early detection of toxicity.
- Instruct the patient to take lithium with meals or milk to prevent GI distress.
- Advise the patient who is taking lithium to withhold one dose and report to the health care provider when evidence of toxicity is present.
- Caution the patient to avoid performing tasks that require alertness, such as driving, until the drug response is known.
- Instruct the patient to maintain a normal diet, including salt and a fluid intake of 2000 to 3000 mL during the dose-stabilization period and 1500 mL per day afterward.
- Warn the patient that prolonged exposure to sunlight can lead to dehydration. Advise the patient to report continued thirst and dilute urine (signs of dehydration) to the health care provider.
- Assess the patient for suicidal ideation and neurological status, including level of consciousness, tremors, and gait.
- Monitor the glucose level in the patient with diabetes who is taking lithium because transient hyperglycemia may occur.
- Teach the patient to monitor weight for early detection of weight loss or gain.
- Inform the patient that with normal renal function, 10 to 12 days may be required for lithium to be completely clear of the body.

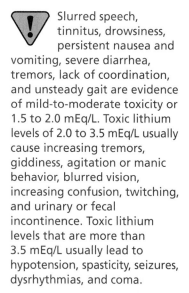

Slurred speech, tinnitus, drowsiness, persistent nausea and vomiting, severe diarrhea, tremors, lack of coordination, and unsteady gait are evidence of mild-to-moderate toxicity or 1.5 to 2.0 mEq/L. Toxic lithium levels of 2.0 to 3.5 mEq/L usually cause increasing tremors, giddiness, agitation or manic behavior, blurred vision, increasing confusion, twitching, and urinary or fecal incontinence. Toxic lithium levels that are more than 3.5 mEq/L usually lead to hypotension, spasticity, seizures, dysrhythmias, and coma.

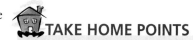

TAKE HOME POINTS

Lithium has an extremely narrow range between therapeutic and toxic levels.

Patients should have lithium blood levels drawn 8 to 12 hours after the initial dose and again 2 to 3 times per week during the first month of therapy. Thereafter, the patient's serum levels should be checked weekly to monthly as indicated by the patient's response to the medication. Lithium decreases reabsorption of sodium in the kidneys, which may result in hyponatremia.

Do You UNDERSTAND?

DIRECTIONS: Indicate in the space provided whether each statement is *true* or *false*. If the answer is false, correct the statement to make it true (using the margin space).

_____ 1. The typical serum lithium level for acute mania is 2.0 mEq/L.

_____ 2. Concurrent administration of thiazide diuretics can increase the rate of lithium excretion and decrease the effectiveness of the medication.

_____ 3. Lithium crosses the placental barrier and, when given during the first trimester of pregnancy, can cause fetal cardiac anomalies.

_____ 4. Lithium undergoes significant metabolism in the liver before excretion via the kidneys.

_____ 5. Concurrent administration of lithium and haloperidol can cause cardiac arrhythmias and cardiovascular collapse.

References

Abrams AC, Lammon CB, Pennington SS: *Clinical drug therapy: rationales for nursing practice*, ed 8, Philadelphia, 2007, Lippincott.

Edmunds MW: *Introduction to clinical pharmacology*, ed 4, St Louis, 2003, Mosby.

Gutierrez K, Queener SF: *Pharmacology for nursing practice*, St Louis, 2003, Mosby.

Hardman JG, Limbird LE: *Goodman & Gilman's the pharmacological basis of therapeutics,* ed 10, New York, 2001, McGraw-Hill.

Hodgson B, Kizior R: *Mosby's 2006 drug consult for nurses, 2006,* St Louis, 2005, Elsevier.

Ignatavicius DD, Workman ML: *Medical-surgical nursing: critical thinking for collaborative care*, ed 5, St Louis, 2006, Elsevier.

Karch AM: *Focus on nursing pharmacology*, ed 3, Philadelphia, 2006, Lippincott.

Kee JL, Hayes ER, McCuistion LE: *Pharmacology: a nursing process approach*, ed 5, Philadelphia, 2006, Elsevier.

Lehne RA: *Pharmacology for nursing care*, ed 5, Philadelphia, 2004, WB Saunders.

Lilley LL, Harrington S, Snyder JS: *Pharmacology and the nursing process,* ed 4, St Louis, 2005, Mosby.

Answers: 1. false; 1.5 mEq/L; 2. false; increases effects of lithium and risk for toxicity; 3. true; 4. false; lithium is not metabolized and is excreted unchanged in kidneys; 5. false; this combination may cause encephalopathy and result in acute extrapyramidal syndromes.

McKenry, LM, Salerno, E: *Mosby's pharmacology in nursing,* ed 21, St Louis, 2003, Mosby.

Smeltzer SC, Bare BG: *Brunner and Suddarth's textbook of medical-surgical nursing*, ed 10, Philadelphia, 2004, Lippincott.

Wilson BA, Shannon MT, Stang CL: *Nurses drug guide,* Upper Saddle River, New Jersey, 2006, Pearson.

NCLEX® Review

Section A

1. An 80-year-old female is taking lorazepam (Ativan) for anxiety. The nurse knows that the beneficial effect of this drug for this patient is that it:
   1 Improves visual ability.
   2 Is less apt to accumulate in the body.
   3 Promotes more wakeful hours of the day.
   4 Causes less GI disturbances.

2. Which adverse effect should the nurse expect from diazepam, a benzodiazepine anxiolytic?
   1 Blurred vision
   2 Increased WBC
   3 Improved memory
   4 Bruising and bleeding

3. A patient is taking buspirone (BuSpar). Which drug may cause an interaction leading to severe hypertension?
   1 MAOI
   2 Alcohol
   3 Opioid
   4 Barbiturate

4. Which patient groups or conditions are contraindications for temazepam and other BZDs?
   1 Elderly
   2 Uncontrolled pain
   3 Acute-angle glaucoma
   4 Debilitated individuals

5. Buspirone should be tapered gradually on discontinuation of therapy to avoid which complication?
   1 Seizure
   2 Laryngospasm
   3 Agranulocytosis
   4 Excessive bleeding

Section B

6. Which is the drug of choice for major depression?
   1 TCA
   2 SSRI
   3 MAOI
   4 Lithium

7. OTC cold medications should not be given concurrently with MAOIs because of which possible drug interaction?
   1. Insomnia
   2. Hypotension
   3 Hypertension
   4 Suicidal tendencies

8. A patient who is taking pheneizine (Nardil). Which food should be avoided?
   1 Fish
   2 Steak
   3 Chocolate
   4 Pineapple

9. A patient is taking bupropion (Wellbutrin). Which drug interaction should the nurse expect when the patient states he is using Zyban?
   1 Seizures
   2 Hyperthermia
   3 Stevens-Johnson syndrome
   4 Neuroleptic malignant syndrome

10. A patient is taking fluoxetine (Prozac). Which adverse effect does the nurse realize is associated with this drug?
    1 Hypothermia
    2 blood dyscrasias
    3 Suicidal tendency
    4 Stevens-Johnson syndrome

Section C

11. A patient is taking chlorpromazine (Thorazine). The nurse should monitor for which adverse effect?
1 Diarrhea
2 Hypotension
3 Bradycardia
4 Excess saliva

12. A patient is taking fluphenazine (Prolixin). The nurse should monitor for which adverse effect?
1 Anemia
2 Thrombocytosis
3 Agranulocytosis
4 Thrombocytopenia

13. A patient is taking an antipsychotic medication. Which nursing intervention is not associated with this category of medications?
1 Monitor for hypertension.
2 Encourage smoking cessation.
3 Warn the patient to use sunscreen and protective clothing when in the sun.
4 Remain with the patient during drug administration to avoid drug hoarding.

14. A patient is taking aripiprazole (Abilify). The nurse realizes this drug is used to:
1 Overcome depression.
2 Manage schizophrenia.
3 Treat mood disorder.
4 Manage severe behavioral problems in children.

15. A patient is taking risperidone (Risperdal). Which drug interaction may occur?
1 Cisapride may lead to NMS.
2 Paroxetine may increase the risk for EPS.
3 Carbamazepine may increase blood levels.
4 Lithium may exacerbate orthostatic hypotension.

Section D

16. A patient who is taking lithium (Eskalith) is having blood drawn to determine lithium levels. Which of the following represents the maximal therapeutic level for lithium?
1 0.6 mEq/L
2 1.2 mEq/L
3 1.5 mEq/L
4 2.5 mEq/L

17. Desired therapeutic effects of lithium include which of the following?
1 Maintaining sleep
2 Controlling a flight of ideas
3 Treating delirious patients
4 Managing schizophrenia

18. Lithium is contraindicated when which condition is present?
1 Dehydration
2 Liver dysfunction
3 Diabetes mellitus
4 Cardiac dysrhythmias

19. Toxic lithium levels may cause all of the following except:
1 Confusion.
2 Twitching.
3 Sedation.
4 Fecal incontinence.

20. A patient is taking lithium. Which teaching does the nurse realize is most associated with this medication?
1 Initially restrict fluid to 1500 mL per day.
2 Withhold one dose when toxicity is present.
3 Warn the patient of potential hypoglycemia.
4 Inform the patient that therapeutic effects may not occur for 2 days.

NCLEX® Review Answers

Section A

1. 2 Short-acting benzodiazepines, such as lorazepam, are preferred for elderly patients because these agents are less likely to accumulate in the body. Benzodiazepines do not improve visual ability. Benzodiazepines lead to insomnia, not wakeful hours. Benzodiazepines do not cause fewer GI disturbances.

2. 1 BZD anxiolytics may cause adverse effects of blurred vision, dry mouth, dizziness, decreased WBCs, and amnesia. Bruising and bleeding are not associated with these drugs.

3. 1 When buspirone is combined with an MAOI, lethal hypertension may occur. CNS depression may occur when buspirone is combined with alcohol, opioids, and barbiturates.

4. 3 BZDs are contraindicated for individuals with acute-angle glaucoma. Short-acting BZDs, such as loracepam and temazepam are preferred for elderly and debilitated patient because these drugs are less likely to accumulate in the body. BZDs are not contraindicated for patients in pain.

5. 1 Buspirone should be tapered gradually on discontinuation of therapy to avoid seizures. Laryngospasms, agranulocytosis, and excessive bleeding are not reasons to taper buspirone gradually.

Section B

6. 2 An SSRI is the drug of choice for major depression. MAOIs, cyclic depressants, and SSRIs are not the drugs of choice.

7. 3 Diuretics, antihistamines, antihypertensives, and ephedrine (frequently found in OTC cold medications) interact with MAOIs to produce hypertension.

8. 3 Chocolate, cheese, smoked meats, coffee, red wines, liver, beer, sour cream, nuts, raisins, and bananas are high in tyramine and when interacting with MAOIs, may lead to hypertensive crisis.

9. 1 Bupropion interacts with smoking cessation medications, producing seizures. Hyperthermia, Stevens-Johnson syndrome, and NMS are not associated with bupropion.

10. 3 Fluoxetine may lead to adverse effects, such as suicidal ideation. Hypothermia, blood dyscrasias, and Stevens-Johnson syndrome are not associated with this drug.

Section C

11. 2 Typical antipsychotics, such as chlorpromazine may cause hypotensive, anticholinergic, and sedative effects. Diarrhea, dry mouth, and bradycardia are not associated with these drugs.

12. 3 Fluphenazine is associated with agranulocytosis. Anemia, thrombocytosis, and thrombocytopenia are not associated with this drug.

13. 1 Antipsychotic drugs tend to cause hypotension, not hypertension. Smoking increases metabolism of some antipsychotics, and the patient should be encouraged to stop smoking. The patient should also be warned to avoid sun exposure. Patients who take antipsychotics commonly hoard medications.

14. 2 Aripiprazole is an atypical antipsychotic used to manage schizophrenia. It is not used as an antidepressant or to treat mood disorders. Haloperidol, a typical antipsychotic, is used to manage severe behavioral problems in children.

15. 2 When risperidone is concurrent with paroxetine, the risk for EPS increases. Concurrent cisapride with atypical antipsychotics may cause dysrhythmias. Concurrent carbamazepine decreases risperidone levels. Lithium is not known to interact nor exacerbate orthostatic hypotension.

Section D

16. 4 The maximal therapeutic level for lithium is 1.5 mEq/L. Levels of 0.6 mEq/L and 1.2 mEq/L are too low, and 2.5 mEq/L is too high.

17. 2 The desired effect of lithium is to prevent and treat acute mania controlling hyperactivity, flight of ideas, restlessness, aggressiveness, and poor judgment. A sedative-hypnotic agent is used to maintain sleep. Typical antipsychotics are used to treat delirious patients. Atypical antipsychotics are used to manage schizophrenia.

18. 1 Lithium is contraindicated for patients with dehydration, renal dysfunction, leukemia, CHF, and organic brain disease. There is no contraindication for liver dysfunction, diabetes mellitus, or cardiac dysrhythmias.

19. 3 Lithium toxicity may cause agitation, blurred vision, tinnitus, confusion, twitching, urinary or fecal incontinence, hypotension, spasticity, seizures, dysrhythmias, and coma. This condition is not associated with sedation.

20. 2 The nurse should teach the patient to withhold one dose and report to the health care provider when evidence of toxicity is present. Other instructions include initially increase fluid intake of 2000 to 3000 mL per day, watch for signs of hyperglycemia, and inform the patient that therapeutic effects may not occur for 5 to 6 days.

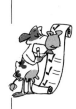 *Notes*

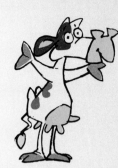

Chapter

6

Drugs Used to Treat Hematologic System Disorders

What You WILL LEARN

After reading this chapter, you will know how to do the following:

- ✔ Contrast the action of anticoagulant and antiplatelet drugs.
- ✔ Identify the laboratory considerations for patients taking anticoagulants and antiplatelet drugs.
- ✔ Explain the role of antiplatelet and anticoagulant drugs in the prevention of stroke and myocardial infarction.
- ✔ Recall the nursing responsibilities for the patient taking an antiplatelet or anticoagulant drug.
- ✔ Discuss drug-drug interactions that are clinically significant for antiplatelet or anticoagulant drugs.
- ✔ Explain the contraindications precautions necessary in the use of thrombolytic drugs.

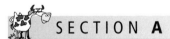

SECTION **A**

ANTIPLATELETS

Coagulation disorders can be treated pharmacologically by preventing formation of intravascular blood clots (**thrombi**) or by dissolving existing thrombi. Antiplatelet, anticoagulant, and thrombolytic drugs are used in the treatment of coagulation disorders. These drugs inhibit platelet aggregation, suppress coagulation, or promote clot dissolution, thereby interfering with normal homeostasis.

Bleeding is stopped in two stages. In stage 1, a platelet plug is formed, followed by coagulation with fibrin reinforcement. After detecting vessel injury, platelets adhere to the injured site. At this time, adenosine diphosphate (ADP) and thromboxane A_2 (TXA_2) are released, causing more platelets to stick to the injured site. Cyclooxygenase is an enzyme required for TXA_2 synthesis.

Coagulation occurs when the fragile platelet plug is reinforced with fibrin through a converging series of reactions called the *intrinsic* and *extrinsic pathways*. The extrinsic pathway is so named because a factor outside of the vascular system—tissue thromboplastin—is necessary for the reaction to occur. The extrinsic pathway responds faster than the intrinsic pathway and begins with tissue damage outside of the blood vessel. All necessary clotting factors for the intrinsic system to respond are present within the blood vessel, and the cascade of reactions begins with vessel injury. The pathways converge at factor X.

Anemia is a decrease in red blood cell number, size, or hemoglobin. Anemia has several causes, including blood loss, hemolysis, and bone marrow dysfunction. Iron deficiency is the most common cause of anemia, but folic acid and vitamin B_{12} deficiencies can also be causative factors for anemia.

What IS an Antiplatelet Drug?

Action

Antiplatelets	Trade Names	Uses
acetylsalicylic acid [ah-SEE-til-sal-ih-SILL-ick]	ASA or aspirin	Reduce the risk for MI, TIA, and CVA
ticlopidine [ti-CLO-pi-deen]	Ticlid	Prevention of CVA
dipyridamole [dye-peer-ID-a-mole]	Persantine	Prevention of thromboembolism
clopidogrel [clo-PI-dro-grel]	Plavix	Prevention of MI, CVA, and vascular death

Antiplatelet drugs interfere with platelet membrane function, prevent the release of platelet constituents, and prolong bleeding time, thereby inhibiting platelet aggregation. Antiplatelet drugs affect the synthesis and release of cyclooxygenase, TXA_2, and ADP.

Aspirin, the most frequently used antiplatelet drug, has an indirect mechanism of action. Aspirin inhibits cyclooxygenase, an enzyme needed by platelets to synthesize TXA_2. TXA_2 acts in two ways to promote hemostasis. TXA_2 acts on platelets to promote aggregation, and on vascular smooth muscles to promote vasoconstriction. When suppression of TXA_2 synthesis occurs, platelet aggregation is inhibited.

Dipyridamole, similar to aspirin, inhibits the formation of TXA_2. Ticlopidine inhibits ADP-mediated platelet aggregation. A single dose of aspirin, ticlopidine, or dipyridamole causes suppression of platelet aggregation. This suppression persists for the life of the platelet, which is 7 to 10 days.

Clopidogrel acts by preventing ADP from binding to its platelet receptor. The action is irreversible; thus bleeding time is prolonged.

Uses

Antiplatelet drugs are used most frequently to prevent arterial thrombosis. Aspirin is indicated for thromboembolic disorders to prevent myocardial infarction (MI), reinfarction, and cerebrovascular accident (CVA) when a transient ischemic attack (TIA) history is present. Ticlopidine is approved only for prevention of thrombotic CVA in patients who are intolerant to aspirin. Dipyridamole is approved only for prevention of thromboembolism following heart valve replacement surgery and as an adjunct for thallium stress testing. Clopidogrel is used in the prevention of MI, CVA, and vascular death in patients with arterial disease.

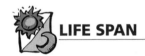

LIFE SPAN

- Antiplatelet drugs are contraindicated for women during pregnancy and lactation.
- Safe and effective use of ticlopidine and dipyridamole in patients under 18 years of age is not established.
- Aspirin use in children and adolescents with influenza-like symptoms or chickenpox is contraindicated because of possible association with Reye's syndrome. Use of aspirin with children under 2 years of age is contraindicated except under the supervision of a health care provider.

What You NEED TO KNOW

Contraindications/Precautions

Antiplatelet drugs are contraindicated for patients with drug hypersensitivity, pathologic bleeding disorders, and severe liver impairment. Aspirin is contraindicated for patients with hypersensitivity to nonsteroidal antiinflammatory drugs (NSAIDs) and in persons with the "allergic triad" (i.e., nasal polyps, aspirin hypersensitivity, and asthma). Patients with vitamin K deficiency, hemophilia, chronic rhinitis, chronic urticaria, or heart failure should not use aspirin.

Drug Interactions

Antiplatelet drugs taken concurrently with anticoagulant drugs may increase the risk for bleeding. When aspirin is given with ammonium chloride and other acidifying drugs, renal elimination of aspirin is decreased and the risk for salicylate toxicity increases. There is an increased risk for hypoglycemia if aspirin doses exceed 2 grams per day. Carbonic anhydrase inhibitors enhance salicylate toxicity, and corticosteroids add to the ulcerogenic effects of aspirin. Low-dose aspirin may antagonize the uric acid–lowering effects of probenecid and sulfinpyrazone. When NSAIDs are given together with clopidrogrel, the risk for bleeding is increased.

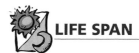

LIFE SPAN

Salicylate toxicity is a primary concern with aspirin use, particularly in older adults because of a decline in serum protein to bind salicylate and a reduced ability to excrete it.

Adverse Effects

Tolerability of antiplatelet drugs is variable. Adverse effects of antiplatelet drugs include rash, purplish red spots **(petechiae)**, bruising, nausea, vomiting, diarrhea, abdominal cramps, anorexia, or flatulence. Hypersensitivity adverse effects include anaphylactic shock, laryngeal edema, bronchospasm, and hives **(urticaria).** Additional adverse effects of aspirin include ulceration, occult blood, GI bleeding, hemolytic anemia, thrombocytopenia, dizziness, drowsiness, confusion, tinnitus, and hearing loss. Dipyridamole may also cause headache, weakness, fainting, a white blood cell deficit or complete lack of white cells **(agranulocytosis),** reduction of all types of blood cells **(pancytopenia),** reduced amount of neutrophils **(neutropenia),** and reduced amount of white blood cells **(leukopenia).** Additional adverse effects of clopidrogrel include back pain, depression, and hypercholesterolemia.

Cautious use of aspirin is advised in patients with renal impairment, gastrointestinal (GI) bleeding, or hypotension, as well as in those who are at risk for bleeding from anticoagulation therapy, bleeding disorders, trauma, or surgery. Caution is also advised in patients with otic diseases, gout, hyperthyroidism, glucose-6-phosphate dehydrogenase (G6PD) deficiency, anemia, and Hodgkin's disease.

What You DO

Nursing Responsibilities

Antiplatelet drugs are usually administered orally but can also be given rectally or intravenously (IV), depending on the purpose for administration and the condition of the patient. Ticlopidine absorption from the GI tract is increased when taken with food.

Aspirin interferes with pregnancy test results; decreases serum cholesterol, potassium, protein-bound iodine (PBI), and T_3 and T_4 concentrations; and falsely deceases plasma theophylline levels. Aspirin may

TAKE HOME POINTS

- Administer antiplatelet drugs with food to reduce gastric irritation associated with aspirin and improve absorption of ticlopidine.
- Monitor the patient for adverse conditions, such as salicylate toxicity.
- Antiplatelet drugs increase the risk for bleeding when given concurrently with anticoagulants.

increase serum T_3 resin uptake, uric acid, and urine vanillylmandelic acid (VMA) values. Aspirin may interfere with test results for urine glucose, urine 5-hydroxyindoleacetic acid (5-HIAA), and phenolsulfonphthalein (PSP) excretion. Liver function abnormalities may cause high plasma salicylate levels.

The nurse who is administering antiplatelet drugs should:
- Evaluate the patient's fluid intake and output.
- Observe the patient who is taking aspirin for tinnitus and muffled hearing because these symptoms frequently indicate chronic salicylate overdose.
- Realize that salicylate hypersensitivity is more common in patients with asthma, hay fever, chronic urticaria, nasal polyps, and perennial rhinitis.
- Monitor the patient for bleeding, such as petechiae, ecchymoses, and bloody urine or stool. Bleeding time is prolonged, and 5 or more grams per day of aspirin prolong prothrombin time.
- Discontinue antiplatelet drugs 1 week before surgery to reduce the risk for bleeding.

Do You UNDERSTAND?

DIRECTIONS: Fill in the blanks with appropriate responses.

1. To ensure safety, the nurse should be aware of the increased risk for neurologic adverse effects with the use of aspirin. They are

   _____, _____, _____,

   _____.

2. Both _____ and _____ age groups are at increased risk for salicylate toxicity should they become dehydrated.

3. To promote safe administration, the nurse should be aware that ticlopidine acts as an antiplatelet drug by inhibiting _____ release.

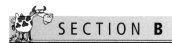

SECTION B

ANTICOAGULANTS

What IS an Anticoagulant?

Anticoagulants	Trade Names	Uses
warfarin [WAR-far-in]	Coumadin	Prevention and treatment of thrombus or embolism
heparin [HEP-a-rin]	Heparin	Prevention and treatment of thrombus or embolism
enoxaparin [e-NOX-a-pa-rin]	Lovenox	Prevention and treatment of thrombus or embolism

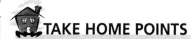

TAKE HOME POINTS

- Warfarin and heparin inhibit the formation of new clots but do not dissolve existing clots.

Action

Anticoagulants are drugs that suppress the production of fibrin, thereby disrupting the coagulation cascade. Both anticoagulants and antiplatelet drugs suppress thrombosis but through different mechanisms. Warfarin indirectly depresses the hepatic synthesis of vitamin K in the liver. Reducing the amount of vitamin K also reduces the dependent coagulation factors II, VII, IX, and X. When warfarin is taken orally, the onset of action is approximately 2 to 7 days. Peak drug action of warfarin is reached in 12 hours to 3 days.

Heparin directly increases the action of antithrombin III. Thus the conversion of prothrombin to thrombin and the conversion of fibrinogen to fibrin are blocked. When heparin is given subcutaneously, the onset of action occurs in 20 to 60 minutes and with an 8- to 12-hour duration of action. IV administration has a rapid onset of 1 to 3 minutes, peak drug action in minutes, and a duration of action of 2 to 6 hours.

Enoxaparin is a low-molecular-weight heparin that blocks factor IIa and inactivates factor Xa, thereby preventing clot formation. Enoxaparin does not bind to protein, tissues, or prothrombin as do the larger molecules of heparin. Enoxaparin has an onset of action of 20 to 60 minutes, peak action in 3 to 5 hours, with a duration of action lasting approximately 12 hours.

Uses

Anticoagulants are used most frequently to prevent venous thrombosis. Warfarin is the drug of choice for long-term prevention of thrombosis. Warfarin is also used in prophylaxis and treatment of pulmonary embolism (PE), atrial fibrillation, and MI.

Heparin is used for prevention and treatment of deep vein thrombosis (DVT), PE, atrial fibrillation with embolization, and diagnosis and treatment of disseminated intravascular coagulation (DIC). Heparin is used to treat acute coronary occlusion and to prevent thromboembolic complications that arise from cardiac or vascular surgery. Heparin is approved for use in preventing the clotting of heparin locks, in blood samples, and during dialysis. Heparin is also used to prevent cerebral thrombosis in evolving ischemic strokes and to prevent stroke and left ventricular thrombi after an MI.

Enoxaparin is used to prevent DVT after abdominal surgery and after hip or knee surgery. Enoxaparin is also used for treatment of DVT in the outpatient setting, and for PE, and acute coronary syndrome in acute care settings.

LIFE SPAN

Heparin may be used during pregnancy because the drug does not cross the placental barrier. Heparin is contraindicated for women during lactation and the postpartum period.

What You NEED TO KNOW

Contraindications/Precautions

Warfarin and heparin are contraindicated in patients with bleeding disorders, vitamin K deficiency, severe hypertension, and advanced renal, kidney, or liver disease. Heparin should also be avoided in patients with severe thrombocytopenia and those at risk for bleeding.

Enoxaparin is contraindicated in patients who are allergic to pork or those who may have religious objections to the consumption of pork products.

Drug Interactions

Concurrent use of low-molecular-weight heparin and spinal-epidural anesthesia or spinal puncture may contribute to epidural or spinal hematomas. Many of the hematomas cause neurologic injury, including long-term or permanent paralysis.

Cautious use of anticoagulants is advised in patients who abuse alcohol, those with hazardous occupations, and those with an indwelling catheter.

Adverse Effects

The principal adverse effect of anticoagulants is bleeding. The risk increases with higher dosages and the addition of antiplatelet drugs. Hypersensitivity reactions are exhibited as dermatitis, urticaria pruritus, fever, and bronchospasm with anaphylactic reaction. Other adverse effects of warfarin include nausea, vomiting, diarrhea, abdominal cramps, or anorexia. Hair loss develops with long-term use of warfarin.

Heparin has similar adverse effects, but these are frequently more severe. Injection site reactions may occur along with transient thrombocytopenia. Large doses of heparin for prolonged periods may suppress renal function, causing osteoporosis, hypoaldosteronism, or hyperkalemia.

What You DO

Nursing Responsibilities

Warfarin is given only by mouth. Heparin can be administered IV or subcutaneously (Sub-Q), depending on the speed of response desired and condition of the patient. The only route for administering enoxaparin is Sub-Q. When administering anticoagulants, the nurse should:

- Monitor the patient's international normalized ratio (INR) values every week for the first month and then as needed based on the patient's individual response. An INR in the target range of 2 to 3 is usually acceptable in reducing the risk for bleeding and providing therapeutic benefits. Higher INRs are associated with a greater risk for bleeding but may be needed in some patients.
- Advise patients taking warfarin to have the INR blood test done in the morning and to take the drug around 5 p.m. This information is important to the health care provider when adjusting anticoagulant dosages and in preventing excessive variation in test results.
- Monitor the partial thromboplastin time (PTT) or activated partial thromboplastin time (APTT) level of the patient who is taking heparin for dosage determination. The therapeutic dose range is usually $1\frac{1}{2}$ to 2 times the normal.
- Adjust heparin dose to achieve desired range of lab values. Unlike heparin, low-molecular-weight heparins such as enoxaparin do not require APTT, PTT, or INR monitoring and can be given on a fixed schedule.

TAKE HOME POINTS

- An INR in the target range of 2 to 3 usually is acceptable.
- Heparin is given parentally based on the PTT or APTT. The therapeutic dose range of heparin is usually $1\frac{1}{2}$ to 2 times the normal.

- Monitor intake and output of the patient who is taking anticoagulants.
- Monitor the patient who is taking anticoagulants for any signs of overt or hidden bleeding.
- Instruct patients and family members to report signs of bleeding (i.e., bleeding gums, unexplained bruising, bloody urine or feces) to the health care provider immediately.
- Realize that anticoagulants may cause elevated results for alanine aminotransferase (ALT), aspartate aminotransferase (AST), and thyroid function. Heparin causes prolonged bromsulphalein (BSP) levels, decreased triglycerides and cholesterol, and an alteration in blood gases.
- Recognize that protamine sulfate is the antidote for heparin and enoxaparin overdose. Protamine sulfate binds to heparin and keeps it from working. Vitamin K is the antidote for warfarin.
- Teach patients to avoid excessive intake of vitamin K–rich foods such as green leafy vegetables (i.e., asparagus, avocado, broccoli, endive, kale, lettuce), canola oil, soybean oil, olive oil, dill pickles, peas, margarine, mayonnaise; sauerkraut, and scallions.

Do You UNDERSTAND?

DIRECTIONS: **Indicate in the space provided whether each statement is** *true* **or** *false***. If the answer is false, correct the statement to make it true (using the margin space).**

_____ 1. Warfarin is the drug of choice for long-term prevention and prophylaxis of thrombosis.

_____ 2. Warfarin is used after abdominal surgery and to prevent DVT after hip or knee surgery.

_____ 3. Heparin blocks factor IIa and factor Xa, thereby preventing clot formation.

_____ 4. Enoxaparin depresses hepatic synthesis of vitamin K.

Answers: 1. true; 2. false; enoxaparin is used after abdominal surgery and to prevent DVT after hip or knee surgery; 3. false; enoxaparin blocks factor IIa and factor Xa, thereby preventing clot formation; heparin increases the action of antithrombin III, blocking prothrombin to thrombin and fibrinogen to fibrin; 4. false; warfarin depresses hepatic synthesis of vitamin K.

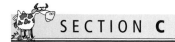

SECTION **C**

THROMBOLYTICS

What IS a Thrombolytic?

Thrombolytics	Trade Names	Uses
streptokinase [strep-toe-KYE-nase]	Streptase	Treatment of thrombosis and embolism of acute MI, PE, DVT
alteplase recombinant [AL-te-plase]	Activase tPA	Treatment of thrombosis and embolism of acute MI, acute ischemic stroke, pulmonary embolism
reteplase [RE-te-plase]	Retavase	Treatment of thrombosis of acute MI
urokinase [euro-KYE-nase]	Abbokinase	Treatment of pulmonary embolism, AV cannula occlusion

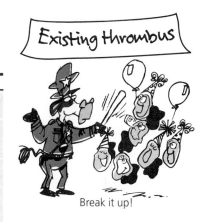

Existing thrombus

Break it up!

Action

Thrombolytics, also known as *fibrinolytics*, break down existing thrombus, rather than preventing thrombi from forming. Thrombolytics work directly or indirectly to convert plasminogen to plastin, an enzyme that acts to digest the fibrin matrix of clots. Plastin is capable of degrading fibrin, fibrinogen, and factors V, VIII, and XII.

Streptokinase is extracted from cultures of streptococci and contains foreign protein, which contributes to allergic reactions and antibody production that neutralize drug effects. Recombinant deoxyribonucleic acid (DNA) technology is used to make reteplase recombinant and alteplase recombinant. These thrombolytics are devoid of foreign proteins and are nonallergic.

Thrombolytic drug action occurs within minutes of IV administration. The half-life of thrombolytics varies from 40 to 80 minutes for streptokinase and to 5 to 20 minutes for alteplase, reteplase, and urokinase.

Uses

Thrombolytic drugs are used to treat acute MI, massive PE, thrombotic strokes, DVT, and arteriovenous cannula occlusion.

What You NEED TO KNOW

Contraindications/Precautions

Thrombolytics are contraindicated for patients with known hypersensitivity, hemorrhagic disorders, severe uncontrolled hypertension, or increased risk for bleeding.

Drug Interactions

When thrombolytics are given concurrently with aspirin, abciximab, dipyridamole, and heparin, the risk for bleeding is increased. Coagulation and fibrinolytic tests are unreliable because of the decrease in plasminogen and fibrinogen. Aminocaproic acid reverses the action of streptokinase.

Adverse Effects

Adverse effects of thrombolytics include hemorrhage and anemia. Hypersensitivity is common (12%) with streptokinase and urokinase and manifests as bronchospasm and anaphylaxis or milder symptoms, such as urticaria, itching, and headache. Adverse effects reported with streptokinase include fever, hypotension, unstable blood pressure, and reperfusion-atrial or ventricular dysrhythmias.

What You DO

Nursing Responsibilities

When administering thrombolytics, the nurse should:
- Explain thrombolytic therapy and possible complications to the patient and family before starting treatment. Instruct the patient to report any adverse effects such as lightheadedness, dizziness, palpitations, or nausea.
- Draw baseline vital signs, hematocrit, platelet count, fibrinogen level, thrombin time, PTT or APTT, and PT/INR before initiating therapy. Abnormalities in these values may prevent the patient from being considered as a candidate for therapy. During therapy, there will be

an increase in the thrombin time, PTT or ATT, and PT/INR, which should normalize within 12 to 24 hours. There will be a decrease in fibrinogen and plasminogen levels.

- Monitor patients for allergic reactions (i.e., rash, dyspnea, fever, changes in facial color, swelling around the eyes, and wheezing) and bleeding. Drug discontinuation may be indicated.
- Evaluate the patient's intake and output, electrocardiogram, and neurologic signs.

Do You UNDERSTAND?

DIRECTIONS: Match Column A with Column B.

Column A

_____ 1. Streptokinase

_____ 2. Alteplase recombinant

Column B

a. Increased risk for dysrhythmias

b. Devoid of foreign proteins or nonallergics

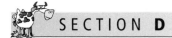

SECTION **D**

ANTIANEMICS

What IS an Antianemic Drug?

Refer to page 619 for a discussion of antianemic drugs such as iron and to page 615 for a discussion of vitamin B_9 (folic acid) and vitamin B_{12} (cyanocobalamin).

References

Arcangelo VP: *Pharmacotherapeutics for advanced practice: a practical approach*, Philadelphia, 2001, Lippincott.

Gutierrez K, Queener S: *Pharmacology for nursing practice*, Philadelphia, 2004, Mosby.

Lehne R: (2004). *Pharmacology for nursing care*, ed 5, Philadelphia, 2004, WB Saunders.

Lewis SM, Heitkemper MM, Dirksen SR: *Medical-surgical nursing: assessment and management of clinical problems*, ed 6, St Louis, 2004, Mosby.

Lilley L, Harrington S, Snyder J: *Pharmacology and the nursing process*, ed 4, St Louis, 2005, Mosby.

McCance K, Huether S: *Pathophysiology: the biologic basis for disease in adults and children*, ed 4, St Louis, 2002, Mosby.

NCLEX® Review

1. Which of the following is an adverse effect of heparin?
   1 Central nervous system depression
   2 Increased seizure activity
   3 Thrombocytopenia
   4 Lens opacity

2. Which of the following is an adverse effect of thrombolytics?
   1 Central nervous system depression
   2 Increased seizure activity
   3 Leukocytopenia
   4 Bleeding

3. Alteplase recombinant is approved as a thrombolytic for which of the following conditions?
   1 Viral gastroenteritis
   2 TIAs
   3 Thrombotic stroke
   4 Angina

4. Which of the following is a symptom of salicylate overdose?
   1 Tinnitus
   2 Bruising
   3 Nausea
   4 Bradycardia

5. Which of the following is a therapeutic PTT value during heparin therapy?
   1 Half of normal
   2 Equal to normal
   3 1½ to 2 times of normal
   4 3 to 3½ times of normal

6. Which of the following is a therapeutic INR value during warfarin therapy?
   1 2-3
   2 3-4
   3 5-6
   4 7-8

NCLEX® Review Answers

1. **3** Heparin may cause an adverse effect of thrombocytopenia. Central nervous system depression, seizures, and lens opacity are not adverse effects of heparin.

2. **4** Thrombolytics may cause bleeding as an adverse effect. Central nervous system depression, seizures, and leukocytopenia are not adverse effects of thrombolytics.

3. **3** tPA is approved for use in thrombotic stroke because it breaks down an existing thrombus. No thrombus exists in viral gastroenteritis, TIAs, or angina.

4. **1** Tinnitus is the most common symptom of salicylate overdose. Bruising and nausea are adverse effects of aspirin but not of aspirin overdose. Bradycardia is not an adverse effect of aspirin.

5. **3** The therapeutic PTT value for the patient on heparin therapy is 1½ to 2 times the normal PTT. Half of or equal to the normal PTT value is too low to be therapeutic, and 3 to 3½ times the normal PTT value is too high to be therapeutic.

6. 1 The therapeutic INR value for the patient on warfarin therapy is 2-3. Occasionally, a patient may have a desired therapeutic value higher than 3, but this is unusual. Other responses are too high to be therapeutic and may in fact contribute to patient bleeding.

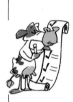

Notes

Drugs Used to Treat Cardio-vascular Disorders

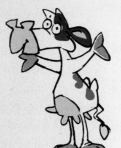

What You WILL LEARN

After reading this chapter, you will know how to do the following:

✔ Contrast the action of an angiotensin-converting enzyme inhibitor, angiotensin receptor blocker, beta-adrenergic blocker, and a calcium channel blocker.

✔ Recall contraindications and nursing responsibilities of antihypertensive administration.

✔ Discuss common adverse effects of antilipidemics.

✔ Explain common adverse effects and appropriate nursing responsibilities for the patient taking an antidysrhythmic drug.

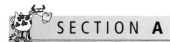 SECTION **A**

ANTIHYPERTENSIVES

This chapter reviews pharmacologic methods that are used to control high blood pressure. Because blood pressure (BP) depends on cardiac output (CO) and peripheral vascular resistance (PVR), pharmacologic interference of either factor can lead to BP control. Body systems that control CO, PVR, and BP involve the vascular, cardiac, renal, and sympathetic nervous systems. Antihypertensive drugs that act on these body systems to lower BP include angiotensin-converting enzyme (ACE) inhibitors, angiotensin II receptor blockers (ARBs), α-adrenergic blockers, β-adrenergic blockers, α-beta blockers, calcium channel blockers, central-acting agents, peripheral adrenergic neuron antagonists, and direct vasodilators. Diuretics decrease fluid volume, the action of which is also helpful in reducing BP. These drugs are discussed in Chapter 11, Section B, of this text.

What IS an ACE Inhibitor?

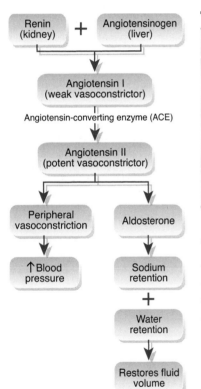

ACE Inhibitors	Trade Names	Uses
captopril [*KAP-toe-prill*]	Capoten	Treatment of hypertension and unresponsive CHF
benazepril [*BEN-AZE-uh-prill*]	Lotensin	Treatment of hypertension
enalapril [*eh-NAL-uh-prill*]	Vasotec	Treatment of hypertension and adjunct therapy in CHF
quinapril [*KWIN-uh-prill*]	Accupril	Treatment of hypertension and adjunct therapy in CHF
ramipril [*RAM-uh-prill*]	Altace	Treatment of hypertension and CHF post MI
lisinopril [*lih-SIN-oh-prill*]	Prinivil, Zestril	Treatment of hypertension and CHF post MI

Action

ACE inhibitors are a classification of antihypertensive medications that interfere with the renin-angiotensin-aldosterone system (RAAS), thereby decreasing BP. In the RAAS, an ACE converts angiotensin I to angiotensin II. Normally, angiotensin II is a potent vasoconstrictor and stimulator of aldosterone, which increases vasoconstriction and fluid volume, resulting in PVR. Through the process of blocking the ACE and its conversion of angiotensin I to angiotensin II, vasodilation, fluid volume reduction, and decreased PVR lead to a reduction in BP.

Uses

ACE inhibitors are indicated for early control of mild-to-severe hypertension in patients with normal renal function. Captopril is widely used to treat hypertension in patients with chronic renal failure (CRF).

ACE inhibitors are frequently used as the first drug of choice in the treatment of hypertensive patients with the following conditions: congestive heart failure (CHF), myocardial infarction (MI), peripheral vascular disease (PVD), and diabetes mellitus (DM). ACE inhibitors maintain this "first drug of choice" status because of their cardioprotective effects. ACE inhibitors are effective in monotherapy or in combination with other antihypertensives and thiazide diuretics.

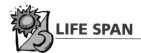

LIFE SPAN

Because of efficiency and tolerability, ACE inhibitors may be used for all age groups.
ACE inhibitors are contraindicated for women during pregnancy and lactation.

What You NEED TO KNOW

Contraindications/Precautions

ACE inhibitors are contraindicated for patients with hypersensitivity, renal artery stenosis, renal dysfunction, and hyperkalemia.

Drug Interactions

Several drugs affect the absorption of other drugs and interact adversely. Antacids decrease the absorption of ACE inhibitors. When tetracycline and ACE inhibitors are taken concurrently, the absorption of tetracycline is decreased. Nonsteroidal antiinflammatory drugs (NSAIDs) and rifampin decrease the ACE action when taken concurrently with ACE inhibitors. Concurrent drugs that increase the hypotensive action of ACE inhibitors include alcohol, nitrates, monoamine oxidase inhibitors (MAOIs), benzodiazepines, probenecid, diuretics, and other antihypertensives. ACE inhibitors can increase the action of other drugs. For example, potassium supplements may cause hyperkalemia, lithium may cause lithium toxicity, and digoxin may cause digoxin toxicity when taken in combination with ACE inhibitors. The risk for hypersensitivity increases when given concurrently with allopurinol.

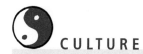

CULTURE

ACE inhibitors have greater effectiveness in young Caucasians than they do in African Americans. Combination therapy with low-dose diuretics can increase the effectiveness of ACE inhibitors in African Americans.

Adverse Effects

The most common adverse effect of an ACE inhibitor is a dry hacking cough—"ACE cough"—which usually subsides within several days after drug discontinuation. The cough is related to an increased sensitivity of the cough reflex induced by bradykinin and prostaglandins. Adverse effects include rash, itching, fatigue, dry mouth, anorexia, nausea, vomiting, abdominal pain, diarrhea, constipation, insomnia, alopecia, paresthesias, neutropenia, agranulocytosis, hyperkalemia, and renal failure. Cardiovascular-related effects include headache, dizziness, tachycardia,

Angioedema is a more common life-threatening adverse effect in African-American patients.

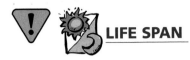

LIFE SPAN

- ACE inhibitors should be used cautiously in patients with CHF, aortic stenosis, and sodium and fluid volume depletion.
- The life-threatening adverse effects of ACE inhibitors include fatal allergic reactions (e.g., anaphylaxis or angio-edema of the face, lips, tongue, glottis, larynx, and the extremities), increased fetal mortality in the second and third trimester of pregnancy, and acute renal failure.

TAKE HOME POINTS

Notify the health care provider when the BP reduction is considered significant (20 mm Hg). Instruct the patient to rise slowly from a lying position and dangle the legs for a few minutes before standing. Orthostatic hypotension is more common in patients with CHF.

palpitations, and first-dose phenomenon (**first-dose syncope**). This phenomenon involves severe hypotension and fainting that can occur within 1 to 4 hours after the initial dose or when the dose is rapidly increased. This severe hypotensive effect may occur with subsequent dosing but is less severe at that time. The phenomenon usually occurs in volume-depleted individuals and those with a sodium level that is less than 130 mmol/L.

What You DO

Nursing Responsibilities

ACE inhibitors are usually administered orally 1 hour before meals. In a hypertensive crisis in the acute care setting, ACE inhibitors are usually given intravenously (IV) for a quick response. Monitoring drug effectiveness in hypertensive crisis may be as frequently as every 5 to 15 minutes until the diastolic BP is less than 90 mm Hg. Monitoring usually continues every 30 minutes until the patient is stable. When administering ACE inhibitors, the nurse should:

- Hydrate patients adequately or discontinue diuretics 2 to 3 days before the initiation of ACE therapy to prevent first-dose phenomenon. The patient may require IV volume expansion when BP reduction is excessive or too rapid.
- Monitor the BP hourly after the first dose or rapid dose increase for early detection of first-dose phenomenon.
- Instruct the patient to lie down for 3 to 4 hours after the first dose or a rapid dose increase.
- Monitor the BP of stable patients in the acute care setting immediately before routine administration of antihypertensives and at least every 4 hours after administration. Patients who are experiencing orthostatic hypotension may require dose reduction or drug discontinuation. The health care provider frequently orders parameters that define an acceptable BP range. When the BP is lower than the parameter, the dose is withheld.
- Ensure that the drug name is correct because several drugs have similar names.
- Teach the patient about appropriate spacing between drug doses. Some medications require that a certain blood level be maintained for effectiveness. When an even blood level is required for a medication,

the nurse should schedule the taking of medications at equally distant times (BID) (e.g., 9:00 AM and 9:00 PM).

- Caution the patient to refrain from activities that require mental alertness (e.g., driving) until the response to the drug is known.
- Inform the patient that if a dose is omitted, the next dose should not be doubled. A patient may take a missed dose of ACE inhibitor when the time before the next dose is greater than 4 hours.
- Instruct the patient to avoid substances that interfere with ACE inhibitors, such as caffeine-containing beverages (e.g., coffee, tea, cola) and over-the-counter (OTC) medications (e.g., cold remedies).
- Encourage the patient to report edema and weight gain greater than 3 pounds per day or 5 pounds per week.
- Evaluate renal and liver function tests and complete blood count (CBC) throughout therapy with ACE inhibitors.
- Monitor CBC every 2 weeks for 3 months and then periodically because neutrophils, hemoglobin, and hematocrit levels may all be reduced with ACE inhibitors.
- Observe potassium levels for early detection of hyperkalemia.
- Monitor the patient's lithium and digoxin levels for potential toxicities.
- Encourage the patient to make lifestyle changes (e.g., weight loss, smoking cessation, reduction of alcohol and salt consumption, and increase exercise).

Do You UNDERSTAND?

DIRECTIONS: Complete the following statements with appropriate responses from the italicized list provided.

1. When a patient is taking potassium concurrently with an ACE inhibitor, the nurse should monitor for potential _____.
2. The most common adverse effect of ACE inhibitors is _____.
3. ACE inhibitors have _____ effects and can safely be given to hypertensive patients with CHF, stable MI, PVD, and DM.

cardioprotective	*hyperkalemia*
detrimental	*cough*
hypokalemia	*seizures*

Answers: 1. hyperkalemia; 2. cough; 3. cardioprotective.

What IS an Angiotensin II Receptor Blocker?

Angiotensin II Receptor Blockers	Trade Names	Uses
losartan [low-SAHR-tan]	Cozaar	Treatment of hypertension
valsartan [val-SAHU-tan]	Diovan	Treatment of hypertension
irbesartan [ir-be-SAHR-tan]	Avapro	Treatment of hypertension
candesartan cilexetil [kan-deh-SAHR-tan sigh-LEX-eh-till]	Atacand	Treatment of hypertension

Action

Angiotensin II inhibitors (**angiotensin II antagonists** or **angiotensin receptor blockers**) selectively block the binding of angiotensin II to specific AT-receptors found in vascular smooth muscle and adrenal glands. ACE inhibitors block the conversion of angiotensin I to angiotensin II, but other enzymes that ACE inhibitors fail to block can form angiotensin II. Therefore, by providing further blockage of the renin-angiotensin system and aldosterone release, angiotensin receptor blockers (ARBs) inhibit vasoconstriction. Blocking vasoconstriction allows vasodilation, which increases renal sodium and water excretion and decreases blood volume. With effective interference of PVR, BP is lowered. Maximal therapeutic reduction of BP from ARBs is usually noted within 3 to 6 weeks after initiating therapy.

Uses

ARBs are beneficial to patients who are unable to tolerate ACE inhibitors but require BP reduction. Losartan is particularly useful in decreasing BP in patients with renal insufficiency without diminishing renal function. ARBs are now recognized as a possible first drug of choice for hypertension.

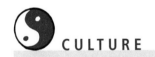

CULTURE

These drugs are effective in all age groups but are less effective in monotherapy for African Americans. For groups other than African Americans, ARBs are effective in monotherapy or combination therapy in the treatment of hypertension.

What You NEED TO KNOW

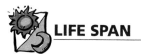 **LIFE SPAN**

Contraindications/Precautions

ARBs are contraindicated for patients with hypersensitivity.

ARBs are contraindicated for women during pregnancy and lactation.

Drug Interactions

The serum level and efficacy of ARBs are reduced when these drugs are given concurrently with phenobarbital. When both drugs are necessary, dose adjustments may be required.

Adverse Effects

ARBs have few adverse effects. Possible effects are headache, dizziness, fainting, weakness, hypotension, rash, dry skin, alopecia, dry mouth, tooth pain, nausea, diarrhea, and abdominal pain. ARBs do not appear to induce cough, angioedema, or significant hyperkalemia as do ACE inhibitors.

Caution should be taken when administering ARBs to patients with hepatic or renal dysfunction and hypovolemia.

What You DO

Nursing Responsibilities

ARBs are given without regard to food. When administering ARBs, the nurse should:

- Ensure that a female patient is not pregnant before beginning therapy.
- Monitor the patient on initiation of ARB therapy for first-dose phenomenon, particularly in volume-depleted patients.
- Encourage the patient to make lifestyle changes (e.g., weight loss, smoking cessation, reduction of alcohol and salt consumption, and increase exercise).
- Monitor the patient's electrolyte levels, as well as hepatic and renal function studies.

Do You UNDERSTAND?

DIRECTIONS: Complete the following statements by selecting the correct word from the italicized choices.

1. ARBs cause _____
   (vasoconstriction, vasodilation).
2. ARBs cause sodium and water _____
   (retention, excretion).
3. ARBs_____angioedema and significant hyperkalemia.
   (cause, do not cause)
4. Monitoring for first-dose phenomenon in the patient taking an ARB is especially important if the patient is _____
   (volume-depleted, hyperkalemic).

What IS an α_1-Adrenergic Blocker?

α_1-Adrenergic Blockers	Trade Names	Uses
prazosin [PRAY-zoe-sin]	Minipress	Treatment of hypertension
doxazosin mesylate [DOX-uh-zoe-sin MEH-suh-late]	Cardura	Treatment of hypertension
terazosin [ter-AZE-oh-sin]	Hytrin	Treatment of hypertension

Action

α_1-Adrenergic blockers (**α_1-blockers, α-adrenergic antagonists,** or **sympatholytics**) selectively block stimulation of postsynaptic α_1-receptors that regulate vasomotor tone. This action inhibits norepinephrine reuptake by smooth muscle cells and reduces vasoconstriction and PVR. The result is vasodilation in both arterioles and veins, leading to a decrease in supine and standing BP. α_1-Blockers trigger the baroreceptor reflex, which causes an increase in heart rate. During long-term therapy, increased renin leads to sodium and water retention in many patients, decreasing the typical postural hypotension.

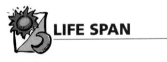

LIFE SPAN

α_1-Blockers are contraindicated for children and for women during pregnancy and lactation.

Uses

α_1-Blockers are used effectively in mild-to-moderate hypertension with monotherapy or in combination therapy with a diuretic or beta blocker (BB). α_1-Blockers are more beneficial in reducing diastolic pressure than they are in reducing systolic pressure.

What You NEED TO KNOW

Contraindications/Precautions

α_1-Blockers are contraindicated for patients with hypersensitivity.

Drug Interactions

When α_1-blockers are taken concurrently with alcohol, the patient will experience increased hypotension. When they are taken with epinephrine and ephedrine, vasoconstriction and hypertension are decreased.

Adverse Effects

Cardiovascular adverse effects of α_1-blockers include the first-dose phenomenon, flushing, headache, dizziness, fainting, weakness, edema, tachycardia, palpitations, and dysrhythmias. Gastrointestinal (GI) adverse effects include dry mouth, nausea, vomiting, abdominal pain, and diarrhea. Other adverse effects include visual disturbances, drowsiness, insomnia, nervousness, confusion, depression, fatigue, paresthesia, nasal congestion, urinary frequency, alopecia, priapism, impotence, and bronchospasm. An advantage of α_1-blockers is that no metabolic or lipid adverse effects are present. Elderly individuals are particularly prone to hypotension and hypothermia effects.

> ⚠ α_1-Blockers should be used cautiously in patients with hepatic impairment, cerebral thrombosis, and in males with the sickle cell trait.

What You DO

Nursing Responsibilities

α_1-Blockers can be taken with milk or meals to minimize GI distress. When administering α_1-blockers, the nurse should:

• Inform the patient that postural hypotension and palpitations usually disappear with continued therapy but may reappear when performing

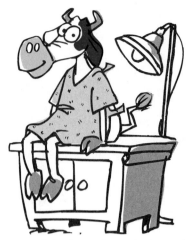

Sit upright for a few minutes and dangle the legs before ambulating to prevent postural hypotension.

strenuous exercise, eating a large meal, or drinking alcohol, or when other conditions that promote vasodilation are present.
- Advise the patient to avoid sudden changes in position.
- Instruct the recumbent patient to sit upright for a few minutes and dangle the legs before ambulating.
- Warn the patient to lie or sit down immediately when dizziness occurs.
- Tell the patient that the therapeutic effect of α_1-blockers usually occurs within 2 weeks after initiating therapy.
- Instruct the patient to report any weight gain or ankle edema.
- Caution the patient to avoid excess caffeine or OTC drugs, particularly cold remedies.
- Encourage the patient to make lifestyle changes (e.g., weight loss, smoking cessation, reduction of alcohol and salt consumption, and increased exercise).
- Instruct the patient to avoid driving 12 to 24 hours after the first dose or an increase in dose.

Do You UNDERSTAND?

DIRECTIONS: **Indicate in the space provided whether each statement is** *true* **or** *false*. **If the answer is false, correct the statement to make it true (using the margin space).**

_____ 1. α_1-Blockers block α_1-receptors, causing vasoconstriction.

_____ 2. α_1-Blockers are used in treating mild-to-moderate hypertension.

Answers: 1. false; the action causes vasodilation; 2. true.

What IS a β-Adrenergic Blocker?

β-Adrenergic Blockers	Trade Names	Uses
propranolol [pro-PRAN-oh-lahl]	Inderal	Treatment of hypertension, angina, MI, and ventricular dysrhythmias
atenolol [ah-TEN-oh-lahl]	Tenormin	Treatment of hypertension, angina, and MI
metoprolol [meh-TOE-proe-lahl]	Lopressor	Treatment of hypertension, angina, and MI
nadolol [nay-DOE-lahl]	Corgard	Treatment of hypertension, angina, and MI

Action

β-Adrenergic blockers (**beta blockers, β-adrenergic antagonists, or sympatholytics**) block both cardiac and bronchial receptors or β-receptors, which compete with epinephrine and norepinephrine for available β-receptor sites. Blocking the sympathetic nervous system's catecholamines results in reduced renin and aldosterone release, as well as decreased fluid volume. By inhibiting β_1-receptors, the heart rate, contractibility (negative inotrope), myocardial oxygen demand, automaticity, and conduction decrease. Blocking β_2-receptors causes vasodilation of the arterioles and a reduction of PVR and BP.

Uses

Beta blockers are used in patients with normal PVR, normal blood volume, high plasma-renin levels, angina, or previous MI, as well as in the initial treatment of uncomplicated hypertension. BBs increase exercise tolerance for the patient with stable angina and also decrease oxygen requirements. Therefore BBs are used in the long-term prevention of angina but not for the immediate relief of an acute anginal attack. In recent years, BBs have also been used to preserve the myocardium, to treat dysrhythmias, and to reduce the cardiac workload that is associated with cardiac ischemia, MI, severe heart failure (particularly diastolic failure), and cardiomyopathy. Propranolol and esmolol are used to suppress sinus and atrial tachydysrhythmias.

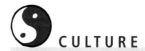

TAKE HOME POINTS

Blocking β_2-receptors causes bronchoconstriction, which is an adverse rather than a therapeutic effect.

CULTURE

BBs are effective in reducing BP in young Caucasian hypertensive patients with high CO.

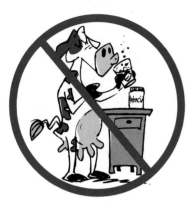

Avoid the antacid!

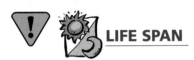

- BBs should be used with caution in women during pregnancy and lactation.
- Caution should be taken in patients with acute bronchospasm, chronic obstructive pulmonary disease (COPD), asthma, depression, PVD, sick sinus syndrome, bradycardia, heart block, valvular heart disease, and systolic heart failure.

What You NEED TO KNOW

Contraindications/Precautions

BBs should be used with caution in patients with DM, thyrotoxicosis, cerebrovascular insufficiency, and hepatic and renal dysfunction.

Drug Interactions

Administering BBs in combination with other drugs that have similar effects results in additive effects. For example, calcium channel blockers also decrease heart rate and BP and thus may result in bradydysrhythmias or hypotension. Antacids decrease absorption of BBs in the GI tract when these drugs are given together. NSAIDs reduce the hypotensive effects of BBs, whereas cimetidine, prazosin, and terazosin may increase severe hypotensive effects of the first BB dose. When BBs are given concurrently with insulin and sulfonylureas, the signs of hypoglycemia and hyperglycemia may be masked. The use of BBs with high doses of tubocurarine may exacerbate neuromuscular blockade. Tricyclic antidepressants and atropine may block bradycardia when given concurrently with BBs. β-Adrenergic agonists increase the effect of BBs.

Adverse Effects

Common adverse effects associated with BBs include headache, flushing, dizziness, bradycardia, postural hypotension, fatigue, drowsiness, confusion, bronchospasm, and bronchoconstriction. GI adverse effects include taste alteration, nausea, vomiting, and diarrhea. Other adverse effects include insomnia, cough, wheezing, dyspnea, malaise, lethargy, hypoglycemia, impotence, peripheral vasoconstriction, dysrhythmias, heart block, and heart failure. Rare adverse effects include bizarre dreams, depression, and blood dyscrasias.

What You DO

Nursing Responsibilities

When administering BBs, the nurse should:

- Assess BP and heart rate before BB administration and monitor closely, particularly when administered with a calcium channel blocker or other similar agents.
- Instruct the patient to report any weakness, dizziness, or fainting because these may be indicative of hypotension and bradycardia.
- Delay the BB dose and notify the health care provider when the patient's systolic BP is less than 90 mm Hg or the apical pulse is less than 60 beats per minute.
- Instruct the patient to take BBs before meals because food delays peak effects.
- Assess the breathing pattern frequently of the patient who is taking BBs to detect bronchoconstriction and bronchospasms.
- Instruct the patient with diabetes who is taking BBs to monitor blood glucose levels regularly and to expect dose changes in the insulin or oral hypoglycemics.
- Caution the patient to avoid substances that interfere with BBs, such as caffeine-containing beverages (e.g., coffee, tea, and cola) and OTC medications (e.g., cold remedies).
- Tell the patient to report edema and weight gain that is greater than 3 pounds per day or 5 pounds per week.
- Encourage the patient to make lifestyle changes (e.g., weight loss, smoking cessation, reduction of alcohol and salt consumption, and increased exercise).
- Monitor the patient's CBC, potassium, renal and liver functions tests, and triglycerides. BBs may decrease high-density lipoprotein cholesterol and increase blood urea nitrogen (BUN) levels in patients with severe heart disease.
- Assess the patient's lungs for fine crackles in the posterior bases for early detection of acute heart failure that is the result of excess myocardial depression and immediately notify the health care provider.
- Teach the patient the proper way to gradually reduce the dose over a 1- to 2-week period when discontinuing BBs after long-term use.

TAKE HOME POINTS

- When treatment is being transferred to an alternative BB, weaning is unnecessary, because the patient may be transferred directly to comparable doses without treatment interruption.
- Administer BBs with equally distant spacing between doses to prevent hypotension and hypertension.

Abrupt withdrawal of BBs can lead to rebound sympathetic overactivity. The patient in a rebound effect may experience reflex tachycardia and vasoconstriction with severe headache, palpitations, trembling, sweating, malaise, rebound hypertension, angina, dysrhythmias, and MI.

Do You UNDERSTAND?

DIRECTIONS: **In the spaces provided, indicate the appropriate direction: increased (I) or decreased (D).**

BBs cause:

_____ 1. renin release

_____ 2. fluid volume

_____ 3. BP

_____ 4. CO

_____ 5. bronchoconstriction

_____ 6. dizziness

_____ 7. pulse

_____ 8. myocardial contractility

_____ 9. vasodilation

What IS an α-Beta Blocker?

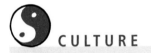

CULTURE

α-Beta blockers have greater effectiveness in African Americans than do BBs.

α-Beta Blockers	Trade Names	Uses
labetalol [la-BET-uh-lahl]	Trandate, Normodyne	Treatment of hypertension
carvedilol [car-ve-DIE-lahl]	Coreg	Treatment of hypertension

Action

α-Beta antagonists (**α-beta adrenergic antagonists, α- and β-adrenergic blocking agents,** or **α-beta blockers**) combine the blocking of selective α-receptors and nonselective blocking of β-receptors. Blockage of α-receptors affects vasomotor tone and results in vasodilation and decreased PVR. Blockage of β-receptors leads to a reduction of heart rate, a delay in atrioventricular (AV) conduction, and a depressed cardiac contractility. BP is reduced primarily because of a decrease in PVR.

Uses

α-Beta blockers are used in stage 1 or 2 of hypertension. These agents may be used alone or in combination with a thiazide or loop diuretic. Labetalol, when given IV, can decrease BP rapidly and is used in the treatment of hypertensive emergencies.

Answers: 1. D; 2. D; 3. D; 4. D; 5. I; 6. I; 7. D; 8. D; 9. I.

What You NEED TO KNOW

Contraindications/Precautions

α-Beta blockers are contraindicated for patients with severe bradycardia, heart block, asthma, shock, and uncontrolled CHF.

Drug Interactions

Drug interactions with α-beta blockers include increased effects when given with cimetidine and halothane. Decreased antihypertensive effects occur when these drugs are given with glutethimide and rifampin. β-Agonists, MAOIs, phenothiazines, and tricyclic antidepressants antagonize the hypotensive effects of α-beta blockers. Carvedilol may increase digoxin levels and may enhance hypoglycemic effects of oral hypoglycemic agents and insulin. Alcohol intensifies the orthostatic hypotension and sedative effect of α-beta blockers.

Adverse Effects

Common adverse effects of α-beta blockers include headache, dizziness, fainting, orthostatic hypotension, drowsiness, dyspnea, fatigue, diarrhea, impaired ejaculation, and edema with weight gain. Other adverse effects include visual disturbances, confusion, cough, nasal congestion, rhinitis, rash, alopecia, hypoglycemia, insomnia, tremors, paresthesias, and depression. GI adverse effects include dry mouth, anorexia, nausea, vomiting, and flatulence. More serious effects include dysrhythmias, CHF, pulmonary edema, cerebral vascular accident (CVA), bronchospasm, and bronchial obstruction.

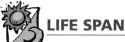

LIFE SPAN

- α-Beta blockers should be used with caution in patients with DM, PVD, COPD, pheochromocytoma, hepatic dysfunction, and bronchospasm.
- α-Beta blockers should be used cautiously in older adults because these individuals are especially susceptible to hypotension.

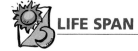

LIFE SPAN

- Edema with weight gain is a common adverse effect, particularly in older adults or those with limited cardiac reserve.
- α-Beta blockers are also contraindicated for women during pregnancy and lactation.

What You DO

Nursing Responsibilities

When IV administration of this drug is given, the patient should be lying supine. The position should be maintained for 3 hours after administration. The patient should return upright slowly. The peak of postural hypotension is 2 to 4 hours after therapy. When administering α-beta blockers, the nurse should:

- Take a baseline BP before α-beta blocker administration and monitor throughout therapy.

- Administer IV α-beta blockers over 2 minutes for a 20-mg dose.
- Monitor the patient who is receiving IV α-beta blockers carefully, q5m for 30 minutes, then q30m for 2 hours, and then q1h for 6 hours.
- Administer α-beta blockers with or immediately after meals because food decreases the risk for orthostatic hypotension. Monitor the patient's intake and output.
- Monitor the BP after the patient has been standing for 10 minutes because dose titration is based on the standing BP reading.
- Warn the patient to withdraw α-beta blockers gradually over a 1- to 2-week period.
- Monitor the patient's glucose levels frequently because α-beta blockers mask the signs of hypoglycemia.
- Evaluate hepatic and renal tests to determine adequate function of the related organs.
- Monitor digoxin levels when carvedilol is given concurrently because digoxin levels may increase.
- Instruct the patient to use caution in operating hazardous equipment after receiving an α-beta blocker until the individual's response to the drug is known.
- Tell the patient to lie down or sit down immediately when feeling dizzy, weak, or faint.
- Advise the patient to report a weight gain of 2 or more pounds in 24 hours.
- Encourage the patient to make lifestyle changes (e.g., weight loss, smoking cessation, reduction of alcohol and salt consumption, and increased exercise).
- Counsel the patient that prolonged standing, hot baths or showers, hot weather, alcohol consumption, and strenuous physical exercise intensify orthostatic hypotension.
- Warn the patient that diarrhea may be explosive and embarrassing.

Do You UNDERSTAND?

DIRECTIONS: Provide answers to the following questions.

1. What is the best time to check a standing BP?

_____

2. In which patients are α-beta blockers used?

_____

_____

_____

What IS a Calcium Channel Blocker?

Calcium Channel Blockers	Trade Names	Uses
diltiazem [dill-TYE-uh-zem]	Cardizem	Treatment of essential hypertension and angina
verapamil [veh-RAP-uh-mill]	Calan	Treatment of hypertension and angina
amlodipine [am-LOW-dih-peen]	Norvasc	Treatment of hypertension and angina
felodipine [feh-LOW-dih-peen]	Plendil	Treatment of hypertension
nifedipine [nye-FED-ih-peen]	Procardia	Treatment of mild-to-moderate hypertension and angina

Action

Calcium channel blockers (**calcium antagonists**) inhibit the influx of calcium into muscle cells through slow calcium channels during membrane depolarization. Calcium is blocked in intracellular sites of vascular smooth muscle, myocardium, and the cardiac conduction system. Extracellular calcium must move into the cell through calcium channels for the contraction of cardiac and smooth muscle to occur. Without this calcium influx coronary and peripheral vasoconstriction, myocardial contractility, automaticity, and conduction velocity are depressed in both cardiac and smooth muscle. The result is a relaxation of the smooth muscle of small arteries and a decrease in PVR. The normal

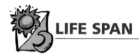

LIFE SPAN

- In older adults with diminished reflexes, this protective vasoconstriction is decreased and occasionally leads to excessive hypotension.
- CCB monotherapy is more effective compared with other antihypertensive classifications in older adults because these patients usually have low CO, decreased blood volume, high PVR, and high catecholamine or low renin levels.

adrenergic response to calcium channel blockers (CCBs) is a reflexive vasoconstriction, which decreases the hypotensive drug effect.

Uses

CCBs are effective in monotherapy for mild-to-moderate hypertension. When CCBs fail to reduce BP adequately, effectiveness is usually increased with BBs or diuretics. CCBs are beneficial and safe in patients with COPD, dysrhythmias, angina, hyperlipidemia, DM, and renal dysfunction. However, CCBs are not used in the immediate relief of an angina attack. Diltiazem and verapamil slow sinoatrial (SA) and AV conduction and are effective in decreasing the rate of paroxysmal atrial tachycardia, atrial flutter, and atrial fibrillation. Diltiazem and verapamil, as class IV antidysrhythmias, are occasionally effective in converting tachydysrhythmias to a normal sinus rhythm.

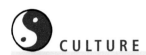

CULTURE

CCBs monotherapy are beneficial and safe in African-American and Chinese patients, in whom renin levels are usually low.

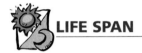

LIFE SPAN

- CCBs are also contraindicated for women during pregnancy and lactation.
- Verapamil may cause hypotension, particularly in older patients, when given at a faster-than-normal rate.

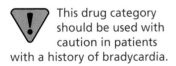

This drug category should be used with caution in patients with a history of bradycardia.

What You NEED TO KNOW

Contraindications/Precautions

CCBs are contraindicated for patients with severe hypotension, heart block, sick sinus syndrome, and hepatic or renal dysfunction. Diltiazem is contraindicated for patients with acute MI and pulmonary congestion. Verapamil is contraindicated for patients with severe left ventricular dysfunction and cardiogenic shock because of the profound vasodilation effect and its ability to compromise cardiac performance.

Drug Interactions

Serum digoxin levels are increased when digoxin is given concurrently with CCBs, which results in increased bradycardia and depression of the AV conduction. Cimetidine decreases the hepatic clearance of the CCB, which prolongs the action. Calcium and vitamin D decrease the action of CCBs. The interaction between CCBs and BBs causes additive effects with myocardial depression and bradycardia. Similarly, quinidine may cause excess hypotension when given together with CCBs. The action of carbamazepine, cyclosporine, and nondepolarizing blockers is exacerbated when given with CCBs.

Adverse Effects

Common adverse effects that are associated with CCBs include primarily vasodilating effects, such as flushing, headache, dizziness, weakness, dysrhythmias, and bradycardia. Other adverse effects include photosensitivity, rash, itching, nasal congestion, nausea, vomiting, diarrhea, muscle fatigue and cramps, hyperglycemia, sexual dysfunction, mood changes, persistent peripheral edema, and orthostatic hypotension. More serious adverse effects include heart block hepatic damage, thrombocytopenia, and Stevens-Johnson syndrome.

What You DO

Nursing Responsibilities

When administering CCBs, the nurse should:
- Administer oral CCBs before meals. However, CCBs may be taken with food when GI distress occurs.
- Give diltiazem IV initially with a bolus over 2 minutes followed by a continuous infusion on a volumetric pump through microdrip tubing to ensure accurate dose administration. Before weaning and discontinuing administration, a regimen of oral diltiazem is usually initiated.
- Monitor BP and heart rate before CCB administration. When the heart rate is less than 60 beats per minute, systolic BP is less than 90 mm Hg, diastolic BP is less than 60 mm Hg, or the parameter ordered, the dose should be delayed and the health care provider should be contacted.
- Instruct the recumbent patient to sit upright for a few minutes and dangle the legs before ambulating. Patients should change positions slowly when taking CCBs. Supervise ambulation until the response is known.
- Monitor the patient's renal and hepatic function for early signs of impairment.
- Monitor the patient's glucose, electrolytes, and intake and output.
- Taper CCBs over a 2-week period when discontinuing because abrupt withdrawal may cause severe reactions.
- Counsel the patient to avoid participating in activities that require alertness until response to the drug is known.

TAKE HOME POINTS

- Do not administer CCBs within a few hours of BBs because the result may cause depressed myocardial contractility and AV conduction, marked hemodynamic deterioration, and ventricular fibrillation.
- Keep the patient in the recumbent position for at least 1 hour after the first CCB dose.

- Caution the patient to check with the health care provider before taking any OTC medications because cold or allergy drugs interfere with CCBs.
- Instruct the patient to report edema and weight gain greater than 3 pounds per day or 5 pounds per week.
- Warn the patient to avoid substances that interfere with CCBs, such as caffeine-containing beverages (e.g., coffee, tea, cola).
- Encourage the patient to make lifestyle changes (e.g., weight loss, smoking cessation, reduction of alcohol and salt consumption, and increased exercise).

Do You UNDERSTAND?

DIRECTIONS: **Complete the following statements appropriately.**

1. _____ response weakens the hypotensive drug effect of CCBs.
2. When patients fail to respond to CCB monotherapy, _____ _____ or _____ are usually added.

What IS a Central α-Adrenergic Agonist?

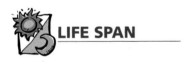

LIFE SPAN

Methyldopa is typically preferred for hypertension during pregnancy.

Central α-Adrenergic Agonists	Trade Names	Uses
methyldopa [meth-ill-DOE-puh]	Aldomet	Treatment of hypertension
clonidine [KLOE-nih-DEEN]	Catapres	Treatment of hypertension
guanabenz [GWAHN-uh-benz]	Wytensin	Treatment of hypertension

Action

Central α-adrenergic agonists (**central agonists** or **sympatholytics**) stimulate central α_2-receptors. α_2-Stimulation decreases the sympathetic outflow from the central nervous system brainstem to the heart, kidneys, and peripheral vessels. The hemodynamic result is an inhibition of vasomotor and cardiac centers, causing a decrease in PVR and a slight decrease in CO. Decreased vascular resistance allows systolic and diastolic BP reduction while only slightly lowering the heart rate.

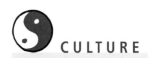

CULTURE

CAAs are used in African Americans, Caucasians, and those in all age groups.

Uses

Central α-adrenergic agonists (CAAs) can be used for treating mild-to-moderate hypertension. Generally, CAAs are not used as a first-line drug option for hypertension. These agents have been used in monotherapy or in combination with other antihypertensive drugs.

CAAs are contraindicated for women during pregnancy and lactation. Guanabenz is contraindicated for children under 12 years of age.

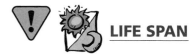

LIFE SPAN

CAAs should be used with caution in older adults because these patients are more prone to fainting and sedation.

What You NEED TO KNOW

Contraindications/Precautions

Methyldopa is contraindicated for patients with mild hypertension, active hepatic disease, blood dyscrasias, or pheochromocytoma, those who are concurrently using MAOIs, and those with hypersensitivity to this drug or to sulfites. Clonidine is also contraindicated for patients with systemic lupus erythematosus (SLE), scleroderma, and polyarteritis.

Drug Interactions

CAAs exacerbate the action of other CNS depressants (e.g., analgesics, opiates, sedatives, barbiturates, anesthetics, alcohol). Tricyclic antidepressants inhibit the hypotensive effect of clonidine. When CAAs are given concurrently with other antihypertensives, the hypotensive effect is increased.

Adverse Effects

Common adverse effects from CAAs include nasal congestion, dry mouth, constipation, impotence, decreased libido, headache, dizziness, drowsiness, weakness, fatigue, and orthostatic hypotension. Sodium retention

Clonidine and guanabenz should be used with caution in patients with a recent MI, severe coronary insufficiency, and cerebrovascular disease. Methyldopa and clonidine should be used cautiously in patients with mental depression. Methyldopa should also be used with caution in patients with angina pectoris. Methyldopa and guanabenz should be given cautiously to patients with hepatic dysfunction. Caution should be used with clonidine administration in patients with Raynaud's disease or Berger's disease. This category should be used cautiously in patients with renal dysfunction.

with weight gain usually occurs after initial administration but persists for only 3 to 4 days. Other adverse effects include rash, restlessness, nervousness, forgetfulness, vivid dreams, hallucinations, anorexia, vomiting, abdominal pain, depression, dyspnea, bradycardia, and rebound hypertension (with abrupt discontinuation). Potentially serious adverse effects include blood dyscrasias and hepatic dysfunction. Guanabenz may cause decreased fluid retention.

What You DO

Nursing Responsibilities

When administering CAAs, the nurse should:

- Inform the patient that orthostatic hypotension is intensified with prolonged standing, hot baths or showers, hot weather, alcohol consumption, and strenuous physical exercise.
- Instruct the patient to avoid more than 4 cups of caffeinated coffee, tea, or cola per day.
- Caution the patient that CAAs should be taken at bedtime to avoid drowsiness or interference with driving or operating hazardous equipment.
- Caution the patient to withdraw slowly over 2 to 4 days when the drug is being discontinued to avoid rebound hypertension.
- Encourage the patient to make lifestyle changes (e.g., weight loss, smoking cessation, reduction of alcohol and salt consumption, and increased exercise).

Do You UNDERSTAND?

DIRECTIONS: Complete the following statements by selecting the correct word from the italicized choices.

1. The best time of day to administer CAAs is _____ _____ *(midmorning, bedtime)*.
2. CAAs should be withdrawn over _____ _____ *(2 to 4 days, 2 weeks)*.
3. CAAs alter the heart rate by causing _____ _____ *(bradycardia, tachycardia)*.
4. The preferred antihypertensive during pregnancy is _____ _____ *(methyldopa, clonidine)*.

What IS a Peripheral Adrenergic Neuron Blocker?

Peripheral Adrenergic Neuron Blockers	Trade Names	Uses
reserpine [re-SER-peen]	Serpasil	Treatment of mild hypertension
guanadrel [GWAHN-uh-drell]	Hylorel	Treatment of hypertension
guanethidine [gwahn-ETH-ih-deen]	Ismelin	Treatment of moderate and severe hypertension

Action

Peripheral adrenergic neuron antagonists block the exit of norepinephrine (neurotransmitter) from storage granules, thereby inhibiting the activity of the sympathetic nervous system. These agents act in adrenergic neurons to deplete norepinephrine stores. Decreasing norepinephrine and vasoconstriction promotes vasodilation, which results in decreased PVR, CO, and BP.

Answers: 1. **bedtime;** 2. **2 to 4 days;** 3. **bradycardia;** 4. **methyldopa.**

Uses

Peripheral adrenergic neuron antagonists are used primarily to treat hypertension and are usually administered concurrently with other medications for efficacy. Reserpine is used as adjunctive therapy in severe hypertension. Guanadrel is used to treat hypertension when the patient is unresponsive to thiazide diuretics.

⚠ Caution must be used in patients with DM, renal or hepatic impairment, peptic ulcer disease, asthma, recent MI, or heart failure, and in those who are taking MAOIs.

What You NEED TO KNOW

Contraindications/Precautions

Peripheral adrenergic neuron antagonists are contraindicated for patients with hypersensitivity, depression, and pheochromocytoma.

Drug Interactions

Other antihypertensives, diuretics, and alcohol increase the hypotensive effect. Tricyclic antidepressants, phenothiazines, and other sympathomimetics block the uptake of peripheral adrenergic neuron antagonists and block or reverse the hypotensive effect. Oral contraceptives may reduce the hypotensive effects. MAOIs antagonize the hypotensive effect when given concurrently. MAOIs should be discontinued at least 1 week before administering peripheral adrenergic neuron antagonists. When this drug category is given concurrently with cardiac glycosides, the patient requires careful monitoring because both drugs decrease heart rate.

Adverse Effects

Common adverse effects associated with peripheral adrenergic neuron antagonists include shortness of breath, fatigue, lethargy, headache, drowsiness, dizziness, diarrhea, impaired ejaculation, and profound orthostatic hypotension. Adverse effects related to the respiratory system include nasal congestion, bronchospasm, and respiratory depression. Psychologic and neurologic adverse effects include paresthesia, seizures, decreased libido, nightmares (with high doses), tardive dyskinesia, inability to perform complex tasks, and severe suicidal depression. Other adverse effects include insomnia, visual disturbances, weakness, GI distress, peripheral edema, leg cramps, hypothermia, bradycardia, and heart failure. Peptic ulcer disease may be exacerbated because reserpine may increase gastric acid secretion.

What You DO

Nursing Responsibilities

When administering peripheral adrenergic neuron antagonists, the nurse should:

- Monitor the patient for seizures and respiratory depression.
- Evaluate the patient's BP and heart rate status. Following large IV doses of reserpine, a transient sympathomimetic effect with a small increase in BP may occur.
- Inform the patient that the full hypotensive effect of peripheral adrenergic neuron antagonists may take 3 weeks to achieve.
- Encourage the patient to make lifestyle changes (e.g., weight loss, smoking cessation, reduction of alcohol and salt consumption, and increased exercise).
- Caution the patient that an increased orthostatic hypotension risk exists with exposure to a hot environment, prolonged standing, and exercise.
- Tell the patient that this drug should be discontinued at the first sign of depression.
- Assess the BP periodically to ensure that the BP surge upon arising has been adequately eased.

Do You UNDERSTAND?

DIRECTIONS: **Indicate in the space provided whether each statement is** *true* **or** *false*. **If the answer is false, correct the statement to make it true (using the margin space).**

_____ 1. Depleting catecholamines increases norepinephrine and causes vasoconstriction.

_____ 2. Reserpine increases gastric acid secretion, which predisposes the patient to peptic ulcer disease.

What IS a Direct Vasodilator?

Direct Vasodilators	Trade Names	Uses
hydralazine [high-DRAL-uh-zeen]	Apresoline	Treatment of essential hypertension
minoxidil [min-OX-ih-dill]	Loniten	Treatment of severe hypertension

Action

Direct vasodilators relax vascular smooth muscles in the arterioles and decrease PVR. Some direct vasodilators affect both the arterial and venous systems, reducing both preload and afterload. As a result of arteriole dilation, decreased PVR, and reduced BP, the baroreceptors are stimulated to release catecholamines. This action leads to an increase in heart rate, fluid retention, CO, cardiac contractility, and cardiac workload. β-Adrenergic blocking agents may reduce increased cardiac workload.

Uses

Hydralazine is used in the treatment of moderate-to-severe hypertension. Minoxidil is used to manage severe hypertension associated with organ damage. Although direct vasodilators are highly effective antihypertensives, they are not used as initial monotherapy. Because minoxidil dilates renal arterioles, it can be used in cases of severe refractory hypertension or renal insufficiency.

What You NEED TO KNOW

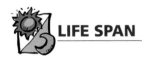

LIFE SPAN

Direct vasodilators are also contraindicated for women during pregnancy.

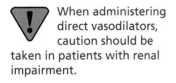

When administering direct vasodilators, caution should be taken in patients with renal impairment.

Contraindications/Precautions

Direct vasodilators are contraindicated for patients with hypersensitivity, coronary artery disease, and mitral valve heart disease.

Drug Interactions

NSAIDs decrease the therapeutic effects of direct vasodilators. BBs decrease tachycardia that results from hydralazine. The therapeutic effects of hydralazine are increased when given together with alcohol, other antihypertensives, MAOIs, nitrates, and general anesthetics. When direct vasodilators are taken concurrently with corticosteroids, estrogen, progesterone, and phenytoin, the risk for hyperglycemia is increased.

Adverse Effects

Common adverse effects that are associated with direct vasodilators include throbbing headache, profuse hirsutism on face and body, sodium and water retention, palpitations, and reflex tachycardia. Other adverse effects include nasal congestion, excess lacrimation, dizziness, flushing, anxiety, drowsiness, syncope, weakness, lethargy, restlessness, GI distress, constipation, tremors, euphoria, edema, weight gain, and impotence. More serious adverse effects include atrial and ventricular dysrhythmias, blood dyscrasias, leukopenia, agranulocytosis, temporary hearing loss, hyperglycemia, hematuria, nocturia, proteinuria, azotemia, severe rebound hypertension, pulmonary edema, and heart failure. Hydralazine (particularly with doses greater than 200 mg per day) can cause a syndrome resembling drug-induced SLE or rheumatoid arthritis, which involves fever, arthralgia, malaise, edema, myalgia, and the presence of antinuclear antibodies (ANAs). These drugs rarely cause orthostatic hypotension.

What You DO

Nursing Responsibilities

Hydralazine is usually administered orally. When a rapid decrease in BP is needed or the patient is unable to take an oral dose, hydralazine may be given intramuscularly (IM) or IV. The patient should remain recumbent for at least 1 hour after injection. Oral administration should replace parenteral therapy as soon as possible. Because of the excessive hair growth, minoxidil is not usually ordered for women, except in rare cases of severe hypertension that is resistant to multiple drug therapy. Additional nursing responsibilities include the following:

- Monitor intake and output, decreased urine output, edema, and weight gain for the patient who is taking direct vasodilators.
- Auscultate lungs frequently for early detection of pulmonary edema.
- Monitor renal and liver function tests, CBC, and ANA titer in patients throughout direct vasodilator therapy.

- Monitor the patient's BP in sitting and standing positions to determine orthostatic hypotension.
- Encourage the patient to make lifestyle changes (e.g., weight loss, smoking cessation, reduction of alcohol and salt consumption, and increased exercise).

Do You UNDERSTAND?

DIRECTIONS: Fill in the blanks with appropriate responses.

1. The most common adverse effects of minoxidil are _____ _____ and _____.
2. To determine orthostatic hypotension, the position of the patient should be _____ when the nurse assesses his or her BP.

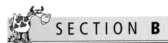

SECTION B

DRUGS AFFECTING CARDIAC OUTPUT

This section reviews the pharmacologic methods that are used to affect cardiac output (CO). Antianginal medications that improve myocardial supply and decrease the demand for oxygen include nitrates, beta blockers, and calcium channel blockers. An inotropic agent that affects CO is a medication that increases the force of myocardial contractility. Inotropics that are discussed in this section include cardiac glycosides and phosphodiesterase inhibitors.

Answers: 1. excessive hair growth; fluid retention; 2. sitting and standing after 10 minutes.

What IS a Nitrate?

Nitrates	Trade Names	Uses
nitroglycerin [nye-troe-GLIH-suh-rin]	Nitrobid, Nitrostat	Treatment of acute angina
isosorbide dinitrate [EYE-sos-ORE-bide die-NYE-trate]	Isordil	Prevention and treatment of angina
isosorbide mononitrate [EYE-sos-ORE-bide MAH-no-NYE-trate]	ISMO, Imdur	Prevention and treatment of angina

Action

Nitrates are antianginal agents that use direct relaxation action on vascular smooth muscles to dilate healthy coronary arteries that atherosclerotic plaque has not encompassed and to improve blood supply to the myocardium, thereby relieving chest pain. Although nitrates act on arterial, venous, and capillaries, they act primarily on the venous system, causing considerable venous vasodilation. Because nitrates dilate veins, less blood is returned to the heart, which decreases preload (e.g., the amount of blood volume in the ventricles at the end of diastole). Because diastole is the period during which the myocardial muscle fibers lengthen and the heart cavities fill with blood, nitrates reduce stretching and wall tension, thereby reducing the myocardial size and oxygen requirements that are required to pump blood out of the ventricles. The vasodilation effect and relaxation of vessels from nitrates decreases the resistance of blood flow that the heart has to pump against (afterload). Reduction of arterial resistance and the energy requirements for each myocardial contraction decreases myocardial oxygen requirements balancing supply and demand again.

Uses

Nitrates are indicated in the immediate relief or prevention of anginal pain. These agents are the drugs of choice in the treatment of acute chest pain and myocardial ischemia because of their ease of administration, rapid absorption, quick onset of action, and low cost. Nitrates can be used in monotherapy or multiple drug therapy with beta blockers or calcium channel blockers.

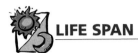

LIFE SPAN

Nitrates are contraindicated for women during pregnancy and lactation.

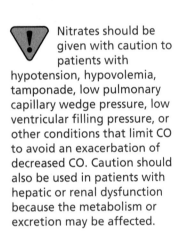

Nitrates should be given with caution to patients with hypotension, hypovolemia, tamponade, low pulmonary capillary wedge pressure, low ventricular filling pressure, or other conditions that limit CO to avoid an exacerbation of decreased CO. Caution should also be used in patients with hepatic or renal dysfunction because the metabolism or excretion may be affected.

What You NEED TO KNOW

Contraindications/Precautions

Nitrates are contraindicated for patients with known hypersensitivity, severe anemia, acute myocardial infarction (MI), head trauma, cerebral hemorrhage, and cardiomyopathy.

Drug Interactions

Nitrates decrease the action of heparin. Severe hypotension can result from drug interaction of nitrates with alcohol, other antihypertensives, phenothiazines, antihistamines, diuretics, haloperidol, and tricyclic antidepressants. Antihistamines, antidepressants, and phenothiazines decrease the absorption of buccal and sublingual nitrate forms. The risk for hypertension increases when taken with ergot derivatives.

Adverse Effects

The most common adverse effects of nitrates involve vasodilation and include flushing, headache, dizziness, fainting, weakness, and orthostatic hypotension. Other adverse effects include nausea, vomiting, sweating, incontinence, reflex tachycardia, and palpitations. Most adverse effects following nitrate administration disappear when the dose is reduced. Large, continuous doses of nitrates may cause blurred vision, dry mouth, peripheral edema, and methemoglobinemia. Additionally, isosorbide mononitrate may cause anxiety, agitation, confusion, loss of coordination, insomnia, tremor, blurred vision, photophobia, and blood dyscrasias. Transdermal preparations of nitrates may cause local skin irritation. Alcohol intoxication can occur with large doses of IV nitroglycerin resulting from the alcohol preservative that is used in the ampule or vial storage of this drug. The most outstanding signs of alcohol intoxication following IV nitroglycerin are hypotension and reduced myocardial contractility. Other serious adverse effects include respiratory depression and cardiovascular collapse.

What You DO

Nursing Responsibilities

Because of the high vascularity of the oral mucosa, nitrates are absorbed rapidly and almost completely when given by sublingual, buccal, or chewable tablets, by translingual spray, or by lingual aerosols. The onset of action from sublingual and a transmucosal tablet is 2 to 5 minutes. Oral capsules or sustained-release tablets are absorbed easily through the GI tract. However, absorption is less predictable with topical ointment and transdermal patch because these depend on the amount of cutaneous circulation. Nitrates may also be given IV. When administering nitrates, the nurse should:

- Instruct patients with angina pectoris to carry nitrates with them at all times for an unexpected anginal attack.
- Teach patients the proper way to store nitrates: away from heat and in a light-protected, dark container. The cotton filler should be discarded because cotton can absorb the drug.
- Tell the patient to replace the nitrate tablet supply every 3 months for freshness.
- Instruct the patient to avoid drinking alcoholic beverages during nitrate therapy to prevent excessive vasodilation, hypotension, and fainting.
- Instruct the patient to sit or lie down before administering the initial oral nitrate dose, and monitor the patient's pulse and blood pressure (BP).
- Caution the patient to sit for a few minutes before standing to prevent orthostatic hypotension.
- Inform the patient that the sustained release tablet should be swallowed and not chewed or crushed to ensure that the capsule reaches the GI tract.
- Encourage the patient to avoid swallowing the sublingual nitrate tablet but allow it to absorb sublingually to ensure effectiveness in an emergency situation.
- Teach the patient to place translingual spray under the tongue for effectiveness.
- Instruct the patient to place a sublingual nitrate under the tongue or in the buccal pouch to relieve an acute anginal attack. The dose may be repeated twice at 5-minute intervals when chest pain is unrelieved for a total of 3 doses.

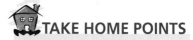

TAKE HOME POINTS

The normal sublingual dose range is 0.3 to 0.6 mg, with a maximum of three tablets given at 5-minute intervals over a 15-minute period.

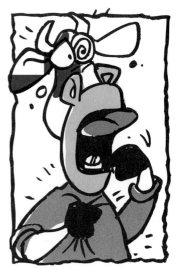

Don't swallow, just let it dissolve.

- Instruct the patient to notify the health care provider when pain persists after three nitrates.
- Instruct the patient to use a plastic wrap cover over a transdermal patch to avoid clothing stains.
- Encourage the patient to rotate the sites of topical application to reduce the risk for skin abrasion.
- Inform patients that tolerance to nitrates may develop within 10 days to 2 weeks, particularly after high-dose, long-term therapy. Using the lowest effective dose and following an intermittent dose schedule can minimize nitrate tolerance.
- Tell the patient not to discontinue nitrate abruptly but taper gradually after long-term therapy.
- Monitor the patient's BP and pulse every 5 to 15 minutes while titrating the IV nitroglycerin dose, then every hour thereafter.
- Use the IV tubing that the manufacturer supplied when administering IV nitroglycerin to ensure efficacy because standard IV tubing absorbs nitroglycerin.
- Use an infusion pump when administering IV nitroglycerin and carefully calculate the dose according to manufacturer's tables.

Inform the patient that nitrates should be gradually tapered on discontinuation of long-term therapy because abrupt withdrawal may cause an MI.

Do You UNDERSTAND?

DIRECTIONS: **Indicate in the space provided whether the statement is *true* or *false*. If the answer is false, correct the statement to make it true (using the margin space).**

_____ 1. Nitrates increase preload and afterload, thereby acting as antianginals.

_____ 2. Nitrates may be taken for immediate relief or prevention of anginal pain.

What IS a Calcium Channel Blocker?

Refer to page 245 for the discussion of calcium channel blockers.

Answers: 1. false; nitrates decrease preload and afterload; 2. true.

What IS a Beta Blocker?

Refer to page 239 for the discussion of β-adrenergic antagonists.

What IS a Cardiac Glycoside?

Cardiac Glycoside	Trade Name	Uses
digoxin [dih-JOX-in]	Lanoxin, Lanoxicaps	Treatment of CHF, atrial dysrhythmias, and cardiogenic shock

Action

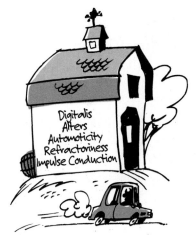

Cardiac glycosides, also known as inotropic or cardiotonic agents are naturally occurring substances found in foxglove plants and in certain toads. These drugs affect the mechanical and electrical action of the heart. The mechanical effect increases the force of myocardial contractility. Digitalis alters the electrical activity in noncontractile tissue and ventricular muscle, which includes the sinoatrial (SA) node, atrioventricular (AV) node, and the Purkinje fibers. Digitalis has the ability to alter automaticity, refractoriness, and impulse conduction. Automaticity refers to the automatic or involuntary functioning of cardiac muscle that occurs because the autonomic nervous system is responsible for controlling cardiac muscular activity. Refractoriness refers to the brief period of repolarization of neuron or muscle fibers when excitability is depressed. The cell may respond at this time when stimulated, but a stronger-than-normal stimulus is required. Impulse conduction refers to electrical impulses transmitted through the conduction system of the heart.

The mechanical effects of cardiac glycosides involve a positive inotropic action on the heart (e.g., an increase in the force of ventricular contractility). Digitalis inhibits an enzyme known as sodium-potassium-ATPase **(Na-K-ATPase),** thereby accomplishing a positive inotropic action. Inhibition of the Na-K-ATPase enzyme blocks the entry of potassium into a cardiac cell and forces sodium out. With each successive action after digitalis alteration, the cardiac cell level of potassium decreases and sodium increases. An increase in sodium leads to an increase in calcium. The calcium accumulation acts to increase the contractile force of the cardiac tissue via proteins, actin, and myosin. Mechanically increasing myocardial contractility increases CO. Results from digitalis-induced increase in CO include decreased sympathetic tone (reducing the heart rate and allowing more ventricular filling time), decreased arterial constriction (allowing greater ventricular emptying), and decreased venous constriction (allowing a reduction in pulmonary congestion and peripheral edema). Another result of a digitalis-induced increase in CO, which improves renal flow, is an increase in urine production, allowing a loss of water and blood volume. Finally, the third result of a digitalis-induced increase in CO is a decrease in renin release, allowing a decrease in the renin-angiotensin-aldosterone system (RAAS), a decrease of vasoconstriction, and a decrease of sodium and water retention.

The electrical effects of digitalis involve inhibiting the Na-K-ATPase enzyme and enhancing the vagal influence on the heart. Because inhibiting Na-K-ATPase decreases the potassium level and increases the sodium and calcium levels in cardiac cells, this ion redistribution alters electrical cell responsiveness. This digitalis-induced alteration in ion distribution and increase in central nervous system stimulation of vagal fibers innervating the heart cause decreased automaticity of the SA node, decreased conduction through the AV node (which prolongs the refractory period), and increased automaticity in the Purkinje fibers.

Uses

Cardiac glycoside is used for treating heart failure (HF) because the actions of digitalis reverse its harmful effects. The reversal of harmful effects includes improving CO, decreasing heart rate and size, reducing vasoconstriction, and reducing water retention and blood volume, thereby reducing peripheral and pulmonary edema. Cardiac glycosides are also used in treating atrial fibrillation, atrial flutter, paroxysmal atrial tachycardia, supraventricular dysrhythmias, and cardiogenic shock.

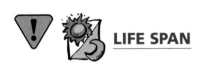 **LIFE SPAN**

- Cardiac glycosides should be used cautiously in patients with hypokalemia, hypothyroidism, advanced heart disease, acute MI, and renal insufficiency.
- Cardiac glycosides should also be used cautiously in premature infants, children, older adults, debilitated patients, pregnancy, and lactation.

What You NEED TO KNOW

Contraindications/Precautions

Digitalis is contraindicated for patients with a hypersensitivity, ventricular tachycardia or fibrillation, sick sinus syndrome, heart block, acute MI, electrolyte abnormalities, and renal dysfunction.

Drug Interactions

The therapeutic effects of cardiac glycosides are decreased when taken concurrently with antacids, neomycin, sulfasalazine, barbiturates, phenytoin, rifampin, metoclopramide, kaolin, pectin, cholestyramine, and methotrexate. Giving BBs, succinylcholine, and thyroid preparations with cardiac glycosides may lead to excessive bradycardia and other dysrhythmias. Giving verapamil, amiodarone, anticholinergics, quinidine, spironolactone, hydroxychloroquine, erythromycin, tetracycline, itraconazole, omeprazole, and calcium preparations concurrently with cardiac glycosides may lead to digitalis toxicity. Additionally, when amphotericin B, steroids, and potassium-wasting diuretics are given with cardiac glycosides, hypokalemia and digitalis toxicity may occur.

Adverse Effects

The adverse effects of cardiac glycosides include dizziness, drowsiness, headache, confusion, mental depression, hallucinations, malaise, fatigue, muscle weakness, paresthesia, diaphoresis, agitation, visual changes, anorexia, nausea, vomiting, diarrhea, hypotension, and dysrhythmias. Cardiac glycosides have a narrow therapeutic range; thus they may lead to digitalis toxicity. Conditions that may predispose a patient to digitalis toxicity include hypokalemia, hypomagnesemia, hypothyroidism, hypoxemia, hypercalcemia, increased vagal tone, and myocardial ischemia.

The most frequent early signs of digitalis toxicity include anorexia, nausea, vomiting, and diarrhea. Typically, the subsequent signs of toxicity include visual disturbances of blurred vision, visual illusions (e.g., yellow-green halos around objects), blind spots, flashing lights, diplopia, and photophobia. Bradycardia (e.g., a pulse less than 60 per minute) is a common sign of digitalis toxicity, in addition to premature ventricular contraction and first-degree, second-degree, or complete heart block. The antidote for severe digitalis toxicity is digoxin immune Fab (Digibind). This agent binds with digoxin to form complex molecules that are excreted in the urine.

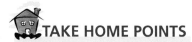

TAKE HOME POINTS

Drugs that reduce digitalis absorption (e.g., antacids, kaolin, pectin) should not be given concurrently.

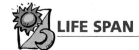

LIFE SPAN

Advanced age may also predispose an individual to digitalis toxicity.

What You DO

Nursing Responsibilities

To avoid waiting for weeks for a desired therapeutic concentration, cardiac glycosides are initially begun with loading doses. After the loading dose raises the digitalis blood concentration level rapidly, a smaller dose that maintains the drug concentration in a therapeutic range is given on a regular schedule. When administering cardiac glycosides, the nurse should:

- Monitor digoxin serum levels throughout digitalis treatment.
- Ensure that the digitalis level has been drawn at least 8 hours after the last dose to avoid falsely elevated serum levels. Preferably, the blood should be drawn immediately before administering the daily dose, which allows 24 hours since the last dose. The normal therapeutic range is 0.8 to 2.0 ng/mL. A serum level of 2.0 ng/mL or more is considered toxic.
- Teach patients to take their own pulse and report a pulse rate that is less than 60 per minute, changes in regularity, or signs of digitalis toxicity.
- Encourage the patient to eat foods that are high in vitamin K, such as orange juice, bananas, apples, prunes, raisins, dates, cantaloupe, watermelon, beans, potatoes, and squash, unless the patient is taking a vitamin K supplement.
- Instruct patients to consult with their health care provider before taking any other medication, including OTC drugs.
- Assess the apical heart rate and rhythm before administering digitalis. When the pulse is less than 60 beats per minute for an adult, less than 90 beats per minute in an infant, or a change in rhythm is noted, the nurse should withhold the drug and retake the pulse in 1 hour. If the heart rate does not meet criteria at this time, notify the health care provider.
- Administer an IV digitalis dose slowly over 5 minutes.
- Instruct patients who are taking digitalis to avoid taking an extra dose when a dose is missed; instead, they should notify their health care provider.

Do You UNDERSTAND?

DIRECTIONS: Provide appropriate responses to the following questions.

1. What is the best time to draw digoxin blood level?

_____

2. What is the normal therapeutic range for digoxin blood level?

_____

3. What important nursing intervention should the nurse carry out before administering digoxin administration?

_____

What IS a Phosphodiesterase Inhibitor?

Phosphodiesterase Inhibitors	Trade Names	Uses
amrinone lactate *[AM-rih-nohn LAK-tate]*	Inocor	Short-term treatment of congestive heart failure
milrinone lactate *[MILL-rih-nohn LAK-tate]*	Primacor	Short-term treatment of congestive heart failure

Action

Phosphodiesterase inhibitors exert an inotropic effect on the heart, thereby increasing the force of myocardial contractility. These agents also dilate arteries and veins, which decreases preload and afterload. Inhibiting cyclic adenosine monophosphate phosphodiesterase (cAMP) activity in cardiac and vascular muscle tissue helps accomplish this action. Because cAMP serves as a second control of intracellular calcium and myocardial contraction, interference of cAMP by phosphodiesterase inhibitors leads to the inhibition of cAMP degradation. This action causes a rise in intracellular adenosine monophosphate, leading to increased contractility, increased CO, decreased systemic vascular resistance, decreased venous return, reduced ventricular filling pressure, and reduced pulmonary capillary wedge pressure (PCWP).

Uses

Phosphodiesterase inhibitors are indicated in short-term management of HF (up to a 48-hour infusion). Milrinone has been used to increase cardiac function before heart transplantation. Because this drug class has been associated with development of potentially fatal ventricular dysrhythmias, its use is limited to severe situations.

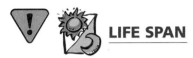 LIFE SPAN

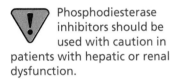

Caution should be used when administering phosphodiesterase inhibitors to women who are pregnant or lactating and to older adults.

Phosphodiesterase inhibitors should be used with caution in patients with hepatic or renal dysfunction.

What You NEED TO KNOW

Contraindications/Precautions

Phosphodiesterase inhibitors are contraindicated for patients with acute MI, hypokalemia (until corrected), fluid volume deficit, ventricular dysrhythmias, or hypersensitivity. Amrinone is also contraindicated for patients who are hypersensitive to bisulfites.

Drug Interactions

Few drug interactions occur with phosphodiesterase inhibitors. When phosphodiesterase inhibitors are given concurrently with disopyramide, excessive hypotension may result.

Adverse Effects

Adverse effects of phosphodiesterase inhibitors include headache, anorexia, nausea, vomiting, abdominal cramps, hypotension, and dysrhythmias. Amrinone also may cause thrombocytopenia. Other serious adverse effects include hepatotoxicity and nephrogenic diabetes insipidus.

What You DO

Nursing Responsibilities

Because phosphodiesterase inhibitors are administered IV, the patient must be monitored carefully. When giving phosphodiesterase inhibitors, the nurse should:
• Evaluate the BP, cardiac rhythm and rate, CO, and PCWP during and for several hours after administration because of the potential risk for severe hypotension and dysrhythmias.

- Slow or stop the phosphodiesterase inhibitor IV solution immediately in the presence of significant hypotension and dysrhythmias.
- Titrate drug doses for maximal hemodynamic effect according to prescribed parameters.
- Monitor the blood level of these drugs. The normal therapeutic amrinone level is 0.5 to 7.0 mcg/mL.
- Evaluate the platelet count before treatment for a baseline and frequently during treatment because of potential thrombocytopenia. When the platelet count drops below 150,000/mm^3, the nurse should immediately report this information to the health care provider.
- Realize that the natural color of amrinone is a clear yellow. When amrinone is discolored or contains a precipitate, it should be discarded.

Do You UNDERSTAND?

DIRECTIONS: **Place a check next to each statement that correctly applies to phosphodiesterase inhibitors.**

- _____ 1. Increased preload
- _____ 2. Long-term therapy
- _____ 3. Monitor cardiac status, rhythm, pulse, BP, CO, heart rate, and PCWP
- _____ 4. Stop infusion for significant hypotension or dysrhythmias

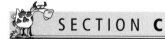 **SECTION C**

ANTILIPIDEMICS

This section reviews the pharmacologic methods used to treat hyperlipidemia, which is an increase in lipids in the blood. Antilipidemics are agents that lower lipids, including cholesterol, triglycerides, and low-density lipoproteins (LDLs). Cholesterol is a sterol\ lipid found in many body tissues, such as brain, spinal cord, kidneys, adrenal glands, and liver.

Answers: 3 and 4.

It is important for metabolism and steroid hormones. Triglycerides constitute a large portion of lipids in the blood. LDLs deliver cholesterol to nonhepatic tissues and are responsible for the greatest contribution of cholesterol to coronary atherosclerosis.

Investigations have established that cardiovascular morbidity and mortality is directly related to elevated total cholesterol, triglycerides, and LDL levels, in addition to inversely lowered high-density lipoprotein (HDL) levels. Therefore the primary goal of cholesterol-lowering drugs is to decrease total cholesterol and LDL levels and to increase HDL levels. Reducing LDL levels may arrest or reverse atherosclerosis, thereby reducing morbidity and mortality in cardiovascular disease. The selected antilipidemic groups that are discussed include HMG-CoA reductase inhibitors, bile acid sequestrants, fibric acid derivatives, and other selected antilipidemic agents.

What IS an HMG-CoA Reductase Inhibitor?

HMG-CoA Reductase Inhibitors	Trade Names	Uses
lovastatin [loe-vah-STAT-in]	Mevacor	Treatment of moderate hypercholesterolemia
simvastatin [sim-vah-STAT-in]	Zocor	Treatment of hypercholesterolemia
atorvastatin [a-tor-vah-STAT-in]	Lipitor	Treatment of elevated cholesterol, LDL levels, and triglycerides
pravastatin [pra-vah-STAT-in]	Pravachol	Treatment of hypercholesterolemia
rosuvastatin [ross-uh-vah-STAT-in]	Crestor	Treatment of elevated cholesterol, LDL levels, and triglycerides

Action

HMG-CoA reductase inhibitors (**statins**) selectively inhibit the enzyme HMG-CoA reductase, which is the rate-limiting enzyme in cholesterol synthesis. HMG-CoA reductase inhibitors block the production of cholesterol, which decreases LDL cholesterol, total cholesterol, very low-density lipoprotein (VLDL) cholesterol, and triglycerides. These inhibitors also increase HDL cholesterol levels. The mechanism of the LDL-lowering effect leads to a decreased production or increased catabolism of LDLs.

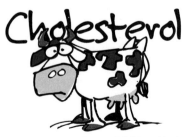

Let HMG-CoA reductase inhibitors block its production.

Uses

HMG-CoA reductase inhibitors are used to treat hypercholesterolemia and dyslipidemia when dietary restrictions and other nonpharmacologic measures have been inadequate. These agents are also used to prevent atherosclerosis, coronary artery disease, and MI.

What You NEED TO KNOW

Contraindications/Precautions

HMG-CoA reductase inhibitors are contraindicated for patients with hypersensitivity, unexplained elevated liver function studies, and active liver disease.

Drug Interactions

Drug interactions of HMG-CoA reductase inhibitors include an increased risk for myopathy and rhabdomyolysis when given concurrently with cyclosporine, gemfibrozil, and erythromycin. Elevated creatine phosphokinase (CPK or CK) levels and renal dysfunction are usually associated with rhabdomyolysis.

Adverse Effects

The majority of adverse effects of HMG-CoA reductase inhibitors are usually mild and transient. Adverse effects include fever, fatigue, dizziness, fainting, palpitations, headache, photosensitivity, blurred vision, anxiety, insomnia, orthostatic hypotension, hypertension, nosebleeds, and tinnitus. GI adverse effects of these agents include increased appetite, dry mouth, alteration in taste, anorexia, nausea, vomiting, diarrhea, constipation, abdominal cramping, GI ulcerations, hepatitis, and pancreatitis. Other adverse effects include skin discoloration, sweating, hives, acne, petechiae, anemia, hyperglycemia, hypoglycemia, decreased libido, breast enlargement, gout, urinary frequency and retention, urgency, incontinence, and muscle pain. More serious adverse effects include facial paralysis, deafness, glaucoma, cataract development, memory loss, depression, thrombocytopenia, renal calculi, angioedema, dyspnea, dysrhythmias, rhabdomyolysis, and Stevens-Johnson syndrome.

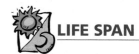

LIFE SPAN

HMG-CoA reductase inhibitors are contraindicated for women during pregnancy and lactation.

HMG-CoA reductase inhibitors should be used with caution in renal dysfunction, and doses may be decreased. Rhabdomyolysis is a fatal disease involving skeletal muscle destruction.

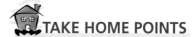

TAKE HOME POINTS

Instruct the patient who is taking HMG-CoA reductase inhibitors to:
- Discontinue these drugs immediately when becoming pregnant to avoid harmful effects to the fetus.
- Report unexplained muscle pain, tenderness, or weakness, particularly when fever or malaise occurs.

What You DO

Nursing Responsibilities

The peak therapeutic response of antilipidemics occurs within 4 to 6 weeks and is maintained throughout therapy. HMG-CoA reductase inhibitors are more effective when taken in the evening compared with other times of the day because cholesterol is synthesized mostly at night. These agents may be taken without regard to meals. However, when combination therapy is used, HMG-CoA reductase inhibitors should be given at least 2 hours after a bile acid sequestrant. When administering HMG-CoA reductase inhibitors, the nurse should:

- Teach the patient to take HMG-CoA reductase inhibitors at bedtime for increased effectiveness.
- Encourage the patient to avoid prolonged sunlight and ultraviolet light exposure and to take safety measures of wearing protective clothing and using sunscreens.
- Instruct the patient to report unexplained muscle pain or weakness, particularly when accompanied by fever or dark red-brown urine, which may indicate rhabdomyolysis.
- Monitor CPK levels carefully for early detection of rhabdomyolysis and possible drug discontinuation.
- Obtain baseline liver function studies before initiating therapy, again at 6 and 12 weeks, and at 6-month intervals thereafter for early detection of liver dysfunction.
- Reevaluate patients monthly to determine any dose adjustments.
- Encourage the patient to have frequent ophthalmic examinations for early detection of cataracts.
- Encourage the patient in lifestyle changes, such as low cholesterol diet.
- Teach the female patient to use barrier contraceptives because the risk for severe fetal abnormalities is great.

Do You UNDERSTAND?

DIRECTIONS: Provide the appropriate responses to the following statements.

1. Rhabdomyolysis is an adverse effect of HMG-CoA reductase inhibitors characterized by what five symptoms?

2. What is the best time of day to take HMG-CoA reductase inhibitors?

3. Circle any of the following that are adverse effects of HMG-CoA reductase inhibitors.

   Hypertension   Hyperglycemia
   Hypotension   Hypoglycemia

What IS a Bile Acid Sequestrant?

Bile Acid Sequestrants	Trade Names	Uses
cholestyramine *[koe-less-TEAR-a-meen]*	Questran	Adjunct treatment of hypercholesterolemia
colestipol *[koe-LESS-ti-pole]*	Colestid	Adjunct treatment of hypercholesterolemia

Action

Bile acid sequestrants (**bile acid-sequestering resins** or **bile acid-binding resins**) bind bile in the intestine to form an insoluble complex that is excreted in the feces. This action results in the partial removal of bile salts, preventing their reabsorption. The loss of bile salts leads to a decrease in LDL and serum cholesterol levels. These drugs increase

Answers: 1. muscle pain, tenderness, weakness, fever, malaise; 2. evening; 3. all of the choices.

hepatic synthesis of cholesterol but decrease plasma cholesterol levels, resulting from an increased clearance rate of cholesterol lipoproteins.

Uses

Bile acid sequestrants agents are used to reduce elevated serum cholesterol in patients with hypercholesterolemia and elevated LDLs. These agents are usually initiated when other nonpharmacologic measures are inadequate.

What You NEED TO KNOW

Caution should be used when administering bile acid sequestrants to children and to women who are pregnant or lactating.
Bile acid sequestrants should be used with caution in patients with bleeding disorders, GI disorders, and hemorrhoids.

Contraindications/Precautions

Bile acid sequestrants are contraindicated for patients with hypersensitivity and complete biliary obstruction.

Drug Interactions

Drug interactions that involve bile acid sequestrants include a decreased anticoagulant effect when given together with anticoagulants. Cholestyramine may enhance the elimination of piroxicam when these drugs are given concurrently. Cholestyramine and colestipol may reduce the absorption of ursodiol. Malabsorption of fat-soluble vitamins A, D, E, and K may occur when given concurrently with bile acid sequestrants.

Adverse Effects

The most common adverse effect of bile acid sequestrants is diarrhea or constipation, leading to fecal impaction and the aggravation of hemorrhoids. Other less frequent adverse effects include headache, dizziness, anxiety, tinnitus, fainting, fatigue, drowsiness, insomnia, chest pain, tachycardia, anemia, increased prothrombin time, hypersensitivity, muscle and joint pain, dysuria, hematuria, weight loss or gain, increased libido, edema, and paresthesia. GI adverse effects include anorexia, abdominal pain, distention, flatulence, heartburn, nausea, vomiting, taste alteration, ulceration, and bleeding.

What You DO

Nursing Responsibilities

After initiating treatment with bile acid sequestrants, LDL levels decline in 4 to 7 days and serum cholesterol levels decrease in 1 month. When administering bile acid sequestrants, the nurse should:

- Advise patients to take bile acid sequestrants at mealtimes.
- Instruct the patient to mix powder forms with fluids and avoid taking the medicine dry. This process helps avoid accidental inhalation or esophageal distress.
- Monitor cholesterol and triglyceride levels frequently during the first few months of therapy and periodically thereafter to ascertain efficacy.
- Teach patients with coronary artery disease to take a laxative, stool softener, and increased fluid or fiber to avoid straining because bile acid sequestrants may cause constipation and fecal impaction.

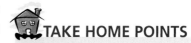

TAKE HOME POINTS

Instruct the patient to increase daily fluid intake.

Do You UNDERSTAND?

DIRECTIONS: Indicate in the space provided whether each statement is *true* or *false*. If the answer is false, correct the statement to make it true (using the margin space).

_____ 1. During bile acid sequestrants therapy, malabsorption of vitamins B, C, and K may occur.

_____ 2. The most common adverse effect of bile acid sequestrants is diarrhea.

Fibric acid derivatives should be used cautiously in patients with biliary disease, peptic ulcer disease, hypothyroidism, and cardiovascular disease. Gemfibrozil should be used with caution in patients with DM.

What IS a Fibric Acid Agent?

Fibric Acid Agents	Trade Names	Uses
clofibrate [kloe-FY-brate]	Atromid-S	Adjunct therapy in hyperlipidemia
fenofibrate [fen-oh-FIE-brate]	Tricor	Treatment of elevated triglyceride levels
gemfibrozil [gem-FI-broe-zil]	Lopid	Treatment of elevated triglyceride levels

Action

The action of fibric acid derivatives is unknown; however, the triglyceride-lowering effect seems to be a result of accelerated catabolism of VLDL to LDL and reduced hepatic synthesis of VLDL. Cholesterol formation is inhibited early in the process, and excretion of cholesterol is increased. Both of the fibric acid derivatives decrease serum triglycerides, cholesterol, LDLs, and VLDLs. Gemfibrozil also increases HDL levels.

Uses

Clofibrate is used to treat severe hyperlipidemia. Gemfibrozil is used to treat severe hypertriglyceridemia.

What You NEED TO KNOW

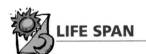 **LIFE SPAN**

Fibric acid derivatives are contraindicated for children under 14 years of age and for women during pregnancy and lactation.

Contraindications/Precautions

These agents are contraindicated for patients with renal or hepatic dysfunction.

Drug Interactions

Clofibrate and gemfibrozil interact with oral anticoagulants, increasing the risk for bleeding. Probenecid increases the action of clofibrate when given together. When clofibrate is given concurrently with sulfonylureas, hypoglycemia is increased. When gemfibrozil and lovastatin are given together, the risk for myopathy and rhabdomyolysis is increased. When clofibrate is given concurrently with sulfonylureas, the hypoglycemic effects are enhanced.

Adverse Effects

The adverse effects of fibric acid derivatives include headache, dizziness, flatulence, nausea, vomiting, diarrhea, abdominal pain, rash, itching, hives, myalgia, muscle soreness, weakness, eosinophilia, anemia, neutropenia, leukopenia, agranulocytosis, renal dysfunction, elevated liver enzymes, or hepatic dysfunction. Additionally, clofibrate may cause drowsiness, gastritis, decreased libido, and impotence. Gemfibrozil may cause blurred vision, arthralgia, hypokalemia, and moderate hyperglycemia.

What You DO

Nursing Responsibilities

A therapeutic response usually occurs within 1 to 2 months. A rebound effect may occur in the second or third month, followed by a further decrease in lipids. When administering fibric acid derivatives, the nurse should:

- Instruct the patient who is taking gemfibrozil to take the drug 30 minutes before morning and evening meals, unless GI distress develops; gemfibrozil may then be taken with meals.
- Monitor patients for gastric pain, nausea, vomiting, and pulmonary edema.
- Evaluate baseline LDL, VLDL, triglyceride, and total cholesterol levels before therapy, again every 2 weeks during the first few months of therapy, and at monthly intervals thereafter.
- Monitor CBC, glucose, electrolytes, prothrombin time (PT), and renal and hepatic function studies frequently throughout fibric acid derivative therapy.
- Instruct the patient to report any bleeding, bruising, epistaxis, and hematuria.
- Counsel patients to avoid operating hazardous machinery until the drug effect is known.
- Warn patients to avoid self-dosing with OTC drugs without consulting the health care provider.

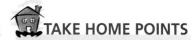

TAKE HOME POINTS

Instruct the patient to report influenza-like symptoms of muscle soreness and weakness. This action facilitates differentiation of adverse effects from viral or bacterial disease.

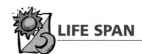

LIFE SPAN

Teach women of childbearing age about the importance of a birth control regimen. When clofibrate is given, the drug should be discontinued at least 2 months before conception.

Do You UNDERSTAND?

DIRECTIONS: **Indicate in the space provided whether each statement is *true* or *false*. If the answer is false, correct the statement to make it true (using the margin space).**

_____ 1. When gemfibrozil is combined with lovastatin, the risk for rhabdomyolysis is increased.

_____ 2. Fibric acid derivatives are ideal antihyperlipidemics for patients with renal and hepatic dysfunction.

What IS a Miscellaneous Antilipidemic Agent?

Miscellaneous Antilipidemic Agents	Trade Names	Uses
niacin, nicotinic acid [NYE-a-sin]	Novo-Niacin	Treatment of hyperlipidemia
fenofibrate [fen-o-FI-brate]	Tricor	Treatment of elevated triglycerides
ezetimibe [eh-ZEH-tih-myb]	Zetia	Treatment of elevated cholesterol levels

Action

The exact action of niacin (**nicotinic acid** or **vitamin B$_3$**) is unknown; however, niacin inhibits lipolysis in adipose tissue, decreases triglyceride esterification in the liver, and increases lipoprotein lipase activity. In summary, niacin reduces serum cholesterol, triglyceride, LDL, and VLDL levels and increases HDL levels. Fenofibrate inhibits triglyceride synthesis. This action lowers VLDL production, stimulates catabolism of triglycerides, and increases HDL cholesterol levels. Ezetimibe is the first drug in a new class of antilipidemics called cholesterol absorption inhibitor. This drug inhibits absorption of cholesterol from the small intestine.

Answers: 1. true; 2. false; fibric acid derivatives are contraindicated for patients with renal and hepatic dysfunction.

Uses

Niacin is used to treat hyperlipidemia. Fenofibrate is used to treat elevated triglyceride levels when patients fail to respond adequately to nonpharmacologic measures.

What You NEED TO KNOW

Contraindications/Precautions

Niacin is contraindicated for patients with hypersensitivity, hepatic dysfunction, severe hypotension, bleeding, and active peptic ulcers. Fenofibrate is contraindicated for patients with hypersensitivity, hepatic or renal dysfunction, gallbladder disease, and thrombocytopenia.

Drug Interactions

The risk of hypotension is increased when antihypertensives are given with niacin. Absorption may be decreased when fenofibrate is given with cholestyramine and colestipol. When combined with HMG-CoA reductase inhibitors, the risk for rhabdomyolysis or acute renal failure is increased. The combination of fenofibrate and cyclosporine may increase the risk for nephrotoxicity.

Adverse Effects

The adverse effects of niacin include flushing, warmth, headache, dizziness, hypotension, fatigue, tingling in extremities, fainting, nervousness, blurred vision, loss of central vision, dry skin, rash, itching, jaundice, flatulence, nausea, vomiting, peptic ulcers, hyperglycemia, hyperuricemia, hypoprothrombinemia, and hypoalbuminemia. Dysrhythmias are rare adverse effects. Additional adverse effects of fenofibrate include arthralgia, paresthesia, insomnia, increased appetite, diarrhea, cough, rhinitis, sinusitis, decreased libido, and eye floaters.

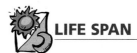 **LIFE SPAN**

Niacin, ezetimibe, and fenofibrate are contraindicated for women during pregnancy and lactation and for children.

Fenofibrate should be used cautiously in patients who are taking HMG-CoA reductase inhibitors and oral anticoagulants together.
Fenofibrate also should be used cautiously in patients with renal impairment, history of bleeding disorders, and myelosuppression (reduced bone marrow function), as well as in older adults.

Niacin should be used cautiously in patients with a history of gallbladder, liver, or coronary artery disease, peptic ulcers, glaucoma, DM, or gout.

What You DO

Nursing Responsibilities

This group of agents should not be given with hot beverages, but rather, with cold water to facilitate swallowing. The absorption is increased with food. However, when bile acid sequestrants are given concurrently, niacin should be separated and given 1 hour before or 4 to 6 hours after bile acid sequestrants. When administering nicotinic acid agents, the nurse should:

* Monitor lipid levels, liver function studies, and CBC periodically for patients who are taking niacin.
* Monitor the glucose level in the patient with diabetes for necessary dose adjustments because of the risk for hyperglycemia.
* Observe patients for hepatic dysfunction (e.g., itching, jaundice, dark urine, light-colored stools).
* Monitor the PT of patients who are taking niacin and Coumadin concurrently.
* Warn the patient who is taking niacin that transient flushing in the face, ears, and neck may occur within 2 hours after oral administration. Relief of transient flushing may be obtained with dose reduction or changing to a sustained-release form of niacin.
* Instruct the patient to report muscle pain, tenderness, and weakness. When muscle pain is present, the CPK should be monitored.
* Explain to the patient the importance of reporting any visual disturbances.

TAKE HOME POINTS

* Assess the patient who is taking niacin and antihypertensives for hypotension.
* Instruct the patient to take niacin agents with *cold* rather than hot beverages. Cold liquids will decrease the risk for persistent flushing. Inform the patient that taking aspirin 30 minutes before niacin may reduce the persistent flushing. Instruct the patient to report any visual disturbances.

Do You UNDERSTAND?

DIRECTIONS: Fill in the blanks with appropriate responses.

1. Visual disturbances from niacin include _____ _____.

2. The patient should be monitored for evidence of hepatic dysfunction, which includes _____.

Answers: 1. blurred vision, loss of central vision, or eye floaters; 2. itching, jaundice, dark urine, and light-colored stools.

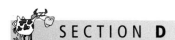

SECTION D

ANTIDYSRHYTHMICS

A dysrhythmia is defined as any deviation from the normal heart rhythm; usually a rapid, irregular rhythm. Antidysrhythmic drugs suppress irregular heart rhythms using one or a combination of actions. These drugs may depress automaticity, decrease conduction, or increase the refractoriness to premature stimulation. The dysrhythmia may develop in any of the cardiac structures, including the SA or AV nodes, atria, bundle branches, ventricles, or myocardial tissue. Dysrhythmias may develop as a result of imbalances in acid-base or electrolytes, smoking, caffeine intake, infections, heart lesions, myocardial infarction, or ventricular hypertrophy related to heart failure. Dysrhythmias are found in 90% to 95% of patients who have had a myocardial infarction and can be mild or severe, acute or chronic, episodic or continuous in nature.

Some drugs are more effective than are others against atrial or ventricular dysrhythmias or both. Antidysrhythmics are classified according to the effect on the heart's electrical conduction. Classes I, II, III, and IV. Class I is subdivided into three categories; A, B, and C. Antidysrhythmic drugs that do not fall into the four classes are referred to as miscellaneous antidysrhythmics.

What IS a Class IA Antidysrhythmic?

Class IA Antidysrhythmics	Trade Names	Uses
moricizine [mor-I-ci-zeen]	Ethmozine	Treatment of sustained ventricular tachycardia and premature ventricular contractions
quinidine [KWIN-ih-deen]	Quinidex	Treatment of atrial fibrillation with cardioversion
procainamide [pro-CANE- uh-mide]	Pronestyl	Treatment of ventricular tachycardia refractory to lidocaine; treatment of ventricular fibrillation; rate control in atrial fibrillation
disopyramide [DIE-so-PIR-uh-mide]	Norpace	Treatment of life-threatening ventricular dysrhythmias

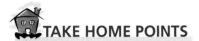

TAKE HOME POINTS

Antidysrhythmics, regardless of the class, are considered myocardial depressants.

Action

Most class IA antidysrhythmic drugs act by restricting the flow of sodium into the myocardial cell, thereby decreasing contractility. They suppress automaticity by lowering the action potential needed to trigger spontaneous depolarization. Class IA drugs prolong the effective refractory periods and have membrane stabilizing effects. Low dosages speed AV conduction via vagolytic effect. High dosages block AV conduction. In a sense, they can be considered a cardiac specific local anesthetic. Class I drug effects on the ECG in general include prolonged PR, QRS, and QT intervals.

Moricizine shares the properties of class IA, IB, and IC. It decreases the rapid current that is carried inward by sodium ions, has local anesthetic activity, and stabilizes the myocardial membrane. Moricizine shortens repolarization, leading to decreased action potential and an effective refractory period.

Uses

Moricizine is used in the treatment of sustained ventricular tachycardia and premature ventricular contractions. Quinidine sulfate is used in the treatment of atrial fibrillation with cardioversion.

Procainamide is used to treat ventricular tachycardia refractory to lidocaine and to treat ventricular fibrillation. It is also used in conjunction with cardioversion for rate control in atrial fibrillation. Disopyramide is used to suppress PVCs and ventricular tachycardia but is used primarily for its unlabeled use of treating supraventricular tachycardias, such as paroxysmal atrial tachycardia, atrial flutter, and atrial fibrillation.

What You NEED TO KNOW

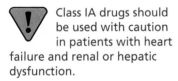

Class IA drugs should be used with caution in patients with heart failure and renal or hepatic dysfunction.

Contraindications/Precautions

Class IA drugs are contraindicated for patients who have second- or third-degree AV block, bradycardia, cardiogenic shock, and bundle branch block, unless a pacemaker is present. Because the drug prolongs the PR and QT intervals, heart blocks may be worsened. Procainamide and quinidine are contraindicated in patients who have myasthenia gravis.

Drug Interactions

Cimetidine increases the serum levels of class IA drugs. Moricizine decreases levels of theophylline. Additive anticholinergic effects occur when class IA drugs are given with antihistamines or tricyclic antidepressants.

Disopyramide and quinidine sulfate can exacerbate the anticoagulation effects of warfarin. Rifampin, phenobarbital, and phenytoin decrease the serum levels of disopyramide and quinidine sulfate. Procainamide and quinidine enhance the effects of neuromuscular blocking drugs. Antihypertensive drugs and nitrates may increase the hypotensive effect of procainamide and quinidine. Procainamide and quinidine reduce the effects of cholinesterase inhibitors.

Disopyramide should not be given within 48 hours before or 24 hours after the calcium channel blocking drug verapamil because this combination causes excessive prolonging of conduction and decreased cardiac output. Procainamide can cause central nervous system (CNS) toxicity when given with lidocaine. Quinidine and trimethoprim increase the effects of procainamide. Quinidine increases digoxin levels, and amiodarone increases quinidine levels. Foods that alkalinize the urine may increase quinidine serum levels and cause toxicity.

Adverse Effects

Common CNS adverse effects of class IA drugs include dizziness, headache, fatigue, and nervousness. Common GI adverse effects include nausea, vomiting, and diarrhea. Diarrhea is particularly common with quinidine, which is frequently the reason it is seldom used. Other adverse effects of quinidine include hemolytic anemia and thrombocytopenia. Signs and symptoms of quinidine toxicity include tinnitus, hearing loss, visual disturbances, headache, nausea, and dizziness.

Moricizine may worsen dysrhythmias and actually cause ventricular tachycardia or PVCs. Adverse effects of procainamide include seizures, confusion, leukopenia, agranulocytosis, and thrombocytopenia. Signs of procainamide toxicity include confusion, dizziness, drowsiness, nausea, vomiting, and tachydysrhythmias.

The most common and dangerous adverse effects of class IA drugs are the cardiovascular adverse effects. Class IA drugs may slow conduction excessively, resulting in second- or third-degree AV block, a widened QRS, prolonged PR or QT intervals, or asystole. Procainamide, particularly when given IV, tends to widen the QRS complex, causes AV blocks, and produces hypotension in some patients. Class IA drugs can excessively depress the myocardium and precipitate acute heart failure.

A rare but serious cardiovascular adverse effect of class IA drugs is the occurrence of torsades de pointes dysrhythmia. This dysrhythmia, which may occur with subtherapeutic dosages, is an atypical rapid ventricular tachycardia that may be self-limiting or progress to ventricular fibrillation.

What You DO

Nursing Responsibilities

When administering class IA drugs, the nurse should:

- Realize that procainamide is the only class IA antidysrhythmic that may be given IV. A volumetric pump with microdrip tubing should be used to ensure accurate dose administration. Follow administration instructions carefully to reduce the risk for hypotension, heart block, and asystole. A loading dose of the dysrhythmic drug is usually given, followed by a continuous infusion. The patient should have electrocardiographic monitoring.

- Discontinue procainamide immediately and notify the health care provider if the QRS complex widens by 50%, the PR interval is prolonged, or hypotension develops.

- Realize that procainamide infusions should not be weaned or discontinued until 1 to 1 1/2 hours after an oral dose of procainamide is given to prevent the recurrence of the dysrhythmia.

- Monitor N-acetylprocainamide (NAPA) and serum procainamide levels for patients taking procainamide. Procainamide is converted in the liver to NAPA, which is an active antidysrhythmic metabolite. The therapeutic range is 4 to 8 mcg/mL. Toxicity occurs when serum levels reach 8 to 16 mcg/mL.

- Administer oral class IA drugs 1 hour before or 2 hours after meals because they are absorbed better on an empty stomach and are absorbed poorly with food.

- Instruct patients taking oral formulations of class 1A drugs to take all doses as prescribed and not to double up doses if forgotten.

- Caution patients who are taking quinidine to avoid all fruits (except cranberries, prunes, and plums), all vegetables, and milk to reduce alkalinization of the urine and subsequent toxicity.

- Monitor quinidine levels for patients who are taking quinidine. The therapeutic range is 2 to 6 mcg/mL. Toxicity results when levels exceed 8 mcg/mL.

- Monitor renal and hepatic function studies for the patient who is taking class IA drugs. Dosages of moricizine should be reduced in the presence of hepatic or renal failure.

- Monitor the CBC and platelet counts for patients who are taking quinidine or procainamide.

> ⚠ Discontinue procainamide and immediately report to the health care provider if the patient develops bradycardia, AV block, widening of the QRS complex by 50%, prolonged PR or QT interval, or hypotension.

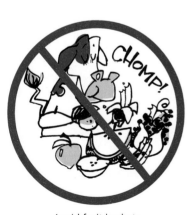

Avoid fruit baskets.

- Report any signs and symptoms of heart failure (e.g., crackles in the lung bases) immediately to the health care provider.
- Advise patients to carry identification that lists all drugs taken, including over-the-counter drugs and herbal preparations.
- Teach patients to report any shortness of breath, irregular heartbeats, or palpitations.
- Warn patients to avoid participating in activities that require alertness until response to the medication is determined.
- Teach patients about the proper way to take their pulse and to report to their health care provider if the pulse is less than 60 beats per minute.

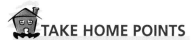

TAKE HOME POINTS

Immediately report any worsening of ventricular dysrhythmias or signs and symptoms of heart failure to the health care provider.

Do You UNDERSTAND?

DIRECTIONS: Complete the following statements with the appropriate terms from the italicized list provided.

1. Foods that alkalinize the urine can increase serum levels of _____ _____.

2. _____ should not be given within 48 hours before or 24 hours after verapamil.

3. _____ can cause central nervous system toxicity when used concurrently with lidocaine.

4. _____ increases quinidine levels.

5. _____ is contraindicated for a patient with third degree AV block.

amiodarone   *procainamide*   *moricizine*
disopyramide   *quinidine*

Answers: 1. quinidine; 2. disopyramide; 3. procainamide; 4. amiodarone; 5. moricizine.

What IS a Class IB Antidysrhythmic?

Class IB Antidysrhythmics	Trade Names	Uses
lidocaine [LIE-doe-cane]	Xylocaine	Treatment of ventricular fibrillation and wide-complex ventricular tachycardia
mexiletine [MEX-ih-leh-teen]	Mexitil	Treatment of life-threatening ventricular dysrhythmias
phenytoin [FEN-ih-toe-in]	Dilantin	Treatment of ventricular tachycardia
tocainide [TOE-cane-ide]	Tonocard	Treatment of life-threatening ventricular dysrhythmias

Dysrhythmias
http://www.
americanheart.org/
presenter.jhtml?identifier

Action

Class IB antidysrhythmics decrease automaticity and the spontaneous depolarization of ventricles during diastole, thereby suppressing ventricular dysrhythmias. These drugs also decrease the duration of the action potential and the refractory period in the conduction system.

Uses

Class IB drugs are used to treat ventricular dysrhythmias. They are ineffective against atrial dysrhythmias. Lidocaine is used in the treatment of ventricular fibrillation and wide-complex ventricular tachycardia. However, according to the American Heart Association's (AHA) Advanced Cardiac Life Support (ACLS) guidelines (2003), amiodarone, a class III antidysrhythmic, is the first-line drug used to treat ventricular fibrillation and ventricular tachycardia.

Phenytoin is primarily an anticonvulsant drug and, in rare cases, is used to treat ventricular dysrhythmias associated with digoxin toxicity. Mexiletine and tocainide are oral class IB drugs used to treat life-threatening ventricular dysrhythmias, such as ventricular tachycardia.

Be careful not to confuse lidocaine formulations used for dental and local anesthetic procedures with lidocaine used for antidysrhythmic purposes.

What You NEED TO KNOW

Contraindications/Precautions

Lidocaine, phenytoin, and tocainide should be used with caution in patients with renal or hepatic dysfunction and heart failure. Lidocaine should be given with caution in patients with respiratory depression, shock, and in those with myasthenia gravis. Lidocaine is contraindicated in patients who have a hypersensitivity to amide anesthetics, blood dyscrasias, supraventricular dysrhythmias, severe SA or AV heart block, and Stokes-Adams syndrome.

Phenytoin should be used with caution in patients with hypotension, alcoholism, blood dyscrasias, bradycardia, and diabetes mellitus. Phenytoin is contraindicated for patients with bradycardia, complete or incomplete heart block, and Stokes-Adams syndrome.

Tocainide is contraindicated in patients with second- and third-degree AV block, hypokalemia, or myasthenia gravis. Mexiletine is contraindicated for patients with severe bradydysrhythmia, severe ventricular heart failure, and cardiogenic shock.

Drug Interactions

Rifampin, phenobarbital, and phenytoin may decrease the blood level of mexiletine, and cimetidine may increase mexiletine blood levels. Rifampin and cimetidine may decrease the serum levels of tocainide. Phenytoin may cause excessive sedation when given with CNS depressants. Phenytoin serum levels can increase when the drug is given with disulfiram, alcohol, amiodarone, isoniazid, chloramphenicol, sulfonamides, fluoxetine, benzodiazepines, omeprazole, metronidazole, ketoconazole, fluconazole, miconazole, estrogens, succinimides, halothane, salicylates, methylphenidate, phenothiazines, tolbutamide, trazodone, and felbamate. Myocardial depression can result when phenytoin is given with lidocaine or BBs.

Foods that alkalinize the urine can increase levels of mexiletine and cause toxicity. Foods that alkalinize the urine include all fruits except cranberries, prunes, and plums; all vegetables; and milk. Opioids, atropine, and antacids may slow the absorption of mexiletine, whereas metoclopramide increases its absorption.

Adverse Effects

CNS effects are the most common adverse effects that occur with class IB drugs. Confusion, excitation, dizziness, and nervousness may occur with tocainide, mexiletine, and lidocaine. Adverse effects of phenytoin include ataxia, agitation, dizziness, drowsiness, and extrapyramidal symptoms. Seizures can result from tocainide and lidocaine. Signs and symptoms of lidocaine toxicity include confusion, excitation, blurred vision, nausea, vomiting, ringing of ears, tremors, twitching, convulsions, dizziness, and bradycardia.

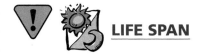

LIFE SPAN

- Class IB drugs should be given with caution in older or debilitated patients and in those who have renal or hepatic dysfunction. Older patients who are taking lidocaine are particularly sensitive to the CNS adverse effects.
- Class IB antidysrhythmic drugs are contraindicated during pregnancy and lactation and in children.

⚠ Lidocaine should be discontinued immediately and the health care provider notified if heart block, bradycardia, or sinus arrest develop. The nurse must differentiate between the two types of prefilled lidocaine syringes because it can be lethal if the prefilled 2 g of lidocaine is given to a patient as a bolus!

Serious cardiovascular adverse effects from class IB drugs include hypotension, bradycardia, dysrhythmias, and cardiac arrest. Mexiletine may also cause palpitations and edema. Tachycardia can result from phenytoin, particularly when it is given IV at a rate that exceeds 50 mg/min. Other cardiovascular adverse effects of tocainide include palpitations, tachycardia, and heart failure.

Mexiletine and tocainide can cause hepatic dysfunction. Hematologic adverse effects can occur with all class IB drugs (except lidocaine). Mexiletine, phenytoin, and tocainide can cause thrombocytopenia. Leukopenia can result from phenytoin and tocainide. Phenytoin can also cause aplastic anemia.

What You DO

Nursing Responsibilities

When administering class IB drugs, the nurse should:
- Follow a loading dose of the class 1B dysrhythmic drug by a continuous infusion.
- Follow administration instructions carefully to reduce the risk for hypotension, heart block, and asystole.
- Monitor the patient electrocardiographically.
- Report any dysrhythmias and hypotensive episodes to the health care provider.
- Administer a continuous lidocaine infusion on a volumetric pump through microdrip tubing to ensure accurate dose administration. Some lidocaine formulations come in prefilled syringes for both the bolus and continuous IV infusion.
- Realize that the earliest signs of lidocaine toxicity involve CNS (e.g., confusion).
- Administer IV phenytoin at the recommended rate to prevent CNS depression, hypotension, and cardiovascular collapse. IV phenytoin is compatible only with 0.9% normal saline solution.
- Monitor CBC and platelet count for patients who are taking mexiletine, phenytoin, or tocainide.
- Monitor renal and hepatic function studies for patients who are receiving mexiletine or tocainide.
- Monitor phenytoin and mexiletine serum levels for early detection of toxicity.

- Instruct the patient to take all doses as prescribed and to avoid trying to catch up on missed doses by doubling.
- Advise patients to carry identification that lists all drugs taken, including over-the-counter drugs and herbal preparations.
- Warn patients to avoid participating in activities that require alertness until response to the drug is known.
- Advise patients to report any shortness of breath, unusual bruising, and irregular heartbeats.
- Teach patients the proper way to take their pulse and to report to their health care provider if the pulse is less than 60 beats per minute.
- Teach the patient who is taking mexiletine to avoid foods that alkalinize the urine.

Do You UNDERSTAND?

DIRECTIONS: Indicate in the space provided whether the statement is *true* or *false*. If the answer is false, correct the statement to make it true (using the margin space).

_____ 1. Phenytoin is used primarily as an antidysrhythmic drug.

_____ 2. Tocainide is given IV for ventricular arrhythmias.

_____ 3. Class IB drugs decrease the action potential.

_____ 4. Class IB drugs are used to treat only ventricular arrhythmias.

_____ 5. The same formulation of lidocaine used for antidysrhythmic purposes can be used as a local anesthetic also.

Answers: 1. false; phenytoin is primarily an anticonvulsant drug; 2. false; tocainide is given orally; 3. true; 4. true; 5. false; the antidysrhythmic formulation of lidocaine is different than a lidocaine local anesthetic formulation and should not be confused.

What IS a Class IC Antidysrhythmic?

Class IC Antidysrhythmics	Trade Names	Uses
flecainide [fleh-CANE-ide]	Tambocor	Prevention of life-threatening ventricular dysrhythmias, paroxysmal atrial fibrillation and flutter, and paroxysmal supraventricular tachycardias
propafenone [pro-PA-fan-one]	Rythmol	Prevent reoccurrence of atrial fibrillation and flutter

Action

Class IC antidysrhythmics alter the transport of ions across cell membranes, thereby slowing conduction. Flecainide slows conduction velocity and increases ventricular refractoriness. Propafenone reduces spontaneous automaticity and suppresses ventricular tachycardia, which stabilizes action on myocardial membranes.

Uses

Class IC drugs are administered orally to treat life-threatening ventricular dysrhythmias, particularly ventricular tachycardia. Flecainide is used to prevent paroxysmal atrial flutter or fibrillation and paroxysmal supraventricular tachycardias. Propafenone is used to prevent the reoccurrence of atrial fibrillation and flutter.

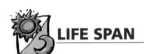

LIFE SPAN

Class IC drugs are contraindicated in nursing mothers. Flecainide is contraindicated during pregnancy and in children under 18 years of age. Propafenone should be used with caution during pregnancy and in children and older adults.

Class IC drugs should be used with caution in patients with renal dysfunction. Flecainide should be used with caution in patients with heart failure. Propafenone should be given cautiously to patients with hepatic dysfunction.

What You NEED TO KNOW

Contraindications/Precautions

Class IC drugs are contraindicated for patients in cardiogenic shock. Flecainide is also contraindicated for patients with second- or third-degree AV block and severe hepatic dysfunction. Propafenone is contraindicated for patients with severe heart failure, SA or AV block, severe hypotension, bradycardia, emphysema, and electrolyte imbalances.

Drug Interactions

There is an increased risk for dysrhythmias when flecainide is taken with other antidysrhythmics (e.g., calcium channel blockers, disopyramide, beta blockers). Amiodarone increases the serum level of flecainide by 50%. Flecainide increases digoxin levels; thus the risk for digoxin toxicity increases.

Foods that alkalinize and acidify the urine affect the blood level of flecainide. Alkalinizing foods promote reabsorption thereby increasing flecainide serum levels. Acidifying foods (e.g., cheese, cranberries, eggs, fish, grains, meat, plums, poultry, and prunes) increase renal elimination of flecainide.

Propafenone increase serum levels of propranolol, metoprolol, and digoxin. Propafenone increases the effects of warfarin and serum levels of cyclosporine. Rifampin decreases blood levels of propafenone.

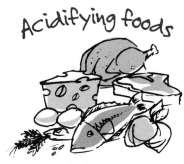

Acidifying foods

Watch what you eat!

Adverse Effects

The adverse effects of class IC drugs primarily involve the cardiovascular and CNS. Flecainide can cause dysrhythmias, chest pain, and heart failure. Propafenone can cause atrial and ventricular dysrhythmias, conduction disturbances, bradycardia, and hypotension. CNS adverse effects include dizziness, shaking, weakness, headache, depression, and tremors.

What You DO

Nursing Responsibilities

When administering class IC drugs, the nurse should:

- Monitor cardiac rhythm, particularly during the initial doses, to assess whether the drug is effective in terminating the dysrhythmia; report any dysrhythmias, hypotension episodes, and any CNS adverse effects (e.g., dizziness, headache, depression, tremors) to the health care provider.
- Realize that dosages of class IC drugs should be decreased for patients with renal or hepatic dysfunction.
- Monitor blood levels of flecainide for early detection of toxicity.
- Advise patients to carry identification that lists all drugs taken, including over-the-counter drugs and herbal preparations.
- Warn patients to avoid participating in activities that require alertness until response to the drug is known.
- Advise patients to report any shortness of breath and irregular, fast, or slow heartbeat to their health care provider.

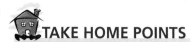

TAKE HOME POINTS

Notify the health care provider immediately of any adverse cardiovascular or CNS-related effects.

- Teach patients the proper way to take their pulse and to report to their health care provider if the pulse is less than 60 beats per minute.
- Instruct the patient to take all doses as prescribed and to avoid trying to catch up on missed doses by doubling.
- Caution patients who are taking flecainide to avoid foods that alkalinize or acidify the urine.

Do You UNDERSTAND?

DIRECTIONS: Complete the following statements with the appropriate terms from the italicized list provided.

1. _____ increases the serum level of flecainide by 50%.
2. The renal elimination of _____ is increased by foods that acidify the urine.
3. _____ increases the effects of warfarin.
4. _____ increases the risk for arrhythmias when taken with flecainide.

propafenone   *disopyramide*
amiodarone   *flecainide*

What IS a Class II Antidysrhythmic?

Class II antidysrhythmics are the beta blockers that are also used in the treatment of hypertension. Refer to page 239 for a discussion of the beta blockers. The desired outcome of treatment with beta blockers is a decreased heart rate, increased PR interval, and decreased QT interval.

Answers: 1. amiodarone; 2. flecainide; 3. propafenone; 4. disopyramide.

What IS a Class III Antidysrhythmic?

Class III Antidysrhythmics	Trade Names	Uses
amiodarone [A-MEE-oh-duh-rone]	Cordarone	Treatment of wide-complex tachycardia, ventricular tachycardia, pulseless ventricular tachycardia and fibrillation, and supraventricular tachycardia; conversion of atrial fibrillation
bretylium [breh-TILL-ee-uhm]	Bretylol	Second-line drug in the treatment of refractory ventricular tachycardia and ventricular fibrillation
ibutilide [ih-BYOO-tih-lide]	Corvert	Treatment of atrial flutter or atrial fibrillation
sotalol [SOTT-uh-lahl]	Betapace	Treatment of atrial fibrillation conversion

Action

Amiodarone prolongs the action potential and the refractory period and inhibits adrenergic stimulation. Bretylium initially releases norepinephrine and then blocks its release. Bretylium increases the fibrillation threshold and therefore is effective in treating and preventing ventricular fibrillation. Ibutilide activates the slow inward current of sodium in cardiac tissue, resulting in delayed repolarization and prolonged action potential. Ibutilide also increases the refractory period. Sotalol is a beta blocker that inhibits the β_1-receptors of the heart. The result of treatment with a class III drug includes prolonged PR, QRS, QT intervals. Sinus bradycardia is possible.

Uses

Amiodarone, bretylium, and sotalol are used to treat life-threatening ventricular dysrhythmias. Amiodarone is also frequently used for its unlabeled use of treating atrial tachydysrhythmias. Ibutilide and sotalol pharmacologically cardiovert a patient with recent onset of atrial fibrillation and atrial flutter to a normal sinus rhythm.

The revisions of the AHA-developed ACLS guidelines in 2003 resulted in several changes in the recommendations regarding antidysrhythmics. Amiodarone is the first-line drug for the treatment of ventricular fibrillation and ventricular tachycardia. Bretylium has been removed as a first-line drug from the guidelines for treatment of ventricular fibrillation.

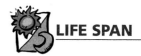 **LIFE SPAN**

Amiodarone, bretylium, and ibutilide are contraindicated during pregnancy and lactation and in children under 18 years of age.

⚠️ Amiodarone should be given with caution to patients with thyroid dysfunction, heart failure, lung disease, or iodine hypersensitivity, as well as in those who have had heart surgery. Ibutilide should be used cautiously in patients with heart failure, recent MI, hepatic dysfunction, or prolonged QT intervals. Ibutilide should not be given within 4 hours of administering amiodarone, disopyramide, procainamide, quinidine, and sotalol because excessive prolonging of the refractory period may occur. Sotalol should also be used cautiously within 14 days of administration of an MAOI to prevent acute hypertension.

What You NEED TO KNOW

Contraindications/Precautions

Amiodarone and sotalol are contraindicated for patients with cardiogenic shock, bradycardia, and heart block. Sotalol is also contraindicated for patients with heart failure. Ibutilide is contraindicated in patients with hypokalemia or hypomagnesia.

Drug Interactions

When digoxin is given with amiodarone, digoxin levels are increased by 50%. Amiodarone increases serum levels of cyclosporine, dextromethorphan, methotrexate, phenytoin, and theophylline when given concurrently. Amiodarone also enhances the anticoagulation effects of warfarin. Bradydysrhythmias may occur when amiodarone is taken with beta blockers or calcium channel blockers. Cholestyramine decreases amiodarone levels, and cimetidine increases amiodarone levels.

Bretylium increases the actions of dopamine and norepinephrine. Bretylium can worsen digoxin toxicity. Phenothiazines, tricyclic and tetracyclic antidepressants, antihistamines, and H_2-receptor blocking drugs increase the risk for dysrhythmias with ibutilide.

Phenytoin and verapamil may cause further myocardial depression and resultant heart failure when given with sotalol. Bradycardia may occur when sotalol is taken with digoxin. Antihypertensive drugs, nitrates, and alcohol taken with sotalol may cause hypotension. Sotalol and insulin together prolong hypoglycemia. Sotalol also decreases the effectiveness of theophylline.

Adverse Effects

Adverse effects of amiodarone include constipation, anorexia, hypotension, bradycardia, worsening of dysrhythmias, heart failure, and hepatic dysfunction. Amiodarone can also cause the CNS adverse effects, which include dizziness, malaise, fatigue, headache, tremor, poor coordination, and paresthesia. Common adverse effects of bretylium include postural hypotension, dizziness, and fainting. Nausea and vomiting also are common when the bolus dose is given at a rate that exceeds 8 minutes.

Ibutilide can cause ventricular tachycardia during infusion and up to 4 hours after administration. The adverse effects of sotalol include fatigue, dizziness, drowsiness, weakness, depression, and mental changes. Cardiovascular adverse effects of sotalol include bradycardia, hypotension,

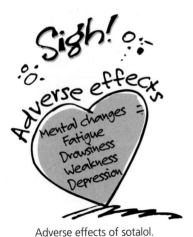

Adverse effects of sotalol.

heart failure, cardiogenic shock, and heart block. Impotence and decreased libido may also result.

What You DO

Nursing Responsibilities

When administering class III antidysrhythmics, the nurse should:

- Monitor cardiac rhythm, particularly during the initial doses, to assess whether the drug is effective in terminating the dysrhythmia; report any dysrhythmias or hypotension to the health care provider.
- Realize that all class III antidysrhythmic drugs must be administered on a volumetric infusion pump through microdrip tubing to ensure accurate dosage administration.
- Dilute infusions that exceed 2 hours in a glass bottle or a nonpolyvinyl chloride bag to prevent the drug from adhering to the plastic. Polyvinyl chloride tubing does not affect absorption.
- Dilute IV amiodarone in D_5W.
- Avoid weaning or discontinuing IV amiodarone until after the oral dose is given to prevent recurrence of the dysrhythmia.
- Realize that when defibrillation and lidocaine are ineffective in the treatment of ventricular fibrillation, bretylium may be used. A bolus dose is given over a period of 10 minutes or more to decrease adverse effects, followed by a continuous infusion.
- Monitor the cardiac rhythm while ibutilide is administered and for 4 hours after administration because sustained ventricular tachycardia can develop. Because of the risk for sustained tachycardia, a defibrillator-cardioverter should be available at the bedside.
- Realize that dosages of class III antidysrhythmics must be reduced in patients with hepatic or renal dysfunction
- Monitor BUN, potassium, triglyceride, lipoprotein, and uric acid levels of patients receiving sotalol.
- Monitor blood glucose levels of patients who are taking insulin and sotalol for detection of hypoglycemia.
- Monitor hepatic function tests in patients who are taking amiodarone.
- Instruct patients to take all doses as prescribed and to avoid trying to catch up on missed doses by doubling.
- Advise patients to carry identification that lists all drugs taken, including over-the-counter drugs and herbal preparations.

Nurses should use caution to avoid confusing amiodarone with another drug that has the similar name of amrinone. Amrinone is a phosphodiesterase inhibitor drug used for the short-term management of heart failure in patients who have not responded to diuretics, digoxin, or vasodilating drugs.

- Warn patients to avoid participating in activities that require alertness until response to the drug is known.
- Advise patients to report any shortness of breath and irregular, fast, or slow heartbeat to their health care provider.
- Teach patients the proper way to take their pulse and to report to their health care provider if the pulse is less than 60 beats per minute.
- Instruct patients who are taking sotalol to avoid consuming alcohol because hypotension may result.

Do You UNDERSTAND?

DIRECTIONS: Complete the following statements with the appropriate terms from the italicized list provided.

1. _____ is contraindicated for patients with CHF and cardiogenic shock.
2. The most common adverse effect of _____ _____ is hypotension.
3. _____ increases digoxin levels by 50%.
4. _____ should not be given within 4 hours of administering procainamide.

amiodarone   *ibutilide*
bretylium   *sotalol*

What IS a Class IV Antidysrhythmic?

Class IV antidysrhythmics are calcium channel blockers also used in the treatment of hypertension. Refer to page 245 for a discussion of these drugs. The outcome of using a class IV antidysrhythmic is a decreased heart rate and increased pulse rate.

Answers: 1. sotalol; 2. bretylium; 3. amiodarone; 4. ibutilide.

What IS a Miscellaneous Antidysrhythmic?

Miscellaneous Antidysrhythmics	Trade Names	Uses
adenosine [ah-DEN-oh-seen]	Adenocard	Treatment of paroxysmal supraventricular tachycardia, Wolff-Parkinson-White syndrome, atrial fibrillation, and ventricular tachycardia
digoxin [dih-JOX-in]	Lanoxin	Treatment of atrial flutter and fibrillation, paroxysmal atrial tachycardia, and cardiogenic shock
isoproterenol [eye-so-pro-TER-uh-nahl]	Isuprel	Treatment of shock

Action

Each miscellaneous antidysrhythmic has a unique action that is effective in treating dysrhythmias. Adenosine restores a normal sinus rhythm by interrupting reentrant pathways in the AV node, causing conduction to slow at the AV node, and is thereby effective in suppressing atrial tachydysrhythmias. Because adenosine causes transient asystole, the SA node is allowed to take over and initiate a normal sinus rhythm.

Digoxin prolongs the refractory period of the AV node and decreases conduction in the SA and AV nodes. Isoproterenol stimulates the β_1-receptors, causing an increase in the heart rate. The increase in heart rate shortens the QT interval, which suppresses the occurrence of torsades de pointes.

Uses

Miscellaneous antidysrhythmics are those drugs used to treat dysrhythmias that are not identified in any of the standard antidysrhythmic classes. Adenosine and digoxin are used to treat atrial tachydysrhythmias. Adenosine is effective, but its duration of action is short (1 to 2 minutes); thus the dysrhythmia frequently returns. A longer-acting antidysrhythmic (e.g., digoxin) should also be used to prevent recurrence of the dysrhythmia. Isoproterenol used as an antidysrhythmic treats only the life-threatening ventricular tachycardia called torsades de pointes. This is a dangerous type of ventricular tachycardia because it does not usually produce a pulse. Torsades de pointes may occur when the serum level of a class IA drug becomes subtherapeutic.

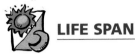

- Adenosine should be used with caution during pregnancy. Digoxin should be used with caution during pregnancy and lactation, as well as in children, older adults, and debilitated patients. Isoproterenol should be used cautiously in older adults and debilitated patients; it is contraindicated during pregnancy.
- Adenosine should be used with caution in patients with renal or hepatic dysfunction and asthma. Digoxin should be used cautiously in patients with hypokalemia, hypothyroidism, lung disease, severe heart disease, incomplete AV block, and renal dysfunction. Isoproterenol should be used cautiously in patients with hypertension, cardiovascular disorders, tuberculosis, hyperthyroidism, glaucoma, diabetes mellitus, and renal dysfunction.

TAKE HOME POINTS

Expect a short run (3 to 6 seconds) of asystole after administration of adenosine. Decrease the infusion rate or temporarily discontinue isoproterenol when heart rate is at or above 110 beats per minute.

What You NEED TO KNOW

Contraindications/Precautions

Adenosine is contraindicated for patients with AV block, second- or third-degree AV block, sick sinus syndrome, atrial flutter or fibrillation, and ventricular tachycardia. Digoxin is contraindicated for patients with ventricular tachycardia or fibrillation and digitalis toxicity. Isoproterenol is contraindicated for patients with tachycardias, ventricular dysrhythmias, digoxin toxicity, heart block, coronary artery disease, and cardiogenic shock.

Drug Interactions

Isoproterenol can have an additive effect on the cardiovascular system. When it is used with adrenergic agonists, tachydysrhythmias may result, including ventricular tachycardia and ventricular fibrillation. Adenosine and carbamazepine increase the risk for developing heart block. Dipyridamole increases the effect of adenosine. Theophylline and caffeine decrease the effect of adenosine. There is an increased risk for digoxin toxicity when digoxin is taken with thiazides, loop diuretics, mezlocillin, piperacillin, ticarcillin, amphotericin B, or glucocorticosteroids. Quinidine, cyclosporine, amiodarone, verapamil, diltiazem, propafenone, and diclofenac also increase serum digoxin levels. There is an increased risk for bradycardia when digoxin and beta blockers are used together. Antacids, kaolin-pectin, cholestyramine, and a high-fiber diet decrease the absorption of digoxin.

Adverse Effects

When adenosine is given IV, a sudden onset of apprehension, dizziness, headache, shortness of breath, chest pain, flushing, transient dysrhythmias, and hypotension may occur. Adverse effects associated with digoxin include fatigue, weakness, headache, dysrhythmias, bradycardia, and thrombocytopenia. Early signs of digoxin toxicity include nausea and vomiting and vision changes. Common adverse effects of isoproterenol include tachydysrhythmias, sinus tachycardia, and chest pain.

What You DO

Nursing Responsibilities

When administering miscellaneous antidysrhythmics, the nurse should:

- Monitor cardiac rhythm, particularly during the initial doses, to assess whether the drug is effective in terminating the dysrhythmia; report any dysrhythmias or hypotension to the health care provider.
- Realize that class IV antidysrhythmic drugs given IV must be administered on a volumetric infusion pump through microdrip tubing to ensure accurate dosage administration.
- Administer adenosine as a rapid bolus IV over 1 to 2 seconds. Adenosine is ineffective when it is given at a slower rate. Follow package instructions for proper administration. Adenosine should be given in the IV port that is closest to the insertion site.
- Give IV digoxin in divided doses over 24 hours.
- Monitor digoxin levels to prevent toxicity. A level greater than 2.0 ng/mL indicates toxicity.
- Titrate isoproterenol slowly when treating torsades de pointes until a heart rate is achieved that suppresses the occurrence of the dysrhythmia. Isoproterenol can trigger ventricular dysrhythmias and tachycardia, which in turn can cause myocardial ischemia and infarction. Discontinue isoproterenol and notify the health care provider immediately when other ventricular dysrhythmias occur or when the patient develops chest pain.
- Instruct the patient taking an oral class IV drug to take all doses as prescribed and to avoid trying to catch up on missed doses by doubling.
- Advise patients to carry identification that lists all drugs taken, including over-the-counter drugs and herbal preparations.
- Warn patients to avoid participating in activities that require alertness until response to the drug is known.
- Advise patients to report any shortness of breath and irregular, fast, or slow heartbeat to their health care provider.
- Teach patients the proper way to take their pulse and to report to their health care provider if the pulse is less than 60 beats per minute.

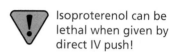 Isoproterenol can be lethal when given by direct IV push!

Do You UNDERSTAND?

DIRECTIONS: **Indicate in the space provided whether the statement is *true* or *false*. If the answer is false, correct the statement to make it true (using the margin space).**

_____ 1. Adenosine is used to treat torsades de pointes.

_____ 2. Digoxin is used to treat atrial tachydysrhythmias.

_____ 3. Isoproterenol inhibits β_1-receptors.

_____ 4. Isoproterenol shortens the QT interval.

References

Abrams AC, Lammon CB, Pennington SS: *Clinical drug therapy: rationales for nursing practice*, ed 8, Philadelphia, 2007, Lippincott.

Arcangelo VP: *Pharmacotherapeutics for advanced practice: a practical approach*, Philadelphia, 2001, Lippincott.

Braunwald E, Zipes DP, Libby P: *Heart disease: a textbook of cardiovascular medicine*, ed 6, Philadelphia, 2001, WB Saunders.

Edmunds MW: *Introduction to clinical pharmacology*, ed 4, St Louis, 2003, Mosby.

Gutierrez K, Queener S: *Pharmacology for nursing practice*, Philadelphia, 2004, Mosby.

Hardman JG, Limbird LE: *Goodman & Gilman's the pharmacological basis of therapeutics*, ed 10, New York, 2001, McGraw-Hill.

Hodgson B, Kizior R: *Saunders nursing drug handbook 2005*, St Louis, 2005, Elsevier.

Karch AM: *Focus on nursing pharmacology*, ed 3, Philadelphia, 2006, Lippincott.

Kee JL, Hayes ER, McCuistion LE: *Pharmacology: a nursing process approach*, ed 5, Philadelphia, 2006, Elsevier.

Khan MG: *Cardiac drug therapy*, ed 5, Philadelphia, 2000, WB Saunders.

Lehne R: *Pharmacology for nursing care*, ed 5, Philadelphia, 2004, WB Saunders.

Lewis SM, Heitkemper MM, Dirksen SR: *Medical-surgical nursing: assessment and management of clinical problems,* ed 6, St Louis, 2004 Mosby.

Lilley L, Harrington S, Snyder J: *Pharmacology and the nursing process*, ed 4, St Louis, 2005, Mosby.

McCance K, Huether S: *Pathophysiology: the biologic basis for disease in adults and children*, ed 4, St Louis, 2002, Mosby.

McKenry LM, Salerno E: *Mosby's pharmacology in nursing*, ed 21, St Louis, 2003, Mosby.

Opie LH, Gersh BJ: *Drugs for the heart,* ed 6, Philadelphia, 2005, WB Saunders.

Wilson BA, Shannon MT, Stang CL: *Nurses drug guide*, Upper Saddle River, New Jersey, 2006, Pearson.

Answers: 1. false; isoproterenol is used; 2. true; 3. false; isoproterenol stimulates β1-receptors; 4. true.

NCLEX® Review

Section A

1. A patient is taking benazepril (Lotensin). Which adverse effect is most associated with this medication?
   1 Seizures
   2 Hemorrhage
   3 Dysrhythmias
   4 First-dose phenomenon

2. When initiating valsartan (Diovan), maximal therapeutic BP reduction is expected within which time frame?
   1 24 hours
   2 3 to 4 days
   3 3 to 6 weeks
   4 2 months

3. A patient is taking doxazosin (Cardura). Which desired effect is most associated with this drug?
   1 Reduction of diastolic pressure
   2 Reduction of systolic pressure
   3 Adverse effect of seizures
   4 Adverse effect of constipation

4. Metoprolol (Lopressor) is most associated with which adverse effect?
   1 Tachycardia
   2 Bronchospasm
   3 Hyperglycemia
   4 Constipation

5. A patient is taking felodipine (Plendil). Which adrenergic response to CCBs is considered normal?
   1 Reflex vasoconstriction
   2 Reflex vasodilation
   3 Risk for hyperactivity
   4 Increased bone density

Section B

6. Which drug would be most beneficial for immediate relief of an acute anginal attack?
   1 Verapamil
   2 Propranolol
   3 Sublingual nitroglycerin
   4 Sustained-released isosorbide mononitrate

7. Which adverse effect has a direct relationship with vasodilation?
   1 Dizziness
   2 Depression
   3 Bradycardia
   4 Hypoglycemia

8. A patient who is taking digoxin (Lanoxin) is having blood drawn to evaluate his digoxin level. Which is the normal therapeutic range of digoxin?
   1 0.8 to 2.0 ng/mL
   2 0.6 to 3.5 ng/mL
   3 3.5 to 5.0 ng/mL
   4 3.0 to 8.0 ng/mL

9. A patient is taking milrinone (Primacor). Which therapeutic action does the nurse expect?
   1 Decreased contractility
   2 Increased PVR
   3 Increased PCWP
   4 Increased CO

10. The nurse teaches the patient to take nitroglycerin sublingually in an anginal attack, repeat the procedure when the chest pain continues, and notify the physician when chest pain continues after ____ tablet(s).
    1 One
    2 Two
    3 Three
    4 Four

Section C

11. A patient is taking lovastatin (Mevacor). The nurse knows that detection of _____ may indicate rhabdomyolysis.
1 Tinnitus
2 Muscle pain
3 Palpitations
4 Photosensitivity

12. When rhabdomyolysis is suspected, what further laboratory test should be evaluated?
1 Red blood cell count
2 CK level
3 White blood cell count
4 PT time assessment

13. Antilipidemics are contraindicated or used with caution in patients with which disorder?
1 Seizures
2 Depression
3 Hypertension
4 Renal and liver dysfunction

14. Which assumption can be made when giving HMG-CoA reductase inhibitors and bile acid sequestrants combination therapy?
1 They may be given at the same time.
2 They must both be given early in the morning.
3 Bile acid sequestrants should be taken without fluids.
4 The HMG-CoA reductase inhibitor should be given at least 2 hours after the bile acid sequestrant.

15. Which agent is unlikely to increase the risk for bleeding?
1 Niacin
2 Bile acid sequestrants
3 HMG-CoA reductase inhibitor
4 Fibric acid derivative

Section D

16. Which of the following drugs would be most beneficial for the treatment of atrial fibrillation with cardioversion?
1 Moricizine
2 Mexiletine
3 Quinidine
4 Disopyramide

17. Disopyramide should not be given within 48 hours before or 24 hours after _____ is given to avoid a drug interaction.
1 Rifampin
2 Quinidine
3 Verapemil
4 Procainamide

18. Which of the following is the normal therapeutic range of quinidine?
1 0.8 to 2.0 mcg/mL
2 0.6 to 1.5 mcg/mL
3 2.0 to 6.0 mcg/mL
4 6.0 to 8.0 mcg/mL

19. Which antidysrhythmic can be lethal when given direct IV push?
1 Lidocaine
2 Amiodarone
3 Procainamide
4 Isoproterenol

20. Which antidysrhythmic would the nurse expect a 3 to 6 second run of asystole to follow?
1 Adenosine
2 Moricizine
3 Mexiletine
4 Propafenone

21. A class IA antidysrhythmic may cause torsades de pointes under which of the following circumstances?
1 When it is taken with food
2 When it is taken with verapamil
3 When its serum level becomes toxic
4 When its serum level is below therapeutic level

22. Which of the following drugs, when taken with flecainide, causes an increased risk for dysrhythmias?
1 Digoxin
2 Lidocaine
3 Warfarin
4 Calcium channel blockers

23. Which drug may cause hypotension in a patient who is taking a class II antidysrhythmic?
    1 Dopamine
    2 Alcohol
    3 Dobutamine
    4 Norepinephrine

24. Which of the following adverse effects may occur during or after administering adenosine?
    1 Torsades de pointes
    2 Atrial tachycardia
    3 Chest pain
    4 Ventricular tachycardia

25. The nurse should discontinue isoproterenol and notify the health care provider immediately when the patient develops which of the following complications?
    1 Bradycardia
    2 Chest pain
    3 A heart rate of 90 beats per minute
    4 A systolic BP of 130 mm Hg

NCLEX® Review Answers

Section A

1. **4** After initiation of ACE therapy or a rapid increase in doses, the first-dose phenomenon with severe hypotension and fainting is common. Seizures, hemorrhage, and dysrhythmias are not adverse effects of ACE inhibitors.

2. **3** Maximal BP reduction following angiotensin II inhibitors occurs in 3 to 6 weeks. The time frames of 24 hours and 3 to 4 days are insufficient to gauge BP reduction. Two months is well past the optimal time to record maximal BP reduction.

3. **1** α_1-Adrenergic blockers, such as doxazosin are more effective in reducing diastolic BP, not systolic BP. Seizures and constipation are not adverse effects of α_1-adrenergic blockers. Diarrhea is an adverse effect.

4. **2** BBs, such as metoprolol may cause bronchospasm, bradycardia, hypoglycemia, and diarrhea.

5. **1** The normal adrenergic response to CCBs, such as felodipine is reflex vasoconstriction. In the older adult patient with diminished reflexes, this protective vasoconstriction is decreased and occasionally leads to excessive hypotension. Reflex vasodilation is incorrect because the effect is directly opposite. Hyperactivity is incorrect because CCBs usually cause weakness. CCBs do not increase bone density.

Section B

6. **3** Sublingual nitroglycerin is the drug of choice in an acute anginal attack because of the rapid onset of action. Verapamil is incorrect because CCBs are not used in the immediate relief of angina attacks or to prevent expected attacks. Propranolol, a BB, is used in long-term prevention of angina, not for immediate relief of acute angina. Sustained-release isosorbide mononitrate is a drug that provides coverage in a time-released manner, not immediately.

7. **1** The adverse effect that is most closely related to vasodilation is dizziness. When vessels dilate, flushing, headache, dizziness, fainting, weakness, tachycardia, and orthostatic hypotension are expected. Depression, bradycardia, and hypoglycemia are not expected.

8. **1** The normal therapeutic range of digoxin is 0.8 to 2.0 ng/mL. All of the remaining options (0.6 to 3.5 ng/mL, 3.5 to 5.0 ng/mL, and 3.0 to 8.0 ng/mL) are excessive therapeutic ranges for digoxin.

9. **4** Phosphodiesterase inhibitors, such as milrinone exert an inotropic effect on the heart, which causes increased myocardial contractility and CO. Decreased contractility is incorrect. Increased PVR is incorrect because phosphodiesterase inhibitors dilate arteries and veins, thereby decreasing PVR. PCWP is decreased, not increased, by phosphodiesterase inhibitors.

10. **3** The nurse should teach the patient the proper way to relieve an acute anginal attack by taking sublingual or buccal nitroglycerin tablets according to established protocol. The dose may be repeated twice at 5-minute intervals if chest pain is unrelieved. When pain persists after three

nitrates, the health care provider should be notified.

Section C

11. 2 Rhabdomyolysis is a fatal disease that causes acute destruction of skeletal muscle. Initial evidence includes muscle pain. Tinnitus, palpitations, and photosensitivity are adverse effects but are not evidence of rhabdomyolysis.

12. 2 Rhabdomyolysis may be accompanied by renal damage and is associated with elevated CK levels. Rhabdomyolysis are not associated with elevated red or white blood cell counts or elevated PT time.

13. 4 Antilipidemics are contraindicated or used with caution in patients with renal and liver dysfunction. Antilipidemics are not contraindicated or to be used cautiously for patients with seizures, depression, or hypertension.

14. 4 When HMG-CoA reductase inhibitors and bile acid sequestrants are given, HMG-CoA reductase inhibitors should be given at least 2 hours after the bile acid sequestrant; thus they may not be given at the same time. HMG-CoA reductase inhibitors should not be given early in the morning because they are more effective when taken in the evening because cholesterol is synthesized mostly at night. Bile acid sequestrants may be taken without regard to meals.

15. 4 Fibric acid derivatives do not increase the chance of bleeding. An increased risk for bleeding occurs when giving fibric acid derivatives, bile acid sequestrants, and HMG-CoA reductase inhibitors. Niacin may lead to hypoprothrombinemia, bile acid sequestrants may increase prothrombin time and GI bleeding, and HMG-CoA reductase inhibitors may cause nosebleeds and thrombocytopenia.

Section D

16. 3 Quinidine is used in the treatment of atrial fibrillation with cardioversion. Moricizine is used to treat ventricular tachycardia and PVCs.

Mexiletine and disopyramide are used to treat life-threatening ventricular dysrhythmias.

17. 3 Disopyramide should not be given within 48 hours before or 24 hours after the calcium channel blocking drug verapamil because an interaction causes prolonged conduction and decreased cardiac output.

18. 3 The normal therapeutic range of quinidine is 2 to 6 mcg/mL.

19. 4 Isoproteranol can be lethal when given direct IV push.

20. 1 Following adenosine administration, the nurse should expect a 3 to 6 second run of asystole.

21. 4 A class IA antidysrhythmic drug may cause torsades de pointes when its serum level is subtherapeutic, not at a toxic level. Class IA antidysrhythmics are poorly absorbed with food and should be taken on an empty stomach. Class IA drugs should not be given with verapamil. Giving class IA drugs and verapamil together may cause excess prolonging of conduction time and decreased cardiac output.

22. 4 An increased risk for dysrhythmias occurs when flecainide is taken with a calcium channel blocker. Digoxin levels are increased by flecainide when taken with a class IC antidysrhythmic. Lidocaine and warfarin have no drug interaction with flecainide.

23. 2 Alcohol, nitrates, and antihypertensives may cause hypotension when taken with a class II antidysrhythmic. Dopamine, dobutamine, and norepinephrine increase blood pressure.

24. 3 An adverse effect of adenosine that may occur during or after administration is 3 to 6 seconds of asystole, which leads to ischemia and chest pain. Torsades de pointes may occur when a class IA antidysrhythmic level is subtherapeutic. Tachycardia does not occur with class IA drugs.

25. **2** When the patient develops chest pain while receiving isoproterenol, the nurse should discontinue the drug and notify the health care provider immediately. Isoproterenol can trigger ventricular dysrhythmias, hypotension, and tachycardia. Therefore bradycardia, a pulse of 90 beats per minute, and a systolic blood pressure of 130 mm Hg are incorrect.

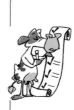

Notes

Chapter

8

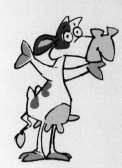

Drugs Used to Treat Respiratory System Disorders

What You WILL LEARN

After reading this chapter, you will know how to do the following:

- ✔ Contrast the action of an antitussive, decongestant, expectorant, antihistamine, and mucolytic.
- ✔ Discuss the contraindications for antitussives, decongestants, and antihistamines.
- ✔ Describe the adverse effects of a decongestant and an antihistamine.
- ✔ Contrast the nursing responsibilities of antihistamines.

Antitussives, decongestants, expectorants, and mucolytics are used to treat upper respiratory tract disorders. These pharmacologic agents are available as both prescription and over-the-counter (OTC) preparations. Antitussives may be nonnarcotic (**nonopioid),** narcotic (**opioid),** and combination agents.

When multiple symptoms are present, a combination form of these medications may be used. The medication that contains ingredients appropriate for relief of the patient's symptoms should be chosen when multiple symptoms exist. Most medications contain an analgesic (e.g., acetaminophen), antihistamine (e.g., diphenhydramine, chlorpheniramine), and a nasal decongestant (e.g., pseudoephedrine). Other medications may contain an expectorant (e.g., guaifenesin) or an antitussive (e.g., dextromethorphan). When only one symptom exists, using a single-ingredient preparation to individualize the action is best.

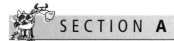

SECTION A

ANTITUSSIVES, DECONGESTANTS, EXPECTORANTS, AND MUCOLYTICS

What IS an Antitussive?

Antitussives	Trade Names	Uses
Opioids		
codeine [KOE-deen]	Codeine	Treatment of cough
hydrocodone bitartrate [HIGH-droe-KOE-done by-TAR-trate]	Hycodin	Treatment of cough
Nonopioids		
benzonatate [ben-ZOE-na-tate]	Tessalon Perles	Treatment of cough
dextromethorphan [DEX-troe-meth-OR-fan]	Robitussin DM, Benylin DM	Treatment of cough

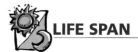

LIFE SPAN

Opioid antitussives are contraindicated during pregnancy, in nursing mothers, and for children under 1 year of age.

Action

Antitussives act either centrally or locally to decrease the frequency and intensity of a cough while the patient retains the protective cough reflex. Centrally acting antitussives inhibit the cough response receptors in the cough center of the medulla of the brain, thereby suppressing the cough. A locally acting antitussive acts directly on the cough production at the site of irritation.

Uses

An antitussive is an agent that is generally used to suppress a persistent, dry, or ineffective cough that prevents restful sleep. Benzonatate is frequently used in procedures (e.g., bronchoscopy, thoracentesis) when coughing should be avoided.

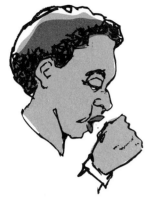

Dextromethorphan is contraindicated with asthma, chronic/productive cough, and hepatic dysfunction.

Cautious use of opioid antitussives is indicated in patients with hepatic or renal dysfunction, history of drug abuse, prostatic hypertrophy, alcoholism, chronic pulmonary disease, hypothyroidism, head injury, and increased intracranial pressure.

Dextromethorphan should be used with caution in patients with prostatic hypertrophy or chronic pulmonary disease or those who are taking monoamine oxidase inhibitors (MAOIs).

The life-threatening adverse effects of antitussives include respiratory depression and anaphylactic reaction.

What You NEED TO KNOW

Contraindications/Precautions

Opioid antitussives are contraindicated for patients with asthma or a hypersensitivity to codeine or morphine derivatives. Contraindications of nonopioid agents vary. Use of dextromethorphan is contraindicated for patients with asthma, productive or chronic cough, and hepatic dysfunction.

Drug Interactions

Concurrent use with central nervous system (CNS) depressant agents and alcohol may increase the action, causing further sedation. The opioid antitussives may increase the effects of MAOIs. Dextromethorphan may cause excitation, fever **(hyperpyrexia),** and hypotension when given concurrently with MAOIs. Dextromethorphan, the only antitussive with research-proven efficacy, is comparable to codeine but without addictive or respiratory depressive effects.

Nonopioid antitussives are contraindicated for women during pregnancy and for nursing mothers. Dextromethorphan is contraindicated for children under 2 years of age and for women during the first trimester of pregnancy.

Adverse Effects

Opioid antitussives, given at high doses, have the adverse effects of CNS depression and dependency. At low doses, the risk for dependency and adverse effects are reduced. The adverse effects of antitussives range from common (e.g., dizziness, drowsiness, nausea, constipation, pruritus) to life-threatening (e.g., respiratory depression, anaphylactic reaction).

Other CNS adverse effects include lightheadedness, euphoria, sedation, and dysphoria. In addition to pruritus, hypersensitivity reactions may be manifested as diffuse erythema, rash, urticaria, excessive perspiration, facial flushing, or shortness of breath. Additional adverse effects that are observed with the use of opioid antitussives include palpitation, hypotension, orthostatic hypotension, bradycardia, tachycardia, circulatory collapse, vomiting, urinary retention, abnormal pupil constriction **(miosis),** lethargy, agitation, convulsions, and unconsciousness **(narcosis).**

The adverse effects of the nonopioid agents vary. Benzonatate has a low incidence of adverse effects, including drowsiness, sedation, headache, mild dizziness, constipation, nausea, skin rash, and pruritus. Adverse effects of dextromethorphan include dizziness, drowsiness, nausea, vomiting, and stomach pain.

What You DO

Nursing Responsibilities

When administering opioid antitussives, the nurse should:

- Evaluate the patient's vital signs, especially the respiratory status, before administering the medication and during treatment for early detection of adverse effects.
- Instruct the patient who is taking benzonatate perles to avoid breaking the soft capsule or allowing it to dissolve in the mouth to prevent an anesthetic or choking effect.
- Monitor bowel elimination and nausea accompanied by vomiting. When vomiting persists, the medication may need to be changed to another antitussive.
- Observe the patient's intake and output for early detection of urinary retention.
- Encourage the intake of fluids to prevent constipation when they are not contraindicated because of the patient's condition.
- Caution the patient to take codeine with milk or food to decrease gastrointestinal (GI) upset.
- Warn the patient to avoid driving or performing tasks that require mental alertness because of the sedative properties of opioid antitussives.
- Instruct patients to notify their health care provider of any cough that lasts longer than 1 week.

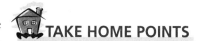

TAKE HOME POINTS

Be aware that naloxone (Narcan) is the antidote for overdose of opioids.

Do You UNDERSTAND?

DIRECTIONS: **Match Column A with Column B.**

	Column A	Column B
_____	1. An agent used to suppress coughs that interfere with sleep.	a. Choking
_____	2. An adverse effect when a benzonatate perle breaks in the mouth.	b. Decrease
		c. Increase
_____	3. Site of action of centrally acting antitussive.	d. Medulla
		e. Site of irritation
_____	4. The effect of opioid antitussives on the action of MAOIs.	f. Antitussive

What IS a Decongestant?

Decongestants	Trade Names	Uses
ephedrine hydrochloride [eh-FED-rin]	Efedron	Relief of nasal congestion
naphazoline [naf-AZ-oh-leen]	Allerest, VasoClear	Relief of nasal congestion and minor eye irritation
phenylephrine HCl [fen-ill-EFF-rin]	Neo-Synephrine, Sinex	Relief of nasal congestion and minor eye irritation
pseudoephedrine [SUE-doe-eh-FED-rin]	Sudafed, Novafed	Relief of nasal congestion

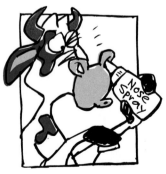

Speedy delivery.

Action

Nasal decongestants in the form of topical sprays or drops are rapidly absorbed through the nasal mucosa. Decongestants act on the sympathetic nerve endings and the smooth muscle of the respiratory tract, causing vasoconstriction of arterioles. This vasoconstriction causes a decrease in blood flow, a reduction of fluid exudate, and shrinkage of edematous mucous membranes, resulting in decreased nasal congestion.

Answers: 1. f; 2. a; 3. d; 4. c.

Uses

Decongestants are agents used to relieve congestion in the nasal passages and eustachian tubes resulting from allergies, the common cold, rhinitis, and sinusitis. Phenylephrine is also used for pronounced dilation of pupil (**mydriasis**) in ophthalmoscopy examinations or surgery.

What You NEED TO KNOW

Contraindications/Precautions

Concomitant use of MAOIs and adrenergic decongestants are contraindicated. Decongestants are contraindicated during pregnancy and lactation. Adrenergic decongestants should be used with caution in patients with a history of hypertension, cardiac disease, diabetes mellitus, hyperthyroidism, or narrow-angle glaucoma.

Drug Interactions

Concurrent use of ephedrine with MAOIs, tricyclic antidepressants, guanethidine, and furazolidone may increase the α-adrenergic effects (e.g., fever, headache, and hypertension). Epinephrine and norepinephrine increase the sympathomimetic effects of ephedrine. When ephedrine or phenylephrine is given with α- and β-blockers, the effects of each are antagonized or counteracted. Tricyclic antidepressants, ergot alkaloids, reserpine, and guanethidine may elevate the blood pressure (BP) when taken with phenylephrine.

MAOIs may cause hypertensive crisis when given concurrently with phenylephrine or pseudoephedrine, and oxytocin may cause persistent hypertension when taken with phenylephrine. Concurrent use of pseudoephedrine with reserpine, methyldopa, and guanethidine increases the risk for hypertension. Urinary acidifiers cause a decrease in the decongestant effects. Urinary alkalinizer medications cause increased decongestant effects.

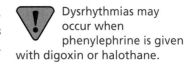 Dysrhythmias may occur when phenylephrine is given with digoxin or halothane.

Adverse Effects

Decongestants may cause mild CNS stimulation, such as euphoria, sneezing, restlessness, tremors, nervousness, headache, blurred vision, thirst, sweating, or insomnia. With higher doses, tachycardia, palpitations, dysrhythmias, dizziness, nausea, or vomiting may occur, particularly

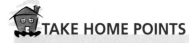**TAKE HOME POINTS**

Because of the short duration and rapid effect, nasal decongestants may become habit forming.

when the patient is hypersensitive to adrenergic drugs. Adverse effects following the use of adrenergic decongestants are less likely to occur with topical use.

The use of topical nasal decongestant drops or sprays may cause stinging, burning, or excessive drying of the nasal mucosa. Prolonged use of more than 3 to 5 days may cause rebound nasal congestion, chronic rhinitis, and possible ulceration of nasal mucosa. Rebound congestion is not observed with pseudoephedrine.

What You DO

Nursing Responsibilities

When administering decongestants, the nurse should:

- Monitor the patient's pulse and BP before administering adrenergic decongestants, particularly in patients with a history of cardiac disease.
- Tell the patient to avoid taking a decongestant within 2 hours of bedtime to reduce CNS stimulation.
- Advise the patient to avoid using nasal sprays for longer than 3 to 5 days to decrease the likelihood of rebound congestion.
- Instruct the patient in the use of topical nasal decongestants. The nurse should first instruct the patient to gently blow the nose before using nose drops or sprays to ensure open passages.
- Instruct the patient to position the head laterally with the head down to keep the medication from entering the throat for the instillation of nose drops.
- Instruct the patient to bend the head slightly forward with the nasal spray nozzle inserted in the nostril (being careful not to occlude the nostril) and to sniff briskly to inhale when spraying. After use, rinse the dropper or spray tip with hot water to prevent contamination of the solution.

Instruct patient to avoid chewing or crushing sustained-release medications. Doing so will cause excessive absorption of the medication in the body at one time, rather than the steady dose over time as intended.

Do You UNDERSTAND?

DIRECTIONS: Match Column A with Column B.

<table>
<tr><td colspan="2">**Column A**</td><td>**Column B**</td></tr>
<tr><td>_____</td><td>1. The action that results in decreased nasal congestion.</td><td>a. swallow</td></tr>
<tr><td>_____</td><td>2. Instruction to the patient taking sustained-release forms of medications.</td><td>b. take orally
c. do not chew
d. topically</td></tr>
<tr><td>_____</td><td>3. Adverse effect caused by prolonged use.</td><td>e. vasoconstriction
f. rebound congestion</td></tr>
<tr><td>_____</td><td>4. Route that may cause stinging or burning.</td><td></td></tr>
</table>

What IS an Expectorant?

Expectorant	Trade Name	Uses
guaifenesin [GWHY-fen-ah-sin]	Robitussin, Anti-Tuss	Treatment of dry, nonproductive cough

Action

An expectorant decreases the thickness (**viscosity**) of the sputum and stimulates productive coughing. The liquefied respiratory tract fluids are then easier to expel (**expectorate**) through coughing. Guaifenesin is a common ingredient of OTC cold medications.

Uses

An expectorant is used in the treatment of dry coughs and when the patient is unable to expectorate mucus that is present in the respiratory tract. The cause of the cough may be a cold or a minor upper respiratory tract infection.

Answers: 1. e; 2. c; 3. f; 4. d.

What You NEED TO KNOW

Contraindications/Precautions

Guaifenesin is contraindicated in the treatment of chronic coughs, such as those resulting from asthma, emphysema, smoking, and copious or productive coughs.

Drug Interactions

Concurrent use of heparin may increase the risk for hemorrhage because guaifenesin inhibits platelet adhesiveness.

Adverse Effects

The use of guaifenesin presents a low incidence of adverse effects. However, GI upset, nausea, vomiting, drowsiness, urticaria, and rash may occur.

What You DO

Nursing Responsibilities

When administering expectorants, the nurse should:
- Advise the patient to increase fluid intake to 2 to 3 L per day to decrease mucus viscosity.
- Warn the patient to avoid driving or performing tasks that require mental alertness because drowsiness from guaifenesin may occur.
- Instruct patients to notify their health care provider when the cough lasts longer than 1 week or when a rash, fever, or persistent headache develops.
- Warn the patient that some OTC combination preparations may contain alcohol and should not be taken by individuals with a history of alcohol intolerance or abuse.

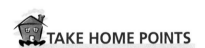

TAKE HOME POINTS

Instruct the patient to follow each dose with a full glass of water to aid in thinning the secretions.

Do You UNDERSTAND?

DIRECTIONS: **Indicate in the space provided whether the statement is *true* or *false*. If the answer is false, correct the statement to make it true (using the margin space).**

_____ 1. The patient's fluid intake should be increased to 2 to 3 liters per day.

_____ 2. Drowsiness is not an adverse reaction of guaifenesin.

_____ 3. Guaifenesin is a common ingredient of OTC cold medications.

_____ 4. An expectorant increases the viscosity of the sputum.

What IS a Mucolytic?

Mucolytic	Trade Name	Use
acetylcysteine [ass-cee-till-SIS-teen]	Mucomyst	Treatment of viscous mucous secretions

Action

Acetylcysteine, administered through inhalation or instillation, is rapidly absorbed through the mucosa of the respiratory tract. The action of a mucolytic involves the disruption of the chemical bonds between the mucoprotein molecules of the respiratory secretions. The result is liquefaction of the mucus.

Administer acetylcysteine with compressed air for nebulization, not with a hand nebulizer.

Uses

Mucolytics are used to facilitate the removal of viscous, tenacious mucus secretions in the respiratory tract. Sodium chloride solution also has mucolytic actions. Oral acetylcysteine is also used as the antidote for acetaminophen overdose.

Answers: 1. true; 2. false; drowsiness may occur with the use of guaifenesin; 3. true; 4. false; an expectorant decreases the viscosity of the sputum.

What You NEED TO KNOW

Contraindications/Precautions

Hypersensitivity and risk for gastric hemorrhage contraindicates the use of mucolytics. Cautious use is recommended for patients with asthma.

Drug Interactions

Mucolytics are incompatible with antibiotics and must be administered separately, not in the same nebulizer. Charcoal decreases the antidote effect.

Adverse Effects

Adverse effects of acetylcysteine include nausea, vomiting, stomatitis, rhinorrhea, rash, fever, drowsiness, chest tightness, bronchoconstriction, respiratory tract irritation, and an increased amount of bronchial secretions. The likelihood of bronchospasm is increased in patients with asthma.

What You DO

Nursing Responsibilities

When administering mucolytics, the nurse should:

- Counsel the patient that mucolytics have a disagreeable odor that soon disappears.
- Warn the patient that acetylcysteine may cause stickiness on the face when administered by facemask or nebulizer.
- Instruct the patient to wash the face with water to remove stickiness.

LIFE SPAN

Caution should be used with mucolytic administration in debilitated or older patients.

Discontinue the mucolytic when bronchospasm occurs and notify the health care provider immediately.

TAKE HOME POINTS

Suction equipment should be made available for the removal of excessive secretions to maintain an open airway when the patient is unable to expectorate.

Do You UNDERSTAND?

DIRECTIONS: **Indicate in the space provided whether the statement is** *true* **or** *false*. **If the answer is false, correct the statement to make it true (using the margin space).**

_____   1. Mucolytics are used to facilitate bronchodilation.

_____   2. Oral acetylcysteine is given as the antidote for acetaminophen toxicity.

_____   3. Acetylcysteine given by inhalation may cause a stickiness on the face.

_____   4. Patients who have asthma are likely to experience bronchospasm with acetylcysteine.

SECTION **B**

ANTIHISTAMINES

In the treatment of coughs that are associated with the common cold or irritants, diphenhydramine (Benadryl), an antihistamine, may also be used.

Two types of antihistamines have been classified: histamine H_1-receptor antagonists and histamine H_2-receptor antagonists. The H_1 antihistamines are used primarily to control symptoms associated with respiratory and allergic responses, particularly seasonal and allergic rhinitis. The H_2 receptor antagonists act primarily on the GI tract. Additionally, selected antihistamines are used as antiparkinsonism agents; other antihistamines are used as antiemetics for the treatment of vertigo and motion sickness.

The six subclasses of antihistamines are alkylamines, ethanolamines, ethylenediamines, phenothiazines, piperidines, and piperazines. Among the subclasses, varying degrees of sedative, antiemetic, anticholinergic, GI, or antipruritic effects are produced. First-generation antihistamines have more sedative effects and are also referred to as *sedating* antihistamines. The second-generation antihistamines produce less sedative effects, because they do not cross the blood-brain barrier. These agents are also referred to as *nonsedating* antihistamines.

Answers: 1. false; mucolytics are used to facilitate the removal of viscous, tenacious mucus secretions in the respiratory tract; 2. true; 3. true; 4. true.

First-Generation Antihistamines

What IS a First-Generation Antihistamine?

First-Generation Antihistamines	Trade Names	Uses
Alkylamines		
chlorpheniramine [klor-fen-EAR-ah-meen]	Chlor Trimeton, Teldrin	Treatment of allergy and cough
Ethanolamines		
clemastine fumarate [kleh-MAS-teen]	Tavist	Treatment of allergic rhinitis
diphenhydramine [dye-phen-HIGH-dra-meen]	Benadryl	Treatment of allergic reactions, nausea, vomiting, motion sickness, antitussive, insomnia, pruritus
Piperidines		
cyproheptadine [si-proh-HEP-tah-deen]	Periactin	Treatment of hypersensitivity reactions and allergic rhinitis

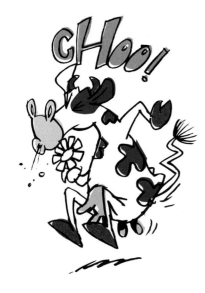

Action

Alkylamines, ethanolamines, ethylenediamines, and phenothiazines are first-generation, or sedating, antihistamines. Piperidines may be first- or second-generation antihistamines. Alkylamines, ethanolamines, and piperidines competitively block the H_1-receptor sites on effector cells and impede histamine-mediated responses. Ethylenediamines are H_1-receptor antagonists that compete with histamine at the receptor sites. Phenothiazines are antipsychotic drugs that block histamine effects at the H_1-receptor sites.

Uses

First-generation antihistamines are used for the treatment of symptoms associated with respiratory and allergic conditions (perennial and allergic rhinitis), for transfusion reactions, and as an adjunct in anaphylactic reactions. Ethanolamines and phenothiazines are used for the treatment of mild urticaria and angioedema. Diphenhydramine is used in the treatment of motion sickness, vertigo, parkinsonian conditions, and insomnia.

What You NEED TO KNOW

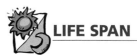

Contraindications/Precautions

Alkylamines, ethanolamines, ethylenediamines, and phenathiazines are contraindicated for patients with narrow-angle glaucoma, sensitivity to antihistamines, GI obstruction, bladder neck obstruction, and prostatic hypertrophy. Alkylamines, ethanolamines, and ethylenediamines are also contraindicated for patients with asthma. Phenothiazines are also contraindicated for patients with bone marrow depression, severe CNS depression, and coma. First-generation piperidines are contraindicated for use in patients with hypersensitivity to H_1-receptor antagonists and those who are undergoing MAOI therapy.

Drug Interactions

Use of CNS depressants or alcohol with first-generation antihistamines increases the sedative effects of these drugs. Concurrent use of MAOIs may increase and prolong the drying (**anticholinergic**) effects of these agents.

Adverse Effects

The most common adverse effects of first-generation antihistamines are drowsiness and dry mouth. Alkylamines are potent antihistamines that have minimal sedative effects, moderate anticholinergic effects, and no antiemetic effects. Other adverse effects of alkylamines include dizziness, epigastric distress, thickening of bronchial secretions, and urinary retention.

Ethanolamines have moderate-to-high sedative effects, considerable anticholinergic and antiemetic effects, and a low rate of occurrence of GI effects. Adverse reactions of these agents include dizziness, epigastric distress, and the thickening of bronchial secretions. Blurred vision, hypotension, increased appetite, weight gain, urinary retention and rash are other adverse effects. Additional adverse effects of diphenhydramine include palpitations and tachycardia.

Ethylenediamines frequently cause more GI distress than do other antihistamines. Ethylenediamines also have moderate sedative effects and minimal anticholinergic and antiemetic effects. Other common adverse reactions of these agents include epigastric distress, anorexia, nausea,

Alkylamines, ethanolamines, and ethylenediamines are contraindicated for women during pregnancy and lactation. First-generation piperidines are contraindicated for use in children under 12 years of age.

- Alkylamines and ethanolamines should be used with caution in women during pregnancy and in older patients. Safe use of ethylenediamines has not been determined for use in women during pregnancy, nursing mothers, or neonates. Cautious use of phenothiazines should be maintained in the treatment of older and debilitated patients. Caution with first-generation piperidines should be used for patients who are pregnant, nursing, older, or debilitated.
- Ethanolamines are to be used with caution for patients with a history of asthma, hypertension, hyperthyroidism, cardiovascular disease, and diabetes.

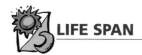

Older patients may experience increased sedation, dizziness, and hypotension because of an increased sensitivity to alkylamines and ethylenediamines. Patients thus require assistance with ambulation to prevent falls.

Diphenhydramine should be used with caution for patients with convulsive disorders. Use ethylenediamines with caution for patients with a history of asthma, cardiovascular disease, diabetes, hypertension, hyperthyroidism, or increased intraocular pressure. Use phenothiazines with caution in patients with impaired hepatic function, asthma, cardiovascular disease, hypertension, and respiratory impairment. Use first-generation piperidines with caution in patients with narrow-angle glaucoma, bladder neck obstruction, prostatic hypertrophy, history of asthma or chronic obstructive pulmonary disease (COPD), cardiovascular disease, and hypertension.

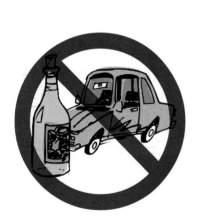

vomiting, and constipation. Blurred vision, headache, mild hypotension or hypertension, urinary hesitancy or retention, dizziness, nervousness, and rash are included as other adverse effects.

Phenothiazines have potent antihistamine actions, with strong sedative, anticholinergic, and antiemetic effects. Promethazine usually produces no extrapyramidal symptoms (EPS), whereas the other phenothiazine derivatives often do. Other adverse CNS effects include blurred vision, confusion, dizziness, tremors, and impaired coordination. Mild hypotension or hypertension, anorexia, photosensitivity, urinary retention, and leukopenia are included as other adverse effects.

First-generation piperidines have moderate antihistamine activity, low-to-moderate sedative effects, moderate anticholinergic effects, and no antiemetic effects. Other adverse reactions to first-generation piperidines include epigastric distress, anorexia, nausea, vomiting, constipation, blurred vision, headache, mild hypotension, palpitations, tachycardia, urinary retention, dizziness, nervousness, rash, and thickening of respiratory secretions. Cyproheptadine has the adverse effect of appetite stimulation and may cause weight gain.

What You DO

Nursing Responsibilities

A major responsibility of the nurse, when administering first-generation sedating antihistamines, is patient teaching. The nurse should:

- Encourage patients to increase their fluid intake to 2000 to 3000 mL per day.
- Teach the patient the importance of avoiding other CNS depressants and alcohol in any form when taking oral first-generation antihistamines to avoid additive CNS depression (e.g., sedation, apnea, coma, death).
- Warn the patient to avoid driving or performing tasks that require mental alertness because of the sedative effects.
- Caution the patient to consult the health care provider before taking any OTC preparations to avoid adverse interactions. OTC allergy and cold preparations frequently contain alcohol.
- Instruct the patient to take first-generation antihistamines with food or milk to decrease GI adverse effects.

- Instruct the patient to chew gum or suck hard candy to relieve symptoms of dry mouth.
- Warn the patient to avoid prolonged exposure to sunlight and use sunscreen protection to decrease photosensitivity reactions.
- Instruct the patient to void before taking the ethanolamines to reduce urinary hesitancy.
- Assist the patient with ambulation as a prevention of falls because piperidines frequently produce hypotension or sedation.
- Instruct the patient in cyproheptadine therapy to notify the health care provider of any significant weight gain.
- Inform the patient that unless first-generation antihistamines are discontinued 4 days before allergy skin testing procedures, false negative results may occur.

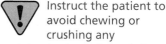
Instruct the patient to avoid chewing or crushing any sustained-release formulations.

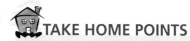
TAKE HOME POINTS

Increased fluid intake helps thin respiratory secretions.

Do You UNDERSTAND?

DIRECTIONS: Complete the crossword puzzle.

Across

1. Antihistamines are mainly excreted in _____.
5. Antihistamines are metabolized by the _____.
7. An adverse GI reaction to ethylenediamines.
9. Administer at this time to lessen GI effects.
11. Days to stop antihistamines before allergy testing.
12. Use of these depressants will increase sedation.
13. Before meals.
16. Antihistamines are _____ in the GI tract.

Down

1. _____ of ethylenediamines is contraindicated during pregnancy.
2. This patient may be more sensitive to the normal dose.
3. Geriatric patients may experience more of this adverse effect.
4. H_1-receptor antagonists compete with histamine here.
6. Drowsiness is this type of reaction to antihistamines.
8. Increases CNS depressant effects and should be avoided.

10. An anticholinergic effect caused by antihistamines.
12. Concurrent _____ depressants with first-generation antihistamines increase sedative effects.
14. Instruct the patient not to _____ sustained-release formulations.
15. Route of most antihistamines.
17. This form of medication should be swallowed whole.

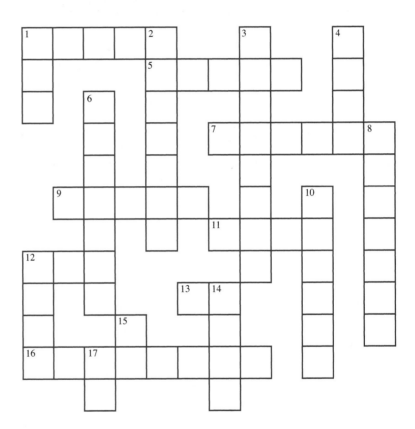

Second-Generation Antihistamines

What IS a Second-Generation Antihistamine?

Second-Generation Antihistamines	Trade Names	Uses
fexofenadine [fex-oh-FEN-ah-deen]	Allegra	Treatment of allergic rhinitis
loratadine [loh-RAH-tih-deen]	Claritin	Treatment of allergic rhinitis
desloratadine [des-lor-AH-tah-deen]	Clarinex	Treatment of allergic rhinitis
cetirizine [see-TIH-rah-zeen]	Zyrtec	Treatment of allergic rhinitis

Action

Second-generation antihistamines competitively block the H_1-receptor sites on effector cells and impede histamine-mediated responses.

Uses

Second-generation antihistamines are used primarily for the treatment of symptoms associated with allergic conditions, particularly seasonal and allergic rhinitis and chronic urticaria.

What You NEED TO KNOW

Contraindications/Precautions

Second-generation antihistamines are contraindicated for patients hypersensitive to the drug. These agents are contraindicated for patients with hypersensitivity to H_1-receptor antihistamines or hydralazine.

Use second-generation antihistamines with caution in patients with impaired hepatic or renal function.

Drug Interactions

Concentrations of loratadine and desloratidine may increase when taken concurrently with ketoconazole, fluconazole, clarithromycin, and erythromycin. Concurrent use of CNS depressants or alcohol with cetirizine

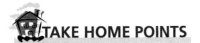

TAKE HOME POINTS

Cetirizine should be taken orally once a day. Meals do not affect this medication.

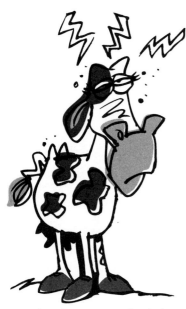

Fexofenadine can cause headaches.

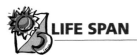

LIFE SPAN

The liquid form of cetirizine may be used for children when needed. Older patients are highly sensitive to the sedative effects of second-generation antihistamines.

may increase sedation and drowsiness. There are no known drug interactions with fexofenadine.

Adverse Effects

Second-generation agents have moderate-to-high antihistamine activity, low to no sedative effects, low to no anticholinergic effects, no antiemetic effects, and fewer adverse effects. The most common adverse effect of fexofenadine is headache. Other adverse effects of second-generation agents include dry mouth, drowsiness, fatigue, nausea, dyspepsia, and throat irritation. Adverse effects are uncommon with loratadine. Children may experience paradoxical reactions, such as nervousness, insomnia, tremors. Elderly patients are more likely to experience sedation, dizziness, and confusion.

What You DO

Nursing Responsibilities

When administering second-generation antihistamines, the nurse should:
- Give loratadine on an empty stomach, either 1 hour before or 2 hours after a meal.
- Inform the patient to increase fluid intake, chew gum, or suck hard candy to help relieve dry mouth.
- Caution the patient to avoid alcohol and the use of other CNS depressants because these substances may increase sedative effects.
- Instruct the patient to avoid taking piperazines concurrently with OTC antihistamines.
- Warn the patient to avoid driving or performing tasks that require mental alertness because drowsiness, dizziness, or blurred vision may occur with these agents.
- Tell the patient that H_1-receptor antagonists interfere with allergy skin testing when the tests are taken within 4 days of the last dose and may produce false results.
- Monitor the patient for paradoxical effects and sedation.

Do You UNDERSTAND?

DIRECTIONS: Match Column A with Column B.

Column A

_____ 1. Common side effect of first-generation piperidines.

_____ 2. Action not observed with piperidine therapy.

_____ 3. An adverse effect of cyproheptadine.

Column B

a. Antiemetic

b. Appetite stimulation

c. Drowsiness

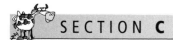

SECTION C

ANTIASTHMATICS AND BRONCHODILATORS

Antiasthmatic and bronchodilator drugs are used for the treatment of obstructive respiratory disorders as a result primarily of inflammation and bronchoconstriction. These disorders include asthma, emphysema, and COPD. The medications used in the treatment and prevention of these disorders are primarily antiinflammatory agents and bronchodilators. The drug classes of antiinflammatory and bronchodilator agents discussed in this section include inhaled corticosteroids, β-agonists, leukotriene antagonists, xanthine derivatives, and anticholinergics.

What IS an Inhaled Corticosteroid?

Inhaled Corticosteroids	Trade Names	Uses
beclomethasone [be-kloh-METH-ah-zone]	Beconase	Treatment of seasonal or perennial rhinitis
dexamethasone [dex-ah-METH-ah-zone]	Decadron, Decaspray	Treatment of allergic conditions
fluticasone [flu-TIH-kah-sone]	Flonase, Flovent	Treatment of seasonal or perennial rhinitis; prevention and treatment of asthma
triamcinolone [try-am-SIN-oh-lone]	Azmacort, Nasacort	Treatment of allergic rhinitis and asthma

Action

Inhaled corticosteroids inhibit the inflammatory response in the airways and decrease edema of the airway mucosa. These agents also increase the number and sensitivity of bronchial β_2-receptors, promote smooth muscle relaxation, and decrease hyperresponsiveness of the airways, which combine to decrease the production of mucus.

Uses

Inhaled corticosteroids are used as prophylaxis and for treatment of asthma. These agents are also used in the treatment of steroid-dependent chronic bronchial asthma and as adjunctive treatment of asthma that nonsteroidal bronchodilators are unable to control. Inhaled corticosteroids should be avoided as treatment of an acute asthmatic attack because they do not provide immediate symptomatic relief. Intranasal inhaled corticosteroids are used in the treatment of seasonal and perennial rhinitis. Oral inhalation is used in the treatment of asthma. Beclomethasone and triamcinolone are also used intranasally to prevent recurrence of polyps after surgery for the removal of nasal polyps.

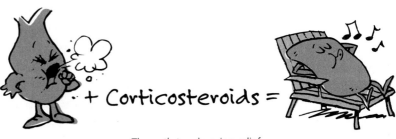

The path to wheezing relief.

What You NEED TO KNOW

Contraindications/Precautions

Contraindications for the use of inhaled corticosteroids are nonasthmatic bronchitis.

Drug Interactions

When inhaled corticosteroids are administered in the recommended doses, no significant interactions with other drugs occur. The concurrent use of corticosteroids and salicylates reduces salicylate effectiveness.

Adverse Effects

Inhaled corticosteroids have minimal systemic absorption; thus they decrease the risk for adverse effects. Common adverse reactions to the oral inhalant corticosteroids are fungal infections (e.g., *Candida albicans, Aspergillus niger*) of the oropharynx and larynx, hoarseness, dry mouth, and sore throat. Adverse effects of nasal inhalant corticosteroids include nasopharyngeal dryness, irritation, burning, itching, and ulceration. Other adverse effects include sneezing, epistaxis, headache, nausea, and vomiting. With the excessive administration of doses (overdosage), Cushing's syndrome or suppression of hypothalamic-pituitary-adrenal (HPA) function may occur as a result of systemic absorption.

 Inhaled oral corticosteroids should be used with caution in patients who are undergoing systemic corticosteroid treatment and patients with ocular herpes simplex or active respiratory infections because serious illness may result because of the antiinflammatory effects. Nasal inhalant corticosteroids should be cautiously used in patients with nasal septal ulcers, nasal trauma, or surgery.

What You DO

Nursing Responsibilities

Respiratory tissues rapidly absorb inhaled oral and nasal corticosteroids. Inhaled corticosteroids must be administered on a routine schedule to prevent asthma attacks. Inhaled corticosteroids are available as metered-dose inhalers (MDIs), which are hand-held canisters that deliver a measured dose of drug with each puff (inhalation). This action facilitates the opening of the airways and allows the corticosteroid to penetrate deeper into the lungs. When the prescribed dose is two puffs (inhalations), allow at least 1 minute between inhalations to allow absorption of the medication. When administering inhaled corticosteroids, the nurse should:

- Teach the patient the correct technique for using an MDI or nasal inhaler.

TAKE HOME POINTS

- Corticosteroids are not intended for emergency use because the medication takes 2 to 3 weeks to reach effective levels. Corticosteroids do not provide immediate symptomatic relief.
- Allow at least 1 minute between puffs or inhalations. When both a bronchodilator and corticosteroid inhaler are prescribed, administer the bronchodilator 5 minutes before using a corticosteroid inhaler to allow opening of airways and deeper lung penetration.

- Instruct the patient who is using intranasal inhalers to use decongestant nose drops first when nasal passages are blocked.
- Advise the patient to avoid using more doses than is prescribed and not to stop using the inhaler without consulting the health care provider.
- Counsel the patient to rinse the mouth with water after each use of a corticosteroid MDI to reduce or prevent the occurrence oropharyngeal fungal infections, hoarseness, or dry cough.
- Instruct the patient to rinse the mouthpiece and cap of the MDI (or the tip of the nasal inhaler) daily with warm, running water, and allow them to air dry before the next use.
- Instruct the patient to clean the mouthpiece and cap of the MDI weekly with warm water and mild dishwashing soap. Cleaning minimizes bacterial exposure and maintains patency.
- Instruct the patient to float the inhalant canister (MDI) in a bowl of water to determine whether the MDI is full or empty. When empty, the canister will float; when full, the canister will sink to the bottom of the bowl.

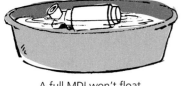

A full MDI won't float.

Do You UNDERSTAND?

DIRECTIONS: Complete the following statements with the appropriate terms from the italicized list provided.

1. Inhaled corticosteroids are used primarily for the treatment of _____.
2. _____ is an intranasal corticosteroid that is used after a nasal polypectomy.
3. Excessive use of corticosteroids may result in _____.
4. A contraindication for the use of inhaled corticosteroids is _____.

   status asthmaticus　　　　*beclomethasone*
   asthma　　　　　　　　*adrenal insufficiency*

What IS a β_2-Agonist?

β_2-Agonists	Trade Names	Uses
albuterol [al-BYOO-ter-ohl]	Proventil, Ventolin	Prevention and treatment of asthma or bronchospasm
metaproterenol [met-ah-proh-TER-ih-nahl]	Alupent	Prevention and treatment of asthma or bronchospasm
terbutaline [ter-BYOO-tah-leen]	Brethine	Prevention and treatment of asthma or bronchospasm
salmeterol [sal-MET-er-ole]	Serevent	Prevention and treatment of asthma or bronchospasm

Action

β_2-Agonists (β_2-**selective adrenergic agonists**) are sympathomimetic agents that stimulate the β_2-receptors to relax the smooth muscles in the bronchioles of the lungs, thereby relaxing bronchospasms and producing bronchodilation. β_2-Agonists also inhibit histamine release from mast cells, decrease airway reaction to allergens, and increase ciliary motility, thereby facilitating expectoration of pulmonary secretions. Inhaled β_2-agonists are absorbed in the lungs; oral β_2-agonists are absorbed in the GI tract.

Uses

β_2-Agonists are available as oral, inhaled short-acting, and inhaled long-acting preparations. The oral and long-acting preparations are used for patients who have frequent asthma attacks. An increased response is achieved when the medication is taken on a fixed schedule. The short-acting preparations (e.g., albuterol, bitolterol, metaproterenol, pirbuterol, terbutaline) are used to treat acute exacerbation of asthma, for short-term relief of bronchoconstriction that is associated with bronchitis and emphysema, and as a prophylaxis for exercise-induced bronchospasm. The only long-acting β_2-agonist available is salmeterol, which is used for prophylaxis of bronchospasm and for the prevention of exercise-induced asthma.

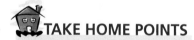

TAKE HOME POINTS

Salmeterol is not useful in the treatment of active bronchospasms.

What You NEED TO KNOW

Cautious use of β₂-agonists should be observed in patients with cardiovascular disease, hypertension, thyroid disease, diabetes mellitus, and sensitivity to sympathomimetics.

Contraindications/Precautions

Cautious use of β_2-agonists should be observed in patients with cardiovascular disease, hypertension, thyroid disease, diabetes mellitus, and sensitivity to sympathomimetics.

β_2-Agonists are contraindicated for use during pregnancy and lactation. Bitolterol, metaproterenol, pirbuterol, salmeterol, and terbutaline are contraindicated for use in children under 12 years of age.

Drug Interactions

Few drug interactions occur with the β_2-agonists, but those that occur are significant. Concurrent use of beta blockers and the β_2-agonists may negate the therapeutic effects of the β_2-agonist. The use of MAOIs or tricyclic antidepressants concurrently with β_2-agonists may exacerbate action on the vascular system. The use of other sympathomimetic bronchodilators may cause additive effects that may lead to hypertensive crisis.

Adverse Effects

Less adverse effects occur with inhalants than with oral preparations. Tremor is the most common adverse effect associated with oral administrations of β_2-agonists. Other adverse effects include anxiety, nervousness, restlessness, tremors, convulsions, weakness, dizziness, vertigo, hallucinations, blurred vision, dilated pupils, headache, hoarseness, palpitations, hypertension, hypotension, bradycardia, reflex tachycardia, nausea, vomiting, muscle cramps, and hypersensitivity reaction. Salmeterol may cause hypokalemia and hyperglycemia.

What You DO

Nursing Responsibilities

β_2-Agonists are available as oral medications, nasal sprays, MDIs, and nebulizer. Patients who require long-term use usually self-administer the drug by inhalation for direct delivery to the constricted bronchial site. Short-acting β_2-agonists provide immediate relief. Inhalation onset of action is 1 minute, whereas the oral onset is 15 minutes. When administering β_2-agonist agents, the nurse should:

- Monitor arterial blood gases and pulmonary function tests periodically during treatment with β_2-agonists.
- Monitor the patient's respiratory status and vital signs.
- Instruct the patient in the correct technique of using an MDI or nasal spray.
- Teach the patient to rinse the mouthpiece and cap of the MDI (or the tip of the nasal spray container) daily with warm, running water, and allow to air dry before the next use. The mouthpiece and cap should be cleaned weekly with warm water and mild dishwashing soap. Cleaning minimizes bacterial exposure and maintains patency.
- Advise the patient to avoid using more than the prescribed doses.
- Tell the patient to notify the health care provider immediately when no response to the usual dose occurs or when the symptoms worsen because the dose may need to be increased.
- Encourage the patient to avoid using OTC medications without approval of the health care provider.

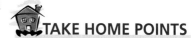

TAKE HOME POINTS

Oral preparations may be given with food to minimize GI adverse effects. Any palpitations, hypotension or hypertension, or any tachycardia should be reported to the health care provider.

Do You UNDERSTAND?

DIRECTIONS: Complete the following statements with the appropriate terms from the italicized list provided.

1. _____ is the only long-acting β_2-agonist available.
2. _____ is an example of a short acting β_2-agonist.
3. β_2-Agonists are used for the treatment of _____.
4. Cautious use of β_2-agonists should be observed in patients with
   _____.

cardiovascular disease   *albuterol*
acute bronchospasms   *salmeterol*

What IS a Leukotriene Antagonist?

Leukotriene Antagonists	Trade Names	Uses
montelukast [mon-te-LOO-cast]	Singulair	Prevention and treatment of asthma
zafirlukast [zah-FIR-loo-cast]	Accolate	Prevention and treatment of asthma
zileuton [zye-LOO-ton]	Leutrol, Zyflo	Prevention and treatment of asthma

Action

Leukotriene receptor antagonists are drugs that inhibit bronchoconstriction. Leukotrienes are inflammatory agents that induce bronchoconstriction and mucus production associated with the inflammatory process of asthma. Zileuton inhibits the enzyme required to start leukotriene synthesis, thereby blocking leukotriene formation. Zafirlukast selectively blocks leukotriene D_4 and E_4 receptors, components of slow-reacting substance of anaphylaxis (SRS-A); montelukast is the receptor antagonist of leukotriene D_4.

Uses

Leukotriene receptor antagonists are used for the prophylaxis and treatment of asthma. Zileuton and zafirlukast are contraindicated for use during lactation.

Montelukast, zileuton, and zafirlukast should be used with caution during pregnancy. Montelukast should be used with caution in children under 6 years of age. Zafirlukast should be used with caution in patients 65 years or older. Safe use of zafirlukast or zileuton has not been established for children under 12 years of age.

What You NEED TO KNOW

Contraindications/Precautions

Leukotriene antagonists are contraindicated for patients with hypersensitivity. Zileuton is contraindicated for use in patients with liver disease. Zafirlukast and montelukast are contraindicated during acute asthma attacks.

Drug Interactions

Concurrent use of zafirlukast or zileuton with warfarin may increase the prothrombin time (PT). Erythromycin decreases the bioavailability of zafirlukast. The theophylline levels may be doubled, resulting in increased toxicity, when used with zileuton. Concurrent use of beta blockers (particularly propranolol) and zileuton may cause hypotension and bradycardia. Concurrent use of zileuton and terfenadine may cause prolonged Q-T intervals. Montelukast has decreased bioavailability and effects when taken concurrently with phenobarbital or rifampin.

Adverse Effects

The most common adverse effects of leukotriene antagonists include headache and dyspepsia. Other adverse effects include weakness **(asthenia),** fever, headache, dizziness, altered taste, anorexia, abdominal pain, diarrhea, nausea, vomiting, insomnia, and liver dysfunction. Additional adverse effects of zileuton include pruritus, conjunctivitis, hypertonia, lymphadenopathy, vaginitis, urinary tract infection (UTI), and leukopenia. Other adverse effects of montelukast include nasal congestion, cough, influenza, laryngitis, pharyngitis, sinusitis, rash, and pyuria.

What You DO

Nursing Responsibilities

Zafirlukast should be administered 1 hour before meals or 2 hours after meals because food decreases the bioavailability of zafirlukast. Montelukast should be administered in the evening for maximal effectiveness. Administer zileuton with meals and at bedtime. When administering leukotriene antagonist agents, the nurse should:

- Evaluate the BP and heart rate for excessive beta blockage and dysrhythmias when the patient is taking propranolol and zileuton.
- Monitor the PT and international normalized ratio (INR) closely in patients who are concurrently taking zafirlukast or zileuton with warfarin.
- Check the complete blood count (CBC) and blood chemistries periodically while undergoing zileuton therapy.
- Monitor liver function tests monthly for the first 3 months of zileuton and zafirlukast therapy, then every 2 to 3 months for the first year, and periodically thereafter.
- Monitor the theophylline levels closely for patients who are taking concurrent zileuton and theophylline therapy for appropriate dosing.
- Monitor the phenytoin level with concurrent zafirlukast or zileuton and phenytoin therapy.

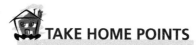

TAKE HOME POINTS

Theophylline levels may be doubled, resulting in increased toxicity, when theophylline and zileuton are used concurrently.

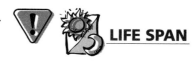

LIFE SPAN

- Montelukast and zafirlukast should be used with caution in patients with severe liver disease.
- Children's chewable tablets of montelukast should not be swallowed whole.
- Chewable montelukast tablets contain phenylalanine and should be administered with caution to patients with phenylketonuria.

- Tell the patient not to crush enteric-coated or sustained-release tablets or capsules.
- Warn the patient that leukotriene antagonists are not to be taken for acute asthma attacks.
- Instruct the patient to take the medication regularly as prescribed and to avoid taking OTC medications without consulting the health care provider to avoid any adverse effects.
- Advise patients to avoid any activities that require alertness and to use caution when driving when they experience any dizziness.
- Instruct patients to notify their health care provider when they experience any acute asthma attacks or influenza-like symptoms.
- Encourage the patient to wear MedicAlert identification.

Do You UNDERSTAND?

DIRECTIONS: **Indicate in the space provided whether the statement is** *true* **or** *false.* **If the answer is false, correct the statement to make it true (using the margin space).**

_____ 1. Children's chewable montelukast tablets may be chewed or swallowed whole.

_____ 2. Patients taking warfarin and zileuton have an increased risk for bleeding.

_____ 3. Leukotriene antagonists are recommended for treatment of status asthmaticus.

What IS a Xanthine Derivative?

Xanthine Derivatives	Trade Names	Uses
theophylline [thee-OFF-ih-lin]	Theo-Dur	Prevention and treatment of asthma and bronchospasm
dyphylline [DYE-fi-lin]	Dilor	Prevention and treatment of asthma and bronchospasm
oxtriphylline [ox-TRYE-fi-lin]	Choledyl	Prevention and treatment of asthma and bronchospasm

Answers: 1. false; children's chewable montelukast tablets should not be swallowed whole; 2. true; 3. false; leukotriene antagonists are used for the prophylaxis and treatment of asthma.

Action

Xanthine derivatives or methylxanthine are agents that relax bronchial smooth muscle cells and suppress airway response to stimuli, thereby producing bronchodilation. The primary effects of methylxanthines are stimulation of the CNS and bronchodilation. Other effects of methylxanthines include cardiac stimulation, vasodilation, and diuresis.

Uses

Xanthine derivatives are used for prophylaxis, for the treatment of chronic asthma, and for the treatment of bronchospasm related to chronic bronchitis and emphysema. Xanthine derivatives are used less frequently than they were in the past because more effective and safer medications (e.g., inhaled corticosteroids, β-agonists) are now available. In the treatment of asthma, theophylline is the primary xanthine derivative that is used.

What You NEED TO KNOW

Contraindications/Precautions

Xanthine derivatives are contraindicated for patients with hypersensitivity to xanthines. Oxtriphylline is contraindicated for patients with cardiac disease and renal and liver disease.

Drug Interactions

Concurrent use of xanthine derivatives with beta blockers, cimetidine, tacrine, zileuton, quinolones, macrolide antibiotics, high-dose allopurinol (more than 600 mg), and caffeine may increase theophylline levels. Concurrent use of theophylline or theophylline salts with lithium increases the excretion of lithium, thereby lowering lithium levels. Concurrent use of dyphylline and beta blockers may antagonize the bronchodilating effects. Use of halothane with dyphylline may increase the risk for cardiac dysrhythmias. Use of probenecid decreases the elimination of dyphylline.

Adverse Effects

Adverse effects associated with plasma theophylline levels less than 20 mcg/mL are few. Levels of 20 to 25 mcg/mL may cause restlessness, nausea, vomiting, diarrhea, headache, and insomnia and levels greater than 30 mcg/mL may cause severe dysrhythmias, seizures, or death. Other common adverse effects of xanthine derivatives include nervousness,

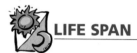

LIFE SPAN

Xanthine derivatives are contraindicated during pregnancy and lactation.

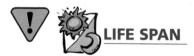

LIFE SPAN

Xanthine derivatives should be used with caution in neonates, young children, and older adults.

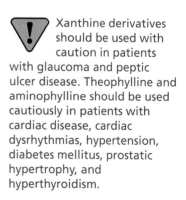

Xanthine derivatives should be used with caution in patients with glaucoma and peptic ulcer disease. Theophylline and aminophylline should be used cautiously in patients with cardiac disease, cardiac dysrhythmias, hypertension, diabetes mellitus, prostatic hypertrophy, and hyperthyroidism.

Theophylline should also be used with caution in patients with seizure disorders. Aminophylline should also be used with caution in patients with renal or hepatic dysfunction, fibrocystic breast disease, COPD, or acute influenza, as well as those who are receiving influenza vaccine. Dyphylline should be used with caution in patients with severe cardiac disease, hypertension, renal or hepatic dysfunction, and hyperthyroidism. Oxtriphylline should be used with caution in patients with prostatic hypertrophy and diabetes mellitus.

TAKE HOME POINTS

Instruct the patient to take medicine at the same time every day for maximal effectiveness. A dose of 156 mg of oxtriphylline is equivalent to 100 mg of theophylline. All doses should be based on ideal body weight. The rate of aminophylline infusion should not exceed 25/mg/min, diluted or undiluted. The therapeutic theophylline plasma level is 10 to 20 mcg/mL.

flushing, dizziness, anorexia, palpitations, hypotension, fever, dehydration, bradycardia, tachycardia, hyperglycemia, hyperreflexia, decreased clotting time, and increased WBC (**leukocytosis**).

What You DO

Nursing Responsibilities

Xanthines should be administered routinely at the same times every day to maintain therapeutic levels. The dosing guidelines for aminophylline are the same as those for theophylline. When administering xanthine derivatives, the nurse should:

- Instruct the patient that the capsule may be swallowed or opened, with the contents sprinkled on a small amount of soft food (e.g., pudding, ice cream) before ingestion.
- Administer aminophylline and dyphylline 1 hour before or 2 hours after meals with a full glass of water to enhance absorption. When GI distress occurs, these agents may be given after meals to reduce GI adverse effects.
- Encourage the patient to drink at least 2000 mL of fluids daily to thin respiratory secretions.
- Advise the patient to avoid caffeine (e.g., colas, chocolate, coffee) to control cardiovascular and CNS adverse effects.
- Instruct the patient to avoid charbroiled foods because they decrease theophylline effectiveness. A high-protein, low-carbohydrate diet will increase theophylline elimination.
- Instruct the patient to take the medication only as prescribed, to avoid exceeding the prescribed dose, and to avoid using OTC drugs without the health care provider's approval. Many common OTC preparations for colds, allergies, and cough contain other sympathomimetics, caffeine, ephedrine, or other xanthines.
- Advise the patient to avoid smoking because cigarette and marijuana smoking decrease theophylline plasma concentration by 50%.
- Realize that aminophylline is the only xanthine that can be administered IV and is rarely used orally.
- Examine the parenteral preparations for any precipitate before using, and avoid using these preparations when clumping occurs.
- Monitor vital signs and intake and output of urine when the patient is receiving IV aminophylline.

- Monitor theophylline drug levels routinely for evidence of toxicity (greater than 20 mcg/mL) for patients who are receiving theophylline.
- Withhold theophylline and measure the theophylline level to rule out toxicity in any patient who develops nausea and vomiting. Theophylline levels are of no use in patients who are taking dyphylline because dyphylline is not metabolized to theophylline, as are the other xanthines. A therapeutic dyphylline blood level is 12 mcg/mL.

> ⚠ Sustained-action capsules of theophylline should not be chewed or crushed. Rapid infusion of intravenous (IV) aminophylline may cause cardiac arrest. A sudden, sharp, unexpected rise in the heart rate is a clinical indicator of IV aminophylline toxicity.

Do You UNDERSTAND?

DIRECTIONS: **Fill in the blanks with the appropriate responses to complete the following statements.**

1. The therapeutic theophylline plasma level is _____.
2. Common adverse effects of xanthine derivatives are nervousness, _____, and tachycardia.

What IS an Anticholinergic?

Anticholinergic	Trade Name	Uses
ipratropium [eye-prah-TROH-pee-um]	Atrovent	Treatment of bronchitis, asthma, and emphysema

Action

Anticholinergics are agents that block muscarinic cholinergic receptors in the bronchi and inhibit vagal-mediated responses (bronchospasms), thereby facilitating bronchodilation. The anticholinergic that affects the respiratory system is ipratropium.

Uses

Ipratropium is used for the maintenance treatment of chronic asthma and bronchospasm associated with COPD, including emphysema and chronic bronchitis. The intranasal spray is used for the treatment of perennial rhinitis and rhinorrhea.

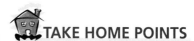

TAKE HOME POINTS

Ipratropium is not used for the treatment of an acute bronchospasm attack.

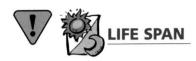

LIFE SPAN

- Ipratropium should be used cautiously in women during pregnancy and lactation.
- Ipratropium should be used cautiously for patients with narrow-angle glaucoma, bladder neck obstruction, or prostatic hypertrophy.

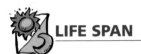

LIFE SPAN

Ipratropium is contraindicated for use in children under 12 years of age.

What You NEED TO KNOW

Contraindications/Precautions

Ipratropium is contraindicated for use as primary treatment in patients with hypersensitivity to atropine and acute bronchospasm episodes.

Drug Interactions

No drug interactions are noted for anticholinergic agents.

Adverse Effects

The most common adverse effects of ipratropium are cough and headache. Other adverse effects include blurred vision, eye pain, exacerbation of narrow-angle glaucoma, bitter taste, dry mouth, hoarseness, exacerbation of respiratory symptoms, nervousness, dizziness, fatigue, palpitations, nasal dryness, rash, urticaria, and urinary retention.

What You DO

Nursing Responsibilities

Ipratropium is available as nasal sprays and MDIs. When administering anticholinergics, the nurse should:

- Auscultate the patient's lungs before and after inhalations, and monitor the respiratory status.
- Instruct the patient to void before administration of the medication to avoid urinary retention.
- Instruct the patient to allow 1 minute between inhalations when the dose is two inhalations for maximal effectiveness. When the patient is taking other inhalants, instruct the patient to wait 5 minutes between inhalations.
- Teach the patient the correct technique for using an MDI or nasal spray.
- Instruct the patient to rinse the mouthpiece and cap of the MDI (or the tip of the nasal spray container) daily with warm, running water, and allow them to air dry before the next use.
- Instruct the patient to clean the mouthpiece and cap weekly with warm water and mild dishwashing soap. Cleaning minimizes bacterial exposure and maintains patency.

- Suggest to the patient who is using MDIs to rinse the mouth after use to decrease the bitter taste.
- Instruct patients to take medication as directed and to notify the health care provider when respiratory symptoms worsen.
- Warn the patient to avoid spraying the medication into the eyes. Blurred vision or eye pain may result.

Do You UNDERSTAND?

DIRECTIONS: Complete the crossword puzzle.

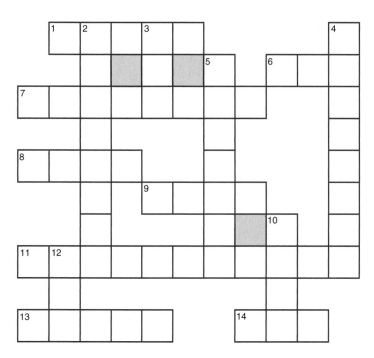

Across

1. Oral inhalation may cause this to be bitter.
6. Minutes to wait between inhalations of ipratropium.
7. Ipratropium is a derivative of this drug.
8. Wait this many minutes before using another inhaler.
9. A 0.06% spray is treatment for the common one of these.
11. MDIs are this type of canister.

13. Ipratropium is excreted in this.
14. Hand-held canister for oral inhalation.

Down

2. An anticholinergic drug used for asthma.
3. After use of nasal spray, rinse this.
4. A common adverse reaction.
5. Route for treatment of asthma.
10. To avoid urinary retention, have the patient do this before taking the drug.
12. Painful when spray gets here.

References

Abrams AC, Lammon CB, Pennington SS: *Clinical drug therapy: rationales for nursing practice,* ed 8, Philadelphia, 2007, Lippincott.

Adams MP, Josephson DL, Holland LN Jr: *Pharmacology for nurses: a pathophysiologic approach,* Upper Saddle River, New Jersey, 2005, Pearson.

Gutierrez K, Queener SF: *Pharmacology for nursing practice,* St Louis, 2003, Mosby.

Hardman JG, Limbird LE: *Goodman & Gilman's the pharmacological basis of therapeutics,* ed 10, New York, 2001, McGraw-Hill.

Hodgson B, Kizior R: *Saunders nursing drug handbook 2005,* St Louis, 2005, Elsevier.

Ignatavicius DD, Workman ML: *Medical-surgical nursing: critical thinking for collaborative care,* ed 5, St Louis, 2006, Elsevier.

Karch AM: *Focus on nursing pharmacology,* ed 3, Philadelphia, 2006, Lippincott.

Kee JL, Hayes ER, McCuistion LE: *Pharmacology: a nursing process approach,* ed 5, Philadelphia, 2006, Elsevier.

Lehne RA: *Pharmacology for nursing care,* ed 5, Philadelphia, 2004, WB Saunders.

Lilley LL, Harrington S, Snyder JS: *Pharmacology and the nursing process,* ed 4, St Louis, 2005, Mosby.

McKenry, LM, Salerno, E: *Mosby's pharmacology in nursing,* ed 21, St Louis, 2003, Mosby.

Smeltzer SC, Bare BG: *Brunner and Suddarth's textbook of medical-surgical nursing,* ed 10, Philadelphia, 2004, Lippincott.

Wilson BA, Shannon MT, Stang CL: *Nurses drug guide,* Upper Saddle River, New Jersey, 2006, Pearson.

Answers: *Across:* 1. taste; 6. one; 7. atropine; 8. five; 9. cold; 11. metered dose; 13. feces; 14. MDI. *Down:* 2. atrovent; 3. tip; 4. headache; 5. inhaled; 10. void; 12. eye.

NCLEX® Review

Section A

1. Which drug is an example of an opioid antitussive?
   1 Pseudoephedrine (Sudafed)
   2 Naphazoline (Allerest)
   3 Hydrocodone (Hycodan)
   4 Benzonatate (Tessalon)

2. OTC combination preparations commonly contain which substance?
   1 Acetylcysteine (Mucomyst)
   2 Guaifenesin (Robitussin)
   3 Codeine (Paveral)
   4 Hydrocodone (Vicodin)

3. Dextromethorphan (Benylin DM), when given concurrently with MAOIs, may cause which adverse effects?
   1 Drowsiness and lethargy
   2 Excitation and hyperpyrexia
   3 Hypertension and nausea
   4 An anesthetic effect and choking

4. Which drug is the antidote for an opioid overdose?
   1 Acetylcysteine (Mucomyst)
   2 Diphenhydramine (Benadryl)
   3 Naloxone (Narcan)
   4 Acetaminophen (Tylenol)

5. Rebound congestion may result from nasal decongestants that are used longer than which time frame?
   1 That which is less than prescribed
   2 24 hours
   3 1 to 2 days
   4 3 to 5 days

Section B

6. Which classification of antihistamines is referred to as nonsedating?
   1 Alkylamines
   2 Ethylenediamines
   3 Phenothiazines
   4 Piperazines

7. Before skin test procedures for allergy, clemastine fumarate (Tavist) should be discontinued at least how many days before administration to avoid false results?
   1 1
   2 2
   3 4
   4 10

8. Concurrent use of MAOIs with H_1-receptor antagonists (ethanolamines) may prolong or increase which type of effects of antihistamines?
   1 Emetic
   2 Anticholinergic
   3 Antiemetic
   4 Hypnotic

9. Because of the life-threatening adverse effects present with overdose, recommendations are that children should not be given which medication?
   1 Sustained-release tripelennamine (PBZ-SR)
   2 Oral brompheniramine (Dimetane)
   3 Oral diphenhydramine (Benadryl)
   4 Rectal promethazine (Phenergan)

10. Most H_1-receptor antagonists are contraindicated in patients with which condition?
    1 Anxiety disorders
    2 Narrow-angle glaucoma
    3 Skin infections
    4 Elevated temperature

Section C

11. Which action decreases the edema and mucus production of the airways as part of the action of inhaled corticosteroids?
    1 Inhibiting protein synthesis
    2 Blocking α-adrenergic receptors
    3 Inhibiting the inflammatory response
    4 Blocking the opiate receptors

12. A patient is taking fluticasone (Flonase). The nurse realizes that excessive use of corticosteroids may cause which result?
    1 Adrenal insufficiency
    2 Status asthmaticus
    3 Sudden death
    4 Vaginal bleeding

13. Montelukast is classified as a _____.
    1 β-Agonist.
    2 Corticosteroid.
    3 Leukotriene antagonist.
    4 Xanthine derivative.

14. Which drug is a long-acting β₂-agonist?
    1 Bitolterol
    2 Metaproterenol
    3 Salmeterol
    4 Terbutaline

15. Which range is considered the therapeutic level of theophylline?
    1 0 to 5 mcg/mL
    2 5 to 10 mcg/mL
    3 10 to 20 mcg/mL
    4 25 to 30 mcg/mL

NCLEX® Review Answers

Section A

1. **3** Hydrocodone is an opioid antitussive. Pseudoephedrine and naphazoline are decongestants. Benzonatate is a nonopioid antitussive.

2. **2** Guaifenesin is commonly found in OTC cold preparations. Acetylcysteine requires a prescription. Codeine and hydrocodone are controlled substances that also require a prescription.

3. **2** Excitation and hyperpyrexia may occur when dextromethorphan is given concurrently with an MAOI. Drowsiness, lethargy, hypertension, and nausea are not adverse effects of dextromethorphan. An anesthetic effect and choking are adverse effects of benzonatate.

4. **3** Naloxone is the antidote for an opioid overdose. Acetylcysteine is the antidote for acetaminophen, not opioid overdose. Diphenhydramine and acetaminophen are not antidotes.

5. **4** Rebound congestion may result from nasal decongestants that are used longer than 3 to 5 days. Rebound congestion occurs with the overuse or abuse of nasal decongestants, not with short-term use. Therefore taking less than prescribed, taking the medication for 24 hours, or taking for 1 to 2 days do cause rebound congestion.

Section B

6. **4** The second-generation antihistamines produce low to no CNS adverse effects of sedation, do not cross the blood-brain barrier, and are called nonsedating. Piperazines are second-generation antihistamines. The most common adverse effect of alkylamines is drowsiness. Ethylenediamines and phenothiazines are first-generation antihistamines.

7. **3** Clemastine fumarate should be discontinued at least 4 days before skin testing to avoid false results. Discontinuing antihistamines 1 day, 2 days, or 10 days before skin testing is inappropriate.

8. **2** Use of MAOIs with H₁-receptor antagonists may prolong or intensify anticholinergic effects because MAOIs interfere with the detoxification of antihistamines and phenothiazines. Taking MAOIs with H₁-receptor antagonists does not cause emetic, antiemetic, or hypnotic effects.

9. **1** The sustained-release form of tripelennamine is not recommended for use in children because overdose may cause hallucinations, convulsions, coma, and cardiovascular collapse. Brompheniramine and diphenhydramine are incorrect because they are not contraindicated in children. Promethazine is contraindicated only in acutely ill, dehydrated children.

10. 2 Most ethanolamines (H_1-receptor antagonists) are contraindicated in patients with narrow-angle glaucoma. Antihistamines, particularly ethanolamines, are not contraindicated in patients with anxiety disorders, skin infections, or an elevated temperature.

Section C

11. 3 Inhaled corticosteroids inhibit the inflammatory process, thereby decreasing edema and mucus production of the airways. Inhaled corticosteroids do not inhibit protein synthesis, block α-adrenergic receptors, or block opiate receptors.

12. 1 Excessive use of corticosteroids, such as fluticasone may result in adrenal insufficiency. Excessive use of corticosteroids does not cause status asthmaticus, sudden death, or vaginal bleeding.

13. 3 Montelukast is classified as a leukotriene antagonist, not as a β_2-agonist, corticosteroid, or a xanthine derivative.

14. 3 Salmeterol is the only long-acting β_2-agonist available. Bitolterol, metaproterenol, and terbutaline are short-acting β_2-agonists.

15. 3 The therapeutic level of theophylline is 10 to 20 mcg/mL. Levels of 0 to 5 mcg/mL and 5 to 10 mcg/mL are subtherapeutic. A level of 25 to 30 mcg/mL is a toxic range.

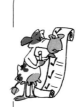

Notes

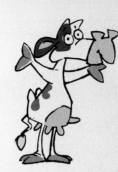

Chapter 9

Drugs Used to Treat Endocrine System Disorders

What You WILL LEARN

After reading this chapter, you will know how to do the following:

- ✔ Identify the pharmacodynamics of drugs used to treat pituitary disorders.
- ✔ Discuss the adverse effects and contraindications for drugs used to treat adrenal disorders.
- ✔ Explain the laboratory considerations for drugs used to treat thyroid and parathyroid disorders.
- ✔ Describe the onset, peak, and duration of rapid-acting, short-acting, intermediate-acting, long-acting, and constant-acting insulin.
- ✔ Differentiate the action of a sulfonylurea, α-glucosidase inhibitor, biguanide, thiazolidinedione, and a meglitinide.

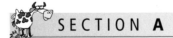

SECTION A

PITUITARY AND ADRENAL HORMONES

This section discusses drugs used to treat patients with altered function of the anterior and posterior pituitary gland and the cortex of the adrenal gland. The pituitary gland is composed of the anterior and posterior lobes.

The anterior lobe of the pituitary gland secretes hormones that regulate the growth, development, and proper functioning of other endocrine glands. Anterior pituitary hormone drugs are used to treat patients with conditions characterized by hormone deficiency. Nerve cells in the hypothalamus produce two hormones that the posterior pituitary gland secretes: antidiuretic hormone (**vasopressin**) and oxytocin.

Posterior pituitary hormone drugs are used to treat diabetes insipidus, a condition that results from a deficiency of antidiuretic hormone (ADH). Patients with diabetes insipidus are unable to control the amount of water lost in the urine and have a large urinary output (**polyuria).**

The adrenal cortex produces two classes of hormones: corticosteroids and androgenic steroids. All adrenal hormones are steroids with similar chemical structures but different physiologic effects. Corticosteroids (**adrenocortical hormones** and **adrenocorticosteroids**) are divided into two groups: glucocorticosteroids (e.g., cortisol, cortisone, corticosterone) and mineralocorticoids (e.g., aldosterone, desoxycorticosterone). When adrenal cortex function is compromised, synthetic adrenal hormones can be used to replace those that are naturally produced. In rare cases, hormones from the adrenal cortex may exceed body requirements. When appropriate, adrenal hormone–inhibiting drugs are used to suppress the production of excess hormones.

What IS an Anterior Pituitary Hormone Replacement Drug?

Anterior Pituitary Hormone Replacements	Trade Names	Uses
somatropin [so-mah-TROH-pin]	Humatrope	Treatment of growth hormone deficiency
somatrem [SO-mah-trem]	Protropin	Treatment of growth hormone deficiency
corticotropin [kor-tih-koh-TROH-pin]	ACTH	Diagnosis and treatment of adrenal insufficiency
cosyntropin [koh-SIN-troh-pin]	Cortrosyn	Diagnosis of adrenocortical insufficiency

Action

Somatropin and somatrem are human growth hormone–like drugs that facilitate the transport of amino acids across cell membranes. These drugs

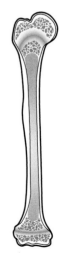

Somatropin and somatrem encourage skeletal growth.

increase cell size and encourage skeletal growth, particularly the epiphyseal plates of long bones. Somatropin and somatrem also decrease the transport of glucose into cells and reduce the amount of glucose that is used, thereby causing an increase in blood glucose levels. This action produces a diabetic-like state in the patient. Additionally, the movement of amino acids increases nitrogen balance and decreases urea production.

Somatropin and somatrem also prompt the release of free fatty acids from fat tissue, leading to increased fat storage in the liver and making more fatty acids available for energy. This action is referred to as **ketogenesis** because it results from fat breakdown leading to the conversion of fatty acids to ketone bodies. When somatropin and somatrem are given to adults with adult-onset pituitary deficiency, a marked increase in high-density lipoproteins (HDL), known as "good" cholesterol, occurs. Low-density lipoprotein (LDL) levels, known as "bad" cholesterol, remain unchanged.

Corticotropin and cosyntropin stimulate the adrenal cortex to release glucocorticosteroids and mineralocorticoids. Corticotropin and cosyntropin are effective only when the adrenal cortex can respond to stimulation. The physiologic effects include increased energy levels and stabilized fluid and electrolyte balance.

Uses

Somatrem and somatropin promote anabolic tissue growth in patients with a deficiency of human growth hormone, a condition known as dwarfism.

Corticotropin and cosyntropin are used diagnostically to stimulate the synthesis of glucocorticosteroids, mineralocorticoids, and androgens. The corticotropin stimulation test helps differentiate primary from secondary adrenal cortex insufficiency. In patients with secondary insufficiency, plasma cortisol levels will rise after an injection of corticotropin. Corticotropin is also used as an antiinflammatory or immunosuppressant drug when conventional glucocorticosteroid therapy fails. Additionally, corticotropin is occasionally used to help manage adrenal crisis.

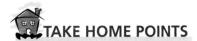

TAKE HOME POINTS

Anterior pituitary hormone replacements are ineffective when impaired growth results from other causes or when used after puberty, during which the ends of long bones have closed.

What You NEED TO KNOW

Contraindications/Precautions

Corticotropin is contraindicated in patients with an excess production of adrenal cortex hormones. Because it exacerbates symptoms, corticotropin is also contraindicated in patients with psychoses. Corticotropin use should be avoided in patients with active tuberculosis or acquired immunodeficiency syndrome (AIDS) because immunity is decreased and the risk for gastrointestinal (GI) perforation and hemorrhage is increased. Corticotropin is also contraindicated for patients with peptic ulcer disease, scleroderma, osteoporosis, systemic fungal infections, as well as for those who are sensitive to pork and pork products.

Drug Interactions

A decrease in growth may result when somatrem and somatropin are given concurrently with glucocorticosteroids or corticotropin. Conversely, when these drugs are given with anabolic steroids, estrogens, and thyroid hormones, an increase in growth may result.

Corticotropin may increase metabolism of glucocorticosteroids when taken concurrently with barbiturates, phenytoin, and rifampin. Estrogens and oral contraceptives block the metabolism of corticotropin when given together. Salicylates increase the risk for GI bleeding. Patients taking insulin or oral hypoglycemic drugs may require increase dosage when these drugs are given with corticotropin. Amphotericin B, carbonic anhydrase inhibitors, mezlocillin, piperacillin, and ticarcillin increase the risk for hypokalemia and subsequent cardiac glycoside toxicity.

Blood or blood products may render cosyntropin inactive when given together. Cosyntropin increases the metabolism of glucocorticosteroids when given concurrently.

Adverse Effects

Locally, somatrem and somatropin cause pain and swelling at the injection site. An additional adverse effect includes a slipped femoral epiphysis. Either drug can cause edema of the hands and feet. Somatrem depresses thyroid function and insulin production and may cause insulin resistance.

The adverse effects of corticotropin appear most frequently with chronic use of doses exceeding 40 units per day. The most common

Generally, anterior pituitary drugs cause elevated serum glucose levels (**hyperglycemia**) in susceptible individuals; thus these drugs are used with caution in patients with a family history of diabetes. Somatropin and somatrem are used cautiously in patients with growth hormone deficiency resulting from lesions in the brain or those who have a coexisting adrenocorticotropic hormone (ACTH) deficiency. These drugs are also used with caution in patients with thyroid dysfunction. Cautious use of corticotropin is warranted in patients with hypertension or heart failure resulting from sodium and water retention. Corticotropin should be used cautiously with patients with myasthenia gravis because muscle weakness is increased. The drug should be used cautiously in patients who are taking salicylates and other nonsteroidal antiinflammatory drugs because of the risk for peptic ulcers.

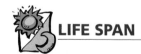

LIFE SPAN

Safe use of anterior pituitary replacements during pregnancy and lactation has not been established.

adverse effects of corticotropin include depression, nausea, and superficial capillary bleeding (**petechiae**), sodium retention (**hypernatremia**), and adrenal suppression. Drug effects of corticotropin on the central nervous system (CNS) include seizure, vertigo, headache, personality changes, euphoria, mood swings, and psychosis. Impaired wound healing, thinning of the skin, bruising (**ecchymosis**), facial redness, increased sweating (**diaphoresis**), and hyperpigmentation may occur. Additionally, the patient may experience hypertension, fluid volume overload, heart failure, low serum calcium levels (**hypocalcemia**), low serum potassium levels (**hypokalemia**), alkalosis, and a negative nitrogen balance. Long-term use of corticotropin suppresses pituitary release of corticotropin causing an overgrowth of adrenal cortex tissue (**adrenocortical hyperplasia**), decreased glucose tolerance, muscle weakness, and stunting of growth in children.

The adverse effect of cosyntropin is hypersensitivity, including anaphylaxis. Patients who are sensitive to pork or pork products may have an allergic response to corticotropin.

What You DO

Nursing Responsibilities

When administering pituitary and adrenal hormones, the nurse should:

- Refrigerate somatropin and somatrem before and after reconstitution with bacteriostatic water for injection. Reconstituted solutions should be clear and used within 14 days.
- Give somatropin injections at least 48 hours apart. Sub-Q injections are preferred and most frequently given because they are less painful. Corticotropin is given Sub-Q because the drug is a protein substance that proteolytic enzymes destroy in the GI tract if taken orally.
- Evaluate bone growth and growth rate, as well as height and weight, every 3 to 6 months. Reevaluate patients who continue to lose weight after the first 2 weeks of treatment.
- Monitor thyroid function throughout therapy because these drugs may decrease thyroid hormone levels, iodine uptake, and thyroxine-binding capacity. When thyroid deficiency (**hypothyroidism**) becomes apparent, concurrent thyroid hormone replacement will be necessary for the growth hormone to be effective.

- Realize that dosages are titrated based on patient response because individual absorption rates vary widely.
- Monitor blood glucose levels periodically for the patient who has diabetes throughout somatrem, somatropin, or corticotropin therapy for possible dose increase of insulin.
- Clarify to the patient the importance of routine monitoring of drug and hormone levels.
- Evaluate hematologic values and electrolytes routinely for patients who are undergoing prolonged corticotropin therapy.
- Monitor inorganic phosphorous, alkaline phosphatase, and parathyroid hormone levels because somatropin may cause an increase in these levels.
- Inform the patient who is receiving anterior pituitary drugs about the consequences of abruptly discontinuing treatment.
- Instruct the patient to report physical changes to the health care provider, including fever, sore throat, muscle weakness, sudden weight gain, and edema.
- Teach the patient about sodium-restricted diets that are high in vitamin D, protein, and potassium.
- Inform the patient that somatropin and somatrem have a great potential for misuse, primarily because of the real and perceived chance of increasing muscle mass and decreasing body fat. Enhanced athletic performance is the most commonly desired result.
- Advise patients who are taking anterior pituitary hormones to wear or carry MedicAlert identification and to check with the health care provider before using over-the-counter (OTC) drugs.
- Instruct patients who are taking anterior pituitary hormones to avoid immunizations that use live vaccines (e.g., mumps, measles, and rubella) because this decreases immunity.

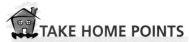

TAKE HOME POINTS

Do not shake the vial when reconstituting somatropin and somatrem; instead, swirl gently. Serum growth hormone levels are greater after a subcutaneous (Sub-Q) abdominal injection compared with a Sub-Q injection in the thigh. Growth hormone drugs are useless for stimulating linear growth in adults because of the closure of the long bones.

Do You UNDERSTAND?

DIRECTIONS: Unscramble each of the following anagrams to find the pituitary drug name(s). Describe the drug's action and its effects or use.

1. Tricorn coop it:

   Action: _____

   Effects: _____

2. I am protons and toms mare:

   Action: _____

   Effects: _____

3. Onions crypt:

   Action: _____

   Use: _____

What IS a Posterior Pituitary Hormone Replacement Drug?

Posterior Pituitary Hormone Replacements	Trade Names	Uses
desmopressin acetate [des-moh-PRESS-in]	DDAVP	Prevention and treatment of diabetes insipidus, enuresis, acute epistaxis
lypressin [lye-PRESS-in]	Diapid	Prevention and treatment of diabetes insipidus
vasopressin [vay-so-PRESS-in]	ADH, Pitressin	Treatment of diabetes insipidus

Action

Vasopressin and its analogs (desmopressin and lypressin) increase the reabsorption of water from the distal renal tubules, which in turn decreases urine formation and controls water balance in the body. In large doses,

Answers: 1. corticotropin. Action: stimulates adrenal cortex to release glucocorticosteroids, mineralocorticoids, and androgens. Effects: increased energy levels and stabilized fluid and electrolyte balance; 2. somatropin and somatrem. Action: stimulates growth via effects on most body tissues, particularly long bones. Effects: increased bone growth and rate; 3. cosyntropin. Action: stimulates adrenal cortex to release glucocorticosteroids, mineralocorticoids, and androgens. Use: diagnosis of ACTH deficiency.

desmopressin and lypressin stimulate smooth muscle contraction, particularly of the arterioles. The vasoconstriction decreases blood flow to the splenic, mesentery, coronary, GI, pancreatic, skin, and muscular systems and raises blood pressure. It is important to note that the amount of drug necessary to promote water conservation is seldom sufficiently high enough to produce widespread effects on blood pressure. These drugs also increase peristalsis of the large bowel and contraction of the gallbladder and urinary bladder. Some oxytocic activity may also occur, causing uterine contractions. The mechanism by which desmopressin enhances platelet function is unknown. Vasopressin is prepared from the pituitary glands of cattle or pigs.

Uses

With the exception of oxytocin, posterior pituitary hormones are used to treat diabetes insipidus, a condition characterized by thirst and the elimination of large amounts of extremely dilute urine. Vasopressin and lypressin are used primarily to control neurogenic diabetes insipidus. Desmopressin is used to treat nephrogenic diabetes insipidus and is useful in treating bedwetting **(enuresis)**. Desmopressin is also indicated to control acute nosebleeds **(epistaxis)** when administered in the nose and GI hemorrhage when administered intravenously (IV).

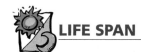

LIFE SPAN

Safe use of posterior pituitary replacements during pregnancy and lactation has not been established.

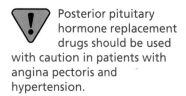

Posterior pituitary hormone replacement drugs should be used with caution in patients with angina pectoris and hypertension.

What You NEED TO KNOW

Contraindications/Precautions

Vasopressin, desmopressin, and lypressin are contraindicated for patients with known hypersensitivity and platelet-type von Willebrand's disease.

Drug Interactions

Chlorpropamide, clofibrate, carbamazepine, and fludrocortisone enhance the antidiuretic response to desmopressin when given concurrently. Lithium, norepinephrine, heparin, and alcohol reduce the antidiuretic response to desmopressin when given together. Ganglionic-blocking drugs, barbiturates, and cyclopropane increase the vasopressor effects of desmopressin.

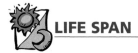

LIFE SPAN

In patients with coronary artery disease, even small doses have been found to precipitate angina, particularly in older adults.

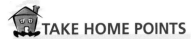

TAKE HOME POINTS

Should fluid overload develop, the drug should be withdrawn and the patient's fluid intake restricted until the urine specific gravity is at least 1.015 (normal: 1.010 to 1.030). Weigh the patient daily and assess for edema. Caution the patient to adhere to the prescribed dose of nasal spray.

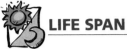

LIFE SPAN

Because of the age-related decline in hepatic and renal function, older adults are at an increased risk for drug overdose.

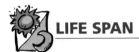

LIFE SPAN

Because children are susceptible to fluid volume disturbances, drug therapies should be carefully chosen. An air-filled syringe may be attached to the rhinyle (flexible calibrated plastic tube) for children, infants, or obtunded patients.

Adverse Effects

The adverse effects of small doses of vasopressin are usually mild. The most common adverse effects include circumoral pallor, abdominal cramps, nausea, sweating, tremor, and severe headache. Uterine cramping and diarrhea may develop because of the stimulant effects of vasopressin. Shifts in fluid volume occur with initial therapy. Large doses of vasopressin can cause blood pressure elevations, anginal pain, dysrhythmias, and myocardial infarction (MI). The pressor effects of vasopressin are not usually evident with the dose used to manage diabetes insipidus. The adverse effects of desmopressin and lypressin, which are infrequent and mild, include conjunctivitis, runny nose, local irritation and congestion of nasal passages, headache, and heartburn.

What You DO

Nursing Responsibilities

Posterior pituitary hormones, whether in natural or synthetic form, are proteins that, when taken orally, gastric enzymes will destroy. These drugs are therefore administered either parenterally or via nasal sprays. When administering posterior pituitary hormone replacement drugs, the nurse should:

- Shake the oil formulation of vasopressin vigorously to disperse the ingredients before administration.
- Give the patient one or two glasses of water at the time the injection is given to minimize the GI adverse effects.
- Monitor for signs of fluid overload. Reevaluate patients who continue to lose weight after the first 2 weeks of treatment.
- Assess the patient for symptoms of dehydration (e.g., excessive thirst, dry skin and mucous membranes, tachycardia, poor skin turgor).
- Monitor older adults and patients who have difficulty tolerating the fluid shifts associated with initial vasopressin therapy. The signs and symptoms of water toxicity include confusion, drowsiness, headache, weight gain, difficulty urinating, seizures, and coma.

- Administer desmopressin via a flexible nasal catheter (**rhinyle**) that is used to measure the drug. After the drug is drawn into the catheter, one end is placed in the patient's nose and the other end in the patient's mouth. The patient then blows into the catheter to deposit the drug in the nasal passages. The tube should be rinsed after each use.
- Administer lypressin by holding the bottle upright with the patient sitting upright and the head tipped slightly backward. No more than three sprays should be taken at any one time.
- Instruct the patient that if a dose is missed, the missed dose should be taken as soon as it is remembered, except when it is nearly time for the next dose. Doubling the dose and transferring any remaining drug to another bottle should be avoided.
- Contact the health care provider if the patient has increased urine output, runny nose, nasal irritation, or an upper respiratory infection for possible dose adjustment.
- Monitor hepatic and renal function tests for patients who are taking a posterior pituitary drug, particularly older patients.
- Monitor the patient's urine specific gravity, urine volume, and serum electrolytes throughout therapy.
- Advise patients to avoid using OTC drugs without checking with the health care provider and to wear or carry MedicAlert identification.

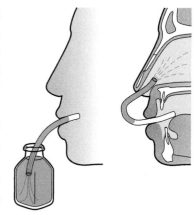

How to administer desmopressin.

Do You UNDERSTAND?

DIRECTIONS: **Unscramble each of the following anagrams to find the posterior drug or a term associated with posterior pituitary drug use.**

1. screen test dame soap it
2. bedsides unit spa ii
3. prison vases
4. entropy shine
5. salan
6. nyrelih

a. vasopressin
b. desmopressin acetate
c. hypertension
d. rhinyle
e. nasal
f. diabetes insipidus

What IS a Glucocorticosteroid?

Glucocorticosteroids	Trade Names	Uses
cortisone [KOR-tih-zone]	Cortone	Treatment of adrenocortical insufficiency
dexamethasone [dex-ah-METH-ah-zone]	Decadron	Treatment of adrenocortical insufficiency
hydrocortisone [hye-droh-KOR-tih-zone]	Hydrocortone	Treatment of adrenocortical insufficiency
prednisone [PRED-nih-zone]	Deltasone	Treatment of adrenocortical insufficiency
triamcinolone [try-am-SIN-oh-lone]	Aristospan	Treatment of adrenocortical insufficiency

Action

A glucocorticosteroid is any substance that increases the synthesis of glucose from noncarbohydrate sources, such as amino acids and glycerol (**gluconeogenesis**). Glucocorticosteroids also increase the breakdown of proteins to amino acids and oxidize and mobilize fatty acids. These drugs mimic the activity of naturally occurring steroid hormones.

The corticotropin-releasing hormone (CRH) from the hypothalamus triggers the initial release of glucocorticosteroids from the adrenal cortex. The target organ for CRH is the anterior lobe of the pituitary gland. Reacting to the presence of CRH, the anterior lobe releases ACTH, which, in turn, stimulates the release of glucocorticosteroids from the adrenal cortex.

When present in large amounts, cortisol inhibits the release of histamine and counteracts potentially destructive activities of the immune system. Because the immune response can damage body cells, as well as those of foreign substances, the protective mechanisms of cortisol help preserve body cells at the site of the inflammatory response. Glucocorticosteroids decrease the migration and accumulation of white blood cells (**leukocytes**) at the site, thereby suppressing the inflammatory response.

Additionally, glucocorticosteroids prevent the release of prostaglandins, leukotrienes, and macrophages, which are important to the inflammatory response. Other cellular factors that increase vascular permeability are inhibited. Glucocorticosteroids also reduce the number of T cells, while impairing the ability of antibodies (**immunoglobulins**) to bind with cell surface receptors, which reduces cell-mediated immune responses.

Uses

Glucocorticosteroids are used for many disorders and for the long-term management of numerous chronic inflammatory conditions, such as rheumatoid arthritis, systemic lupus erythematosus (SLE), asthma, and other chronic airway limitation and airway obstruction disorders. Glucocorticosteroids are helpful in managing idiopathic thrombocytopenic purpura (ITP), psoriasis, hemolytic anemia, multiple sclerosis, tuberculosis, ulcerative colitis, suppression of inflammatory responses during organ transplantation, and some neoplastic diseases.

Glucocorticosteroids are helpful in the short-term management of acute exacerbations of inflammation associated with the eye, dermatitis, urticaria, bronchitis, infectious diseases, sensitivity reactions, and Stevens-Johnson syndrome. Patients with head or spinal cord injuries may be helped because of the antiinflammatory effects of glucocorticoids. Glucocorticoids are also used in the treatment of adrenal insufficiency and other disorders when naturally occurring adrenal hormones are not present in sufficient quantities to sustain life.

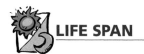 **LIFE SPAN**

Safe use of glucocorticosteroids during pregnancy and lactation has not been established. Safe use of cortisone, dexamethasone, hydrocortisone, and triamcinolone for children has not been established.
Long-term glucocorticosteroid use causes growth suppression in children.

What You NEED TO KNOW

Contraindications/Precautions

Glucocorticosteroids are contraindicated in patients with systemic fungal infections because they may worsen.

Drug Interactions

Phenobarbital, phenytoin, rifampin, antidiabetic drugs, isoniazid, and oral anticoagulants enhance elimination, thereby decreasing serum levels of glucocorticosteroid when given together. Ketoconazole, oral contraceptives, and salicylates increase serum levels of glucocorticosteroids. Glucocorticosteroids increase the effects of cyclosporin, digoxin, diuretics, amphotericin B, and theophylline and increase the risk for potassium loss. Glucocorticosteroids may increase intraocular pressure when given with tricyclic antidepressants, anticholinergics, and adrenergic drugs. Salicylates increase the risk for gastric ulcers when given concurrently with glucocorticosteroids.

Caution is necessary when using glucocorticosteroids for long-term therapy because of the risk for adrenal suppression. Glucocorticosteroids are used with caution in patients who have diabetes mellitus or peptic ulcers and for those with immunosuppression from cancer, kidney disease, or HIV.

A severe, life-threatening condition is treated through IV administration for quick action.

TAKE HOME POINTS

- Do not administer vaccinations containing live viruses to patients taking glucocorticosteroids because the inflammatory response is suppressed.
- The normal adult adrenal gland secretes an average of 20 mg of cortisol per day. Administration of high-dose glucocorticosteroids turns off the normal negative-feedback loop that exists between the adrenal and pituitary glands. When the drug is suddenly discontinued, the patient's circulating levels of cortisol fall dramatically because the adrenal gland is unable to secrete sufficient quantities to sustain body needs. This action places the patient at risk for a life-threatening, permanent adrenal suppression **(Addison's disease).** Adrenal suppression is dose-dependent and can last from months to years.

Adverse Effects

Muscle wasting and weakness, facial redness, impaired wound healing, hypertension, menstrual irregularities, Cushing's syndrome, cataract formation, GI bleeding, pancreatitis, peptic ulcer disease, psychosis, and osteoporosis are adverse effects that have been noted with the long-term use of glucocorticosteroids. Hypokalemia, alkalosis, negative nitrogen balance, weight gain, edema, abdominal distention, facial erythema, bruising, electrocardiogram (ECG) changes that are secondary to hypokalemia, headache, seizures, and opportunistic infections (e.g., candidiasis) are also likely adverse effects.

What You DO

Nursing Responsibilities

Glucocorticosteroids are available in oral, IV, IM, and topical formulations. The doses vary with the reason for use. The selected route varies with the severity of the patient's illness or condition. Oral and topical forms are used most frequently in patients with allergies or disorders that can be treated in a clinic or office. When administering glucocorticosteroids, the nurse should:

- Administer the lowest effective dose of glucocorticosteroids for the shortest period.
- Administer glucocorticosteroids in a pattern that mimics the natural hormone surges of the body. For example, two thirds of the daily dose may be administered in the morning with the remaining one third given in the late afternoon.
- Monitor the patient's fluids and electrolytes, particularly potassium, on a regular basis because these drugs cause sodium and fluid retention and potassium loss.
- Monitor glucose levels regularly because high-dose glucocorticosteroids increase serum levels.
- Instruct patients to take the drug with food to reduce gastric irritation and upset.
- Instruct patients to take their drug as prescribed and to avoid suddenly discontinuing therapy.
- Teach the patient the symptoms of glucocorticosteroid withdrawal syndrome (e.g., exhaustion, fever, diffuse musculoskeletal pain).

- Taper therapy after the patient's condition stabilizes; the dose given on the first day of therapy should be gradually reduced over a period of 1 to 2 weeks. Provide written instructions to the patient regarding the taper regimen.

Do You UNDERSTAND?

DIRECTIONS: **Indicate in the space provided whether the statement is *true* or *false*. If the answer is false, correct the statement to make it true (using the margin space).**

_____ 1. Physiologic doses of glucocorticosteroids help maintain normal nerve excitability.

_____ 2. Glucocorticosteroids cause excretion of sodium and increase the retention of calcium and potassium.

_____ 3. High doses of glucocorticosteroids decrease serum glucose levels.

_____ 4. Cortisol levels vary greatly throughout the day, with peak levels found at approximately 4:00 PM to 5:00 PM and the lowest levels at dawn.

_____ 5. Prednisone suppresses proliferation of lymphocytes and thus reduces the immune component of inflammation.

What IS an Adrenal Hormone–Inhibiting Drug?

Adrenal Hormone–Inhibiting Drugs	Trade Names	Uses
aminoglutethimide [ah-mi-noe-glue-TETH-ih-mide]	Cytadren	Treatment of Cushing's syndrome
mitotane [MY-toe-tane]	Lysodren	Treatment of adrenocortical carcinoma
metyrapone [me-TIE-ra-pone]	Metopirone	Diagnostic of pituitary function

Answers: 1. true; 2. false; sodium retention and calcium and potassium excretion; 3. false; increase serum glucose levels; 4. false; 6:00 pm to 8: 00 pm and midnight; 5. true.

Action

Adrenal hormone–inhibiting drugs act primarily to inhibit activity of the adrenal cortex. In turn, the synthesis of all adrenal steroids is inhibited. Mitotane exerts a direct killing effect on the mitochondria of the adrenal cortex cells.

Uses

Adrenal hormone–inhibiting drugs are used as a temporary means of decreasing excessive glucocorticosteroid production in patients who are waiting for more definitive therapy (e.g., surgery). Aminoglutethimide has also been used to produce a so-called medical adrenalectomy in patients with advanced breast cancer and in those with metastatic cancer of the prostate gland. Mitotane is used in the treatment of inoperable adrenocortical cancer. Metyrapone is used in a test of pituitary activity.

What You NEED TO KNOW

Metyrapone and mitotane are used with caution in patients with liver disease.

Contraindications/Precautions

Aminoglutethimide, metyrapone, and mitotane are contraindicated in patients with hypersensitivity. Metyrapone and mitotane should not be used for patients in shock or those who have experienced trauma.

Drug Interactions

Aminoglutethimide decreases the effects of medroxyprogesterone, theophylline, oral anticoagulants, glucocorticosteroids, and digoxin when given together. The actions of aminoglutethimide, mitotane, and metyrapone are enhanced when given with alcohol. When given concurrently, phenytoin and estrogens increase the metabolism of metyrapone. When mitotane is given concurrently with barbiturates, oral anticoagulants, and phenytoin, the effects of the drugs are decreased. Additive CNS depression may occur when mitotane is given with CNS depressants. Spironolactone blocks the action of mitotane.

Adverse Effects

Adverse effects of adrenal hormone–inhibiting drugs include nausea, abdominal distress, headaches, drowsiness, dizziness, and a measles-like rash (**morbilliform**). Additional adverse effects include hematologic abnormalities, hypothyroidism, muscle pain, and fever. Masculinization can occur in women, and precocious sexual development may occur in men who are taking these drugs.

What You DO

Nursing Responsibilities

Adrenal inhibitor drug therapy requires multiple daily dosing. Doses vary depending on the drug used. Patients are started on small doses, with titration upward as necessary until vital signs stabilize, serum electrolytes and glucose levels return to normal, and emotional changes are less disruptive. When administering adrenal inhibitors, the nurse should:

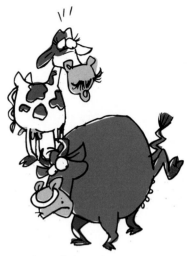

Masculinization in women.

- Teach patients the importance of taking their drug regularly as prescribed.
- Inform patients about the signs and symptoms of adrenal insufficiency. Warn patients of the occasional erratic nature of the signs and symptoms and the possibility of recurrence of adrenal hormone excess.
- Monitor 24-hour urine samples of 17-hydroxyglucocorticosteroids and 17-ketogenic steroids, which reveal increased elimination of glucocorticosteroid byproducts to validate drug efficacy.

Do You UNDERSTAND?

DIRECTIONS: Fill in the blanks with the appropriate responses to complete the following statements.

1. Adrenal hormone–inhibiting drugs inhibit or promote the metabolism of synthetic _____.
2. Aminoglutethimide is used as a temporary means of decreasing excessive _____ production in patients who are awaiting more _____.
3. Corticosteroid-inhibiting drugs can produce signs and symptoms that are associated with adrenal _____.

Answers: 1. adrenal hormones; 2. cortisol, definitive therapy; 3. insufficiency (Addison's disease).

What IS a Mineralocorticoid Drug?

Mineralocorticoids	Trade Names	Uses
fludrocortisone [flew-droh-KOR-tih-zone]	Florinef	Treatment of adrenocortical insufficiency
desoxycorticosterone [des-OX-e-kor-tih-co-steer-one]	DOCA	Treatment of adrenocortical insufficiency

Action

Mineralocorticoid drugs are any of a group of hormones from the adrenal cortex, thus named because of their effects on sodium, chloride, and potassium concentrations in extracellular fluid. The primary mineralocorticoid hormone—aldosterone—is essential to the maintenance of extracellular and intracellular fluid volume, normal cardiac output, and adequate levels of blood pressure. Without mineralocorticoids, diminished cardiac output and fatal shock can quickly occur.

Desoxycorticosterone acetate and fludrocortisone (aldosterone-like drugs) promote the reabsorption of sodium and water and the excretion of potassium and hydrogen ions via the renal tubules. The secondary effects are related to the reabsorption of water, serum levels of sodium and potassium, anion reabsorption, and the secretion of hydrogen ions. The result is maintenance of fluid and electrolyte balance and therefore adequate cardiac output.

Uses

Mineralocorticoids are used primarily as replacement therapy for patients with adrenal insufficiency and with salt-losing forms of congenital adrenal hyperplasia. Fludrocortisone is the drug of choice for chronic mineralocorticoid therapy. However, in most cases, a glucocorticosteroid must also be administered for adequate control. Cortisone and hydrocortisone are the drugs of choice for replacement because they promote both mineralocorticoid and glucocorticosteroid activity.

What You NEED TO KNOW

Contraindications/Precautions

Mineralocorticoids are contraindicated for patients with systemic fungal infections or hypersensitivity to the drug.

Drug Interactions

Aminoglutethimide, carbamazepine, phenobarbital, phenytoin, and rifampin increase the metabolism of the mineralocorticoids when given concurrently. Fludrocortisone decreases the effectiveness of diuretics and potassium supplements. Fludrocortisone increases the metabolism of isoniazid and salicylates when given together.

Adverse Effects

At normal physiologic levels, the mineralocorticoids have no adverse effects or contraindications. When the dose is excessive, sodium and water are retained, and potassium is lost. The effects on water and sodium result in expansion of fluid volume, hypertension, edema, cardiac enlargement, and hypokalemia. Bruising, sweating, hives, and an allergic rash have been reported. Desoxycorticosterone (DOCA) may produce hypertensive changes in mental functioning and permanent brain damage in susceptible patients.

The drugs should be used cautiously in patients with hypothyroidism, cirrhosis, ocular herpes simplex, emotional instability, psychotic tendencies, ulcerative colitis, diverticulitis, peptic ulcer disease, renal insufficiency, hypertension, osteoporosis, and myasthenia gravis.

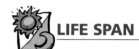

LIFE SPAN

Mineralocorticoids are used with caution in children because these drugs can cause suppression of the hypothalamic-pituitary-adrenal (HPA) axis.

What You DO

Nursing Responsibilities

Fludrocortisone is administered by mouth on a variable schedule, ranging from twice daily to three times weekly, depending on patient response. Supplemental doses may be required during physiologic stress resulting from serious illness, trauma, or surgery. When administering mineralocorticoids, the nurse should:

- Monitor the patient for significant weight gain, edema, hypertension, or severe headaches.
- Realize that fludrocortisone therapy increases serum sodium levels and decreases potassium levels.

- Teach the patient to recognize the signs and symptoms of electrolyte imbalance (e.g., muscle weakness, paresthesia, numbness, fatigue, anorexia, nausea).
- Instruct the patient to report altered heart rhythm, mental status, increased urination, severe or continuing headaches, unusual weight gain, and swelling of the feet to the health care provider.

Do You UNDERSTAND?

DIRECTIONS: Fill in the blanks with the appropriate responses to complete the following statements.

1. The net result of reabsorption of sodium and water and the excretion of potassium and hydrogen ions is the maintenance of _____ and therefore _____ output.

2. Monitor the patient who is taking fludrocortisone for significant _____, _____, _____, or severe _____.

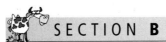

SECTION B

THYROID AND PARATHYROID DRUGS

The endocrine system, which includes the hypothalamus, pituitary, thyroid, parathyroid glands, pancreas, adrenals, ovaries, and testes, participates in the regulation of all essential body activities. Hormones produced in each of these glands are secreted and act as chemical influences on distant organs. This section will discuss specific antithyroid drugs, thyroid hormones, hypocalcemic drugs, and hypercalcemic drugs.

What IS an Antithyroid Drug?

Antithyroid Drugs	Trade Names	Uses
propylthiouracil [pro-puhl-thigh-oh-YOU-rah-sill]	PTU	Treatment of hyperthyroidism and thyrotoxic crisis
methimazole [meth-IM-a-zole]	Tapazole	Treatment of hyperthyroidism
strong iodine solution	Lugol's Solution	Preparation for thyroidectomy
potassium iodide solution	SSKI	Short-term treatment of Grave's disease and thyrotoxic crisis

Action

Antithyroid drugs are pharmacologic preparations used to treat hyperthyroidism. Hyperthyroidism results when an oversecretion of thyroid hormone is present. The abundance of this hormone greatly increases metabolism and may induce a toxic state. Antithyroid drugs decrease the production or release of thyroid hormones.

Thioureylene drugs such as propylthiouracil, methimazole, and iodide solutions are used to inhibit the production or secretion of thyroid hormone. These drugs are not chemically related but both help decrease the blood levels of thyroid hormone.

Uses

Antithyroid drugs are used to treat the oversecretion of thyroid hormone **(hyperthyroidism);** thus they may be given in preparation for a thyroidectomy, in conjunction with radioactive iodine therapy, and in the case of thyroid storm or thyrotoxic crisis. Antithyroid drug therapy is usually continued until the patient is euthyroid for 6 to 12 months.

What You NEED TO KNOW

Contraindications/Precautions

Contraindications for thioureylene drugs include any known sensitivity to an antithyroid drug. The iodine preparations are contraindicated for patients with pulmonary edema and tuberculosis.

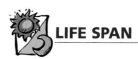
LIFE SPAN

Antithyroid drugs and iodine preparations are contraindicated during pregnancy. Thioureylene drugs should be used cautiously during lactation because of the potential antithyroid effect on the infant.

Drug Interactions

When potassium iodide solution is given with lithium, an increased hypothyroid action may result. Hyperkalemia may occur when potassium iodide solution is given with potassium supplements, potassium-sparing diuretics, and ACE inhibitors.

Adverse Effects

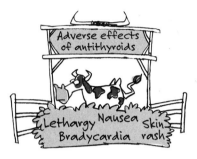

Adverse effects of antithyroid drugs are those associated with thyroid suppression (e.g., lethargy, bradycardia, nausea, skin rash). Propylthiouracil in particular is associated with GI disturbances.

Adverse effects of the iodine solutions, in addition to hypothyroidism, include iodism (e.g., metallic taste, stomach upset, diarrhea, discomfort of the mouth, teeth, and gums). Staining of the teeth, skin rash, and goiter may also occur.

What You DO

Monitor frequent laboratory tests of patients who are taking methimazole for early detection of bone marrow suppression.

Nursing Responsibilities

When administering antithyroid drugs, the nurse should:

- Evaluate patients for allergy to any antithyroid drug.
- Instruct patients who are receiving propylthiouracil to divide the dose and take the drug around the clock to ensure consistent levels.
- Monitor patients who are receiving iodine solutions for signs of iodism and immediately report these signs to the health care provider when they occur.
- Teach patients who are undergoing iodine solution therapy to take the medicine orally through a straw to prevent staining of teeth.
- Inform patients that they will undergo laboratory tests to evaluate the effectiveness of the antithyroid drug.
- Monitor patients for signs of adverse effects, such as anxiety, decreased cardiac output, ECG abnormalities, blood dyscrasias, and skin rash.
- Withdraw antithyroid drug gradually, and perform frequent evaluations to determine the likelihood of the patient remaining euthyroid.

Do You UNDERSTAND?

DIRECTIONS: Fill in the blanks with the appropriate responses to complete the following statements.

1. Iodine solutions are contraindicated during _____.
2. A strong iodine solution is known as _____.
3. Hyperthyroidism is the result of _____.
4. Antithyroid drugs act by _____.
5. Propylthiouracil should be taken _____.
6. Iodine solutions should be taken _____.

What IS a Thyroid Hormone Replacement Drug?

Thyroid Hormone Replacement Drugs	Trade Names	Uses
levothyroxine [lee-voe-thigh-ROX-een]	Synthroid Levoxyl	Treatment of hypothyroidism, myxedema coma
liothyronine [lie-oh-THIGH-row-neen]	Cytomel Triostat	Treatment of hypothyroidism, myxedema, myxedema coma, nontoxic goiter
liotrix [LYE-oh-trix]	Thyrolar	Treatment of hypothyroidism

Action

Thyroid drugs contain natural and synthetic thyroid hormones that control the rate of metabolism and thus significantly influence all bodily functions. Heart, skeletal muscle, liver, and kidneys are especially sensitive to the stimulating effects of these substances. These hormones are essential for normal growth and development. Thyroid hormones are also critical for brain and skeletal maturation. Thyroid hormones increase metabolic rate of body tissues, thereby increasing oxygen utilization. Carbohydrate and fat metabolism are increased under the influence of thyroid hormones.

Answers: 1. pregnancy; 2. Lugol's solution; 3. an oversecretion of thyroid hormone occurs; 4. decreasing production or release of thyroid hormone; 5. in divided doses, usually three times a day, around the clock; 6. through a straw to prevent staining of teeth.

Uses

Thyroid hormone drugs are used for replacement therapy in hypothyroidism and in the treatment of myxedema, myxedema coma, goiters, and some thyroid cancers. These hormones are also used when thyroid hormone levels are low or absent and to control the pituitary gland's overproduction of the thyroid-stimulating hormone (TSH).

What You NEED TO KNOW

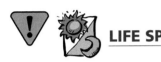 **LIFE SPAN**

During lactation, thyroid replacement drugs should be used with extreme caution.

Contraindications/Precautions

Thyroid replacement hormone drugs are contraindicated in patients with a known allergy or sensitivity to the drugs or their binders. These hormones should not be used during an MI or in patients with hypoadrenal conditions.

Drug Interactions

Decreased absorption of thyroid hormones occurs when the drug is taken with food or cholestyramine. When the patient is taking thyroid hormones and cholestyramine, these drugs must be taken 2 hours apart. Thyroid hormones increase the potency of oral anticoagulants. These hormones may decrease the effectiveness of digitalis. Theophylline clearance is lowered in patients who are hypothyroid.

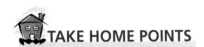 **TAKE HOME POINTS**

Liothyronine has a greater potential for causing cardiac problems and is therefore not recommended for patients with cardiac disease.

Adverse Effects

With appropriate dosaging for replacement therapy, adverse effects of thyroid hormones are few. Adverse effects of thyroid hormones include cardiac dysrhythmia, anxiety, headache, and sleeplessness. Loss of hair and skin reactions may occur, particularly in children during the first months of treatment.

What You DO

Nursing Responsibilities

Thyroid hormones are generally given in a single dose on an empty stomach, about 30 minutes before breakfast. The initial dose is usually increased until desired effects are evident and serum thyroid profile is within a normal range. When administering thyroid replacement drugs, the nurse should:

- Monitor the patient's response to thyroid drugs and any adverse cardiac effect, hypertension, tachycardia, anxiety, or skin rash. The patient's metabolism should gradually increase to a more normal state.
- Instruct the patient taking a thyroid hormone replacement drug to notify the health care provider immediately if adverse signs appear.
- Evaluate specific drug interactions, particularly those related to cholestyramine, digoxin, and theophylline. Monitor digoxin levels; thus adjustments in the dose can be made appropriately.
- Monitor periodic thyroid function blood tests to evaluate effectiveness.
- Recognize that as thyroid function returns to normal, the dose of theophylline should be altered accordingly.
- Realize that thyroid hormones increase cellular metabolism, thus also increasing heat production.
- Warn the patient to avoid discontinuing thyroid hormones without checking with the health care provider.
- Advise the patient that in most instances thyroid hormone replacement therapy is lifelong.

Do You UNDERSTAND?

DIRECTIONS: **Fill in the blanks with the appropriate responses to complete the following statements.**

1. Thyroid hormones _____ heart rate and cardiac output.
2. Thyroid hormones are critical for _____ and _____ maturation.
3. Decreased absorption of thyroid hormone occurs when taken with

   _____.
4. Thyroid hormones may cause decreased effectiveness of _____

   _____.
5. _____ are necessary to evaluate response to thyroid hormone therapy.
6. Thyroid replacement hormones are frequently taken _____

   _____.

What IS a Hypocalcemic Drug?

Vitamin D compounds act therapeutically to regulate the absorption of phosphate and calcium. Vitamin D assists the parathyroid hormone (PTH) and calcitonin in regulating calcium.

Hypocalcemic drugs are used to treat the signs and symptoms of hypocalcemia, such as neuromuscular irritability, which may progress to tetany. In acute severe hypocalcemia, calcium gluconate or calcium chloride may be prescribed. In long-term, less acute situations, oral calcium supplements and vitamin D may be indicated to maintain normal levels of calcium. Vitamin D is frequently used in chronic situations when calcium preparations alone are ineffective in maintaining normal calcium levels. Treatment of hypoparathyroidism consists primarily of vitamin D preparations and calcium supplements.

For discussions of vitamin D and calcium, refer to pages 612 and 619, respectively.

What IS a Hypercalcemic Drug?

Hypercalcemic Drugs	Trade Names	Uses
calcitonin-salmon, calcitonin-human [kal-si-TOE-nin]	Miacalcin	Treatment of osteoporosis, Paget's disease, hypercalcemia
alendronate [a-LEN-dro-nate]	Fosamax	Prevention and treatment of postmenopausal osteoporosis, steroid-induced osteoporosis, male osteoporosis, Paget's disease
etidronate [e-ti-DROE-nate]	Didronel	Treatment of Paget's disease and hypercalcemia associated with malignancy
risendronate [rye-SIN-dron-ate]	Actonel	Treatment of postmenopausal osteoporosis, steroid-induced osteoporosis, Paget's disease
gallium nitrate [GAL-lee-um]	Ganite	Treatment of hypercalcemia associated with malignancy

A hypercalcemic state diminishes the ability of nerves and muscles to respond to stimuli. The problems associated with elevated calcium levels include GI disturbances, such as nausea, vomiting, constipation, abdominal discomfort, lethargy, syncope, hallucinations, and coma. Polyuria, polyphagia, and dysrhythmias may also occur. Calcium deposits in organs

Plate 1

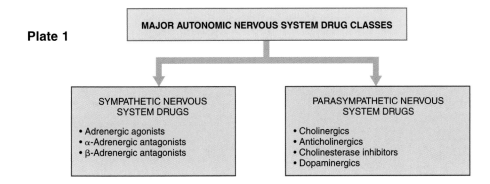

MAJOR AUTONOMIC NERVOUS SYSTEM DRUG CLASSES

SYMPATHETIC NERVOUS SYSTEM DRUGS

- Adrenergic agonists
- α-Adrenergic antagonists
- β-Adrenergic antagonists

PARASYMPATHETIC NERVOUS SYSTEM DRUGS

- Cholinergics
- Anticholinergics
- Cholinesterase inhibitors
- Dopaminergics

Plate 2

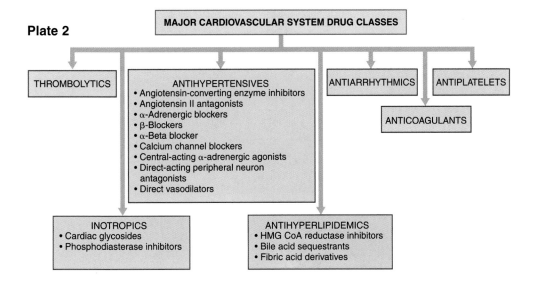

MAJOR CARDIOVASCULAR SYSTEM DRUG CLASSES

THROMBOLYTICS

ANTIHYPERTENSIVES
- Angiotensin-converting enzyme inhibitors
- Angiotensin II antagonists
- α-Adrenergic blockers
- β-Blockers
- α-Beta blocker
- Calcium channel blockers
- Central-acting α-adrenergic agonists
- Direct-acting peripheral neuron antagonists
- Direct vasodilators

ANTIARRHYTHMICS

ANTIPLATELETS

ANTICOAGULANTS

INOTROPICS
- Cardiac glycosides
- Phosphodiasterase inhibitors

ANTIHYPERLIPIDEMICS
- HMG CoA reductase inhibitors
- Bile acid sequestrants
- Fibric acid derivatives

Plate 3

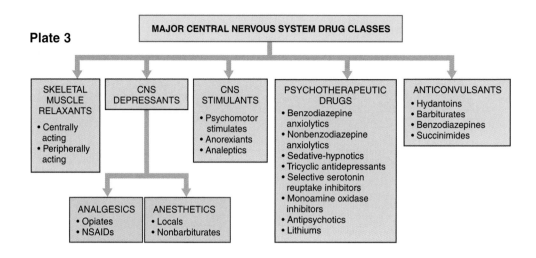

MAJOR CENTRAL NERVOUS SYSTEM DRUG CLASSES

SKELETAL MUSCLE RELAXANTS
- Centrally acting
- Peripherally acting

CNS DEPRESSANTS

CNS STIMULANTS
- Psychomotor stimulates
- Anorexiants
- Analeptics

PSYCHOTHERAPEUTIC DRUGS
- Benzodiazepine anxiolytics
- Nonbenzodiazepine anxiolytics
- Sedative-hypnotics
- Tricyclic antidepressants
- Selective serotonin reuptake inhibitors
- Monoamine oxidase inhibitors
- Antipsychotics
- Lithiums

ANTICONVULSANTS
- Hydantoins
- Barbiturates
- Benzodiazepines
- Succinimides

ANALGESICS
- Opiates
- NSAIDs

ANESTHETICS
- Locals
- Nonbarbiturates

Plate 4

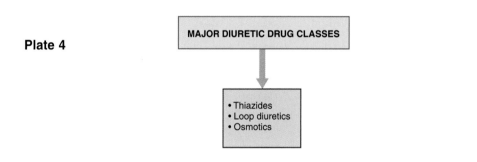

MAJOR DIURETIC DRUG CLASSES
- Thiazides
- Loop diuretics
- Osmotics

Plate 5

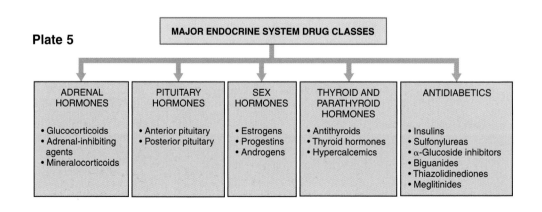

MAJOR ENDOCRINE SYSTEM DRUG CLASSES

ADRENAL HORMONES
- Glucocorticoids
- Adrenal-inhibiting agents
- Mineralocorticoids

PITUITARY HORMONES
- Anterior pituitary
- Posterior pituitary

SEX HORMONES
- Estrogens
- Progestins
- Androgens

THYROID AND PARATHYROID HORMONES
- Antithyroids
- Thyroid hormones
- Hypercalcemics

ANTIDIABETICS
- Insulins
- Sulfonylureas
- α-Glucoside inhibitors
- Biguanides
- Thiazolidinediones
- Meglitinides

Plate 6

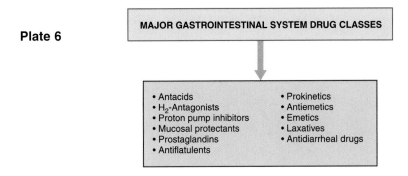

MAJOR GASTROINTESTINAL SYSTEM DRUG CLASSES

- Antacids
- H$_2$-Antagonists
- Proton pump inhibitors
- Mucosal protectants
- Prostaglandins
- Antiflatulents
- Prokinetics
- Antiemetics
- Emetics
- Laxatives
- Antidiarrheal drugs

Plate 7

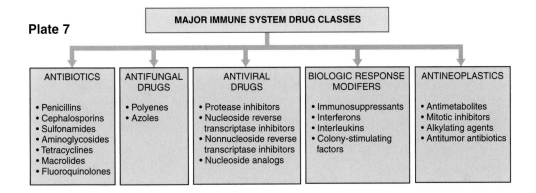

MAJOR IMMUNE SYSTEM DRUG CLASSES

ANTIBIOTICS

- Penicillins
- Cephalosporins
- Sulfonamides
- Aminoglycosides
- Tetracyclines
- Macrolides
- Fluoroquinolones

ANTIFUNGAL DRUGS

- Polyenes
- Azoles

ANTIVIRAL DRUGS

- Protease inhibitors
- Nucleoside reverse transcriptase inhibitors
- Nonnucleoside reverse transcriptase inhibitors
- Nucleoside analogs

BIOLOGIC RESPONSE MODIFERS

- Immunosuppressants
- Interferons
- Interleukins
- Colony-stimulating factors

ANTINEOPLASTICS

- Antimetabolites
- Mitotic inhibitors
- Alkylating agents
- Antitumor antibiotics

Plate 8

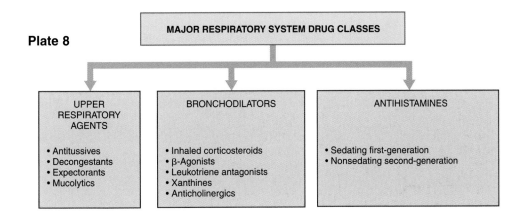

MAJOR RESPIRATORY SYSTEM DRUG CLASSES

UPPER RESPIRATORY AGENTS

- Antitussives
- Decongestants
- Expectorants
- Mucolytics

BRONCHODILATORS

- Inhaled corticosteroids
- β-Agonists
- Leukotriene antagonists
- Xanthines
- Anticholinergics

ANTIHISTAMINES

- Sedating first-generation
- Nonsedating second-generation

Plate 9

Sympathetic Drug Action

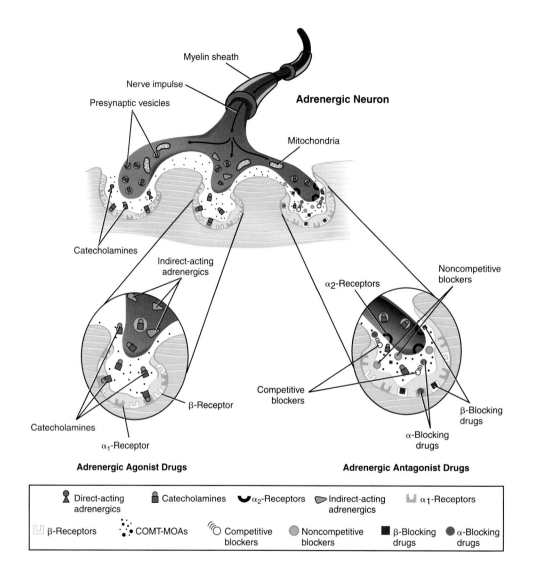

Myelin sheath

Nerve impulse

Presynaptic vesicles

Adrenergic Neuron

Mitochondria

Catecholamines

Indirect-acting
adrenergics

α₂-Receptors

Noncompetitive
blockers

Competitive
blockers

Catecholamines

β-Receptor

β-Blocking
drugs

α₁-Receptor

α-Blocking
drugs

Adrenergic Agonist Drugs

Adrenergic Antagonist Drugs

Direct-acting adrenergics	Catecholamines	α₂-Receptors	Indirect-acting adrenergics	α₁-Receptors
β-Receptors	COMT-MOAs	Competitive blockers	Noncompetitive blockers	β-Blocking drugs
				α-Blocking drugs

Plate 10

Parasympathetic Drug Action

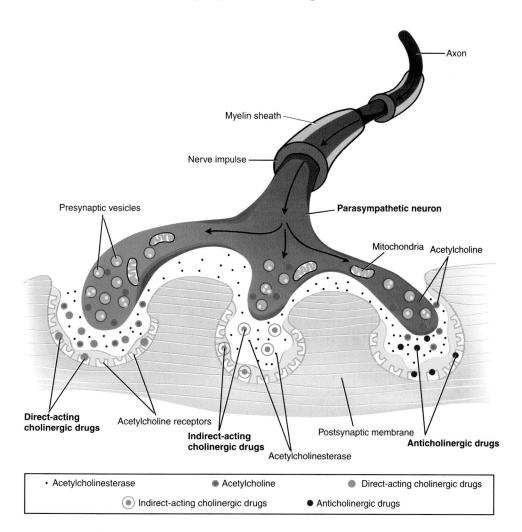

Axon

Myelin sheath

Nerve impulse

Presynaptic vesicles

Parasympathetic neuron

Mitochondria Acetylcholine

**Direct-acting
cholinergic drugs**

Acetylcholine receptors

**Indirect-acting
cholinergic drugs**

Acetylcholinesterase

Postsynaptic membrane

Anticholinergic drugs

- Acetylcholinesterase ● Acetylcholine ● Direct-acting cholinergic drugs
  ◉ Indirect-acting cholinergic drugs ● Anticholinergic drugs

Plate 11 **Pharmacodynamics of Antidepressant Drugs**

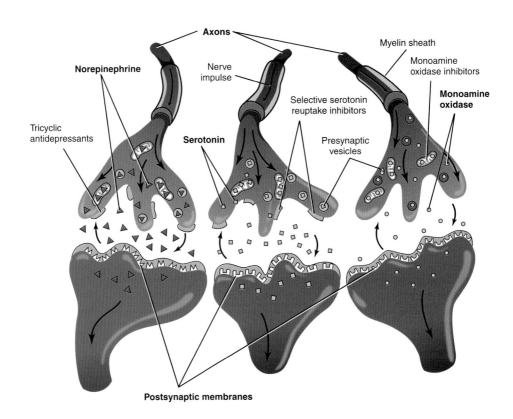

Plate 12   Site and Mechanism of Action of Antibiotics

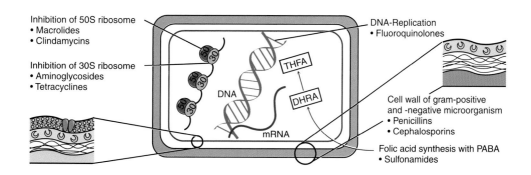

Inhibition of 50S ribosome
- Macrolides
- Clindamycins

Inhibition of 30S ribosome
- Aminoglycosides
- Tetracyclines

DNA

THFA

DHRA

mRNA

DNA-Replication
- Fluoroquinolones

Cell wall of gram-positive and -negative microorganism
- Penicillins
- Cephalosporins

Folic acid synthesis with PABA
- Sulfonamides

Plate 13   Sites of Drug Action on the Renal System

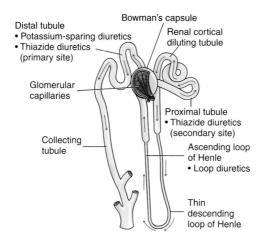

Distal tubule
- Potassium-sparing diuretics
- Thiazide diuretics
  (primary site)

Bowman's capsule

Renal cortical
diluting tubule

Glomerular
capillaries

Proximal tubule
- Thiazide diuretics
  (secondary site)

Collecting
tubule

Ascending loop
of Henle
- Loop diuretics

Thin
descending
loop of Henle

Plate 14

Mechanism of Action of the Four Types of Laxatives

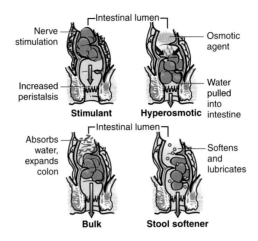

Plate 15

Insulin-Glucose Balance

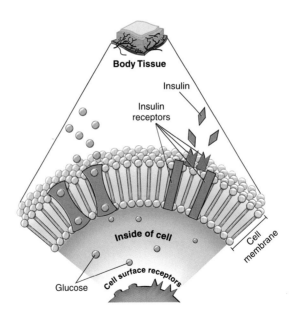

(e.g., kidneys, eyes) may lead to decreased function. Elevated levels of serum calcium may occur in hyperparathyroidism, malignancies, adrenal disorders, immobilization, and with excessive ingestion of vitamin D. The ingestion of estrogen, thiazide diuretics, and lithium may also result in elevated serum calcium levels.

Action

Most hypercalcemic drugs are bisphosphonates that lower serum calcium levels to normal or near-normal levels. These drugs prevent bone resorption by attaching to bone mineral to be absorbed into newly formed bone matrix. However, hypercalcemic drugs do not affect normal bone formation. Gallium inhibits calcium reabsorption from bone, possibly by inhibiting bone turnover.

Uses

Bisphosphonates are used in the prevention and treatment of postmenopausal osteoporosis, Paget's disease, and hypercalcemia secondary to hyperparathyroidism. Calcitonin-salmon, derived from gallium nitrate, is used in the management of hypercalcemia caused by malignancy.

What You NEED TO KNOW

Contraindications/Precautions

Bisphosphonates and gallium are contraindicated for patients with renal dysfunction. Bisphosphonates are also contraindicated for patients with acidosis, heart block, severe hypotension, hypertension, and spinal or epidural anesthesia. Calcitonins are contraindicated for patients with allergies to salmon and fish products. Calcitonin should be used cautiously in patients with osteoporosis, renal dysfunction, and pernicious anemia.

Drug Interactions

The absorption of bisphosphonates is impaired when taken with multiple vitamins, iron, and antacids. The risk for nephrotoxicity increases when gallium is given concurrently with aminoglycosides, vancomycin, or amphotericin B.

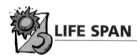

LIFE SPAN

Hypercalcemic drugs are contraindicated during pregnancy and lactation and in children.

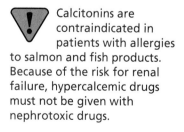

Calcitonins are contraindicated in patients with allergies to salmon and fish products. Because of the risk for renal failure, hypercalcemic drugs must not be given with nephrotoxic drugs.

Adverse Effects

Common adverse effects of hypercalcemic drugs include facial flushing and nausea. Other adverse effects include irritation at the insertion site, hand flushing, skin rash, eye pain, headache, anorexia, vomiting, abdominal pain, diarrhea, temporary increase in bone discomfort associated with Paget's disease, urinary frequency, nocturia, and renal failure. Additional adverse effects of bisphosphonates include a metallic or altered taste in the mouth.

What You DO

Nursing Responsibilities

Hypercalcemic drugs are given orally and IV. Because the absorption of bisphosphonates is impaired when taken with multiple vitamins, iron, and antacids, concurrent administration should be separated by at least 30 minutes. When administering hypercalcemic drugs, the nurse should:

- Instruct the patient to decrease intake of dairy products and other foods and drugs that contain calcium.
- Administer calcitonin at bedtime to decrease discomfort.
- Encourage patients to drink 3000 to 4000 mL of fluids per day to minimize renal dysfunction.
- Observe for the signs of hypercalcemia, such as GI distress, lethargy, syncope, polyuria, and dysrhythmias.
- Monitor ECG changes, such as a shortened QT interval and inverted T wave.
- Evaluate the patient for signs of hypocalcemia with aggressive treatment of hypercalcemia.
- Monitor periodically the patient's calcium levels to determine treatment effectiveness.
- Evaluate renal function and fluid and electrolyte balance for early detection of abnormalities in patients who are receiving hypercalcemics.

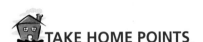

TAKE HOME POINTS

An intradermal skin test should precede calcitonin therapy. Rotate the injection sites when administering injections of calcitonin to decrease risk for inflammation. Follow package instructions for the nasal formulation of calcitonin. Aspirin should not be combined with bisphosphonates because of the increased risk for GI adverse effects.

Do You UNDERSTAND?

DIRECTIONS: Provide the appropriate responses to the following statements or questions.

1. List three drugs that may cause elevated serum calcium levels.

   _____

   _____

   _____

2. Bisphosphonates should not be given concurrently with what three drugs?

   _____

   _____

   _____

3. Calcitonin-human may cause what?

   _____

4. Gallium is contraindicated for patients with what?

   _____

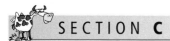

SECTION C

ANTIDIABETICS

Antidiabetic drugs are medications used in managing diabetes mellitus. Insulins are used primarily in the treatment of type 1 diabetes. Insulins are also used in treating patients with type 2 diabetes who are unable to control their blood glucose levels by diet, exercise, and oral hypoglycemic agents. Insulins are also used in treating diabetic ketoacidosis (DKA) and hyperosmotic hyperglycemic nonketotic (HHNK) coma. Insulins are classified by their action times, concentration, and origin.

Oral hypoglycemic agents are used to treat type 2 diabetes. These agents are classified as sulfonylureas, α-glucosidase inhibitors, biguanides, thiazolidinediones, and meglitinides. These agents may be used alone or in combination with other oral antidiabetics or insulin.

What IS Insulin?

Classification	Generic	Brand	Onset	Peak	Duration
Rapid-acting insulin	Insulin lispro	Humalog	Less than 15 min	0.5-1.0 hr	5-7 hr
	Insulin aspart	Novolog	5-10 min	30-60 min	2-3 hr
	Insulin glulisine	Apidra	2-5 min	30-60 min	2-4 hr
Short-acting insulin	Insulin injection	Regular, Humulin R, Novolin R, Regular Iletin II	30-60 min	2-3 hr	5-7 hr
	Insulin zinc suspension prompt	Semilente Insulin, Semilente Purified Pork Insulin	30-60 min	4-7 hr	12-16 hr
Intermediate-acting insulin	Isophane insulin suspension (NPH)	Humulin N, Novolin N	1.0-2.5 hr	7-15 hr	22 hr
	Insulin zinc suspension (Lente)	Humulin L, Lente Iletin II, Lente Purified Pork Novolin L	1-2 hr	8-12 hr	18-24 hr
Long-acting insulin	Insulin zinc suspension extended (Ultralente)	Humulin U	4-8 hr	16-18 hr	36 hr
Constant-acting insulin	Insulin glargine	Lantus R	Immediate	Constant	24 hr

Doses are individualized and dose adjustments are made according to blood glucose levels.

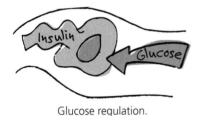

Glucose regulation.

Action

Insulin is a hormone secreted by the pancreas that is necessary for regulating the metabolism and storage of carbohydrates, fats, and proteins. Insulin binds to the insulin receptor sites of the cell membrane, thereby allowing the glucose molecules to cross the cell membrane and lowering the blood glucose concentration. Insulin is active in carbohydrate metabolism, facilitating the uptake and storage of glucose by the cells and promoting the conversion of glucose to glycogen. Insulin also promotes the normal cell's uptake and conversion of amino acids and fatty acids. Insulin is metabolized in the liver and kidneys and excreted in the urine.

Uses

The wide variety of insulin types allows the health care provider to select the insulin best suited for the individual. Choice of insulin and dose must be individualized according to the patient's needs and lifestyle.

Insulins are classed by their action times (onset, peak, and duration) as rapid-acting, short-acting, intermediate-acting, long-acting, and constant-acting. Onset indicates the time after administration that the insulin begins to work. The peak is the time during which the maximal effect of the insulin occurs. Duration is the length of time that the insulin is active in the body.

Insulin is used to maintain normal or near-normal blood glucose levels in the treatment of type 1 and type 2 diabetes. Regular insulin is used in the emergency treatment of DKA and HHNK to regulate glucose levels and in the treatment of severe hyperkalemia to promote the intracellular shift of potassium. In psychiatry, insulin is used to induce hypoglycemic shock as therapy. Insulin is used IV as a secretion-stimulating test for the evaluation of pituitary growth hormone.

What You NEED TO KNOW

Contraindications/Precautions

Insulin is contraindicated for patients with a hypersensitivity to animal insulin protein.

Drug Interactions

Concurrent use of beta blockers, salicylates, anabolic steroids, alcohol, monoamine oxidase inhibitors (MAOIs), sulfinpyrazone, clofibrate, tetracyclines, guanethidine, and oxytetracycline may increase the hypoglycemic effects of insulin. Use of corticosteroids, dextrothyroxine, diltiazem, dobutamine, epinephrine, ethacrynic acid, and estrogens may decrease the hypoglycemic effects of insulin. Thiazide diuretics, furosemide, phenytoin, and thyroid preparations increase blood glucose levels and may require an increase in the insulin dose. Use of beta blockers may mask signs and symptoms of hypoglycemia.

Adverse Effects

Adverse effects of insulin include hypersensitivity, hypoglycemia, lipodystrophy of injection sites, and rebound hyperglycemia. Localized reactions (e.g., itching and erythema at the injection site) or systemic reactions (e.g., dyspnea, tachycardia, angioedema, anaphylaxis) are used to classify hypersensitivity. Evidence of an overdose (**hypoglycemia**) includes

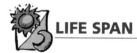
LIFE SPAN

Insulin should be used with caution during pregnancy. Insulin glargine is contraindicated for children under 6 years of age.

profuse perspiration, palpitations, tremulousness, and nausea. Other hypoglycemic adverse effects include tachycardia, hunger, confusion, incoherent speech, irritability, inability to concentrate, headache, blurred or double vision, convulsions, loss of consciousness, and coma.

What You DO

Nursing Responsibilities

Insulin is available in concentrations of 100 units/mL (U100) or 50 units/mL (U50). The origin of insulin preparations may be pork, beef, pork and beef, human, or an analog of human insulin. The most common form of insulin used is the biosynthetic human insulin. When administering insulin, the nurse should:

- Contact the health care provider for dose instructions when breakfast is delayed for diagnostic tests.
- Rotate vial gently prior to insulin withdrawal to ensure uniform suspension without vigorous shaking.
- Instruct the patient that insulin vials should be inspected for any clumping, discoloration, solid deposits, or a granular appearance before use and to discard when any of these are noted.
- Teach the patient the proper technique of mixing two insulins in one syringe. Instruct the patient to always withdraw the short-acting insulin into the syringe before the long-acting insulin ("clear before cloudy"). Rapid- and short-acting insulins are clear solutions. Intermediate- and long-acting insulin solutions appear cloudy. This distinction reduces the risk for the short-acting insulin accidentally being drawn into the long-acting insulin vial and causing an unexpected hypoglycemic reaction. Do not mix glargine with any other insulin.
- Give mixed insulin within 15 minutes.
- Inform the patient that insulin is to be injected at a 90-degree angle to prevent local reactions. Always use an insulin syringe.
- Instruct the patient to store insulin in a cool place away from direct sunlight.
- Inform the patient that predrawn syringes are stable for 1 week when refrigerated.

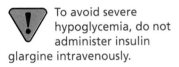

TAKE HOME POINTS

- U100 insulin is the most common concentration used in the United States. Always double-check that the insulin being used is the insulin that was ordered. Rotate insulin injection sites systematically within one area, using all available sites, before moving to the next anatomic area. Massaging the site after insulin injection may alter the rate of absorption. Regular insulin is the only type of insulin that can be given IV.
- Food should be available before administering lispro administration. Glargine should be given at bedtime.

To avoid severe hypoglycemia, do not administer insulin glargine intravenously.

- Monitor the patient closely during times of trauma or severe stress for possible dose adjustments.
- Inform the patient that during insulin therapy, a meal must be eaten regularly every 4 to 5 hours and regular moderate exercise must be carried out to increase cell responsiveness to insulin.
- Rotate insulin injection sites to prevent subcutaneous atophy, muscle damage, and tissue necrosis.
- Instruct the patient to apply gentle pressure to the injection site and to avoid massaging the site after injection.
- Check blood glucose levels at the time of the insulin's peak action to monitor for hypoglycemia. The frequency of blood glucose monitoring is determined according to the health status of the patient and the insulin regime.
- Administer insulin via a parenteral route (Sub-Q or IV) because insulin is a protein and is destroyed in the GI tract.
- Monitor the patient's blood pressure, intake and output, blood glucose level, and ketones every hour when administering IV insulin as a treatment for DKA.
- Instruct the patient to always carry some form of quick-acting complex carbohydrate, such as five to eight Lifesavers candies, other hard candies, or lump sugar, for the treatment of hypoglycemia.
- Teach patients and their family about signs of hypoglycemia and home emergency treatment.
- Advise patients to always carry identification that identifies them as a person with diabetes who is undergoing insulin therapy.
- Counsel the patient to avoid taking OTC medications without consulting the health care provider.
- Inform the patient that blurred vision may occur at the beginning of therapy, but it will usually subside within 6 to 8 weeks.

Do You UNDERSTAND?

DIRECTIONS: Complete the following crossword puzzle.

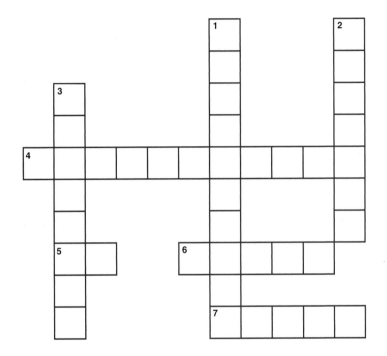

Down

1. Route of insulins.
2. Short-acting insulin.
3. Time that insulin is active in body.

Across

4. Masks signs of hypoglycemia.
5. Only regular insulin can be given this route.
6. Where insulin is excreted.
7. Onset of this insulin is less than 15 minutes.

What IS a Sulfonylurea?

Sulfonylureas	Trade Names	Uses
First-generation		
acetohexamide [a-seat-oh-HEX-ah-mide]	Dymelor	Treatment of type 2 diabetes mellitus
chlorpropamide [klor-PROH-pah-mide]	Diabinese	Treatment of type 2 diabetes mellitus
tolazamide [toll-AZ-ah-mide]	Tolinase	Treatment of type 2 diabetes mellitus
tolbutamide [toll-BYOU-tah-mide]	Orinase	Treatment of type 2 diabetes mellitus
Second-generation		
glipizide [GLIP-ih-zide]	Glucotrol	Treatment of type 2 diabetes mellitus
glyburide [GLYE-byou-ride]	DiaBeta, Micronase	Treatment of type 2 diabetes mellitus
glimepiride [glye-MEH-pye-ride]	Amaryl	Treatment of type 2 diabetes mellitus

Action

Both first and second generations of sulfonylureas are oral antidiabetic agents that lower blood glucose levels. Sulfonylureas bind to the potassium channels on the beta cells of the pancreas, thereby stimulating the pancreas to release insulin. These agents also increase the sensitivity of the peripheral insulin receptors, which increases insulin binding in the peripheral tissues. Sulfonylureas decrease the formation of glucose in the liver, reducing hepatic glucose release. The patient must have functional pancreatic beta cells that are able to produce insulin for sulfonylurea treatment to be effective.

The second-generation sulfonylureas are more potent than are the first-generation sulfonylureas. These agents lower the blood glucose levels with a smaller dose and less drug interactions. Second-generation sulfonylureas have a longer duration of action compared with first-generation sulfonylureas; therefore they are available in once-a-day dosing or twice-a-day dosing. The second-generations are excreted in the urine and bile; therefore they are safer for patients with renal dysfunction.

Uses

Sulfonylureas are used in the treatment of mild to moderately severe type 2 diabetes mellitus when diet and exercise programs fail to maintain glycemic control. Sulfonylureas may be used alone, as an adjunct to diet and exercise, or in combination with other oral antidiabetics or insulin.

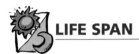

LIFE SPAN

Sulfonylureas are contraindicated during pregnancy.

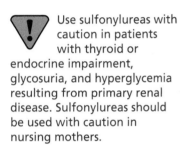

Use sulfonylureas with caution in patients with thyroid or endocrine impairment, glycosuria, and hyperglycemia resulting from primary renal disease. Sulfonylureas should be used with caution in nursing mothers.

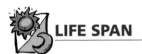

LIFE SPAN

Hypoglycemia is the primary adverse effect in older adults.

What You NEED TO KNOW

Contraindications/Precautions

Contraindications for use of sulfonylureas include hypersensitivity, severe hepatic or renal impairment, type 1 diabetes mellitus, and complications of type 2 diabetes (e.g., HHNK, DKA, severe infections, major surgery, trauma, coma).

Drug Interactions

Use of sulfonylureas with insulin, sulfonamides, chloramphenicol, oxyphenbutazone, phenylbutazone, salicylates, probenecid, MAOIs, oral anticoagulants, alcohol, and clofibrate increases the risk for hypoglycemia. Beta blockers may mask signs of hypoglycemia. Concurrent use of diazoxide and sulfonylureas causes a decrease in effectiveness. An increased risk for hyperglycemia occurs when sulfonylureas are used with thiazides, other diuretics, nicotinic acid, glucocorticoids, thyroid hormone, rifampin, and oral contraceptives. Concurrent use of sulfonylureas and alcohol may produce a disulfiram-like reaction (e.g., facial flushing, sweating, tachycardia, headache, dyspnea), which may last up to 24 hours.

Adverse Effects

Common adverse effects of sulfonylureas include nausea, vomiting, anorexia, epigastric discomfort, heartburn, and hypoglycemia. Hypoglycemia is the primary adverse effect in patients with renal or liver impairment. Other adverse effects of sulfonylureas include diarrhea, jaundice, leukopenia, thrombocytopenia, agranulocytosis, hemolytic anemia, aplastic anemia, photosensitivity, rash, pruritus, and erythema. Chlorpropamide may also cause an antidiuretic adverse effect called the syndrome of inappropriate antidiuretic hormone (SIADH).

What You DO

Nursing Responsibilities

When administering sulfonylureas, the nurse should:

- Instruct the patient of the exact times at which the oral antidiabetic should be taken (e.g., as a single morning dose, 30 minutes before breakfast and dinner, with breakfast) for the maximal effectiveness.
- Monitor laboratory values that are altered by sulfonylureas because these drugs may produce increased blood urea nitrogen (BUN) levels, increased creatinine levels, abnormal thyroid function tests, and reduced radioactive iodine (RAI) uptake.
- Monitor complete blood count (CBC), hemoglobin (HbA$_1$c), electrolyte levels, and liver function tests.
- Monitor the patient closely during pregnancy, trauma, and severe stress for a possible need of insulin coverage.
- Stress to the patient the importance of diet and exercise in the control of diabetes.
- Instruct the patient to monitor and record blood glucose levels at the frequencies the health care provider prescribes when the patient experiences signs or symptoms of hypoglycemia and during illness.
- Warn the patient to avoid using OTC medications or discontinuing this medication without consulting with the health care provider.
- Realize that acetohexamide is the sulfonylurea of choice to treat patients with diabetes who have gout because of its uricosuric properties.
- Realize that second-generation sulfonylureas are more potent, produce fewer adverse reactions, and have longer duration times than do first-generation agents.

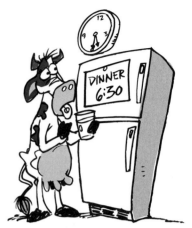

Keep a tight schedule.

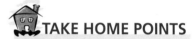

TAKE HOME POINTS

The health care provider individualizes the dose according to the blood glucose levels and the requirements of the patient. Instruct the patient to notify the health care provider of any hypoglycemic episodes or persistently low blood glucose levels.

Do You UNDERSTAND?

DIRECTIONS: Complete the following statements with the appropriate terms from the italicized list provided.

1. Sulfonylureas stimulate the pancreas to _____ insulin.
2. For sulfonylureas to be effective, pancreatic beta cells must be _____.
3. Use of alcohol when taking sulfonylureas may cause a _____ _____ reaction.
4. The primary adverse effect of sulfonylureas is _____.

hypoglycemia	*metabolized*	*hyperglycemia*
functional	*excreted*	*inhibit*
stimulate	*disulfiram-like*	

What IS an α-Glucosidase Inhibitor?

α-Glucosidase Inhibitors	Trade Names	Uses
acarbose [ah-CAR-bohs]	Precose	Treatment of type 2 diabetes mellitus
miglitol [MIG-lih-tohl]	Glyset	Treatment of type 2 diabetes mellitus

TAKE HOME POINTS

α-Glucosidase inhibitors delay the absorption of glucose in the intestines, which lowers blood glucose and glycosylated hemoglobin levels.

Action

An α-glucosidase inhibitor is an oral antidiabetic agent that lowers blood glucose levels after meals. α-Glucosidase inhibitors block an enzyme in the small intestine responsible for breaking down complex carbohydrates into monosaccharides and delay the digestion of glucose. In summary, α-glucosidase inhibitors interfere with the digestion of carbohydrates to glucose.

Uses

Acarbose and miglitol are used to lower blood glucose levels in the treatment of type 2 diabetes. These agents may be used alone, as an adjunct

Answers: 1. release; 2. functional; 3. disulfiram-like; 4. hypoglycemia.

to a diet and exercise regime, or in combination with a sulfonylurea to improve glycemic control.

What You NEED TO KNOW

Contraindications/Precautions

Acarbose and miglitol are contraindicated for patients with inflammatory bowel disease, colon ulcers, partial bowel obstructions, renal dysfunction, and ketoacidosis.

Drug Interactions

Concurrent use of α-glucosidase inhibitors with sulfonylureas may increase the risk for hypoglycemia. Charcoal and digestive enzymes decrease the effectiveness of α-glucosidase inhibitors. Digoxin levels are lowered when taken with acarbose or miglitol. Pancreatin diminishes the effect of miglitol. Miglitol decreases the bioavailability of propranolol and ranitidine.

Adverse Effects

The most common adverse effects of α-glucosidase inhibitors include abdominal pain, diarrhea, flatulence, and hypoglycemia. Other adverse effects include anorexia, nausea, and vomiting. Acarbose may cause additional adverse effects of weakness, dizziness, sleepiness, headache, vertigo, anemia, and increased liver function levels. Miglitol may cause a transient skin rash.

What You DO

Nursing Responsibilities

Acarbose and miglitol should be given with the first bite of each meal. When administering α-glucosidase inhibitors, the nurse should:
- Monitor both fasting and postprandial blood glucose levels and glycosylated hemoglobin levels to evaluate the effectiveness of the medication.
- Monitor the hemoglobin, hematocrit, and liver function studies in patients who are taking acarbose for early detection of adverse effects.

Acarbose should be used with caution in patients with hepatic dysfunction.

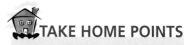 **LIFE SPAN**

Acarbose and miglitol are contraindicated for nursing mothers. Safe use of these agents during pregnancy has not been determined.

TAKE HOME POINTS

Teach the patient to take acarbose and miglitol with the first bite of each meal. Teach patients to take glucose tablets or gelatin caps for hypoglycemia for quicker action.

- Warn the patient to avoid discontinuing the medication without consulting the health care provider.
- Instruct patients to monitor their weight and to report any significant changes because these agents may cause weight loss.
- Advise the patient to notify the health care provider when any severe abdominal pain or distress develops for necessary dose adjustment.
- Instruct the patient that glucose tablets or gelatin caps should be given for hypoglycemia—not candy or sugar—because α-glucosidase inhibitors delay carbohydrate breakdown.

Do You UNDERSTAND?

DIRECTIONS: **Indicate in the space provided whether the statement is *true* or *false*. If the answer is false, correct the statement to make it true (using the margin space).**

_____ 1. Miglitol therapy causes elevated glycosylated hemoglobin.

_____ 2. α-Glucosidase enzyme inhibitors delay the absorption of glucose.

_____ 3. Instruct patient to take acarbose with first bite of each meal.

_____ 4. Give candy to a hypoglycemic patient treated with miglitol.

What IS a Biguanide?

Biguanides	Trade Names	Uses
metformin [met-FOR-min]	Glucophage	Treatment of type 2 diabetes mellitus

Action

A biguanide is an oral antidiabetic agent that decreases blood glucose concentrations. Biguanides increase the binding of insulin at receptor sites, thereby enhancing the action of insulin. These agents inhibit hepatic

Answers: 1. false; miglitol therapy lowers glycosylated hemoglobin by delaying the absorption of glucose in the intestines 2. true 3. true 4. false; when treated with miglitol, give the hypoglycemic patient glucose tablets or gelatin caps because α-glucosidase inhibitors delay carbohydrate breakdown.

glucose production and reduce glucose absorption in the intestines. Biguanides increase the glucose transport across the cell membrane, particularly in skeletal muscle cells, thus increasing glucose utilization. Biguanides have no effect on insulin secretion.

Uses

Biguanides are used in the treatment of type 2 diabetes mellitus when diet and exercise programs fail to maintain glycemic control. Metformin, the only biguanide that is approved for use in the United States, may be used alone or in combination with an oral sulfonylurea.

What You NEED TO KNOW

Contraindications/Precautions

Contraindications for use of biguanides include hypersensitivity, hepatic or renal impairment, alcoholism, metabolic acidosis, and DKA.

Drug Interactions

When biguanides are used concurrently with captopril, furosemide, or nifedipine, the risk for hypoglycemia is increased. Concurrent use of alcohol or glucocorticoids increases the risk for lactic acidosis. Concurrent use of cimetidine increases metformin peak levels.

Adverse Effects

The most common adverse effects of biguanides include nausea, vomiting, diarrhea, flatulence, abdominal pain or bloating, anorexia, and a bitter or metallic taste. Additional adverse effects include headache, dizziness, agitation, fatigue, decreased vitamin B_{12} level, and lactic acidosis.

What You DO

Nursing Responsibilities

When administering biguanide agents, the nurse should:
• Hold metformin for 48 hours before and after diagnostic studies in which the patient is administered iodinated contrast dye to prevent lactic acidosis or renal failure from occurring.

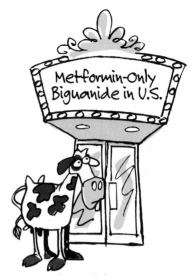

Now playing...

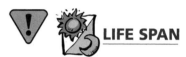
LIFE SPAN

Biguanides should be used with caution during pregnancy. Biguanides are contraindicated during lactation.

Use of metformin with fluconazole, ketoconazole, itraconazole, and oral hypoglycemic drugs may cause severe hypoglycemia. Use of iodinated contrast material (e.g., dyes that are used in radiologic studies) can cause acute renal failure and lactic acidosis.

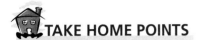

TAKE HOME POINTS

Monitor suspected or known alcoholics for decreased hepatic function.

- Administer metformin with meals to reduce GI side effects.
- Expect the health care provider to reduce the doses of metformin when the patient is undergoing cimetidine therapy.
- Evaluate baseline renal and hepatic function tests because the use of metformin is contraindicated for patients with renal or hepatic insufficiency.
- Monitor CBC, HbA$_1$c, and renal and hepatic function tests periodically.
- Instruct the patient to avoid using OTC drugs without consulting with the health care provider.
- Inform the patient that a bitter or metallic taste may occur but will subside.

Do You UNDERSTAND?

DIRECTIONS: Choose the correct response from each set of italicized choices to fill in the blanks in the following statements.

1. When the patient is on cimetidine therapy, the nurse should expect the metformin dosage to be _____ *(increased, decreased, discontinued, not given).*
2. An adverse reaction of metformin is a _____ *(sour, sweet, tangy, metallic)* taste that usually subsides.
3. Administer metformin immediately before a diagnostic test using iodinated contrast dye. _____ *(true or false).*

What IS a Thiazolidinedione?

Thiazolidinediones	Trade Names	Uses
pioglitazone *[PIE-oh-GLIT-ah-zone]*	Actos	Treatment of type 2 diabetes mellitus
rosiglitazone *[ROH-sih-GLIH-tah-zone]*	Avandia	Treatment of type 2 diabetes mellitus

Answers: 1. decreased; 2. metallic; 3. false.

Action

Thiazolidinediones are oral antidiabetic agents that increase the effects of circulating insulin, thereby lowering the blood glucose concentration. Thiazolidinediones decrease insulin resistance of the tissues, which causes the skeletal muscles and adipose tissue to increase the uptake of glucose. Thiazolidinediones inhibit gluconeogenesis, thereby decreasing the liver's production of glucose. Thiazolidinediones require the presence of insulin to be effective; they do not stimulate the production of insulin.

Uses

Thiazolidinediones are used to lower blood glucose levels in the treatment of type 2 diabetes. These agents may be used alone, as an adjunct to diet and exercise, or in combination with sulfonylurea, insulin, or metformin to improve glycemic control.

What You NEED TO KNOW

Contraindications/Precautions

Thiazolidinediones are contraindicated for patients with hypersensitivity, type 1 diabetes, DKA, and hepatic dysfunction.

Drug Interactions

Pioglitazone may reduce the effectiveness of oral contraceptives. Ketoconazole may increase pioglitazone levels.

Adverse Effects

The common adverse effects of thiazolidinediones include headache, pain, myalgia, infections, and fatigue. Other adverse effects include rhinitis, diarrhea, liver injury, upper respiratory infections, hypoglycemia, hyperglycemia, fluid retention, and weight gain.

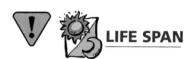

LIFE SPAN

Thiazolidinediones are contraindicated for nursing mothers.
Thiazolidinediones should be used with caution during pregnancy.

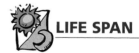

LIFE SPAN

Women who are premenopausal and anovulatory may be at risk for conception because ovulation may resume with thiazolidinedione therapy.

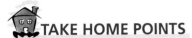

TAKE HOME POINTS

Teach the patient who is taking oral contraceptives to use barrier contraceptives because thiazolidinediones reduce the effectiveness of oral contraceptives.

What You DO

Nursing Responsibilities

Thiazolidinediones may be administered without regard for meals. When administering thiazolidinediones, the nurse should:

- Expect the health care provider to consider a higher dose of oral contraceptives or to suggest an alternative method of contraception for women of childbearing age who are taking thiazolidinediones.
- Evaluate baseline and periodic liver function tests because thiazolidinediones are contraindicated for patients with liver failure.
- Evaluate frequent blood glucose levels to monitor the effectiveness of thiazolidinedione therapy.
- Teach the patient to avoid discontinuing this medication without consulting the health care provider.
- Advise the patient to maintain the prescribed diet and exercise program.

Do You UNDERSTAND?

DIRECTIONS: **Indicate in the space provided whether the statement is *true* or *false*. If the answer is false, correct the statement to make it true (using the margin space).**

_____ 1. Rosiglitazone is a second-generation sulfonylurea.

_____ 2. Thiazolidinediones must be taken with the first bite of the meal.

_____ 3. Thiazolidinediones may be used in combination with other oral antidiabetic agents.

_____ 4. A common adverse effect of thiazolidinediones is headache.

Answers: 1. false; rosiglitazone is not a sulfonylurea but a thiazolidinedione; 2. false; thiazolidinediones may be administered without regard for meals; 3. true; 4. true.

What IS a Meglitinide?

Meglitinides	Trade Names	Uses
repaglinide [re-PAY-gli-nide]	Prandin	Treatment of type 2 diabetes mellitus
nateglinide [nah-TE-gli-nide]	Starlix	Treatment of type 2 diabetes mellitus

Action

A meglitinide is an oral antidiabetic agent that stimulates endogenous insulin production to reduce postprandial glucose levels. This agent stimulates the beta cells of the pancreas to release insulin on demand; thus functioning beta cells must exist for this action to occur. Nateglinide, an α-phenylalanine derivative, stimulates maximal insulin secretion when taken with a meal, exerting a synergistic interaction with blood glucose levels.

Uses

Meglitinides are used to maintain glycemic control in the treatment of type 2 diabetes as an adjunct to diet and exercise. Meglitinides may also be used in combination with metformin.

What You NEED TO KNOW

Contraindications/Precautions

Contraindications for use of meglitinides include hypersensitivity, type 1 diabetes, and ketoacidosis.

Drug Interactions

No noted drug interactions occur with meglitinides.

Adverse Effects

The most common adverse effect of meglitinides is hypoglycemia. Other adverse effects include nausea, vomiting, diarrhea, rhinitis, bronchitis, headache, chest pain, tooth disorder, allergy, arthralgia, back pain, and paresthesia.

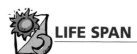
LIFE SPAN

Meglitinides are contraindicated during pregnancy and lactation.

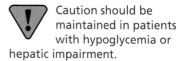
Caution should be maintained in patients with hypoglycemia or hepatic impairment.

What You DO

TAKE HOME POINTS

Meglitinides significantly lower postprandial blood glucose levels. Meglitinides have a rapid onset and short half-life, which prevents hyperinsulinemias and decreases hypoglycemic episodes.

Nursing Responsibilities

Meglitinides should be administered within 30 minutes before meals. When the patient skips a meal, the dose that is scheduled before that meal should also be skipped to decrease the risk for hypoglycemia. When administering meglitinides, the nurse should:

- Monitor the glycosylated HbA1c and blood glucose tests to evaluate the efficacy of meglitinide treatment.
- Monitor liver function tests periodically.
- Instruct the patient that when meglitinide is replacing another oral antidiabetic, it may be started the morning after the last dose of the previous drug.
- Teach the patient to monitor capillary blood glucose routinely and record results for the health care provider for review.
- Advise the patient to maintain the prescribed diet and exercise program to control blood glucose levels.
- Teach the patient signs and symptoms of hypoglycemia and to notify the health care provider of any hypoglycemic occurrences.

Do You UNDERSTAND?

DIRECTIONS: **Indicate in the space provided whether the statement is** *true* **or** *false.* **If the answer is false, correct the statement to make it true (using the margin space).**

_____ 1. Meglitinides may be given safely during pregnancy.

_____ 2. Meglitinides may be administered without regard to meal times.

_____ 3. Type 1 diabetics are treated with meglitinide to maintain glycemic control.

_____ 4. Meglitinides should be administered within 30 minutes before meals.

Answers: 1. false; meglitinides are contraindicated during pregnancy; 2. false; meglitinides should be administered 30 minutes before meals; 3. false; meglitinides are used to maintain glycemic control in the treatment of type 2 diabetes; 4. true.

What IS an Incretin Mimetic?

Incretin Mimetic	Trade Names	Uses
exenatide *[ex-IN-ah-tide]*	Byetta	Improves glucose control in type 2 diabetes mellitus

Action

A incretin mimetic is an injectable antidiabetic agent that increases beta-cell responsiveness, enhances insulin secretion, suppresses glucagon secretion, slows gastric emptying, and reduces food intake. Exenatide, a drug newly approved by the Food and Drug Administration, is the first in its class.

Uses

Exenatide is used to improve glucose control in type 2 diabetes mellitus. This agent has significantly improved A_1C levels and weight loss in many individuals.

What You NEED TO KNOW

Contraindications/Precautions

Contraindications for use of incretin mimetics include diabetic ketoacidosis, severe renal dysfunction, and severe gastrointestinal disease. Exenatide is not a substitute for insulin and should not be administered to patients with type 1 diabetes mellitus.

Drug Interactions

There are no known drug interactions.

Adverse Effects

The most common adverse effects of incretin mimetics include headache, dizziness, jitteriness, nausea, vomiting, and diarrhea.

What You DO

Nursing Responsibilities

When administering an incretin mimetic agent, the nurse should:

- Evaluate baseline renal and hepatic function tests because the use of exenatide is contraindicated for patients with severe renal dysfunction.
- Monitor CBC, HbA$_1$c, and renal function tests periodically.
- Instruct the patient to avoid using OTC drugs without consulting with the health care provider.
- Administer exenatide with the injectable prefilled pen in twice-a-day dosing.

Do You UNDERSTAND?

DIRECTIONS: Fill in the blanks with an appropriate response to complete the following statements.

1. Exenatide should not be administered to patients with _____ _____.

2. An adverse reaction of incretin mimetics is _____.

References

Abrams AC, Lemmon CB, Pennignton SS: *Clinical drug therapy: rationales for nursing practice,* ed 8, Philadelphia, 2007, Lippincott.

Arcangelo VP: *Pharmacotherapeutics for advanced practice: a practical approach,* Philadelphia, 2001, Lippincott.

Black JM, Hawks JH: *Medical-surgical nursing: clinical management for positive outcomes,* ed 7, St Louis, 2005, Elsevier.

Gutierrez K, Queener S: *Pharmacology for nursing practice,* Philadelphia, 2004, Mosby.

Hardman JG, Limbird LE: *Goodman & Gilman's the pharmacological basis of therapeutics,* ed 10, New York, 2001, McGraw-Hill.

Hodgson B, Kizior R: *Mosby's 2006 drug consult for nurses,* 2006, St Louis, 2005, Elsevier.

Answers: 1. type I diabetes; 2. headache, dizziness, jitteriness, nausea, vomiting, or diarrhea.

Karch AM: *Focus on nursing pharmacology,* ed 3, Philadelphia, 2006, Lippincott.

Kee JL, Hayes ER, McCuistion LE: *Pharmacology: a nursing process approach,* ed 5, Philadelphia, 2006, Elsevier.

Lehne R: *Pharmacology for nursing care,* ed 5, Philadelphia, 2004, WB Saunders.

Lewis SM, Heitkemper MM, Dirksen SR: *Medical-surgical nursing: assessment and management of clinical problems,* ed 6, St Louis, 2004, Mosby.

Lilley L, Harrington S, Snyder J: *Pharmacology and the nursing process,* ed 4, St Louis, 2005, Mosby.

McCance K, Huether S: *Pathophysiology: the biologic basis for disease in adults and children,* ed 4, St Louis, 2002, Mosby.

Wilson BA, Shannon MT, Stang CL: *Nurses drug guide,* Upper Saddle River, New Jersey, 2006, Pearson.

NCLEX® Review

Section A

1. A health care provider would evaluate that desmopressin therapy has been effective when which of the following findings is noted during reassessment?
   1 Increased pulse rate
   2 Increased blood glucose
   3 Decreased urinary output
   4 Decreased blood pressure

2. A health care provider who is preparing to administer corticotropin would obtain which of the following pieces of equipment?
   1 Syringe
   2 Glass measuring device
   3 Plastic medicine cup
   4 Medicine dropper

3. A patient is receiving glucocorticosteroid replacement therapy. How should the health care provider administer the total daily dose?
   1 The entire dose is given in the morning.
   2 The entire dose is given in the late afternoon.
   3 One third of the dose is given in the early morning and two thirds given in the late afternoon.
   4 Two thirds of the dose is given in the early morning and one third is given in the late afternoon.

4. The objective of drug therapy for patients with adrenal insufficiency has been met when mineralocorticoids accomplish which of the following results?
   1 Decrease cardiac output
   2 Decrease adrenal steroids
   3 Maintain fluid and electrolyte balance
   4 Counteract destructive activities of the immune system

5. A patient who is taking an adrenal-inhibiting drug should have which of the following tests to monitor determine drug efficacy?
   1 CBC
   2 Blood chemistries
   3 24-hour urine samples
   4 Routine urinalysis tests

Section B

6. Which of the following actions are representative of antithyroid drugs?
   1 Decrease production or release of thyroid hormone
   2 Increase release of parathyroid hormone
   3 Increase production and release of thyroid hormone
   4 Decrease the release of parathyroid hormone

7. Iodine solutions may cause which of the following effects?
   1 Yellow eyes
   2 Staining of teeth
   3 Loss of teeth
   4 Gray hair

8. At what time of the day should propylthiouracil be given?
   1 Only at bedtime
   2 Only as a single dose
   3 Every 2 hours
   4 In divided doses around the clock

9. Which of the following are possible actions of thyroid replacement hormones?
   1 Decrease the potency of oral anticoagulants
   2 Increase the effectiveness of digoxin
   3 Increase the risk for bleeding with oral anticoagulants
   4 Act as an antiinflammatory

10. Bisphosphonate drugs are used most often in the treatment of:
1 Hyperparathyroidism
2 Malignancies
3 Osteoporosis
4 GI disorders

Section C

11. A patient is receiving metformin (Glucophage). When the patient is scheduled for radiologic studies with iodinated dye, for what length of time should metformin be withheld?
1 24 hours before and after the test
2 36 hours before and after the test
3 48 hours before and after the test
4 2 weeks after the test

12. A patient is taking rosiglitazone (Avandia). Which of the following is an action of thiazolidinediones?
1 Increase the effects of circulating insulin
2 Stimulate the production of insulin
3 Increase the production of glucose by the liver
4 Decrease the uptake of insulin by the skeletal muscles

13. A patient is receiving lispro (Humalog). The nurse expects the onset of this insulin to occur in:
1 Less than 15 minutes
2 30 to 60 minutes
3 1 to 2 hours
4 4 to 8 hours

14. A patient with diabetes is being treated with acetohexamide (Dymelor). Which reaction should the nurse expect when this drug is combined with alcoholic beverages?
1 Bradycardic episode
2 Hyperglycemic reaction
3 Disulfiram-like reaction
4 Edema

15. A patient is taking acarbose (Precose). The nurse realizes this drug is contraindicated in patients with diabetes who have:
1 Hypothyroidism
2 Colon ulcers
3 Severe acne
4 Freckles

NCLEX® Review Answers

Section A

1. 3 Desmopressin acts in the distal renal tubules and collecting ducts to increase water reabsorption and decrease urinary output; thus urine volume is reduced and more concentrated. No evidence exists to suggest that desmopressin causes an increased pulse rate and blood glucose level. Desmopressin usually causes a slightly elevated, not decreased, blood pressure.

2. 1 Because replacement hormones are made of protein, they are digested in the GI tract and must therefore be administered parenterally with a syringe. A glass measuring device, plastic medicine cup, and a medicine dropper all indicate oral administration.

3. 4 Two thirds of the dosage is given in the early morning and one third is given in the late afternoon; this routine mimics the body's normal glucocorticoid secretion cycle. The entire dose given in the morning, the entire dose given in the late afternoon, one third of the dose given in the early morning, and two thirds given in the late afternoon do not mimic the body's normal glucocorticoid secretion cycle.

4. 3 Mineralocorticoids exert an effect on sodium, chloride, and potassium and maintain extracellular and intracellular fluid volume; thus they maintain fluid and electrolyte balance. Mineralocorticoids do not decrease cardiac output or adrenal steroid production. Mineralocorticoids do not counteract the destructive activities of the immune system as glucocorticosteroids do.

5. 3 The nurse should monitor 24-hour urine samples of 17-hydroxyglucocorticosteroids and 17-ketogenic steroids, which reveal increased elimination of glucocorticosteroids byproducts to validate drug efficacy. A CBC, blood chemistries, and routine urinalysis are not indicated with adrenal inhibitor drug therapy.

Section B

6. **1** Antithyroid drugs decrease production or the release of thyroid hormone in the treatment of hyperthyroidism. The action of antithyroid drugs does not increase the release of the parathyroid hormone, increase the production and release of the thyroid hormone, or decrease the release of the parathyroid hormone.

7. **2** Iodine solutions may cause staining of the teeth. Iodine solutions do not cause yellow eyes, loss of teeth, or gray hair.

8. **4** Propylthiouracil should be given in divided doses around the clock. Giving propylthiouracil only at bedtime, only as a single dose, or every 2 hours is inappropriate.

9. **3** Thyroid hormones may increase the risk for bleeding if taken concurrently with oral anticoagulants. They do not decrease the effectiveness of anticoagulants or increase the effectiveness of digoxin, but rather increase the risk for digoxin toxicity or act as an antiinflammatory.

10. **3** Bisphosphonate drugs are used most often in the prevention and treatment of osteoporosis. Hypercalcemic drugs will not reduce calcium levels in patients with GI disorders. Hypercalcemic drugs may be given to reduce the calcium levels for patients with hyperparathyroidism, adrenal disorders, and hypercalcemia that are associated with malignancies, although these uses are less common.

Section C

11. **3** Metformin should be withheld for 48 hours before and after radiologic studies during which iodinated dye is administered. Withholding metformin 24 or 36 hours before and after the test or for 2 weeks after the test are inappropriate.

12. **1** The action of thiazolidinediones, such as rosiglitazone increases the effects of circulating insulin. Thiazolidinediones do not stimulate the production of insulin, increase the production of glucose by the liver, or decrease the uptake of insulin by skeletal muscles.

13. **1** The onset of ultra rapid-acting insulin (Lispro) is less than 15 minutes. The remaining options (30 to 60 minutes, 1 to 2 hours, and 4 to 8 hours) do not represent the time at which the onset of rapid-acting insulin occurs.

14. **3** A disulfiram-like reaction may occur when the patient takes sulfonylureas, such as acetohexamide and alcohol together. Sulfonylurea with alcohol does not cause bradycardia, hyperglycemia, or edema. Sulfonylureas may cause hypoglycemia.

15. **2** α-Glucosidases, such as acarbose, are contraindicated in patients with diabetes who have colon ulcers. α-Glucosidases are not contraindicated in patients with hypothyroidism, severe acne, or freckles.

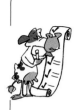

Notes

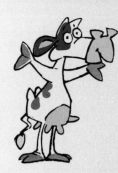

Drugs Used to Treat Gastrointestinal System Disorders

What You WILL LEARN

After reading this chapter, you will know how to do the following:

- ✔ Contrast the action of a laxative, stool softener, and an antiflatulent.
- ✔ Discuss the contraindications for antiemetics, prokinetics, and emetics.
- ✔ Describe the adverse effects of a digestive enzyme and an intestinal flora modifier.
- ✔ Contrast the nursing responsibilities of hyperacidity agents.

This chapter reviews the pharmacologic preparations used to treat gastric motility, flatulence, mucosa, hyperacidity, and digestion. The nurse must provide more consumer education with these gastrointestinal (GI) preparations than they do with any other over-the-counter (OTC) drugs because large quantities of these nonprescription, or OTC, drugs are purchased for self-medication.

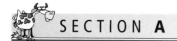

SECTION **A**

ANTIEMETICS

Antiemetic drugs are used to treat gastric mobility disorders, as well as nausea and vomiting. These drugs include phenothiazines, serotonin antagonists, prokinetics, and emetics. The goal of treatment is to relieve symptoms of nausea and prevent serious nutritional and fluid-electrolyte deficits.

What IS a Phenothiazine?

Phenothiazines	Trade Names	Uses
prochlorperazine [pro-klor-PAIR-ah-zeen]	Compazine	Treatment of severe nausea and vomiting
promethazine [pro-METH-uh-zeen]	Phenergan	Treatment of motion sickness and nausea

Action

Phenothiazines block dopamine receptors in the CTZ. The CTZ is responsible for activating the vomiting reflex. Stimulation of the vomiting center produces reflex contraction of abdominal and respiratory muscles, relaxation of the cardiac sphincter in the stomach, and glottis closure. Dopamine, a potent neurotransmitter, is required for the conduction of impulses from excited afferent nerves to stimulate the medullary-vomiting center. Blocking dopamine receptors inhibits the stimulation of the vomiting center, and an antiemetic effect results.

Phenothiazine drugs also block (to varying degrees) the neurotransmitters acetylcholine, histamine, and norepinephrine. Blocking a neurotransmitter or its receptor interrupts conduction of the nerve impulse across the synapse. Blocking acetylcholine, histamine, and norepinephrine receptors and the conduction of central and peripheral nerves across the synapse interrupts the impulse to vomit, resulting in an antiemetic effect.

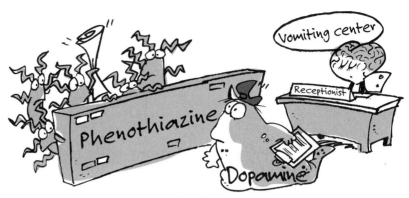

Block dopamine receptors.

Uses

Phenothiazines are indicated for suppression of nausea and vomiting that is associated with varied noxious stimuli. Drugs in this classification are frequently considered first in the prevention and treatment of nausea and vomiting that are associated with anesthesia, antineoplastic therapy, radiation therapy, and motion sickness.

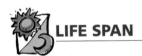

LIFE SPAN

Phenothiazines are contraindicated for women during pregnancy and lactation and for children under 2 years of age.

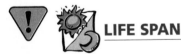

LIFE SPAN

- Caution should be taken when phenothiazines are given to patients with cardiovascular disease, hypertension, asthma, breast cancer, and hepatic dysfunction.
- Phenothiazines should be given with caution to older and debilitated patients.

What You NEED TO KNOW

Contraindications/Precautions

Phenothiazines are contraindicated for patients with known hypersensitivity, depression, glaucoma, GI or genitourinary (GU) obstruction, and coma. Phenothiazines are also contraindicated for acutely ill and dehydrated patients.

Drug Interactions

Alcohol, nitrates, and antihypertensives cause increased hypotension when given with phenothiazines. CNS depressants (e.g., alcohol) produce additive CNS depression when given concurrently with phenothiazines. Antacids and antidiarrheal drugs reduce absorption of phenothiazines from the GI tract. The risk for granulocytosis is increased when phenothiazines are given with antithyroid drugs. Phenothiazines with lithium may present an increased risk for lithium toxicity. Beta blockers may increase the response to prochlorperazine. Phenobarbital increases the metabolism of prochlorperazine, thereby reducing its action. Prochlorperazine antagonizes the antihypertensive action of guanethidine.

Adverse Effects

Common adverse effects of phenothiazines include drowsiness, hypotension, and anticholinergic effects. Anticholinergic effects include dry mouth, flushing, blurred vision, tachycardia, photosensitivity, and constipation. Other adverse effects of phenothiazines include anorexia, hypotension, hypertension, incoordination, weakness, urine retention, darkened urine (pink to brown), respiratory depression, jaundice, leukopenia, agranulocytosis, and thrombocytopenia. Major adverse effects of phenothiazines include extrapyramidal symptoms (EPS), particularly with prolonged therapy. When phenothiazines block dopamine receptors, EPS that occur include prolonged muscle contraction, causing twisting, repetitive movements, or abnormal posture (**dystonia**), slow rhythmical movements (**tardive dyskinesia**), restlessness (**akathisia**), periorbital tremor, and tremors and rigidity (**pseudo parkinsonism**).

What You Do

Nursing Responsibilities

Phenothiazines may be administered orally, rectally, IV, or IM, depending on the desired speed of response and the condition of the patient. When administering phenothiazines, the nurse should:

- Mix oral prochlorperazine with 60 mL of fluids or soft food (e.g., tomato or fruit juice, milk, pudding) to disguise the taste and decrease GI distress.
- Monitor the patient for depressed cough reflex, thickened secretions, respiratory distress, and aspiration.
- Encourage an adequate intake of fluid because dehydrated persons are more likely to experience EPS.
- Teach the patient to rise and change positions slowly to prevent orthostatic hypotension.
- Encourage adequate fluid intake for patients who are taking phenothiazines.
- Warn the patient to report EPS (e.g., tremors, abnormal body movements).

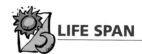
LIFE SPAN

- Children under 12 are at increased risk for extrapyramidal symptoms (EPS), particularly when they become dehydrated, have chickenpox, or have a CNS infection.
- Children and older adults are at an increased risk and should have ongoing assessment for EPS. Provide safety measures in assisting patients with ambulation, particularly older adults.

 Although rare, agranulocytosis is an extremely serious adverse effect of phenothiazines. Extended use of chlorpromazine may lead to opacity of the lens of the eye.

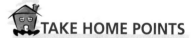
TAKE HOME POINTS

- Tablets of prochlorperazine may be crushed to mix with food or liquids.

- Evaluate complete blood count (CBC) periodically for ongoing phenothiazine therapy because blood dyscrasias may occur.
- Inform the patient that an additive hypotensive effect occurs when taking phenothiazines concurrently with alcohol, antihypertensives, CNS depressants, or nitrates.
- Encourage the patient to have an eye examination every 6 months for early detection of cataracts.
- Auscultate bowel sounds and monitor elimination patterns to prevent constipation.
- Avoid contact of prochlorperazine with the skin to prevent a rash and irritation.
- Instruct the patient to rinse the mouth frequently with water and suck on sugarless candy or ice chips to prevent drying of the oral mucosa.
- Encourage the patient to avoid driving or performing hazardous tasks until the response is known because prochlorperazine has a sedative effect.
- Instruct the patient to use sunscreen as protection against sunlight and to avoid prolonged exposure to prevent photosensitivity.
- Instruct the patient to avoid altering the dose, changing the schedule, or discontinuing phenothiazine therapy without consulting the health care provider.

When skin comes in contact with prochlorperazine, wash hands immediately with soap and water.

Do You UNDERSTAND?

DIRECTIONS: **Fill in the blanks with the appropriate response.**

1. An increased risk for what neurologic problem occurs with the use of phenothiazine? _____
2. What age groups are at increased risk for EPS if they become dehydrated? _____
3. To promote safe administration, what do phenothiazines block, thereby acting as antiemetics? _____
   _____

Answers: 1. EPS, tardive dyskinesia; **2.** children and older adults; **3.** dopamine and, to a varying degree, acetylcholine, histamine, and norepinephrine receptors.

What IS a Serotonin Antagonist?

Serotonin Antagonists	Trade Names	Uses
granisetron [gran-ISS-eh-tron]	Kytril	Prevention of emetogenic chemotherapy
ondansetron [on-DAN-sih-tron]	Zofran	Prevention of emetogenic chemotherapy

Action

Antiemetics act as an antagonist of a selective serotonin receptor (5-HT3). Serotonin 5-HT3 receptors are located centrally in the CTZ and peripherally in the GI tract. When central serotonin receptors in the CTZ are blocked, the vomiting center is not activated, producing an antiemetic effect. Peripheral serotonin 5-HT3 receptors are located on the vagal nerve terminals in the upper GI tract. When serotonin is released from the walls of the small intestine, serotonin receptors transmit impulses on the vagal afferent nerve to initiate the vomiting reflex. Peripheral serotonin-receptor antagonists interrupt vagal impulse transmission, resulting in an antiemetic effect.

Uses

Serotonin antagonists are used to prevent nausea and vomiting associated with emetogenic cancer therapy. These agents are effective for initial and repeated courses of chemotherapy, including high-dose cisplatin. Serotonin antagonists are the most effective antiemetics for highly emetogenic anticancer drugs. Serotonin antagonists can also be used for postoperative nausea and vomiting.

What You NEED TO KNOW

Contraindications/Precautions

Serotonin antagonists are contraindicated for those with known hypersensitivity.

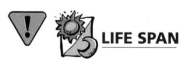
LIFE SPAN

- Granisetron requires cautious use for patients with liver disease.
- Cautious use of serotonin antagonists is advised during pregnancy and lactation.
- Ondansetron requires cautious use in children 2 years of age and younger.

Drug Interactions

An increased risk for EPS is present when serotonin antagonists are taken with phenothiazines. Rifampin decreases ondansetron drug levels when given together.

Adverse Effects

Adverse effects of serotonin antagonists include headaches, drowsiness, fatigue, dizziness, agitation, insomnia, diarrhea, and constipation. Other adverse effects include rash, blurred vision, flushing, tachycardia, hypotension, hypertension, chest pain, dysrhythmias, and EPS. Granisetron may cause elevated liver enzymes. Additional adverse effects of ondansetron include seizures and bronchospasms.

What You DO

Nursing Responsibilities

Oral serotonin antagonist drugs have an onset of action in approximately 30 minutes, and IV has a rapid onset of 1 to 3 minutes. Duration of drug action for oral medications is 4 to 24 hours; the peak is 30 to 90 minutes. The granisetron IV dose regimen is initiated before chemotherapy to prevent the onset of nausea and vomiting. Similarly, orally administered drugs are given 30 to 60 minutes before chemotherapy. When administering serotonin antagonists, the nurse should:

- Monitor the patient's cardiovascular status for early detection of angina and tachycardia.
- Monitor fluid and electrolyte status resulting from diarrhea.
- Evaluate intake and output.
- Discuss methods of managing constipation with patients.
- Inform the patient that headache is a common adverse effect, which may require an analgesic for relief.
- Monitor liver function tests periodically. Elevated aspartate aminotransferase, alanine aminotransferase, or bilirubin levels return to normal within 2 weeks of serotonin antagonist withdrawal.

Do You UNDERSTAND?

DIRECTIONS: **Indicate in the space provided whether the statement is *true* or *false*. If the answer is false, correct the statement to make it true (using the margin space).**

_____ 1. Serotonin antagonists rarely act as an effective antiemetic for highly emetogenic anticancer treatments.

_____ 2. Serotonin receptors of the 5-HT3 type are located centrally in the CTZ and peripherally in the GI tract.

_____ 3. Serotonin antagonists interrupt vagal impulse transmissions to the vomiting center, resulting in an antiemetic effect.

What IS a Miscellaneous Antiemetic?

Miscellaneous Antiemetics	Trade Names	Uses
dimenhydrinate [dye-men-HYE-dri-nate]	Dramamine	Treatment of motion sickness
diphenhydramine [dye-fen-HIGH-drah-meen]	Benadryl	Treatment of motion sickness
hydroxyzine [hye-DROX-ih-zeen]	Vistaril	Treatment of nausea and vomiting
droperidol [droh-PAIR-ih-dol]	Inapsine	Treatment of emetogenic chemotherapy
scopolamine [scoh-POLL-ah-meen]	Transderm-Scop	Treatment of motion sickness, preoperative nausea, and vomiting

Action

Dimenhydrinate depresses the labyrinth and vestibular function to decrease nausea and vomiting. Diphenhydramine competes for H_1-receptor sites, thereby blocking histamine release, prolonging dopamine action, and decreasing cholinergic activity. Hydroxyzine causes CNS depression and anticholinergic effects, the action of which controls emesis. Droperidol is classified as a butyrophenone that blocks dopamine-2 receptors in the CTZ, thereby suppressing emesis. The action of butyrophenones is similar to that of phenothiazines. Scopolamine exerts an anticholinergic effect to stop nausea and vomiting.

Answers: 1. false; serotonin antagonists are used to prevent nausea and vomiting associated with emetogenic cancer therapy; 2. true; 3. true.

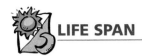

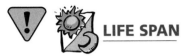

Uses

Several antihistamines are used for motion sickness and nausea control. Droperidol is a potent drug used for the control of chemotherapy-induced vomiting. Scopolamine, an anticholinergic drug, is also used for motion sickness and as a preanesthesia antiemetic.

What You NEED TO KNOW

Contraindications/Precautions

These antiemetics are generally contraindicated for patients with severe hypotension, glaucoma, prostatic hypertrophy, asthma, and GI obstruction.

Drug Interactions

Increased CNS depression may result when alcohol, CNS depressants, and monamine oxidase inhibitors (MAOIs) are taken concurrently with dimenhydrinate and diphenhydramine. The anticholinergic effect is enhanced when tricyclic antidepressants are given together with dimenhydrinate, diphenhydramine, and hydroxyzine.

Adverse Effects

These drugs may lead to adverse effects of drowsiness, dizziness, dry mouth, fatigue, headache, incoordination, blurred vision, restlessness, insomnia, tachycardia, hypotension, hypertension, and urinary frequency. Adverse effects of dimenhydrinate also include euphoria, confusion, anorexia, diarrhea, and constipation. Diphenhydramine may cause thickened secretions. Hydroxyzine may lead to wheezing. Droperidol may cause adverse effects that include EPS, respiratory depression, and bronchospasms.

What You DO

Nursing Responsibilities

When administering miscellaneous antiemetics, the nurse should:
- Provide safety for the patient who is taking these drugs because they cause sedation. Assist the patient with bed rails, and supervise ambulation for safety.

- Instruct the patient to avoid driving or performing hazardous activities because of the sedative effect.
- Advise the patient to avoid alcohol when taking these drugs to prevent oversedation.
- Instruct the patient and family to report EPS effects immediately (e.g., restlessness, facial grimacing, rigidity, tremors, involuntary movements).
- Monitor the patient's vital signs because of the adverse effects affecting blood pressure and heart rate.
- Instruct the patient that when a dose is missed, the missed dose should be taken as soon as possible, except when it is nearly time for the next dose.
- Inform the patient that tablets may be crushed and capsules may be emptied and mixed with food or fluids.
- Warn the patient to check with the health care provider before taking OTC medications.
- Instruct the patient to report anorexia, persistent nausea, diarrhea, excess weight loss, aggression, and suicidal ideation.

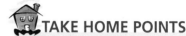

TAKE HOME POINTS

Be prepared to treat EPS with anticholinergic drugs. Be prepared to treat hypotension with fluid therapy. The patient should avoid taking a doubled dose.

Do You UNDERSTAND?

DIRECTIONS: Complete the following statements with the appropriate terms from the italicized list provided.

1. Diphenhydramine is used as an antiemetic primarily for

   _____.

2. Droperidol is used as an antiemetic primarily for

   _____.

3. EPS may be an adverse effect of

   _____.

emetogenic chemotherapy	*diphenhydramine*
motion sickness	*scopolamine*
preoperative nausea and vomiting	*hydroxyzine*
droperidol	

Answers: 1. motion sickness; 2. emetogenic chemotherapy; 3. droperidol.

What IS a Prokinetic?

Prokinetic	Trade Name	Use
metoclopramide [MET-oh-KLOE-pra-mide]	Reglan	Treatment of gastric stasis

Action

Prokinetic GI drugs increase the motion or movement through the GI tract. Metoclopramide is a cholinergic drug that stimulates motility of the upper GI tract without increasing gastric, biliary, or pancreatic secretions. Metoclopramide also increases the tone and force of gastric contractions, relaxes the pyloric sphincter, and increases peristalsis of the duodenum and jejunum. The result is increased transit time and increased gastric emptying time. Metoclopramide also increases esophageal sphincter tone but has little effect on peristaltic movement in the colon. The exact mechanism of action is unknown, but metoclopramide appears to sensitize the GI smooth muscle to acetylcholine. Metoclopramide also has an antiemetic effect that is thought to be a result of blocking stimulation of dopamine receptors in the chemoreceptor trigger zone (CTZ) in the medulla.

Uses

Metoclopramide is indicated in short-term treatment (4 to 12 weeks) of adults with GERD who fail to respond to conventional treatment. Other indications are in patients who require radiographic examinations during which gastric emptying is important, those with symptomatic diabetes with gastric stasis, and postoperative patients with GI hypomotility. Metoclopramide also facilitates small bowel intubation when the tube will not pass the pylorus. Prokinetic GI agents are also useful in patients who are receiving cancer chemotherapy and in the prevention of postoperative nausea and vomiting when gastric intubation and suction is undesirable.

Caution should be used in patients with a history of congestive heart failure, hypertension, renal impairment, mental depression, or Parkinson's disease.

What You NEED TO KNOW

Contraindications/Precautions

Metoclopramide is contraindicated for patients with GI obstruction, hemorrhage, or perforation when stimulation of the GI tract may be dangerous. This agent is also contraindicated for patients with a known hypersensitivity, pheochromocytoma (because of the risk for a hypertensive crisis), epilepsy, and those who are receiving other drugs that are likely to cause EPS.

Drug Interactions

When metoclopramide is given concurrently with alcohol and CNS depressants, sedation may be increased. Phenothiazines may increase the risk for EPS when given with metoclopramide. Anticholinergics and opiate analgesics may antagonize the therapeutic effect of metoclopramide, thereby decreasing GI motility.

Adverse Effects

Adverse effects of metoclopramide increase with higher doses or with prolonged administration. The most common adverse effects include drowsiness, restlessness, fatigue, diarrhea, and EPS, particularly acute dystonic reactions. Other adverse effects include dizziness, visual disturbances, irritability, confusion, depression, bradycardia, insomnia, and suicidal ideation. Galactorrhea, gynecomastia, and menstrual disorders are adverse effects that resolve weeks after drug discontinuation. EPS effects usually subside within 2 to 3 months after discontinuation. Methemoglobinemia in neonates may occur with overdosing.

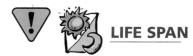

LIFE SPAN

Metoclopramide is contraindicated for women during pregnancy and for children, with the exception of pediatric use in aiding small bowel intubation.

LIFE SPAN

Caution should be used with nursing mothers who are receiving metoclopramide.

Methemoglobinemia in neonates may occur with overdosing.

Chest Medicine On-Line
http://www.gerd.com/
http://www.rxmed.com/
prescribe.html

What You DO

Nursing Responsibilities

Metoclopramide is available in tablets and liquid form for oral administration and as an injectable for intramuscular (IM) or IV use. In diabetic gastroparesis, symptom severity determines the route of administration.

Relief from nausea, vomiting, and anorexia indicate improvement in symptoms. The dose should be decreased by one half in patients with reduced renal function. Metoclopramide may be mixed with parenteral IV solutions. When administering prokinetic GI agents, the nurse should:

- Administer the oral dose 30 minutes before meals and at bedtime.
- Dilute IV doses above 10 mg or more in 50 mL of a parenteral solution and give slowly over 15 minutes or longer; 10 mg or less may be given over 1 to 2 minutes.
- Protect IV metoclopramide from light with aluminum foil or other protective covering.
- Monitor for EPS, which are most likely to occur early in the treatment, at high doses, in patients who are dehydrated, or in pediatric and young patients. Diphenhydramine HCl (Benadryl) or benztropine mesylate (Cogentin) may be given IM to reverse EPS.
- Monitor for tardive dyskinesia symptoms, including involuntary movements of the tongue, mouth or jaw, face, or extremities. Tardive dyskinesia is potentially irreversible. Metoclopramide may mask symptoms, which may make recognition of tardive dyskinesia more difficult. When symptoms occur, withhold metoclopramide and notify the health care provider.
- Encourage patients who are taking prokinetics to have adequate fluid intake.
- Advise the patient to avoid hazardous tasks (e.g., driving) for a few hours after taking metoclopramide because the agent may cause sedation and impair mental and physical abilities.
- Counsel the patient to avoid alcohol and other central nervous system (CNS) depressants, such as sedatives, hypnotics, narcotics, and tranquilizers, all of which may increase sedation.
- Monitor blood sugar and signs and symptoms of hypoglycemia. Insulin dose or administration schedule may require changing when hypoglycemia that is related to rapid transit of food through the GI tract occurs.

Do You UNDERSTAND?

DIRECTIONS: Fill in the blanks with the appropriate response.
1. Metoclopramide increases the tone in the _____.
2. Metoclopramide exerts an effect in the _____,
   thereby preventing nausea and vomiting.
3. EPS occur most frequently with the use of metoclopramide in
   _____.
4. Diphenhydramine HCl (Benadryl) given IM counteracts the symptoms of _____.

What IS an Emetic?

Emetic	Trade Name	Use
ipecac [IP-eh-kak]	Ipecac Syrup	Treatment of oral poisoning or overdose

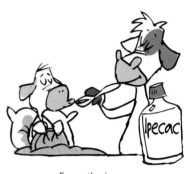

Force the issue.

Action

Ipecac syrup, taken by mouth, is an OTC drug that stimulates the CTZ and acts directly on the gastric mucosa to stimulate vomiting.

Uses

Emetic drugs are used to expel toxic substances that may have been consumed by accident or overdose. The goal is to expel the toxic substance from the body before material is absorbed from the GI tract.

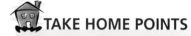

TAKE HOME POINTS

Vomiting should not be induced when caustic substances (e.g., ammonia, bleach, drain opener, lye, battery acid, gasoline, kerosene, lighter fluid) have been ingested.

What You NEED TO KNOW

Contraindications/Precautions

Emetics are contraindicated for patients with cardiac dysfunction, hypersensitivity, severe inebriation, depressed gag reflex, and deep sedation, as well as those in shock and in a coma.

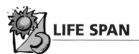

LIFE SPAN

The safe use of emetics in women during pregnancy and nursing mothers has not been established. The use of ipecac in infants under 6 months of age has not been established.

Answers: 1. esophageal sphincter; 2. CTZ; 3. first days of therapy; 4. EPS.

Caution is advised when using an emetic in an anticonvulsant drug overdose victim because convulsions may be precipitated.

CNS stimulation, severe CNS depression, fatal respiratory depression, and circulatory collapse may occur with larger-than-normal doses.

Vomiting with emesis should be avoided when caustic substances have been ingested.

TAKE HOME POINTS

Follow ipecac with one to two glasses of water. Monitor vital signs, use side rails, and caution the patient to avoid ambulating without assistance.

Drug Interactions

Milk and activated charcoal may inactivate ipecac. When ipecac is given together with carbonated beverages, abdominal distention may occur. Vegetable oil may delay the absorption of ipecac.

Adverse Effects

Adverse effects of ipecac include diarrhea, drowsiness, and mild GI upset. Adverse effects that may occur when ipecac is not vomited and is absorbed or when ipecac is overdosed include persistent vomiting, severe myopathy, tremors, cardiotoxicity, dysrhythmias, chest pain, bradycardia, tachycardia, hypotension, fatal myocarditis, depression, and coma.

What You DO

Nursing Responsibilities

The adult dose of ipecac should be followed with 8 to 16 oz of water. The dose may be repeated in 20 minutes as needed. Children over the age of 1 year should follow an oral dose with 6 to 8 oz of water. Children under 1 year of age should follow the dose with 4 to 8 oz of water. The dose may be repeated in 20 minutes in children. Regurgitating caustic substances may cause additional injury to the esophagus. When emesis is contraindicated, activated charcoal may be given. When administering emetics, the nurse should:

- Avoid storing ipecac syrup and ipecac fluid extract together. Ipecac fluid extract is 14 times stronger than ipecac syrup and has caused death when mistakenly given at the same dose as ipecac syrup. When the ipecac dose is not vomited and allowed to absorb, cardiotoxicity may occur. Activated charcoal may inactivate the ipecac.
- Caution parents and patients to be careful about confusing ipecac syrup with ipecac fluid extract.
- Teach families about the proper storage of ipecac, such as keeping it in a safe location and making it inaccessible to children.
- Counsel the patient to phone the emergency department or poison control center before using ipecac. Ipecac should be available in the home.
- Give ipecac *before* activated charcoal, not after.
- Prevent aspiration following emesis by positioning patients on their side.

- Use motion by gently bouncing the pediatric patient to begin emesis. Emesis is reduced when the patient is lying still in a recumbent position.
- Teach parents about the proper procedure after ipecac has been given. When vomiting does not occur within 15 to 20 minutes, the health care provider should be contacted immediately and the dose of ipecac that was given should be recovered using gastric lavage and activated charcoal as needed.

Do You UNDERSTAND?

DIRECTIONS: **Fill in the blanks with the appropriate responses.**

1. List four CNS depression safety precautions.

   _____

   _____

   _____

   _____

2. Instruction on the proper storage of ipecac includes

   _____

   _____

3. Before using ipecac, instruct the patient to phone the emergency department or

   _____

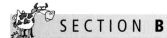

SECTION B

LAXATIVES, STOOL SOFTENERS, AND ANTIFLATULANTS

This section reviews the pharmacologic preparations that are used to treat constipation and gas, thereby influencing GI motility. This section explains stimulant, bulk, lubricant, and hyperosmotic laxatives, as well as stool softeners and antiflatulents.

What IS a Stimulant Laxative?

Stimulant Laxatives	Trade Names	Uses
bisacodyl [BISS-uh-KOE-dill]	Dulcolax	Treatment of constipation and colon evacuation
cascara sagrada [cass-CARE-uh]	Cascara	Treatment of constipation and prevention of straining
senna [SEN-ah]	Senokot	Treatment of constipation and colon evacuation
castor oil	Neoloid	Treatment of constipation
phenolphthalein [fee-nahl-THAY-leen]	Ex-Lax, Correctol	Treatment of constipation

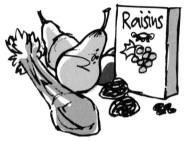

Natural laxatives.

Action

Stimulant laxatives irritate or stimulate the nerve plexus in the mucosa of the small intestine and colon to stimulate peristalsis and increase motility of the intestinal contents. The resulting stools of bisacodyl, phenolphthalein, cascara, and senna tend to be semisoft, whereas castor oil produces a stool of watery consistency. Certain foods in the diet naturally contain organic acids that cause irritation of the intestinal mucosa and stimulation of peristalsis. These foods include prunes, raisins, figs, rhubarb, and pears.

Uses

Because stimulant laxatives produce defecation, they are used to treat constipation or to evacuate the bowel before radiologic examination or surgery. These drugs are frequently used for bowel retraining to reestablish normal elimination patterns in patients with spinal cord injury (SCI) or neurologic disorders. Stimulant laxatives may also be given to prevent straining after a myocardial infarction (MI) or GI surgery.

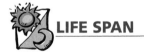

LIFE SPAN

Stimulant laxatives are contraindicated for patients who are pregnant and lactating.

What You NEED TO KNOW

Contraindications/Precautisons

Stimulant laxatives are contraindicated for patients with hypersensitivity, undiagnosed abdominal pain, rectal fissures, ulcerated hemorrhoids, colon spasticity, Crohn's disease, ulcerative colitis, and other chronic inflammatory bowel diseases.

Because cascara sagrada contains alcohol, it should be avoided in patients with a known intolerance to alcohol.

Drug Interactions

The increased intestinal motility of stimulant laxatives allows quick passage and elimination from the GI tract. Increased GI motility reduces the absorption of other concurrently administered drugs, particularly sustained-release drugs.

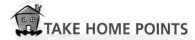 Long-term use of stimulant laxatives may lead to hypokalemia, metabolic acidosis or alkalosis, and tetany.

Adverse Effects

Adverse effects to stimulant laxatives include nausea, vomiting, abdominal cramping, weakness, diarrhea, dehydration, and electrolyte imbalances. A burning sensation may occur after rectal administration of bisacodyl. After intestinal evacuation, a period may follow without bowel movements. This time lapse occurs to allow sufficient accumulation of fecal matter that is required for another evacuation. When large amounts of stimulant laxatives are taken, a potential for toxic absorption exists. The most common adverse effect after administering a stimulant laxative is abdominal cramping resulting from the increased peristalsis. Senokot may color urine and feces to a reddish or yellow-brown.

What You DO

Nursing Responsibilities

All stimulant laxatives can be given orally, although bisacodyl may also be given as a rectal suppository. The quick onset after rectal administration makes bisacodyl the drug of choice when surgery or procedures requiring bowel cleansing need to be scheduled immediately. When administering stimulant laxatives, the nurse should:

- Inform patients that laxatives are to be taken as a short-term treatment, which avoids the development of laxative dependence.
- Counsel the patient about appropriate dietary measures, environmental control, and exercise to encourage the return of normal bowel function.
- Inform the patient that to promote optimal therapeutic action of oral laxatives, these drugs should be taken with a full glass of water and that tablets should not be chewed, but rather, swallowed whole to ensure reaching the GI tract for contact stimulation.

TAKE HOME POINTS

The enteric coating of bisacodyl and phenolphthalein is prematurely removed when taken concurrently within 1 hour of antacids or dairy products.

- Teach the patient to increase fluid intake to at least 8 to 10 glasses per day.
- Instruct the patient to report dizziness, confusion, sweating, or laxative dependence.
- Provide ready access to bathroom facilities and any necessary assistance with ambulation after laxative administration.
- Mix castor oil with fruit juice or carbonated drink to increase palatability.

Do You UNDERSTAND?

DIRECTIONS: **Fill in the blanks with the appropriate response.**
1. What is the expected time frame of action of bisacodyl when given via rectal suppository? _____
2. What is the expected time frame of action of oral cascara? _____
3. Stimulant laxatives produce stools through what action? _____
4. Stimulant laxatives are used to treat patients with what condition(s)? _____

_____

What IS a Bulk Laxative?

Bulk Laxatives	Trade Names	Uses
psyllium [SILL-i-um]	Metamucil	Treatment of chronic constipation
polycarbophil [pol-i-CAR-boe-fill]	FiberCon	Prevention of straining and treatment of diarrhea

Action

Bulk laxatives absorb free water in the intestine to form a gelatinous or viscous mass. The mass causes the colon to distend and stimulate peristalsis. This action increases intestinal motility and decreases stool transit time. Because the resultant stools are soft, they pass through the GI tract easily with no trauma to rectal or anal tissues.

Bulk laxatives are indigestible, mild, and less apt to be habit-forming than are other laxatives. Because bulk laxatives evacuate only the descending colon, sigmoid colon, and rectum, the risk for laxative dependence is greatly reduced. This classification of laxatives does not interfere with the absorption of nutrients.

Uses

Bulk laxatives are useful in short-term treatment of constipation and long-term chronic constipation. Additionally, these agents are used to prevent constipation and straining, particularly after MI or rectal surgery.

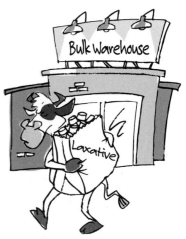

Long-term constipation relief.

What You NEED TO KNOW

Contraindications/Precautions

Bulk laxatives are contraindicated for patients with GI obstruction, acute abdominal pain, fecal impaction, rectal bleeding, and appendicitis, or those who have had bowel surgery or poisoning.

Drug Interactions

When taken concurrently with bulk laxatives, absorption of antibiotics, salicylates, warfarin, nitrofurantoin, and cardiac glycosides may be decreased.

Adverse Effects

Bulk-forming laxatives may produce adverse effects of abdominal fullness, flatulence, and cramps. Hypersensitivity rarely occurs with administration of bulk natural laxatives. Excessive use of bulk laxatives may cause nausea, vomiting, and severe diarrhea. Serious adverse effects from bulk laxatives involve esophageal or intestinal obstruction.

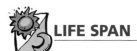

LIFE SPAN

Psyllium and polycarbophil are contraindicated for women during pregnancy and lactation and for children under 3 years of age.

What You DO

Nursing Responsibilities

Bulk laxatives, usually considered as the safest laxative, produce the same natural action as do 6 to 10 grams of dietary fiber per day. Fiber foods include cereals, bran, fresh fruits, and vegetables. When administering bulk laxatives, the nurse should:

- Monitor the patient for diarrhea because adequate hydration should be maintained.
- Teach the patient to increase fluid intake to at least 8 to 10 glasses per day.
- Inform the patient that the laxative effect usually occurs in 12 to 24 hours, therefore 2 to 3 days may be required to establish regularity.
- Monitor blood glucose levels in patients with diabetes who are given bulk laxatives.

TAKE HOME POINTS

Bulk laxative administration must be accompanied with at least an 8-ounce glass of water to prevent esophageal or intestinal obstruction. Bulk laxative preparations contain sugar and may lead to elevated blood glucose levels with prolonged use.

Do You UNDERSTAND?

DIRECTIONS: **Indicate in the space provided whether the statement is *true* or *false*. If the answer is false, correct the statement to make it true (using the margin space).**

_____ 1. Bulk laxatives irritate the intestinal mucosa.
_____ 2. Bulk laxatives should be avoided in patients following an MI.
_____ 3. Bulk laxatives should not be administered with water.

What IS a Lubricant Laxative?

Lubricant Laxative	Trade Name	Uses
mineral oil	Kondremul Plain	Treatment of constipation and fecal impaction; prevention of straining

Answers: 1. false; bulk laxatives expand intestinal feces with water, thereby distending the colon and stimulating peristalsis, which decreases transit time; 2. false; bulk laxatives are used in patients after an MI to prevent straining; 3. false; bulk laxatives should be given with an 8-ounce glass of water.

Action

Lubricant laxatives coat fecal material with a film, which prevents the reabsorption of water through the colon, and they soften the stool and lubricate the intestinal wall, which facilitates the smooth passage of feces. Mineral oil produces semi-soft stools.

Uses

These laxatives are used in the treatment of constipation or fecal impaction and to prevent straining following rectal surgery or an MI.

What You NEED TO KNOW

Contraindications/Precautions

Lubricant laxatives are contraindicated for patients with abdominal pain and intestinal obstruction.

Drug Interactions

Few drug interactions occur with mineral oil and concurrent medications. The absorption of food and fat-soluble vitamins (vitamins A, D, E, and K) may be reduced when administered with a lubricant laxative, which may necessitate vitamin supplements. When stool softeners are given concurrently, the absorption of mineral oil may be increased.

Adverse Effects

The potential adverse effects following mineral oil include anorexia, nausea, vomiting, and nutritional deficiencies. When mineral oil droplets are aspirated, lipid pneumonia can occur. Repeated rectal administration can cause anal irritation from leakage. Prolonged use of mineral oil may lead to bowel-elimination dependence.

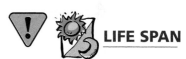 **LIFE SPAN**

Caution should be taken with mineral oil use in older and debilitated patients to avoid lipid pneumonia. Because of the decrease in fat-soluble absorption, mineral oil should be used cautiously during pregnancy.

What You DO

Nursing Responsibilities

When administering lubricant laxatives, the nurse should:

- Administer mineral oil after the evening meal and before bedtime to avoid the loss of fat-soluble vitamins. When mineral oil is administered in the evening, it should be given at least 2 hours after meals to avoid interference with digestion of food. Because aspiration of mineral oil appears to be greatest during sleep, it should be given well before bedtime to prevent aspiration and resultant lipid pneumonia.
- Administer mineral oil to older and debilitated patients after placement in an upright position.
- Warn patients who are taking mineral oil that excessive use (longer than 2 weeks) can decrease absorption of fat-soluble vitamins, such as vitamins A, D, E, and K, and may require supplemental vitamins.
- Advise patients who take repeated rectal enemas of mineral oil that anal leakage can cause pruritus and soiling.

LIFE SPAN

Instruct older and debilitated patients to maintain an upright position for at least 2 hours after administration.

Do You UNDERSTAND?

DIRECTIONS: Fill in the blanks with the appropriate response.

1. The action of a lubricant laxative involves _____ _____.

2. The best time to administer mineral oil is _____ _____.

3. The most serious adverse effect of mineral oil is _____ _____.

What IS a Hyperosmotic Laxative?

Hyperosmotic Laxatives	Trade Names	Uses
magnesium hydroxide glycerin [GLI-ser-in]	Milk of Magnesia Glycerol	Short-term treatment of occasional constipation Treatment of constipation
polyethylene glycol-electrolyte	GoLYTELY	Bowel evacuation solution
lactulose [LAK-tyoo-lose]	Cephulac, Chronulac	Treatment of chronic constipation and reduced ammonia

Action

Hyperosmotic laxatives are hypertonic drugs that draw water from surrounding tissues into the intestine, thereby creating an increased osmotic pressure in the bowel. The fluid moves from extracellular fluid compartments through the intestinal mucosa into the bowel. This additional fluid in the bowel changes stool consistency to liquid, which distends the bowel, stimulates stretch receptors, and stimulates peristalsis. As an osmotic agent, glycerin suppositories soften and lubricate feces and stimulate rectal contraction. Lactulose also promotes outward diffusion and elimination of ammonia in the feces, which promotes the reduction of blood ammonia levels. Lactulose also inhibits absorption of amines and acidifies bowel contents. Glycerin is not absorbed systemically. Lactulose is absorbed only slightly. Polyethylene glycol is nonabsorbable and does not alter electrolyte balance. Hyperosmotic laxatives that are absorbed include the magnesium preparations.

Uses

Hyperosmotic laxatives are used to treat constipation and cleanse the GI tract before surgery or examinations. Glycerin is used in bowel retraining to reestablish normal bowel function. Because of the increased transit time, hyperosmotic laxatives are used as an adjunct treatment for poisoning and to treat parasitic infestations. Lactulose is also used to reduce high blood ammonia levels that are associated with portal system encephalopathy.

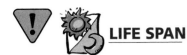

LIFE SPAN

- Glycerin is contraindicated for women during pregnancy and lactation and for children.
- Glycerin should be given cautiously to older and dehydrated patients.
- Glycerin should be given cautiously to patients with diabetes mellitus and cardiac, renal, or hepatic disease.

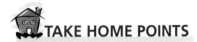

TAKE HOME POINTS

Polyethylene glycol is more palatable when given as a chilled solution. However, because of the large volume of a 4-liter dose, the patient should be monitored for hypothermia.

What You NEED TO KNOW

Contraindications/Precautions

Hyperosmotic laxatives are contraindicated for patients with nausea, vomiting, or undiagnosed abdominal pain. Magnesium preparations are contraindicated for patients with renal impairment. Sodium preparations are contraindicated for those who require sodium restriction (e.g., patients with edema and heart failure).

Drug Interactions

Hyperosmotic laxatives do not interact significantly with other concurrent drugs. Absorption of fluoroquinolones is decreased when given concurrently with magnesium preparations.

Adverse Effects

Adverse effects of glycerin include abdominal cramping, rectal irritation or burning, and hyperemia of rectal mucosa. Lactulose may cause nausea, vomiting, abdominal distention, flatulence, abdominal cramping, diarrhea, hypokalemia, hypovolemia, hyperglycemia, and increased hepatic encephalopathy. Adverse effects from hyperosmotic (**saline**) laxatives include weakness, lethargy, dehydration, hypernatremia, hypovolemia, hypermagnesemia, hyperphosphatemia, hypocalcemia, with resulting cardiac dysrhythmias and hypovolemic shock.

What You DO

Nursing Responsibilities

Oral hyperosmotic laxatives should not be given within 1 hour of other oral medications because the increased transit time of the laxatives will interfere with the absorption of other drugs. Glycerin is given via rectal suppository or enema when treating constipation. When administering hyperosmotic laxatives, the nurse should:

- Administer oral hyperosmotic laxatives with at least 8 ounces of water to prevent nausea.
- Administer polyethylene glycol electrolyte solutions orally over a 3-hour period; they may be administered at a rate of 240 mL every 10 minutes. This administration should begin approximately 4 to

5 hours before the examination or procedure. When the patient is unable to take the polyethylene glycol orally, it may be administered through a nasogastric tube at a rate of 20 to 30 mL per minute.

- Monitor the patient's hydration carefully because of the potential risk for fluid and electrolyte imbalances. Fluids should be replaced as necessary.
- Instruct the patient to avoid activities that require mental alertness when drowsiness, weakness, or lethargy occurs.
- Advise the patient with diabetes who is taking lactulose to be aware of signs of hyperglycemia, which include polydipsia, polyphagia, polyuria, weakness, and drowsiness.
- Dilute lactulose with water or unsweetened juice before administration to decrease the sweetness and prevent nausea.
- Instruct the patient who is taking hyperosmotic laxatives to drink 8 to 13 glasses of fluid per day, unless contraindicated.
- Monitor the patient for hypermagnesemia (e.g., weakness, confusion, sedation).

Do You UNDERSTAND?

DIRECTIONS: Complete the following statements with the appropriate terms from the italicized list provided.

1. The hyperosmotic laxative used primarily for GI cleansing before tests is _____.
2. _____ is absorbed more than any other hyperosmotic laxative.
3. The most common adverse effect of continued use of hyperosmotic laxatives is _____.

glycerin	*magnesium preparations*
GoLYTELY	*fluid overload*
lactulose	*electrolyte imbalance*

Answers: 1. GoLYTELY; 2. magnesium preparations; 3. electrolyte imbalance.

What IS a Stool Softener?

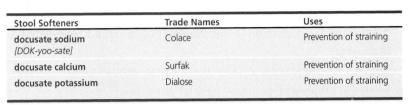

Stool Softeners	Trade Names	Uses
docusate sodium [DOK-yoo-sate]	Colace	Prevention of straining
docusate calcium	Surfak	Prevention of straining
docusate potassium	Dialose	Prevention of straining

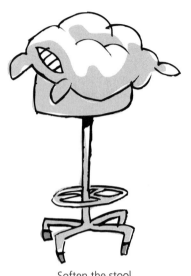

Soften the stool.

Action

Docusate stool softeners are surface-active agents that emulsify and wet the stool by permitting water to penetrate and soften the stool for easier passage. As a surface-active agent, the effect of docusate is local (in the jejunum and colon) rather than systemic. Docusate softens the stool only and does not act as a laxative.

Uses

Stool softeners are drugs that are given to soften the stool to help in elimination. Docusate is indicated for constipation, painful anorectal conditions, cardiac, and other conditions in which it is desirable to avoid straining and when laxatives are contraindicated.

What You NEED TO KNOW

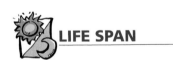

LIFE SPAN

Stool softeners are contraindicated during pregnancy.

Contraindications/Precautions

Stool softeners are contraindicated for patients with abdominal pain, fecal impaction, intestinal obstruction, and inflammatory GI disorders (e.g., ulcerative colitis, diverticulitis). Docusate sodium is contraindicated for patients who are on sodium restriction. Docusate potassium is contraindicated for patients who have renal dysfunction.

Drug Interactions

Docusate may increase the systemic absorption of mineral oil when given together.

Adverse Effects

Few adverse effects occur following stool softener administration. A bitter taste, nausea, and mild abdominal cramping are the most common, although diarrhea occurs infrequently.

What You DO

Nursing Responsibilities

Docusate is available in capsules, tablets, syrup, and liquid. The dose should be adjusted to individual response. Liquid or syrup forms may be mixed with mild juice or infant's formula. Capsules and tablets must be given whole and not chewed or crushed. When administering stool softeners, the nurse should:

- Instruct patient that capsules and tablets should be swallowed whole and not chewed or crushed.
- Instruct patient to take the oral dose with a full glass of water, unless contraindicated.
- Monitor stools because the effect of the drug may take up to 3 days.
- Avoid concurrent use of mineral oil with docusate because systemic absorption of mineral oil may be increased.

Do You UNDERSTAND?

DIRECTIONS: **Indicate in the space provided whether the statement is** *true* **or** *false*. **If the answer is false, correct the statement to make it true (using the margin space).**

_____ 1. Docusate acts by increasing bulk in the stool and increasing peristalsis.

_____ 2. The onset of action of docusate is 15 minutes when given orally.

_____ 3. Docusate may be indicated for the patient after rectal surgery.

_____ 4. Docusate tablets may be crushed and mixed with water to administer via a nasogastric tube.

What IS an Antiflatulent?

Antiflatulents	Trade Names	Uses
simethicone [sigh-METH-ih-cone]	Mylicon	Treatment of flatulence

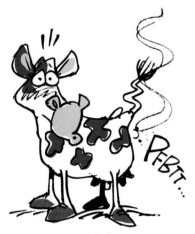

Get rid of gas.

Action

Simethicone changes the surface tension of gas bubbles in the stomach and intestines. The changed surface tension allows gas bubbles to stick together to form larger bubbles. The larger bubbles are easier than are smaller bubbles to pass via peristaltic movement and motility in the GI tract through the mouth by belching or through the anus as flatus.

Uses

Antiflatulents are drugs given to treat the discomfort of excessive gas in the GI tract. Gas is introduced into the body by (1) swallowing air, (2) bacterial action leading to gas as a byproduct, and (3) diffusion of gas from the blood stream into the GI tract. Most of the gas in the stomach

Answers: 1. false; docusate increases the amount of water that is mixed in the stool, thus making the stool softener and easier to pass; 2. false; the onset of oral docusate is 24 to 72 hours and 15 minutes when given as an enema. 3. true; 4. false; docusate capsules and tablets should not be crushed or chewed; liquid docusate may be used.

comes from swallowing air. Intestinal gas results primarily from bacterial action. An average of 7 to 10 liters of gas pass through the GI tract each day, most of which is reabsorbed. The use of simethicone is indicated for the symptoms of excess gas and discomfort particularly in patients who swallow air and cannot expel it or in postoperative patients with gaseous distention.

What You NEED TO KNOW

Contraindications/Precautions
No contraindications are listed.

Drug Interactions
No interactions are listed.

Adverse Effects
No adverse effects are listed.

What You DO

Nursing Responsibilities
Simethicone is given orally and is marketed under several different trade names, each with different amounts of the active ingredient. Some of the forms are combination drugs that may include an antacid or antidiarrheal medication. When administering antiflatulents, the nurse should:

- Mix the liquid forms of simethicone with water, infant formula, or other suitable liquids.
- Shake suspensions thoroughly before pouring.
- Teach the patient that tablets must be chewed thoroughly before swallowing. Gelatin caps should not be chewed.
- Assess bowel sounds for the presence of peristaltic activity, particularly in postsurgical patients before simethicone administration.
- Counsel the patient that activity (e.g., walking) will increase peristalsis.
- Instruct the patient that eating in an upright position and avoiding gas-producing foods or carbonated beverages may help decrease the swallowing of air and encourage gas movement through the GI tract.

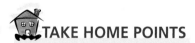

TAKE HOME POINTS

Teach patient that chewable tablets must be chewed and that suspensions should be thoroughly shaken before pouring.

Do You UNDERSTAND?

DIRECTIONS: **Indicate in the space provided whether the statement is** *true* **or** *false*. **If the answer is false, correct the statement to make it true (using the margin space).**

_____ 1. Simethicone liquid may be mixed with water, infant formula, or other liquids before administration.

_____ 2. Antiflatulents break up bubbles into smaller bubbles that can be expelled.

_____ 3. Simethicone tablets must be chewed before swallowing.

_____ 4. Simethicone suspension must be thoroughly shaken before pouring.

_____ 5. Adverse effects of simethicone include diarrhea.

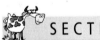

SECTION C

ANTIDIARRHEALS

Antidiarrheals are used to treat diarrhea, as well as nausea and vomiting. These drugs include absorbents and opioid or opioid-derivative agents.

What IS an Absorbent Antidiarrheal?

Absorbent Antidiarrheals	Trade Names	Uses
bismuth subsalicylate [BIS-muth sub-sal-IH-sah-late]	Pepto-Bismol	Prevention and treatment of traveler's diarrhea
kaolin-pectin [KAY-oh-lyn peck-tin]	Kaopectate	Prevention of diarrhea

Action

Absorbent antidiarrheals act by coating the GI mucosa, which absorbs water and toxic substances that cause diarrhea. Bismuth subsalicylate has two additional actions: (1) an added antiinflammatory action that is believed to decrease motility and the secretion of fluid and mucus into the colon by decreasing prostaglandin production and (2) an antimicrobial effect. The absorbent antidiarrheals have a local action with little or none being absorbed systemically, except bismuth subsalicylate, which is absorbed systemically.

Uses

Antidiarrheals are used for diarrhea, a common GI symptom characterized by frequent, watery stools. Diarrhea results from rapid transit of fecal material through the intestines and increased fluid in the stool. Causes of diarrhea include bacterial or viral enteritis, ulcerative colitis, psychogenic diarrhea, overuse of laxatives, Crohn's disease, irritable bowel disease, superinfections, bowel radiation, dietary intolerance, enteral feedings, and short-gut syndrome. Enteritis is the most frequent cause of diarrhea and can lead to fluid loss, dehydration, and electrolyte imbalance.

Absorbents are indicated for the adjunct treatment of diarrhea, in addition to identifying and eliminating the cause of the diarrhea. Bismuth subsalicylate may also be used in combination with antibiotics to treat ulcer disease caused by *Helicobacter pylori*. Indications for use of polycarbophil in diarrhea include patients with acute bowel syndrome, diverticulosis, irritable bowel, diarrhea caused by cholera, or following small-bowel surgery in which diarrhea may be a problem.

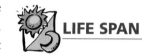 **LIFE SPAN**

Bismuth subsalicylate is contraindicated for pregnant and lactating women. Because bismuth subsalicylate contains salicylate, it is contraindicated for children and adolescents who have or are recovering from viral infections (because of the danger of Reye's syndrome) or in patients with an allergy to aspirin or other salicylates.

What You NEED TO KNOW

Contraindications/Precautions

Use bismuth subsalicylate with caution in patients who are taking anticoagulant, diabetic, or gout medications. Cautious use of all antidiarrheals is indicated when diarrhea continues more than 2 days despite treatment or when a high fever is present with diarrhea.

Drug Interactions

Bismuth subsalicylate may decrease absorption when taken together with tetracyclines and quinolones. Serum salicylate levels are increased when taken with aspirin. Bismuth subsalicylate may increase the risk for

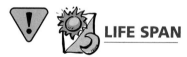 **LIFE SPAN**

- The use of bismuth should be made cautiously in children under 3 years of age.
- Use bismuth subsalicylate with caution in patients who are taking anticoagulant, diabetic, or gout medications. Cautious use of all antidiarrheals is indicated when diarrhea continues longer than 2 days despite treatment or when a high fever is present with diarrhea.

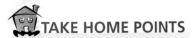

TAKE HOME POINTS

When diarrhea persists longer than 2 days, the health care provider should be consulted. Bismuth may interfere with radiographic examinations of the GI tract because bismuth is radiopaque.

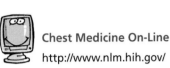

Chest Medicine On-Line
http://www.nlm.hih.gov/
medlineplus/pepticulcer.html
http://niddk.nih.gov/health/digest/
pubs/hpylori/hpylori.htm#7
http://www.mayohealth.org/
mayo/9909/htm/peptic.htm
http://pharminfo.com/pubs/msb/
tritec.html

bleeding when taken with heparin, warfarin, and thrombolytics. Kaolin-pectin may decrease absorption when given concurrently with oral medications.

Adverse Effects

Adverse effects are rare and mild, with abdominal fullness, diarrhea, and vomiting being the most common. Bismuth may cause temporary darkening of the stool.

What You DO

Nursing Responsibilities

Onset of action for the absorbent antidiarrheal agents varies but is generally approximately 1 day. Bismuth may be used prophylactically to prevent traveler's diarrhea in patients who are traveling to areas with poor sanitation. However, prophylactic use should be limited to 3 weeks. When administering absorbent antidiarrheals, the nurse should:

- Administer absorbent antidiarrheal agents at least 2 hours before or after other oral drugs.
- Instruct the patient to avoid using antidiarrheals for longer than 2 days or in the presence of high fever.
- Encourage fluid intake when taking absorbents to prevent dehydration.
- Monitor and record the number and consistency of stools, intake and output, and bowel sounds. Bismuth may cause temporary darkening of stools and mouth. However, darkened stools should not be confused with melena.
- Teach the patient to shake bismuth suspensions thoroughly before administration.
- Inform the patient to chew tablets or dissolve in the mouth before swallowing. Caplets should be swallowed whole. Regular- and extra-strength attapulgite tablets must be swallowed whole. Polycarbophil tablets should be crushed or chewed before swallowing. Mix with fruit juice or chocolate powder to improve the taste.
- Instruct the patient to avoid OTC medications unless directed by the health care provider because many OTC medications contain subsalicylates and may increase salicylate levels.
- Encourage the patient to avoid fried foods and milk products until diarrhea is resolved.

Do You UNDERSTAND?

DIRECTIONS: Match each description in Column A with the correct drug in Column B. You may use an answer more than once.

Column A	Column B
_____ 1. A GI absorbent that is similar to kaolin and pectin combinations	a. Kaopectate
	b. Bismuth (Pepto-Bismol)
_____ 2. Contains subsalicylate	c. Activated charcoal
_____ 3. Is frequently used in combination with other drugs to treat *Helicobacter pylori* infection.	
_____ 4. An absorbent that is most commonly used in poisonings.	

What IS an Opioid and Opioid-Derivative Antidiarrheal?

Opioid and Opioid-Derivative Antidiarrheals	Trade Names	Uses
paregoric (opium tincture) [par-ih-GOR-ik]	Paregoric	Short-term treatment of diarrhea
diphenoxylate with atropine [dye-fen-OX-ih-late]	Lomotil	Treatment of diarrhea
loperamide [low-PER-a-mide]	Imodium	Treatment of diarrhea

Action

Opioid and opioid-derivative antidiarrheals are systemic drugs that decrease GI motility, prolong transit time, decrease fluid secretion into the bowel, and allow fluid and electrolytes to be reabsorbed because of the increased time that the stool remains in the colon. Most of the opioid

Answers: 1. a.; 2. b.; 3. b.; 4. c.

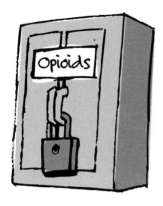

and opioid-derivative antidiarrheals are rapidly and thoroughly absorbed after oral administration, except tincture of opium and loperamide hydrochloride, which have variable absorption. Peak plasma levels occur within 40 minutes to 5 hours, depending on the drug.

Uses

Opioid and opioid-derivative antidiarrheals are the mainstay of treatment for moderate to severe diarrhea. Indications for use include acute diarrhea, acute exacerbations of chronic diarrhea, and for reduction of fecal volume from ileostomies.

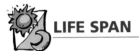

LIFE SPAN

Opioid and opioid-derivative antidiarrheals are contraindicated for children under 2 years of age.

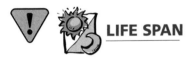

LIFE SPAN

- Caution should be used in women during pregnancy and lactation.
- Caution should be used in patients with prostatic hypertrophy, narrow-angle glaucoma, and liver disease.

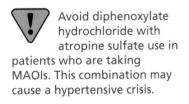

Avoid diphenoxylate hydrochloride with atropine sulfate use in patients who are taking MAOIs. This combination may cause a hypertensive crisis.

What You NEED TO KNOW

Contraindications/Precautions

Contraindications for all types of opioid antidiarrheals are a known sensitivity to the drug, obstructive jaundice, diarrhea in pseudomembranous colitis, and diarrhea associated with microorganisms that penetrate intestinal mucosa, such as *Escherichia coli*, *Salmonella*, or *Shigella*; chronic ulcerative colitis; and acute dysentery.

Drug Interactions

When diphenoxylate is given together with MAOIs, hypertensive crisis may occur. Diphenoxylate may increase the effects of barbiturates, tranquilizers, narcotics, and alcohol when taken together with these drug classifications.

Adverse Effects

Adverse effects of the opioids include nausea, vomiting, dry mouth, dizziness, drowsiness, and headache. Overdosing effects include CNS depression, dryness of the skin and mucous membranes, nystagmus, pinpoint pupils, and respiratory depression. Respiratory depression may not be apparent initially but may occur up to 30 hours after overdose. Nearly all of the opioid and opioid derivatives are controlled substances, with the exception of loperamide. Camphorated opium tincture and tincture of opium remain available for clinical use but are not recommended and are less commonly used than are the synthetic opium derivatives.

What You DO

Nursing Responsibilities

The response to opioid antidiarrheals should be noticeable 48 hours after treatment begins. Opioid antidiarrheal agents are not innocuous drugs and are not intended for prolonged use. When administering opioid antidiarrheals, the nurse should:

- Instruct the patient to reduce the dose after initial control of diarrhea. When no response is apparent, these agents will likely be ineffective and should be discontinued.
- Monitor the patient's vital signs because opiates cause CNS depression.
- Warn patients to follow dose recommendations and to avoid exceeding the maximal daily dose.
- Inform patient that drowsiness may be an adverse effect and that hazardous activities should be avoided.
- Monitor and record the patient's intake and output, number and consistency of stools, and bowel sounds.
- Instruct patient to notify the health care provider when a high fever develops, diarrhea persists, or when blood is noted in the stool.
- Warn the patient to avoid exceeding the recommended daily dose.
- Inform patients that diphenoxylate hydrochloride with atropine sulfate tablet may be crushed.
- Monitor patient with ulcerative colitis for abdominal distention and other GI symptoms, which may indicate toxic megacolon.
- Avoid confusing the two preparations of opium. Deodorized opium tincture contains 25 times more anhydrous morphine than does camphorated opium tincture. Similar to large doses of any narcotic, the respiratory depressant effects of an overdose may last longer than does an antagonist that is given to reverse effects.
- Monitor the patient for respiratory depression!

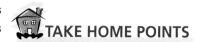

TAKE HOME POINTS

Opioid antidiarrheal agents, with the exception of loperamide, are controlled substances and may have abuse potential that leads to dependence.

Do You UNDERSTAND?

DIRECTIONS: Fill in the blanks with the appropriate response.

1. _____ and
   _____ cross the
   placenta, causing an effect on the fetus.

2. Some of the adverse effects of diphenoxylate HCl (Lomotil) and
   difenoxin (Motofen) are a result of the addition of _____
   _____ sulfate to discourage abuse.

3. Opioid antidiarrheals _____ GI motility and
   _____ water reabsorption in the colon.

4. Adverse effects of opioid antidiarrheals include _____
   _____.

5. Opioid antidiarrheals should be discontinued after _____
   _____ when no improvement in diarrhea is noted.

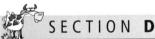

SECTION **D**

HYPERACIDITY AGENTS

This section reviews the pharmacologic preparations used to treat hyperacidity, heartburn, duodenal ulcers, gastric-esophageal reflux disease, and
pathologic hypersecretion of acid. This section discusses nonsystemic
antacids, histamine H_2-antagonists, proton pump inhibitors, mucosal
protectants, and prostaglandins.

What IS a Nonsystemic Antacid?

Nonsystemic Antacids	Trade Names	Uses
aluminum hydroxide	Amphojel	Treatment of hyperacidity
calcium carbonate	Tums, OsCal	Treatment of hyperacidity
magaldrate [MAG-al-drate]	Riopan	Treatment of hyperacidity

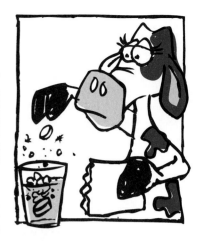

Action

Antacids are alkaline drugs that directly neutralize hydrochloric acid that the stomach secretes. Antacids reduce the corrosive effect of hydrochloric acid on GI mucosa; thus they have a protective and restorative effect. Because the absorption is minimal, the residue of salts from the chemical neutralization of acid is subjected to the normal digestive process. Nonsystemic antacids are eliminated in GI tract via feces.

Uses

Antacids are used to treat peptic ulcers and gastric hyperacidity. Examples of hyperacidity include heartburn, acid indigestion, and gastroesophageal reflux disease (GERD).

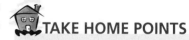**TAKE HOME POINTS**

Antacids neutralize hydrochloric acid through direct chemical reaction in the midportion of the stomach and provide a demulcent or soothing effect on GI mucosa.

What You NEED TO KNOW

Contraindications/Precautions

Antacids are contraindicated for patients with any known allergy to any antacid component.

Drug Interactions

When antacids are taken with enteric-coated medications, antacids tend to disintegrate the coating and release the drug prematurely in the stomach. When antacids are taken with tetracycline and fluoroquinolone antibiotics, both drugs combine chemically and decrease absorption. This activity may indicate a needed change in dose requirements of tetracycline. Calcium and magnesium preparations exacerbate the action of digitalis, which also may require dose adjustments.

Caution should be used when administering antacids to patients who are pregnant or lactating and with any conditions that may be exacerbated by electrolyte or acid-base imbalance, GI obstruction, or renal dysfunction.

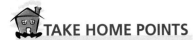

Adverse Effects

The most common adverse effects of antacids are associated with acid-base and electrolyte levels. Rebound acidity is a major concern with antacid administration. When the antacid changes the stomach contents to an alkaline environment, the stomach produces additional acid in response.

Systemic alkaline absorption (particularly aluminum) may result in encephalopathy. With systemic absorption of antacids, severe electrolyte disorders may occur. Some adverse effects of antacids may vary with the preparation that has been administered. Aluminum forms of antacids may cause constipation, delayed gastric emptying, and hypophosphatemia. Calcium forms of antacids may cause constipation, hypercalcemia, milk-alkali syndrome or severe alkalosis, and renal calculi. Magnesium preparations may lead to diarrhea, with resultant hypokalemia, iron deficiency, and hypermagnesemia. The adverse effects of hypermagnesemia following magnesium antacid administration include drowsiness, weakness, and cardiac dysrhythmias, all of which occur more frequently in patients with renal impairment. Sodium antacid preparations may cause a reduction of iron absorption and water retention.

What You DO

Nursing Responsibilities

Antacids are administered orally for their acid-neutralizing capacity (ANC) in liquid or chewable tablet form. The onset of drug action is within 5 to 15 minutes, and the duration is usually 2 hours. When giving antacids, the nurse should:

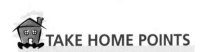

- Administer antacids at least 1 hour before or 2 hours after any other oral drugs to ensure adequate absorption.
- Monitor electrolytes of the patient who is taking antacids for early detection of an electrolyte imbalance.
- Instruct the patient to chew antacid tablets thoroughly and follow with one glass of water to ensure that the medication reaches the stomach for direct action and to avoid the development of intestinal concretions calculi.
- Inform patients that antacids should be stored in a tightly closed container at 15° to 30° C (59° to 86° F).

- Tell the patient to report any shortness of breath, chest pain, darkened or tarry stools, sweating, or recurrent symptoms to the health care provider.
- Teach patients about acid rebound and that repeated use for 1 to 2 weeks might cause a rebound acid stimulation action, quickly leading to the development of a chronic antacid user.
- Inform the patient that antacids should be used for short-term relief only. If symptoms continue, the patient should seek the help of a health care provider.
- Instruct the patient that aluminum antacids may interfere with phosphate metabolism by binding to dietary phosphates causing hypophosphatemia.
- Teach the patient that large quantities of antacids over a prolonged period or a diet that is low in phosphorus (while taking antacids continuously) may develop hypophosphatemia within 2 weeks.

Do You UNDERSTAND?

DIRECTIONS: Fill in the blanks with the appropriate responses to complete the following statements.

1. _____ is a concurrent drug that is administered with antacids that poses a risk for decreased absorption.
2. Two of the most common adverse effects of antacids include _____ and _____.
3. _____ is the substance that antacids neutralize in the stomach.
4. List five conditions that antacids treat: _____, _____, _____, _____, and _____.
5. _____ and _____ are the acceptable timeframes during which an antacid may be administered before and after another drug to avoid absorption interference.

What IS a Histamine H$_2$-Antagonist?

Histamine H$_2$-Antagonists	Trade Names	Uses
cimetidine [sigh-MET-ih-deen]	Tagamet	Treatment of duodenal ulcers, GERD, and pathologic hypersecretion
ranitidine [ran-EYE-tih-deen]	Zantac	Treatment of duodenal ulcers, GERD, and pathologic hypersecretion
famotidine [fuh-MOE-tih-deen]	Pepcid	Treatment of duodenal ulcers, GERD, and pathologic hypersecretion
nizatidine [nigh-ZAT-ih-deen]	Axid	Treatment of duodenal ulcers, GERD, and prevention of heartburn

Action

Histamine H$_2$-antagonists directly block H$_2$-receptors sites to decrease acid production. This classification of GI agents selectively blocks histamine H$_2$-receptors, which are located on the gastric parietal cells. The blockage of histamine receptors prevents gastrin secretion. Because gastrin is responsible for local release of histamine, stimulation of hydrochloric acid and pepsin production is decreased.

Uses

This drug classification is used in the treatment of active gastric or duodenal ulcer maintenance therapy. Stress reduces the production of protective mucus. Histamine H$_2$-antagonists reduce the overall acid level, thereby alleviating discomfort and promoting healing. These agents are also used in the treatment of hypersecretory conditions, such as Zollinger-Ellison syndrome. By blocking the overproduction of hydrochloric acid, the condition is relieved. Histamine H$_2$-antagonists alleviate the discomfort of heartburn, acid indigestion, and GERD. These drugs are also used prophylactically to prevent stress-induced ulcers and acute upper GI bleeding.

What You NEED TO KNOW

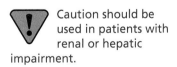 Caution should be used in patients with renal or hepatic impairment.

Contraindications/Precautions

Cimetidine is contraindicated for women who are pregnant and lactating, for children, and for patients with a known allergy and hepatic dysfunction.

Drug Interactions

When histamine H_2-antagonists are taken concurrently with warfarin, phenytoin, β-adrenergic blockers, quinidine, theophylline, chloroquine, benzodiazepines, nifedipine, pentoxifylline, tricyclic antidepressants, procainamide, triamterene, carbamazepine, and alcohol, metabolism is slowed and toxic serum levels may be reached. Nizatidine increases the serum levels of aspirin. Cimetidine may decrease the absorption of iron, tetracyclines, and lidocaine. When administered concurrently with morphine, cimetidine has been known to cause apnea. Antacids decrease the absorption of histamine H_2-antagonists.

Adverse Effects

The most common adverse effects of histamine H_2-antagonists include diarrhea, constipation, blurred vision, headaches, dizziness, fatigue, somnolence, confusion, hallucinations, bradycardia, hypotension, and dysrhythmias. Additional adverse effects that are related to histamine H_2-antagonists include musculoskeletal pain, arthralgia, myalgia, rash, allergic reaction, gynecomastia, breast tenderness, renal impairment, bone marrow depression, and leukocytosis. Famotidine may cause flushing, palpitations, hypertension, and tinnitus. Ranitidine has been known to cause vomiting and abdominal discomfort. Cimetidine may cause reversible impotence. Nizatidine may lead to hyperuricemia and hepatic damage.

What You DO

Nursing Responsibilities

Histamine H_2-antagonists may be administered orally. All but nizatidine are available for intravenous (IV) use. When administering histamine H_2-antagonists, the nurse should:

- Administer oral drug preparations before or with meals and at bedtime to ensure adequate protection when needed.
- Monitor renal and hepatic function tests for early detection of any organ damage.
- Monitor drug levels for potential drug interaction with concurrent administration of histamine H_2-antagonists that might lead to drug toxicity.

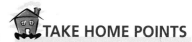

TAKE HOME POINTS

Nizatidine is the only histamine H_2-antagonist that is unavailable in an IV form.

- Teach the patient about the medication to enhance compliance.
- Monitor the patient for cardiac dysrhythmias when given by continuous IV therapy.

Do You UNDERSTAND?

DIRECTIONS: **Select from the italicized choices to indicate the concern when the following drugs are given concurrently with histamine H$_2$-antagonists.**

1. Tetracyclines: _____
   (increased or decreased absorption)
2. Alcohol: _____
   (increased metabolism or increased toxic serum levels)
3. Theophylline: _____
   (increased metabolism or increased toxic serum levels)
4. Antacids: _____
   (increased or decreased absorption)
5. Nifedipine: _____
   (increased metabolism or increased toxic serum levels)

What IS a Proton Pump Inhibitor?

Proton Pump Inhibitors	Trade Names	Uses
omeprazole [oh-MEH- pray-zole]	Prilosec	Treatment of duodenal ulcers, GERD, and pathologic hypersecretion
lansoprazole [lan-SO- pray-zole]	Prevacid	Treatment of duodenal ulcers, esophagitis, and pathologic hypersecretion
pantoprazole [pan-TOW-pray-zole]	Protonix	Treatment of GERD, erosive esophagitis, duodenal ulcers due to *H. pylori*
esomeprazole [es-oh-MEH-pray-zole]	Nexium	Treatment of GERD, erosive esophagitis, duodenal ulcers due to *H. pylori*

Answers: 1. decreased absorption; 2. increased serum levels; 3. increased serum levels; 4. decreased absorption; 5. increased serum levels.

Action

Proton pump inhibitors (**antisecretory agents**) act directly on the secretory surface of the gastric parietal cells at the final step of acid production to decrease acid levels in the stomach. These agents inhibit the hydrogen-potassium-ATPase gastric enzyme system, which catalyzes the final step. Proton pump inhibitors are absorbed rapidly when given orally. Their antisecretory effects last up to 72 hours.

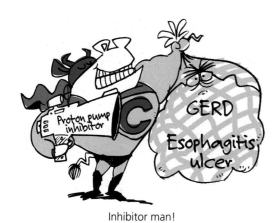

Inhibitor man!

Uses

Proton pump inhibitors are used in the treatment of esophagitis, GERD, peptic ulcers, duodenal ulcers, Zollinger-Ellison syndrome, and other hypersecretory syndromes.

What You NEED TO KNOW

Contraindications/Precautions

Proton pump inhibitors are contraindicated for patients with a known allergy to the medication.

Drug Interactions

The absorption of concurrent drugs may be decreased because of the alteration of gastric pH by proton pump inhibitors, such as iron, digoxin,

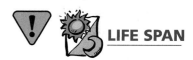 **LIFE SPAN**

Proton pump inhibitors should be given with caution to patients who are pregnant or lactating.

 Caution should be used when giving proton pump inhibitors to patients with hepatic impairment because dose adjustments may be required.

ampicillin, and ketoconazole. Omeprazole inhibits the metabolism and increases the drug level of diazepam, phenytoin, and warfarin, requiring dose adjustments for efficacy.

Adverse Effects

The incidence of adverse effects after administering proton pump inhibitors is low, and those that occur are relatively mild. Common adverse effects from proton pump inhibitors include headache, dizziness, cough, stuffy nose, hoarseness, and epistaxis. Other reported adverse effects include dry mouth, nausea, vomiting, flatulence, diarrhea, constipation, abdominal pain, weakness, vertigo, dream abnormalities, and insomnia. Adverse effects that are less common include rash, dry skin, fever, alopecia, and back pain.

What You DO

Nursing Responsibilities

Pantoprazole and esomeprazole are effective with convenient once-a-day dosing. When administering proton pump inhibitors, the nurse should:

- Instruct the patient to avoid opening, chewing, or crushing capsules. These medications should be swallowed whole for therapeutic effect.
- Teach the patient to take a proton pump inhibitor 30 minutes before meals.
- Encourage the patient to avoid alcohol consumption and smoking because alcohol can increase gastric irritation.
- Instruct the patient to return for follow-up medical treatment when the symptoms are unresolved after 4 to 8 weeks of therapy.

The patient should avoid opening, chewing, or crushing proton pump inhibitor capsules.

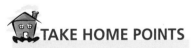

TAKE HOME POINTS

Proton pump inhibitors should be administered before meals to ensure drug efficacy.

Do You UNDERSTAND?

DIRECTIONS: Fill in the blanks with the appropriate response.

1. Is the incidence of adverse effects following proton pump inhibitors high or low? _____

2. List six common adverse effects of proton pump inhibitors:
   _____, _____,
   _____, _____,
   _____, and _____.

3. List four conditions that proton pump inhibitors are used to treat.
   _____
   _____

4. Which time of day is best to administer proton pump inhibitors for better efficacy? _____

5. What instructions regarding ingestion of proton pump inhibitor capsules should the nurse teach the patient? _____
   _____

What IS a Mucosal Protectant?

Mucosal Protectant	Trade Name	Use
sucralfate [soo-CRAWL-fate]	Carafate	Treatment of duodenal ulcer

Action

Mucosal protectants (**cytoprotective agents**) react with gastric acid and proteins at the ulcer site to form a thick paste that covers and sticks to the ulcer site. The paste helps protect the ulcer from gastric acid, pepsin, and bile; its action is local rather than systemic. Sucralfate contains an aluminum complex. The small amount that is absorbed through the GI tract is excreted in the urine of patients with normal kidney function. Ninety percent of the paste is excreted in the feces.

Answers: 1. low; 2. headache, dizziness, cough, stuffy nose, hoarseness, epistaxis; 3. esophagitis, GERD, peptic or duodenal ulcers, Zollinger-Ellison syndrome; 4. before meals; 5. avoid opening, chewing, or crushing capsules; rather, swallow them whole.

Uses

Mucosal protectants are drugs that are given to protect the wall of the GI tract from ulceration or injury from excess acid (**hyperacidity**). Sucralfate is given to prevent or treat ulcer disease and is used for short-term treatment (up to 8 weeks) of duodenal and gastric ulcers.

What You NEED TO KNOW

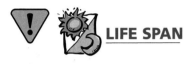

LIFE SPAN

- Sucralfate should be used with caution in patients with chronic kidney failure or those on dialysis.
- Sucralfate should be used with caution in women who are pregnant and nursing and in children.

Contraindications/Precautions

Aluminum blood levels may be extremely elevated because aluminum is not removed via the impaired kidneys or dialysis of patients who may be receiving other drugs with aluminum (e.g., antacids).

Drug Interactions

Sucralfate may decrease the absorption and action of tetracyclines, fluoroquinolones, phenytoin, digoxin, and fat-soluble vitamins.

Adverse Effects

The most commonly reported adverse effect following mucosal protectant administration is constipation. Less frequent side effects include dizziness, drowsiness, dry mouth, nausea, gastric discomfort, and diarrhea.

What You DO

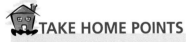

TAKE HOME POINTS

Administer sucralfate 1 hour before meals and at bedtime.

Nursing Responsibilities

Sucralfate is given orally in either tablet or suspension form. When administering mucosal protectants, the nurse should:

- Administer sucralfate on an empty stomach (1 hour before meals or 2 hours after meals and at bed time). Schedule medication administration times to avoid giving sucralfate with other oral medications. Give other oral medications 2 hours before sucralfate.
- Administer other oral medications 2 hours before giving sucralfate to prevent drug interactions. Because sucralfate provides a protective barrier to the GI mucosa, administration with other oral medications

may interfere with absorption and decrease the action of the other drugs.

- Consult the pharmacist to obtain the correct diluent to prevent clogging of the tube when giving sucralfate through a nasogastric tube. Mucosal protectant therapy should continue for 4 to 8 weeks, even when symptoms of the ulcer disappear, unless healing can be confirmed by endoscopy or x-ray film.
- Advise the patient to avoid smoking and spicy foods that might aggravate the ulcer.
- Monitor patients with chronic renal failure for increasing signs and symptoms of aluminum toxicity, such as acute dementia, osteomalacia, and bone pain, with or without fractures.
- Administer antacids 30 minutes before or after sucralfate.
- Instruct the patient that frequent mouth care should be performed to maintain healthy mucous membranes.

Do You UNDERSTAND?

DIRECTIONS: **Indicate in the space provided whether the statement is** *true* **or** *false.* **If the answer is false, correct the statement to make it true (using the margin space).**

_____ 1. Sucralfate forms a thick coating that sticks to the ulcer, thereby protecting the mucosa.

_____ 2. Sucralfate can be administered either orally or IV.

_____ 3. Sucralfate can be given with oral antibiotics.

_____ 4. Administration of sucralfate and other oral medications together may reduce the bioavailability of the medications.

_____ 5. The most common side effects of nausea and vomiting occur in approximately 50% of patients who are taking sucralfate.

What IS a Prostaglandin?

Prostaglandin	Trade Name	Use
misoprostol [MY-so-PRAHST-ole]	Cytotec	Prevention of gastric ulcers

Action

Misoprostol is a synthetic prostaglandin E1 that decreases gastric acid secretion and helps protect the GI mucosa. Misoprostol may be used in patients who are taking nonsteroidal antiinflammatory drugs (NSAIDs), including aspirin, and in those who are at risk for NSAID-induced gastric ulcers. NSAIDs inhibit prostaglandin production, which leads to a decrease in bicarbonate and mucus production. The decrease in bicarbonate and mucus increases the risk for gastric mucosal injury from the NSAIDs. In contrast, misoprostol increases bicarbonate and mucus production, thereby having a protectant effect. Misoprostol also produces uterine contractions.

Uses

Misoprostol is used to prevent NSAID-induced gastric ulcers in patients who are at a high risk for developing ulcers, such as patients with a history of gastric ulcers. The drug is usually used concurrently, as long as the patient is on NSAID therapy. The unlabeled use involves preventing and treating duodenal ulcers.

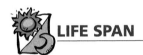

LIFE SPAN

- Misoprostol is used to prevent NSAID-induced gastric ulcers in older adults.
- Misoprostol is contraindicated during pregnancy because partial or complete abortion and uterine bleeding may result. Misoprostol is also contraindicated for nursing mothers and for children.

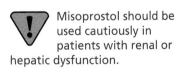

Misoprostol should be used cautiously in patients with renal or hepatic dysfunction.

What You NEED TO KNOW

Contraindications/Precautions

Misoprostol is contraindicated for patients with hypersensitivity to prostaglandins.

Drug Interactions

Antacids may reduce the action of misoprostol.

Adverse Effects

The most common adverse effects are diarrhea and abdominal pain. Diarrhea is usually dose-related, mild, and self-limiting (resolving in approximately 8 days). Other adverse effects include nausea, vomiting, constipation, dysmenorrheal, and hypermenorrhea.

Advise the patient with childbearing potential to avoid pregnancy and to use an effective contraceptive method. When pregnancy occurs, discontinue the therapy and contact the health care provider immediately.

What You DO

Nursing Responsibilities

Misoprostol is an oral medication. No dose reduction is routinely suggested for patients with renal impairment or for older patients, unless the dose is not tolerated. When administering prostaglandins, the nurse should:

- Arrange for a pregnancy test 2 weeks prior to initiating treatment with misoprostol.
- Encourage the patient to use barrier contraceptives during therapy for the prevention of pregnancy.
- Monitor for GI distress, the number and consistency of stools, and signs and symptoms of dehydration.
- Administer misoprostol at mealtime and at bedtime with food to prevent GI discomfort and medication-induced diarrhea.
- Avoid administering misoprostol with magnesium-containing antacids, which may increase the incidence and severity of diarrhea.

Do You UNDERSTAND?

DIRECTIONS: Fill in the blanks with the appropriate response.

1. Misoprostol is indicated for the prevention of _____ _____ ulcers.
2. Misoprostol prevents ulcers by _____.
3. High-risk patients who are using _____ may be candidates for concurrent use of misoprostol.
4. The most common side effect of misoprostol is _____.
5. Misoprostol is contraindicated for use in patients who are _____.

SECTION E

DIGESTIVE ENZYMES AND INTESTINAL FLORA MODIFIERS

This section reviews the pharmacologic preparations used to treat disorders of digestion and explains digestive enzymes and intestinal flora modifiers.

What IS an Acidifier-Digestive Enzyme?

Acidifier-Digestive Enzymes	Trade Names	Uses
pancreatin [pan-kree-AH-tin]	Pancreatin	Replacement therapy for malabsorption syndrome
pancrelipase [pan-kree-LIE-pace]	Pancrease	Replacement therapy for malabsorption syndrome

Action

The action of pancreatic enzymes aids in the digestion of carbohydrate (CHO), fat, and proteins. The pancreas produces four digestive enzymes: lipase, amylase, trypsin, and chymotrypsin.

Pancrelipase is made from hog-porcine protein and is the preferred preparation because its enzyme activity is far greater than that of pancreatin. For example, the pancrelipase lipolytic enzyme activity is 12 times greater than that of pancreatin. Pancrelipase trypsin and amylase enzyme activities are four times greater than that of pancreatin. Enteric-coated preparations are preferred over conventional powders or tablets. Gastric pepsin and acid in the stomach may destroy conventional tablets. Enteric-coated preparations have an increased likelihood of dissolving in the duodenum, where pancreatic enzyme action is needed and most effective.

Uses

Pancreatic enzymes are used as replacement therapy when the body is producing and secreting insufficient amounts of pancreatic enzymes. Causes of deficiencies include disorders of the pancreas, such as pancreatitis, pancreatectomy, obstruction of the pancreatic duct, and cystic fibrosis.

What You NEED TO KNOW

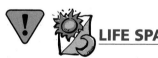 LIFE SPAN

Contraindications/Precautions

Pancrelipase is contraindicated for patients with acute pancreatitis.

Drug Interactions

The activity of pancreatic enzymes is decreased when given with H_2-blockers and calcium and magnesium antacids. Pancreatic enzymes decrease the absorption of iron when given concurrently.

Adverse Effects

Adverse effects of pancreatic enzymes that can occur with high doses include anorexia, ulcerative stomatitis, nausea, cramping, vomiting, diarrhea, and perianal irritation. Hyperuricemia and hyperuricosuria may also develop with high doses because of increased serum uric acid.

- Cautious use of pancreatic enzymes is advised for persons with an allergy to hog protein or enzymes.
- Caution should be used with pancreatic enzymes during pregnancy and lactation.

What You DO

Nursing Responsibilities

The dose of pancreatic enzyme is individualized and adjusted based on the degree of enzyme deficiency and the enzyme preparation that is selected. Pancreatic enzymes can be taken orally with meals. The amount of fat content in the diet determines the dose. Comparing fat intake with the amount of fat excreted in a 24-hour period indicates the effectiveness of treatment. When administering acidifiers, the nurse should:

- Educate patients on the proper use of pancreatic enzymes.
- Caution patients to swallow the medication whole and avoid crushing or chewing enteric-coated preparations. Stomach acid or gastric pepsin may destroy pancreatic enzymes; thus an antacid or histamine-receptor blocker may be given before the enzyme to reduce gastric pH and protect the pancreatic enzyme from inactivation.
- Instruct the patient to follow pancreatic enzymes with a glass of water to ensure complete effectiveness.
- Counsel the patient to monitor weight loss and weight gain, intake and output, and quality of stools. Fatty stools indicate insufficiency of pancreatic enzyme. Adequate replacement decreases the number of bowel movements and improves stool consistency.
- Store pancreatic enzyme medication away from heat and light to protect the medication.
- Instruct patients to avoid changing brands without approval from their health care provider.

> ⚠ Instruct patients to avoid crushing or chewing enteric-coated preparations of pancreatic enzymes.

Do You UNDERSTAND?

DIRECTIONS: Fill in the blanks with the appropriate response.

1. Instruct patients that enteric-coated preparations are not to be

   _____.

2. _____

   may be given before the enzyme to reduce gastric acid pH.

3. _____ indicate

   insufficiency of pancreatic enzyme.

Answers: 1. crushed or chewed; 2. Antacid or histamine-receptor blockers; 3. Fatty stools.

What IS an Intestinal Flora Modifier?

Intestinal Flora Modifier	Trade Names	Uses
Lactobacillus acidophilus [LACK-tol-bah-SILL-us AS-id-off-ill-us]	*Acidophilus Lactobacillus* Lactinex	Prevention and treatment of superinfections

Action

Intestinal flora modifiers are bacterial cultures that contain *lactobacillus acidophilus* or *lactobacillus bulgaricus*. These agents are given to help augment or to replace the usual normal flora and to reestablish intestinal flora balance.

Numerous bacteria are normally present in the GI tract, particularly in the colon. Bacteria in the colon help to digest small amounts of cellulose and help form vitamin K, vitamin B_{12}, thiamin, and riboflavin. An additional byproduct is the production of gases in the bowel. The presence of favorable bacteria helps prevent an overgrowth of unfavorable bacteria in the colon. Following administration of antibiotics or after diarrhea, the normal flora of the intestine may be altered, leading to additional diarrhea and gas.

Uses

Indications for use are to assist in the restoration and maintenance of the normal flora of the oral and intestinal tracts. Unlabeled uses include the treatment of uncomplicated diarrhea, small ulcers of the mouth resulting from antibiotic use or other causes, and herpetic stomatitis.

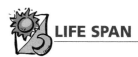

LIFE SPAN

Safe and effective use in children under 3 years of age has not been established.

What You NEED TO KNOW

Contraindications/Precautions

Contraindications include an allergy to milk and sensitivity to lactose.

Drug Interactions

No drug interactions have been notes for *Lactobacillus acidophilus*.

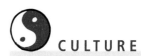

CULTURE

Estimates indicate that 5% to 15% of adult Caucasians are lactose-intolerant, whereas African Americans and Asians have an incidence as high as 80% to 90%.

Adverse Effects

Adverse effects with *Lactobacillus acidophilus* are few. In patients with milk product allergies or intolerance, administration of *Lactobacillus acidophilus* may cause similar symptoms of bloating, cramps, diarrhea, and flatulence. Because *Lactobacillus acidophilus* may cause the same symptoms as those found in lactose-intolerant patients, genetic and cultural differences may be present in adverse effects that are associated with the administration of the supplement.

What You DO

Nursing Responsibilities

Lactobacillus is an OTC oral nutritional supplement and is available in capsules, granules, chewable tablets, or powder. Recommended frequency of administration is one to four times daily. These agents should not be used for more than 2 days or in the presence of high fever, unless directed by health care provider. When administering intestinal flora modifiers, the nurse should:

- Mix granules with cereal, food, milk, fruit juice, or water to increase palatability.
- Check the label or with the pharmacy to determine storage requirements. Most forms must be refrigerated to prevent contamination.
- Instruct the patient to notify the health care provider when bloating, cramps, flatulence, or diarrhea occur.

Do You UNDERSTAND?

DIRECTIONS: Match Column A with Column B.

Column A

_____ 1. *Lactobacillus* may cause this adverse effect in lactose-intolerant patients.

_____ 2. Lactose intolerance occurs frequently in patients of this racial or ethnic group.

_____ 3. *Lactobacillus acidophilus* is indicated for use with patients with this condition.

_____ 4. Prolonged antibiotic therapy may have this effect.

Column B

a. Constipation

b. European

c. Flatulence

d. Decrease of bacteria in the colon

e. Vomiting

f. African American

g. Sore mouth

References

Abrams AC, Lemmon CB, Pennington SS: *Clinical drug therapy: rationales for nursing practice,* ed 8, Philadelphia, 2007, Lippincott.

Black JM, Hawks JH: *Medical-surgical nursing: clinical management for positive outcomes,* ed 7, St Louis, 2005, Elsevier.

Gutierrez K, Queener SF: *Pharmacology for nursing practice,* St Louis, 2004, Mosby.

Hardman JG, Limbird LE: *Goodman & Gilman's the pharmacological basis of therapeutics,* ed 10, New York, 2001, McGraw-Hill.

Hodgson B, Kizior R: *Mosby's 2006 drug consult for nurses, 2006,* St Louis, 2005, Elsevier.

Karch AM: *Focus on nursing pharmacology,* ed 3, Philadelphia, 2006, Lippincott.

Kee JL, Hayes ER, McCuistion LE: *Pharmacology: a nursing process approach,* ed 5, Philadelphia, 2006, Elsevier.

Lehne RA: *Pharmacology for nursing care,* ed 5, Philadelphia, 2004, WB Saunders.

Lewis SM, Heitkemper MM, Dirksen SR: *Medical-surgical nursing: assessment and management of clinical problems,* ed 7, St Louis, 2004, Mosby.

Lilley LL, Harrington S, Snyder JS: *Pharmacology and the nursing process,* ed 4, St Louis, 2005, Mosby.

Wilson BA, Shannon MT, Stang CL: *Nurses drug guide,* Upper Saddle River, New Jersey, 2006, Pearson.

Answers: 1. c; 2. f; 3. g; 4. d.

NCLEX® Review

Section A

1. Phenothiazines act as antiemetics in which way?
   1 Blocking dopamine receptors in the CTZ
   2 Increasing GI motility
   3 Inhibit vomiting center directly
   4 Blocking muscarinic receptors from the cholea

2. Granisetron is approved as an antiemetic for which condition?
   1 Viral gastroenteritis
   2 Radiologic enteral intubation
   3 Cancer chemotherapy nausea
   4 Preoperative and postoperative nausea

3. Absorption or overdose of ipecac syrup can produce which effect?
   1 Cardiotoxicity
   2 Vertigo
   3 Tinnitus
   4 Dermatitis

4. Extrapyramidal reactions are more common with metoclopramide when taken concurrently with which drug?
   1 Phenothiazine
   2 Antacid
   3 Antidysrhythmic
   4 Anticoagulant

5. The nurse assesses a patient who is taking metoclopramide (Reglan) after the nurse's aide notices "something different" about the patient. The nurse notices that the patient is grimacing and her tongue keeps protruding in a rhythmic, repetitive motion. The nurse recognizes this as a sign of which of the following?
   1 Parkinson's disease
   2 Prodrome phase of a seizure
   3 Pain
   4 Tardive dyskinesia

Section B

6. Which laxative is prone to decrease absorption of food and fat-soluble vitamins?
   1 Bisacodyl
   2 Mineral oil
   3 Psyllium
   4 Bismuth subsalicylate

7. A patient is receiving simethicone (Mylicon). The nurse knows that excessive gas in GI tract is caused by all but which of the following?
   1 Swallowing air
   2 Bacterial action
   3 Osmosis from pancreatic secretions
   4 Diffusion of gas from blood circulation

8. A patient is prescribed bisacodyl (Dulcolax) in a rectal suppository form. The nurse teaches the patient to expect the most common adverse effect of:
   1 diarrhea.
   2 sweating.
   3 abdominal cramping.
   4 electrolyte imbalance.

9. A patient who is having a GI surgery is taking magnesium hydroxide (Milk of Magnesia). The nurse expects to monitor for which adverse effect?
   1 Bitter taste
   2 Hyponatremia
   3 Hypomagnesemia
   4 Hyperphosphatemia

10. A patient is taking docusate sodium (Colace). Which is pertinent teaching for this medication?
    1 Swallow the capsules whole and avoid chewing or crushing them.
    2 It may take up to 6. days for a bowel movement to occur with this drug.
    3 Encourage concurrent use of mineral oil for full evacuation effect.
    4 Report symptoms evident of dehydration and electrolyte imbalance.

Section C

11. An 84-year-old female patient is admitted to the hospital with a history of six to eight watery stools per day for the last 3 days. What nursing assessment is most important for this patient?
    1 Her pain level
    2 Intake and output
    3 CBC and blood glucose
    4 Heart rate and rhythm

12. The 84-year-old patient is taking diphenoxylate hydrochloride with atropine sulfate (Lomotil) to treat her diarrhea. While reviewing her current medication history, you find she is taking MAOI tranylcypromine (Parnate). What drug interaction is possible with an MAOI and antidiarrheal?
    1 It may exacerbate the effects of the MAOI.
    2 It may cause a hypertensive crisis.
    3 It may decrease the absorption of the MAOI.
    4 It may increase the risk for bleeding.

13. A 57-year-old man has severe diarrhea and oral ulcers as a result of antibiotic use. What drug would most likely be ordered to treat his diarrhea?
    1 Lactobacillus acidophilus
    2 Polycarbophil (FiberCon)
    3 Deodorized opium tincture
    4 Loperamide (Imodium)

14. A patient is taking bismuth subsalicylate (Pepto-Bismol). The nurse realizes the action of this drug is to:
    1 decrease prostaglandin production.
    2 reestablish intestinal flora balance.
    3 increase fluid and mucus secretion.
    4 increase absorption of water and toxic substances.

15. A patient is taking kaolin-pectin (Kaopectate). The nurse realizes that related teaching should include all except which of the following?
    1 Instruct the patient to avoid this drug when having a high fever.
    2 Teach the patient to take the drug at least 2. hours before or after other oral drugs.
    3 Inform the patient to avoid milk products until the diarrhea is resolved.
    4 Warn the patient not to take atropine sulfate with this drug to avoid hypertensive crisis.

Section D

16. A patient is taking misoprostol (Cytotec). The nurse knows that this drug is used to treat gastric ulcers caused by:
    1 stress.
    2 excessive gastric acid production.
    3 NSAIDs.
    4 *Helicobacter pylori.*

17. The nurse realizes that which of the following is an undesirable drug action of misoprostol (Cytotec)?
    1 Uterine contractions
    2 Blurred vision
    3 Dry mouth
    4 Tardive dyskinesia

18. The drugs that are ordered for a 79-year-old male patient include digoxin 0.25 mg po qid, norfloxacin 400 mg po bid, Dilantin 150 mg po bid, Maalox 2 tsp po qid, and Carafate 1 g po ac and at bedtime. The routine hospital medication administration times for qid are 9 AM, 1 PM, 5 PM, and 9 PM; meals are delivered at 7 AM, 12 PM, and 5 PM. Based on these routines, at what times should the nurse schedule the Carafate?
    1 6 AM, 11 AM, 4 PM, and 9 PM
    2 7 AM, 12 PM, 5 PM, and 9 PM
    3 9 AM, 1 PM, 5 PM, and 9 PM
    4 6 AM, 12 PM, 6 PM, and 12 AM

19. How should proton pump inhibitors be administered?
    1 Chewed
    2 Given before meals
    3 Given after meals
    4 Followed by two glasses of water

20. A 56-year-old man has a recent history of peptic ulcer and *Helicobacter pylori*. Which medication might be taken in combination with other drugs to treat his disease?
    1 Docusate (Surfak)
    2 Mineral oil
    3 Diphenoxylate with atropine
    4 Bismuth subsalicylate

Section E

21. A patient is taking pancrelipase (Pancrease). The nurse knows that _____, when given concurrently, will decrease the activity of pancreatic enzymes.
    1 H_2 blockers
    2 iron preparations
    3 phenothiazines
    4 prostaglandins

22. The nurse teaches the patient taking pancrelipase to:
    1 swallow the medication whole.
    2 take the liquid form with 1 oz of chocolate milk.
    3 crush and mix the granules with food to improve palatability.
    4 take the medication at bedtime, depending on the day's intake of fat content.

23. The nurse knows that the patient taking pancrelipase may develop which adverse effect?
    1 Hypotension
    2 Hyperuricemia
    3 Cardiac dysrhythmias
    4 Reddish or yellow-brown urine or feces

24. A patient is taking lactobacillus acidophilus (Lactinex). The nurse knows that this drug should be given cautiously to all of the following patients *except*:
    1 a patient with an allergy to milk.
    2 a patient with sensitivity to lactose.
    3 a patient with a history of diabetes mellitus.
    4 a child under 3 years of age.

25. The nurse teaches the patient taking lactobacillus acidophilus to:
    1 take the full regimen of 7 days.
    2 take the medication at bedtime only.
    3 continue taking the medication until fever subsides.
    4 refrigerate the medication to prevent contamination.

NCLEX® Review Answers

Section A

1. 1 Phenothiazines act as antiemetics by blocking dopamine receptors in the CTZ, which is responsible for activating the vomiting reflex. The action of phenothiazines does not increase GI motility, directly inhibit the vomiting center, or block muscarinic receptors from the cholea.

2. 3 Granisetron is approved and used as an antiemetic for emetogenic chemotherapy. Granisetron is not approved for use for viral gastroenteritis, radiologic enteral intubation, or preoperative and postoperative nausea.

3. 1 An overdose or absorption of ipecac can produce cardiotoxic effects, such as dysrhythmias, chest pain, bradycardia, and tachycardia. Overdosing of ipecac does not cause vertigo, tinnitus, and dermatitis.

4. 1 EPS reactions are more common with metoclopramide when taken concurrently with phenothiazines. Extrapyramidal reactions are not common when metoclopramides are given with antacids, antidysrhythmics, and anticoagulants.

5. 4 Tardive dyskinesia is a potentially serious adverse effect of metoclopramide. Dyskinesia involves repetitive, rhythmic, uncontrollable movements, usually of the face, mouth, jaw, and tongue. Protrusion of the tongue, jaw movements, facial grimace, or pursing or smacking of the lips may occur. Tardive dyskinesia can become permanent; thus early detection and withdrawal of the medication is necessary. Rhythmic, repetitive tongue movement, and grimacing are not indicative of Parkinson's disease, prodrome phase of a seizure, or pain.

Section B

6. 2 Mineral oil is the laxative that is likely to decrease absorption of food and fat-soluble vitamins. Bisacodyl, psyllium, and bismuth subsalicylate do not decrease the absorption of food and fat-soluble vitamins.

7. 3 Gas is introduced into the body by swallowing air, bacterial action, and diffusion of gas from blood circulation. Excessive gas in the GI tract is not caused by osmosis from pancreatic secretions.

8. 3 The most common adverse effect of bisacodyl is abdominal cramping from the stimulation of peristalsis. Diarrhea and electrolyte imbalance may occur rarely but are not common. Sweating is usually not associated with bisacodyl.

9. 4 Magnesium hydroxide may lead to hyperphosphatemia, hypernatremia, and hypermagnesemia. Bitter taste is not associated with magnesium hydroxide.

10. 1 Docusate sodium capsules and tablets should be swallowed whole and not chewed or crushed. It may take up to 3 days for a bowel movement to occur not 6. Mineral oil should be avoided when taking docusate to prevent its systemic absorption. Dehydration and electrolyte imbalance are not associated with docusate.

Section C

11. 2 Assess her intake and output to determine fluid volume deficit and dehydration, primarily because of her age, which makes her more susceptible to dehydration. A complete assessment is always necessary for your patients and should be performed. However, you should be aware that dehydration is the greatest concern in this case. Electrolytes would also be an important assessment but was not one of the choices. Pain level assessment, CBC and blood glucose assessment, and heart rate and rhythm assessment are incorrect because they are not related to dehydration as closely as is intake and output assessment.

12. 2 The combination of MAOI and opioid antidiarrheal may cause hypertensive crisis.

MAOIs that contain diphenoxylate hydrochloride with atropine sulfate do not enhance the MAOI, decrease MAOI absorption, or increase bleeding.

13. 1 Lactobacillus acidophilus is used to prevent and treat superinfections following antibiotic therapy. Polycarbophil, deodorized opium tincture, and loperamide are not used to treat superinfections.

14. 1 Bismuth subsalicylate decreases prostaglandin production. This medication does not restore intestinal flora balance. Bismuth decreases the secretion of fluid and mucus into the colon not increase. Bismuth does not increase absorption of water and toxic substances.

15. 2 Kaolin-pectin should be taken at least 2 hours before or after other oral drugs. The patient should be instructed to avoid using antidiarrheals for the presence of high fever. The patient should avoid milk products until diarrhea is resolved. This drug has no relationship with atropine.

Section D

16. 3 Misoprostol is indicated for the prevention and treatment of ulcers caused by NSAIDs, including aspirin. NSAIDs decrease prostaglandin production, which decreases bicarbonate and mucus production in the stomach. Misoprostol increases bicarbonate and mucus, which helps protect the gastric lining. Misoprostol is not indicated for ulcers resulting from stress, excessive gastric acid production, or *Helicobacter pylori*.

17. 1 Cytotec is a synthetic prostaglandin E1. Prostaglandins are found in the female reproductive system, as well as other systems in the body (e.g., prostaglandins are abundant in the uterus). When prostaglandins are given to either pregnant or nonpregnant women in sufficient amounts, uterine contractions occur and the cervix softens. Misoprostol does not cause blurred vision, dry mouth, or tardive dyskinesia.

18. 1 Give Carafate at 6:00 AM, 11:00 AM, 4:00 PM, and 9:00 PM. Considerations include the following: Carafate should be given 1 hour before meals and at bedtime; oral medications should be given 2 hours before giving Carafate; antacids must be given 30 minutes before or after

Carafate; and Carafate may decrease absorption of digoxin, Dilantin, and the quinolone antibiotic when they are administered too close together.

19. **2** Proton pump inhibitors should be given before, not after, meals. Proton pump inhibitors should not be chewed or followed by two glasses of water.

20. **4** Bismuth subsalicylate has an antiinflammatory and antimicrobial effect and is frequently used in combination with antibiotics to treat *Helicobacter pylori* infection. Docusate is a stool softener. Mineral oil is a lubricant laxative. Diphenoxylate with atropine is an opioid antidiarrheal. Laxatives, stool softeners, or opioid antidiarrheals are not used to treat *Helicobacter pylori*.

Section E

21. **1** Concurrent H_2-blockers, as well as calcium and magnesium antacids, decrease the activity of pancreatic enzymes. Phenothiazines and prostaglandins do not decrease pancreatic enzyme activity. Pancreatic enzymes decrease absorption of iron when given together.

22. **1** Pancrelipase should be swallowed whole with a glass of water for greater effectiveness and not crushed or chewed. Pancrelipase should be taken orally 1 to 2 hours before meals, with meals, or with food between meals.

23. **2** Hyperuricemia is an adverse effect of pancrelipase. Hypotension, cardiac dysrhythmias, and reddish or yellow-brown urine or feces are not associated with pancrelipase.

24. **3** Lactobacillus acidophilus is contraindicated for individuals with an allergy to milk or a sensitivity to lactose and in children under 3 years of age.

25. **4** Lactobacillus acidophilus should be refrigerated to prevent contamination and taken 1 to 4 times daily. This agent should not be taken for more than 2 days or in the presence of high fever.

Notes

Drugs Used to Treat the Genitourinary Tract and Renal Disorders

What You WILL LEARN

After reading this chapter, you will know how to do the following:

✔ Recall the laboratory considerations for drugs used to treat a urinary tract infection.
✔ Identify the hematologic life-threatening adverse effects of urinary antimicrobial drugs.
✔ Compare the action of loop diuretics, thiazide diuretics, and potassium-sparing diuretics.
✔ Discuss nursing responsibilities of diuretics.
✔ Compare the types of drugs used in the treatment of renal failure and the reasons for their use.

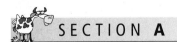

SECTION **A**

URINARY TRACT AGENTS

What IS a Urinary Tract Antimicrobial Antiseptic?

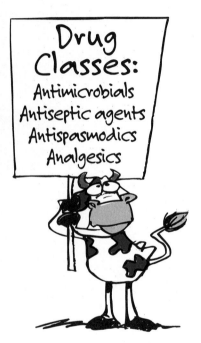

Drug Classes:
Antimicrobials
Antiseptic agents
Antispasmodics
Analgesics

Urinary Tract Antimicrobial Antiseptics	Trade Names	Uses
Urinary tract antimicrobials ciprofloxacin [sip-row-FLOX-ah-sin]	Cipro	Treatment of urinary tract infection
nitrofurantoin [NYE-troh-FYOOR-an-toyn]	Macrodantin	Treatment of urinary tract infection
ofloxacin [oh-FLOX-ah-sin]	Floxin	Treatment of urinary tract infection, prostatitis
sulfisoxazole [sul-fih-SOX-ah-zole]	Gantrisin	Treatment of urinary tract infection
trimethoprim-sulfamethoxazole [tri-METH-oh-prim sul-fa-meth-ox-ah-zole]	Bactrim	Treatment of urinary tract infection
Urinary tract antiseptics methenamine [meh-THEEN-ah-meen]	Urised	Prevention of urinary tract infection
nalidixic acid [nah-lih-DIX-ik]	NegGram	Treatment of urinary tract infection

Action

Urinary tract antimicrobial antiseptic drugs act in various ways and are effective against different organisms. Fluoroquinolone drugs such as ciprofloxacin are potent, broad-spectrum bactericidal drugs that inhibit deoxyribonucleic acid (DNA) gyrase, an enzyme needed for bacterial replication and protein synthesis. These drugs also exhibit postantibiotic effects, meaning that bacterial growth does not occur for several hours after drug exposure and a shorter treatment period can be used in treating a urinary tract infection (UTI).

Sulfonamides are broad-spectrum antiinfectives that have a bacteriostatic effect. These drugs interfere with the synthesis of purines and DNA in the organism. As broad-spectrum antimicrobials, sulfonamides are clinically effective against several pathogens.

Urinary tract antiseptics are bactericidal; they inhibit DNA replication and protein synthesis. Methenamine decomposes into ammonia and formaldehyde within the urine. High levels of formaldehyde kill the bacteria that are present in the urine. Although urinary tract antiseptics exert antibacterial action on the urine, they have little or no systemic antibacterial action.

Uses

Selection of a urinary tract antimicrobial antiseptic drug depends primarily on results of a urinalysis in addition to a culture and a sensitivity test. The primary antimicrobial drugs used to treat UTIs are fluoroquinolones and sulfonamides. Additionally, fluoroquinolones are used for the treatment of lower respiratory tract, skin, bone, joint, and gastrointestinal (GI) infections, as well as gonorrhea.

Sulfonamides are frequently used for treatment of UTIs resulting from community-acquired microorganisms (e.g., *Escherichia coli, Klebsiella, Enterobacter*). Sulfonamides are ideal for patients with a first-time UTI because of their ease of administration, effectiveness, low cost, and safety. Sulfamethoxazole is often combined with trimethoprim (a synthetic anti-infective) and given twice a day for 3 days. The combined drug is also more effective in delaying drug resistance than when the drugs are given separately.

What You NEED TO KNOW

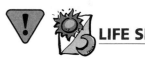 **LIFE SPAN**

Contraindications/Precautions

Antimicrobial antiseptics are contraindicated for patients with hypersensitivity. Sulfonamides are also contraindicated for patients with porphyria, and in patients with gastrointestinal or genitourinary tract obstruction.

Cautious use of antimicrobial antiseptics is advised for patients with hepatic or renal impairment. Caution should be used when using fluoroquinolones in patients who have seizures, a psychosis, or increased intracranial pressure. Sulfonamides should be used with caution for patients with asthma and blood dyscrasias.

Urinary tract antiseptics should be used cautiously for patients with diabetes mellitus, electrolyte imbalances, vitamin B deficiency, and debilitation.

- Antimicrobial antiseptics should be avoided during pregnancy and lactation and in children.
- Hematologic life-threatening adverse effects of antimicrobial antiseptics include aplastic and hemolytic anemia, hypoprothrombinemia, thrombocytopenia, and agranulocytosis.
- Hypersensitivity adverse effects range from mild skin reactions of rash, itching, and burning to severe anaphylactic shock.

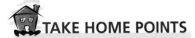

Drug Interactions

Theophylline levels are elevated 15% to 30% when administered with ciprofloxacin. When ciprofloxacin is given with warfarin, the prothrombin time (PT) level is increased; when it is given with phenytoin, the phenytoin level is decreased. Sulfonamides increase the risk for hypoprothrombinemia when given with oral anticoagulants. The risk for hypoglycemia is increased when sulfisoxazole and sulfonylureas are given together. The absorption of nitrofurantoin and ciprofloxacin is decreased when these drugs are given with antacids, sucralfate, and iron. When methenamine is given with acetazolamide and sodium bicarbonate, the conversion into formaldehyde may be inhibited, thereby decreasing the action of methenamine.

Adverse Effects

Adverse effects for most antimicrobial antiseptics include nausea, vomiting, diarrhea, constipation, gastric distress, and crystalluria. Other adverse effects include headache, dizziness, drowsiness, photosensitivity, fatigue, seizures, stomatitis, and a drug-induced hepatitis.

Insomnia, chest pain, edema, hypertension, euphoria, hallucinations, extrapyramidal symptoms, such as repetitive and abnormal movements, restlessness, rigidity, and neuroleptic malignant syndrome (a potentially fatal condition characterized by altered mental status, muscle rigidity, irregular pulse, tachycardia, blood pressure fluctuations, and sweating) have occurred from ofloxacin. Other adverse effects of sulfonamides include pancreatitis, acute psychosis, and Stevens-Johnson syndrome. Pseudomembranous enterocolitis may be an adverse effect of trimethoprim-sulfamethoxazole. Seizures have been noted following nalidixic acid therapy.

What You DO

Nursing Responsibilities

Most antimicrobial antiseptics are administered orally, but several of these drugs can also be given intravenously (IV), depending on the purpose of administration and the condition of the patient. When administering antimicrobial antiseptics, the nurse should:
• Administer antacids, sucralfate, and iron at least 4 hours apart from fluoroquinolones to ensure absorption.

- Assess fluid intake, urine output, and urine pH.
- Administer nitrofurantoin with food to decrease GI distress.
- Monitor theophylline levels for patients who are taking theophylline and ciprofloxacin.
- Monitor renal and hepatic function studies for necessary dose adjustment.
- Assist the susceptible female patient in planning alternative contraception because oral contraceptives may be unreliable when taken with sulfonamides.
- Monitor blood glucose in patients who have diabetes and are taking sulfonamides for detection of hypoglycemia.
- Teach the patient to use sunscreen protection and avoid prolonged exposure to sunlight to prevent photosensitivity.
- Instruct the patient who is taking nalidixic acid to report visual disturbances, particularly during the first few days of therapy. This adverse effect usually disappears with dose reduction or discontinuation.
- Monitor the complete blood count for patients who are taking antimicrobial antiseptic drugs on a chronic basis for early detection of blood dyscrasias (sore throat, fatigue, joint pains, pallor, bleeding, and jaundice). Report these symptoms to the health care provider.
- Monitor the patient who is taking ofloxacin for early detection of extrapyramidal symptoms and neuroleptic malignant syndrome and report these to the health care provider.
- Counsel the patient who is taking nalidixic acid to report vomiting, irritability, headache, insomnia, excitement, drowsiness, and mental depression.
- Instruct the patient who is taking antibiotics to report milky urine, foul-smelling urine, and perineal irritation for early detection of superinfections.
- Warn the patient to avoid alcohol while taking these drugs.

 To prevent staining of teeth, do not crush nitrofurantoin tablets. Do not give theophylline and caffeine within 2 to 4 hours of ciprofloxacin because this drug combination may lead to CNS stimulation (e.g., tachycardia, anxiety, nervousness, insomnia).

Do You UNDERSTAND?

DIRECTIONS: Provide the appropriate responses to the following questions.

1. To ensure safety, the nurse should be aware of the increased risk for what neurologic problems with the use of nalidixic acid?

   _____

2. Absorption of nitrofurantoin and ciprofloxacin is decreased when these drugs taken with what other drug?

   _____

What IS a Urinary Tract Antispasmodic Analgesic?

Urinary Tract Antispasmodic Analgesics	Trade Names	Uses
Urinary tract antispasmodics		
flavoxate [fla-VOX-ate]	Urispas	Treatment of dysuria, nocturia, and incontinence
oxybutynin [ox-ee-BYOO-tih-nin]	Ditropan	Treatment of neurogenic bladder, overactive bladder
tolterodine [toll-tear-o-dine]	Detrol	Treatment of overactive bladder
Urinary tract analgesic		
phenazopyridine [fen-az-oh-PEER-ih-deen]	Pyridium	Treatment of cystitis

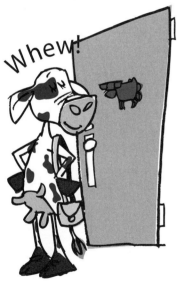

Whew!

No need to rush.

Action

Flavoxate acts on the detrusor muscles in the bladder; thus it is a parasympatholytic drug with papaverine-like activity. The antispasmodic effect increases bladder capacity in patients with bladder spasms. Oxybutynin and tolterodine act as a parasympatholytic drug. These drugs have a prominent antispasmodic effect, directly inhibiting the muscarinic effects of acetylcholine on smooth muscles of the bladder.

Answers: 1. seizure, dizziness, drowsiness; 2. antacids.

The analgesic action for phenazopyridine is unclear. The azo dye of phenazopyridine produces a topical analgesia effect on the urinary mucosa but has little or no antiinfective action.

Uses

Urinary tract antispasmodic drugs are used to treat a variety of symptoms, such as dysuria, urgency, nocturia, suprapubic pain, frequency, and incontinence. Oxybutynin and tolterodine are used to relieve symptoms associated with overactive bladder and to provide relief after transurethral surgery. Urinary tract analgesics are used to relieve the urgency, frequency, and dysuria associated with UTIs. The primary urinary tract analgesic drug is phenazopyridine, which is also used in the treatment of cystitis.

What You NEED TO KNOW

Contraindications/Precautions

Antispasmodic analgesics are contraindicated in patients with glaucoma, gastrointestinal or genitourinary obstruction, and ileus. Flavoxate is contraindicated for patients with GI bleeding. Oxybutynin and tolterodine are contraindicated in patients with glaucoma, myasthenia gravis, severe colitis, megacolon, or cardiovascular disorders. Phenazopyridine is contraindicated for patients with GI inflammation or bleeding, renal impairment, and severe hepatitis. Cautious use is advised when treating older adults.

Drug Interactions

There are no known drug interactions with phenazopyridine. Flavoxate, oxybutynin, and tolterodine interact with digoxin when the drugs are taken concurrently, elevating serum digoxin levels and contributing to digoxin toxicity. These same drugs used in combination with other parasympathomimetic drugs or with cholinesterase inhibitors may cause a decrease in the anticholinergic activity. Cautious use is advised in patients taking antihistamines since the anticholinergic effects may be exaggerated. Constipation can be worsened when these drugs are taken in combination with opioid analgesics.

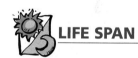

LIFE SPAN

Antispasmodic analgesics are contraindicated during pregnancy and lactation and in children less than 12 years of age.

Flavoxate should be used with caution in patients who have glaucoma. Oxybutynin and tolterodine should be used cautiously in patients who have prostate hypertrophy, autonomic neuropathy, reflex esophagitis, renal or hepatic dysfunction, hyperthyroidism, and cardiovascular disorders.

Adverse Effects

The adverse effects of urinary tract antispasmodic analgesic drugs are drug-specific but in general include headache, dizziness, drowsiness, mental confusion, insomnia, restlessness, nausea, vomiting, dry mouth, constipation, dysuria, hyperpyrexia, heart palpitations, blurred vision, and tachycardia. Flavoxate, oxybutynin, and tolterodine may cause hypersensitivity reactions, urinary hesitancy, retention, and impotence. Other adverse effects from oxybutynin and tolterodine include fatigue, fever, decreased sweating, psychotic behavior, and suppression of lactation. Jaundice and increased intraocular pressure have also been reported. Eosinophilia has occurred from flavoxate. Hemolytic anemia, renal stones, and acute renal failure may result from prolonged use of phenazopyridine.

TAKE HOME POINTS

Teach patients who are taking parasympatholytic drugs such as flavoxate, oxybutynin, and tolterodine to take their apical pulse for 1 full minute and report tachycardia to the health care provider. Inform the patient that phenazopyridine may cause staining of contact lenses. Because of the decreased sweating associated with oxybutynin and tolterodine, fever or heat stroke may occur in a hot environment.

What You DO

Nursing Responsibilities

Antispasmodic analgesics are only given by mouth. Flavoxate may be taken without regard to meals. Phenazopyridine may be taken with meals or after meals to decrease the GI distress. When administering antispasmodic analgesics, the nurse should:

- Confirm a diagnosis of overactive bladder before initiating oxybutynin or tolterodine therapy.
- Monitor vital signs of the patient who is taking flavoxate, oxybutynin, or tolterodine for early detection of adverse effects and alert the health care provider.
- Caution the patient who is taking flavoxate to avoid activities requiring alertness (e.g., driving) until the response is known.
- Discontinue antispasmodic analgesic drugs when dysuria subsides, which is generally 3 to 5 days.
- Instruct the patient to report to the health care provider immediately if jaundice (e.g., yellow skin discoloration) develops, which indicates liver impairment.
- Advise the patient that phenazopyridine changes the urine to an orange-red color and may stain fabrics as well as contact lens. Protective padding may be needed in some patients.

- Monitor the patient's CBC for early detection of blood dyscrasias with chronic use of antimicrobial antiseptics.
- Assess the patient for adequate intake and output.
- Warn the patient who is taking oxybutynin, tolterodine to avoid hot environments to avoid a drop in blood pressure.

Do You UNDERSTAND?

DIRECTIONS: Match Column A with Column B.

	Column A	Column B
_____	1. Route of administration of antispasmodics	a. By mouth
_____	2. Side effect of oxybutynin	b. Subcutaneously
_____	3. Side effect of phenazopyridine	c. Urinary tract obstruction
_____	4. Contraindication of flavoxate	d. Orange-red urine
		e. Abdominal pain

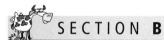

SECTION **B**

DIURETICS

What IS a Loop Diuretic?

Loop Diuretics	Trade Names	Uses
furosemide [fur-OH-see-mide]	Lasix	Treatment of edema, acute CHF, and acute pulmonary edema
bumetanide [byoo-MET-ah-nide]	Bumex	Treatment of edema, acute CHF, and acute pulmonary edema
torsemide [TORE-se-mide]	Demadex	Treatment of hypertension, hepatic cirrhosis, acute pulmonary edema, and chronic renal failure

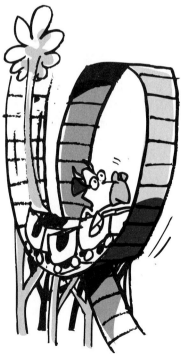

Looping to treat fluid excess.

Answers: 1. a; 2. e; 3. d; 4. c.

Action

Loop diuretics are classified based on their site of action in the nephrons of the kidneys. These drugs (also known as "high-ceiling diuretics") inhibit sodium and chloride reabsorption through direct action primarily in the ascending loop of Henle but also in the proximal and distal tubules. Inhibiting sodium and chloride reabsorption causes potassium and magnesium loss. Phosphate and bicarbonate reabsorption is also inhibited. Loop diuretics cause a greater degree of diuresis than do other diuretics. However, at the usual diuretic doses, loop diuretics produce only mild antihypertensive effects. The bumetanide diuretic action is 40 times greater than the action of furosemide, but it has a shorter duration of action. Torsemide has a longer duration of action and is effective with once-a-day dosing.

Uses

Loop diuretics are used to treat edema that involves fluid volume excess resulting from a number of disorders of the heart, liver, or kidney (e.g., pulmonary edema, CHF, nephrotic syndrome, hepatic cirrhosis). These drugs are effective even when the patient has renal failure.

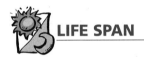

LIFE SPAN

Furosemide and bumetanide are contraindicated during pregnancy and lactation.

What You NEED TO KNOW

Contraindications/Precautions

Loop diuretics are contraindicated for patients with hypersensitivity to sulfonamides in general or to a specific drug, and to those with severe adrenocortical or renal impairment, anuria, progressive oliguria, fluid and electrolyte depletion, or hepatic coma.

Drug Interactions

Digitalis toxicity may result when loop diuretics are given concurrently with digoxin and other potassium-depleting drugs (e.g., corticosteroids, amphotericin B). Lithium toxicity may result from its decreased elimination when given together with loop diuretics. When bumetanide is given with cisplatin and aminoglycosides, the risk for ototoxicity is increased. Nonsteroidal antiinflammatory drugs (NSAIDs) reduce the diuretic and hypotensive activity of loop diuretics. When loop diuretics are given concurrently with anticoagulants, an increased anticoagulation effect may occur.

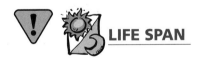

LIFE SPAN

- Cautious use is advised for older adults and infants.
- Cautious use of loop diuretics is advised in patients with gout, severe renal or liver dysfunction, cardiogenic shock, and systemic lupus erythematosus (SLE). These drugs should also be used with caution in patients who are taking digoxin, potassium-depleting steroids, or those who are at risk for hypokalemia.

Adverse Effects

The adverse effects of loop diuretics include ototoxicity, tinnitus, dizziness, hearing loss, muscle spasms, hyperglycemia, hypokalemia, hypocalcemia, alkalosis, hypotension, weakness, photosensitivity, blurred vision, paresthesias, nausea, vomiting, anorexia, constipation, and severe diarrhea. Hematologic effects include agranulocytosis, aplastic anemia, leukopenia, and thrombocytopenia. Renal changes include fluid and electrolyte imbalance, frequency, polyuria, hyperuricemia, irreversible renal failure, and allergic nephritis. Other adverse effects of furosemide include diuresis, circulatory collapse, acute pancreatitis, and SLE.

What You DO

Nursing Responsibilities

Furosemide may be administered orally, IM, or IV, preferably with meals to decrease gastric distress. When administering loop diuretics, the nurse should:

- Monitor adequate intake and output, as well as improvement of edema for effectiveness and adverse effects.
- Notify the health care provider when the patient reports severe diarrhea because the drug may need to be discontinued.
- Teach the patient and family to report evidence of ototoxicity (e.g., dizziness, tinnitus, hearing loss).
- Check the patient's vital signs and weight at the same time each day (in the morning before breakfast) and with the patient wearing the same type of clothing.
- Monitor potassium levels for the patient who is taking loop diuretics. Potassium supplements are usually given for patients who are undergoing long-term loop diuretic treatment.
- Monitor the patient who is taking loop diuretics for tachycardia, hypotension, and dysrhythmias for early detection of hypokalemia.
- Instruct the patient to report dry mouth, thirst, anorexia, weakness, drowsiness, restlessness, muscle cramps, oliguria, nausea, and vomiting.
- Help the patient create a schedule of drug administration to avoid nocturia (e.g., 8 am and 2 pm).

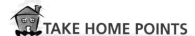

TAKE HOME POINTS

Hearing loss usually lasts a short time (1 to 24 hours). When diuresis is excessively vigorous, the patient may develop rapid and excessive weight loss or acute hypotension. The patient who is taking loop diuretics and digoxin is particularly prone to hypokalemia, and the patient who is taking loop diuretics while on a sodium-restricted diet is particularly prone to hyponatremia. Hypokalemia may result from loop diuretics, particularly in patients with ventricular dysrhythmias.

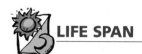

LIFE SPAN

Excessive diuresis may lead to thromboembolic conditions (e.g., pulmonary emboli, cerebral vascular thrombosis), particularly in older adults.

- Monitor renal and hepatic function studies frequently during the first few months and periodically thereafter for potential damage to these organs.
- Monitor the patient's uric acid levels because hyperuricemia is an adverse effect that may precipitate gout.
- Evaluate initial and ongoing CBC for potential blood dyscrasia development.
- Monitor glucose levels closely for patients with diabetes who are taking loop diuretics because these drugs may cause hyperglycemia.
- Advise the patient to use protection (e.g., sunscreen, protective clothing) when exposed to sunlight.
- Teach the patient to change positions slowly to avoid dizziness and falls.

Do You UNDERSTAND?

DIRECTIONS: **Provide appropriate responses for the following questions.**

1. For patients on long-term treatment, what type of diet may be ordered? _____

2. What can hematologic problems include? _____
   _____

3. What is caused by Lasix and the other loop diuretics that requires close monitoring of glucose levels in patients with diabetes? _____
   _____

Answers: 1. potassium supplement diet; 2. agranulocytosis and anemia (aplastic); 3. hyperglycemia.

What IS a Thiazide and a Thiazide-Like Diuretic?

Thiazides and Thiazide-Like Diuretics	Length of Action	Trade Names	Uses
Thiazide diuretics hydrochlorothiazide [HY-droh-klor-ah-THIGH-ah-zide]	Short-acting	Hydro-Diuril, HCTZ	Treatment of edema and hypertension
chlorothiazide [klor-ah-THIGH-ah-zide]	Short-acting	Diuril	Treatment of edema and hypertension
Thiazide-like diuretic metolazone [meh-TOH-lah-zone]	Intermediate-acting	Zaroxolyn	Treatment of hypertension
indapamide [in-DAP-ah-myd]	Long-acting	Lozol	Treatment of hypertension and edema
chlorthalidone [klor-THAL-ih-doan]	Long-acting	Hygroton	Treatment of hypertension, edema, hepatic cirrhosis, and renal dysfunction

Action

Thiazide-like diuretics differ chemically from thiazides in the site of action but share similar use, contraindications, drug actions, precautions, adverse effects, and drug interactions. Although thiazides have some carbonic anhydrase inhibitory action, metolazone has none.

Thiazide and thiazide-like diuretics, acting primarily on the distal collecting tubules and on the proximal tubules as a secondary site, inhibit sodium and chloride reabsorption through direct action on the proximal tubules. Inhibiting sodium and chloride reabsorption causes potassium, magnesium, phosphate, and bicarbonate loss. These diuretics also produce elevated plasma renin activity, antihypertensive effect, uric acid retention, and precipitate diabetes onset in prediabetes patients. Thiazides and thiazide-like diuretics are chemically related to the sulfonamides.

Uses

Thiazide and thiazide-like diuretics are used to treat edema and hypertension. Thiazides are used in the treatment of CHF, hepatic cirrhosis, renal dysfunction, and during corticosteroid and estrogen therapy. These agents (e.g., metolazone) are used to treat hypertension. Metolazone is effective in patients with impaired renal function. Thiazide-like diuretics are less efficient than loop diuretics and not effective in patients with renal failure.

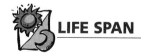

LIFE SPAN

Thiazides and thiazide-like drugs are contraindicated for women during pregnancy and lactation and for children.

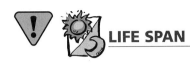

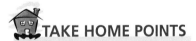

What You NEED TO KNOW

Contraindications/Precautions

Thiazides and thiazide-like drugs are contraindicated for patients with hypersensitivity to sulfonamides and thiazides, hypokalemia, anuria, and concurrent administration of blood or blood products.

Drug Interactions

Alcohol and other CNS depressants exacerbate the sedative effects when taken with thiazide and thiazide-like diuretics. Corticosteroids and amphotericin B may increase hypokalemia when given with chlorothiazide. Because of hypokalemia and hypomagnesemia, the risk for digitalis toxicity is increased when digoxin is taken with thiazide and thiazide-like diuretics. The decreased lithium elimination may increase the risk for lithium toxicity when given with drugs in this classification. When thiazide and thiazide-like diuretics are given with diazoxide, hypoglycemia is increased.

Cimetidine, oral contraceptives, propylthiouracil, and methimazole increase the action of metolazone. Conversely, barbiturates and rifampin decrease the action of metolazone. Metolazone and verapamil taken concurrently increases the risk for heart block. When metolazone is given with verapamil and digoxin, bradycardia may occur.

Adverse Effects

Adverse effects with thiazide and thiazide-like diuretics include fluid and electrolyte imbalance, dehydration, photosensitivity, hypersensitivity, mood changes, drowsiness, weakness, dizziness, renal or hepatic damage, and SLE. GI adverse effects include dry mouth, nausea, vomiting, anorexia, and diarrhea. Hematologic effects include aplastic anemia, agranulocytosis, and leukopenia. Cardiovascular adverse effects include irregular heart rate, weak pulse, and orthostatic hypotension. Hyperglycemia and hyperuricemia are metabolic adverse effects.

What You DO

Nursing Responsibilities

Thiazide and thiazide-like diuretics are given orally, except for chlorothiazide, which can also be given IV. When administering thiazide and thiazide-like diuretics, the nurse should:

- Assess adequate intake and output for evaluating effectiveness. Drug discontinuation may be needed when adverse effects develop.
- Record the patient's weight and vital signs.
- Evaluate initial and ongoing CBC for early detection of blood dyscrasias.
- Check the patient's electrolytes for drug effectiveness and electrolyte imbalance. Patients are usually taking potassium supplements when undergoing long-term treatment.
- Monitor for signs and symptoms of dehydration (e.g., thirst, weakness, muscle cramping, hypotension, tachycardia).
- Review renal and hepatic function studies for early detection of organ damage.
- Monitor glucose levels closely in patients with diabetes because these drugs may cause hyperglycemia.
- Observe the patient's serum uric acid for early detection of hyperuricemia, which may precipitate gout.
- Discontinue thiazides before parathyroid function tests are performed because they tend to decrease calcium excretion.
- Instruct the patient to use protection when exposed to sunlight because thiazide diuretics may cause photosensitivity.

Do You UNDERSTAND?

DIRECTIONS: **Indicate in the space provided whether the statement is *true* or *false*. If the answer is false, correct the statement to make it true (using the margin space).**

_____   1. Thiazide diuretics are classified based on their chemical composition.

_____   2. Inhibiting sodium and chloride reabsorption causes both potassium and magnesium loss.

_____   3. Thiazides do not produce antihypertensive effects.

What IS a Potassium-Sparing Diuretic?

Potassium-Sparing Diuretics	Trade Names	Uses
amiloride [ah-MILL-oh-ride]	Midamor	Treatment of edema and hypertension
spironolactone [speer-on-oh-LAK-tone]	Aldactone	Treatment of edema and hypertension
triamterene [try-AM-ter-een]	Dyrenium	Treatment of edema

Action

Potassium-sparing diuretics have a mild diuretic and antihypertensive effect. Amiloride and triamterene have a direct effect on the distal tubules in the kidney. Presumably, spironolactone competes with aldosterone for cell receptor sites in the distal tubules. Potassium-sparing diuretics induce urinary excretion of sodium and reduce excretion of potassium and hydrogen ions, and they lower BP through an unknown mechanism.

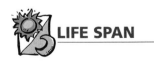

LIFE SPAN

Potassium-sparing diuretics are contraindicated during pregnancy.

Uses

Potassium-sparing diuretics are effective in preventing or treating diuretic-induced hypokalemia in patients with disorders of the heart, liver, kidney, and those with hypertension. These agents are also useful in reducing edema in patients with CHF, significant dysrhythmias, and those who are undergoing digoxin therapy, and they are used in managing primary aldosteronism. Potassium-sparing diuretics may be combined with a thiazide or loop diuretic.

What You NEED TO KNOW

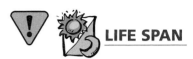

LIFE SPAN

Contraindications/Precautions

Potassium-sparing diuretics are contraindicated for patients with hypersensitivity, anuria, severe renal dysfunction, hyperkalemia (potassium level above 5.5 mEq/L), and those who are taking another potassium-sparing diuretic.

Drug Interactions

When potassium-sparing diuretics are given concurrently with potassium supplements or angiotensin-converting enzyme (ACE) inhibitors, severe hyperkalemia with dysrhythmias or cardiac arrest may occur. NSAIDs decrease the amiloride action when these drugs are given together. Salicylates decrease the diuretic action of spironolactone. Triamterene increases amantadine and cimetidine levels as a result of decreased urine elimination when given together. The drug combination of indomethacin and potassium-sparing diuretics increases the risk for acute renal failure.

Adverse Effects

Potassium-sparing diuretic adverse effects include hyperkalemia, particularly in patients who have diabetes mellitus or renal impairment. Other adverse effects include weakness, dizziness, tinnitus, confusion, depression, headache, drowsiness, insomnia, tremors, paresthesia, and photophobia. Muscle cramps, hyperglycemia, hyperuremia, impotence, blurred vision, nausea, vomiting, anorexia, diarrhea, and constipation have been reported. Unlike other diuretics, amiloride is not associated with hyperuricemia or hyperglycemia, but some association exists with triamterene and spironolactone. Other amiloride adverse effects include chest pain, palpitations, orthostatic hypotension, and dysrhythmias. Hematologic adverse effects of spironolactone and triamterene include agranulocytosis and mild acidosis, whereas amiloride may cause aplastic anemia and neutropenia.

Caution should be used for older adults and infants. Use of spironolactone is controversial during lactation because the drug label states that it is contraindicated during lactation, but the American Academy of Pediatrics considers spironolactone appropriate with breastfeeding.

Avoid concurrent use of potassium-sparing diuretics with potassium supplements or ACE inhibitors.

Caution should be used for patients who are taking digoxin or those who are at risk for hyperkalemia. Cautious use of diuretics is also advised in patients with renal or liver impairment, gout, and diabetes.

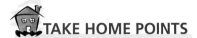

What You DO

Nursing Responsibilities

Potassium-sparing diuretics are given orally. When administering potassium-sparing diuretics, the nurse should:

- Assess for adequate intake and output.
- Evaluate initial and ongoing levels of electrolytes for hyperkalemia.
- Encourage the patient to avoid large amounts of potassium-rich foods (e.g., milk, bananas, apricots, peaches, oranges, grapefruit, cantaloupe, watermelon, tomatoes, potatoes, squash, lima beans, spinach, broccoli, avocados, nuts).
- Instruct the patient to report muscle cramps, weakness, fatigue, severe headache, dry mouth, nausea, and vomiting for early detection of electrolyte imbalances.
- Record the patient's weight and vital signs.
- Monitor uric acid levels for early detection of hyperuricemia, which may precipitate gout.
- Observe blood glucose levels in patients with diabetes who are taking potassium-sparing diuretics because hyperglycemia may require dose adjustment.
- Warn the patient to avoid tasks that require alertness or coordination until the response to the drug is known.
- Inform the patient who is taking a single daily dose to take the drug in the morning to decrease interruption of nighttime sleep.
- Advise the patient to use sun protection and limit exposure to sunlight.
- Instruct the patient to report mouth soreness, sore throat, fever, bruising, or unusual bleeding for early detection of blood dyscrasias.

Do You UNDERSTAND?

DIRECTIONS: **Indicate in the space provided whether the statement is *true* or *false*. If the answer is false, correct the statement to make it true (using the margin space).**

_____ 1. Potassium-sparing diuretics have a strong diuretic and antihypertensive effect.

_____ 2. Amiloride and triamterene have a direct effect on the distal tubules in the kidney.

_____ 3. Spironolactone compete with aldosterone for cell receptor sites in the distal tubules.

_____ 4. Potassium-sparing diuretics induce urinary excretion of sodium and increase excretion of potassium and hydrogen ions.

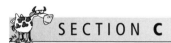

SECTION C

AGENTS USED IN RENAL FAILURE

Several drug classifications are used to maintain adequate body function in patients with renal failure. As the patient's condition deteriorates, dosage adjustments may be required. The drug classifications discussed in this section include ACE inhibitors, antianemic agents, iron and vitamin D supplements, phosphate-binding drugs, cation exchange resins, heavy metal antagonists, and systemic antacids.

What IS an ACE Inhibitor?

Action

Approximately 80% to 90% of patients with chronic renal failure have hypertension, which may be either the cause or the result of their chronic renal failure. Elevated blood pressure is usually a result of sodium and fluid overload, which leads to circulatory overload in a cyclic process,

Answers: **1. false; potassium-sparing diuretics have a mild diuretic and antihypertensive effect; 2. true; 3. true; 4. false; potassium-sparing diuretics induce urinary excretion of sodium and reduce excretion of potassium and hydrogen ions.**

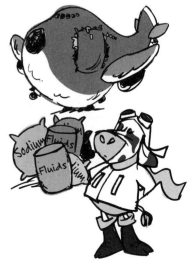

Overload!

further elevating the blood pressure. Elevated blood pressure may also be a result of a malfunction in the renin-angiotensin-aldosterone system, in which failing kidneys do not detect the increase in blood pressure and continue to produce renin. Additional renin furthers the vasoconstriction of vessels from angiotensin and reabsorption of more sodium and fluid from aldosterone stimulation, further elevating blood pressure.

Refer to page 230 for a discussion of ACE inhibitors.

What IS an Antianemic Drug?

Action

Patients who have chronic renal failure develop a decreased erythropoietin levels, which in turn results in anemia, the major hematologic abnormality of renal failure. Erythropoietin, a hormone produced primarily in the kidneys in response to hypoxia, stimulates red blood cell production. Lowered levels of erythropoietin decrease red blood cell production. Erythropoietin elevates the hematocrit of patients with anemia that is secondary to chronic renal failure.

Refer to page 85 for a discussion of the antianemic drug erythropoietin. When the hematocrit rises more than 5 points in 2 weeks, the best nursing action is to notify the health care provider and expect a dose reduction of erythropoietin.

What IS an Iron Supplement?

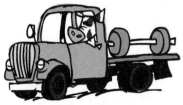

To the marrow!

Action

Iron, a mineral essential for life, is transported to the bone marrow and used in the production of hemoglobin and red blood cells. Normally, iron is absorbed from food in the small intestine and travels in the blood to the bone marrow where 60% to 70% of body iron is used to produce hemoglobin. After forming hemoglobin, iron is used for red blood cell production. After the red blood cell circulates in blood for approximately 120 days, it is destroyed and the iron is used over again.

Refer to page 619 for a discussion of iron supplements. Liquid iron preparations may stain the teeth when not taken with a straw. Iron tablets should not be crushed. Antacids decrease iron absorption. The liquid form should be adequately diluted.

What IS a Vitamin D Supplement?

Action

Vitamin D is a fat-soluble vitamin that is usually deficient in the body of a patient who has nonfunctioning kidneys. This vitamin promotes intestinal absorption of dietary calcium. Vitamin D elevates serum calcium levels, decreases phosphate and parathyroid hormone levels, and decreases bone resorption and mineralization defects, which improves bone density.

Refer to page 612 for a discussion of vitamin D.

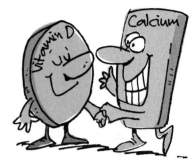

Teamwork is essential.

What IS a Phosphate-Binding Drug?

Phosphate-Binding Drugs	Trade Names	Uses
calcium acetate	Phos-Ex PhosLo	Treatment of hypocalcemia and hyperphosphatemia
calcium carbonate	Caltrate OsCal Tums	Treatment of hypocalcemia and hyperphosphatemia
aluminum hydroxide	Amphojel	Treatment of hypocalcemia and hyperphosphatemia
aluminum carbonate	Basaljel	Treatment of hypocalcemia and hyperphosphatemia

Action

Hypocalcemia resulting from hyperphosphatemia and decreased production of active vitamin D always accompanies renal insufficiency. Phosphate-binding drugs decrease serum phosphate levels, which decreases the incidence and severity of bone disease. These drugs bind with phosphorus in the GI system to form calcium or aluminum phosphate, thereby preventing absorption of dietary phosphorus.

Uses

Phosphate-binding drugs are used to prevent and treat hypocalcemia and hyperphosphatemia resulting from renal failure.

What You NEED TO KNOW

Contraindications/Precautions

Phosphate-binding drugs are contraindicated in patients who have hypersensitivity, hypercalcemia, hypophosphatemia, or ventricular fibrillation. These drugs should be used with caution in patients who are taking digoxin and in those with cardiac, respiratory, or renal disease.

Drug Interactions

Drug interactions with phosphate-binding drugs include reduced absorption of iron, thyroid hormone, salicylates, antimuscarinics, phenothiazines, anticoagulants, diazepam, isoniazid, vitamin A, tetracyclines, and fluoroquinolones. In contrast, glucocorticoids reduce the absorption of oral calcium. Thiazide diuretics decrease the excretion of calcium and may lead to hypercalcemia. Additionally, when calcium compounds are given concurrently with digoxin, the actions of each are intensified, leading to toxic effects and dysrhythmias. This drug interaction is increased particularly when calcium is administered IV.

A large intake of dietary fiber may decrease calcium absorption because of increased GI transit time and formation of calcium-fiber complexes. Calcium acetate may also increase the effects of quinidine. Foods such as rhubarb, spinach, and cereals decrease calcium absorption.

Adverse Effects

The adverse effects of phosphate-binding drugs include flatulence, diarrhea, hypercalcemia, confusion, and renal calculi. As phosphate levels decrease, calcium levels increase. Therefore in the presence of excess calcium, hypophosphatemia, aluminum toxicity, dysrhythmias, osteoporosis, and osteomalacia may occur. Rapid IV administration may lead to hypotension, bradycardia, dysrhythmias, fainting, and cardiac arrest.

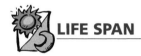

LIFE SPAN

Older patients taking calcium supplements are predisposed to constipation and fecal impaction.

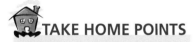

TAKE HOME POINTS

Constipation resulting from vitamin D intake can be managed with a stool softener or laxative. Aluminum hydroxide is to be avoided as a phosphate-binding drug whenever possible because aluminum accumulates in body tissues, causing aluminum toxicity.

What You DO

Nursing Responsibilities

Phosphate-binding drugs are administered orally with meals or within 20 minutes of a meal. Tablets should be chewed thoroughly before they are swallowed with water. When given in liquid form, the solution should be diluted in water or juice and thoroughly shaken. The patient should avoid taking other oral drugs, antacids, or large amounts of fiber-rich foods and drinking large amounts of alcohol or caffeine-containing beverages within 2 hours of taking phosphate-binding drugs. When administering phosphate-binding drugs, the nurse should:

- Monitor the serum calcium and phosphorus levels in the patient who is taking phosphate-binding drugs. Ideally, the calcium level is maintained between 9.0 and 10.4 mg/dL (4.5 and 5.2 mEq/L) and the phosphorus level is maintained between 3.5 and 6 mg/100 dL.
- Be aware that vitamin D is necessary for the absorption of calcium compounds.
- Monitor the patient for hypophosphatemia (e.g., anorexia, muscle weakness, malaise).
- Use aluminum drugs only as a last resort because they can accumulate in the lungs, bones, and nerve tissue.
- Observe the patient for bone disease and dementia, which may indicate aluminum toxicity.

Do You UNDERSTAND?

DIRECTIONS: Provide appropriate responses to the following questions by selecting from the italicized choices.

1. The preferred phosphate-binding drug is composed of what ingredient? _____

   (aluminum, calcium)

2. How long should the patient wait after taking a phosphate-binding drug before taking other oral drugs? _____
   _____ *(30 minutes, 2 hours)*

Answers: 1. calcium; 2. 2 hours.

What IS a Cation-Exchange Resin?

Cation-Exchange Resin	Trade Name	Use
sodium polystyrene sulfonate [pol-ee-STYE-reen]	Kayexalate	Treatment of hyperkalemia

Action

A cation-exchange resin releases sodium in exchange for other cations. Following oral administration, sodium is released from the cation-exchange resin in exchange for hydrogen ions in the acidic stomach environment. When this drug reaches the intestines, hydrogen cations are exchanged for potassium cations. Following rectal administration, sodium ions are released in exchange for other cations that are present (e.g., potassium, calcium, magnesium, iron, organic cations).

Uses

Cation-exchange resins are used in the treatment of hyperkalemia caused by excessive intake or reduced loss of potassium.

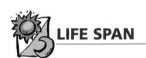

LIFE SPAN

Sodium polystyrene sulfonate should be used cautiously during pregnancy and in older adults to avoid further alterations in electrolyte balance.

What You NEED TO KNOW

Contraindications/Precautions

Sodium polystyrene sulfonate should be used with caution in patients with severe hypertension, heart failure, or marked edema and in those who are unable to tolerate an increase in sodium. Sodium polystyrene sulfonate should also be used with caution in patients who are taking digoxin.

Drug Interactions

When sodium polystyrene sulfonate is given concurrently with cation-donating antacids and laxatives (e.g., magnesium hydroxide, calcium carbonate), a drug interaction may cause metabolic alkalosis in patients with renal impairment.

Adverse Effects

The adverse effects of sodium polystyrene sulfonate include anorexia, nausea, vomiting, diarrhea, constipation, hypokalemia, hypocalcemia, hypomagnesemia, and sodium retention. Intestinal necrosis has occurred with rectal administration.

What You DO

Nursing Responsibilities

When giving cation exchange resins, the nurse should:

- Administer sodium polystyrene sulfonate orally diluted in 20 to 100 mL of fluid.
- Administer a cleansing enema, which should be retained for at least 30 to 60 minutes, prior to rectal administration of sodium polystyrene sulfonate. Following elimination of the sodium polystyrene sulfonate enema, the colon should be irrigated with 1 to 2 quarts of a nonsodium solution. A fresh solution should be prepared for each dose of cation-exchange resin.
- Monitor serum electrolyte levels, particularly sodium, potassium, calcium, and magnesium levels, in patients who are taking sodium polystyrene sulfonate.
- Observe bicarbonate levels at least once a week for early detection of metabolic alkalosis in patients taking sodium polystyrene sulfonate on a regular basis.
- Monitor serum digoxin levels when the patient is taking sodium polystyrene sulfonate and digoxin concurrently.
- Observe the patient who is taking sodium polystyrene sulfonate for confusion, irregular pulse, severe gastrointestinal distress, and constipation.

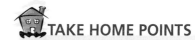

TAKE HOME POINTS

A laxative should be given in conjunction with the cation-exchange resin to facilitate passage of potassium from the body and to prevent constipation. Hypokalemia predisposes a patient to digoxin toxicity when taken concurrently with sodium polystyrene sulfonate.

Do You UNDERSTAND?

DIRECTIONS: **Provide appropriate responses to the following questions.**

1. Which two administration routes are used to administer sodium polystyrene sulfonate? _____

_____

2. The nurse should monitor which electrolytes when sodium polystyrene sulfonate is used? _____, _____, _____, and _____.

What IS a Heavy Metal Antagonist?

Heavy Metal Antagonist	Trade Name	Use
deferoxamine [de-fer-OX-a-meen]	Desferal	Treatment of aluminum toxicity in renal failure

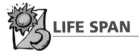

Action

The heavy metal antagonist deferoxamine mesylate chelates iron or aluminum by enclosing the metal and rendering it nonactive and nontoxic. One gram of deferoxamine mesylate is capable of sequestering 85 mg of iron. This action is pH-dependent and is more rapid in an acid pH compared with alkaline pH.

Uses

Deferoxamine is used to treat patients with chronic iron overloads and acute iron or aluminum toxicity.

Deferoxamine encloses the metal, rendering it nontoxic.

LIFE SPAN

Deferoxamine is contraindicated during pregnancy and for children less than 3 years of age.

What You NEED TO KNOW

Contraindications/Precautions

Deferoxamine is contraindicated for patients with severe renal disease or anuria. Caution should be used in the presence of a low ferritin level.

Answers: 1. oral, rectal enema; 2. sodium, potassium, calcium, magnesium.

Drug Interactions

The combination of deferoxamine and ascorbic acid intake may increase the risk for cardiac dysfunction in patients with severe iron overload. Prochlorperazine in combination with deferoxamine may lead to temporary impairment of consciousness. The mechanism of this interaction is unknown.

Adverse Effects

The common adverse effects of deferoxamine include red urine, flushing, urticaria, hypotension, injection site reactions, rash, arthralgia and myalgias, fever, headache, and malaise. Nausea and vomiting, abdominal pain, diarrhea, tachycardia, leg cramps, dizziness, visual disturbances, and tinnitus with hearing impairment have also been reported. Severe adverse effects include anaphylactoid reactions, angioedema, seizures (with iron overload), acute respiratory distress syndrome (ARDS), dialysis encephalopathy and hyperparathyroidism (with aluminum overload), growth retardation (with high dosages), and vision and hearing loss. Adverse effects usually occur with rapid IV infusions.

> ⚠ Deferoxamine should be given cautiously to patients with severe renal disease, low serum ferritin levels, and aluminum overload.

What You DO

Nursing Responsibilities

When administering heavy metal antagonists, the nurse should:
- Reconstitute the drug following package instructions. For IV use, the drug may be added to 0.9% sodium chloride, D_5W, or lactated Ringer's solution.
- Avoid storing solutions that are reconstituted with sterile water at room temperature for longer than 1 week.
- Monitor the patient's vital signs throughout administration.
- Teach the patient who is taking deferoxamine to have ophthalmic and otic examinations every 3 months. When ophthalmic or otic toxicities have developed, the dosage should be temporarily reduced or the drug discontinued.
- Warn patients who are taking deferoxamine that their urine will turn a characteristic reddish color.

Do You UNDERSTAND?

DIRECTIONS: Fill in the blanks with the appropriate response.

1. What two types of examinations should a patient have when taking deferoxamine?

   _____

2. What warning should the nurse give the patient taking deferoxamine about the urine?

   _____

What IS a Systemic Antacid?

Systemic Antacids	Trade Names	Uses
sodium bicarbonate [bye-CAR-bon-ayt]	Citrocarbonate	Correction of metabolic acidosis
sodium citrate [SIH-trate]	Bicitra	Correction of metabolic acidosis

Action

Systemic antacids buffer excess hydrogen ions and elevate blood pH, which reverses acidosis. As renal failure progresses, acid retention increases. The resulting metabolic acidosis requires alkali replacement to neutralize or counteract the acidosis.

Uses

Systemic antacids are used as alkalizing drugs to prevent and treat metabolic acidosis resulting from renal failure. Sodium bicarbonate and sodium citrate are equally effective in treating chronic acidosis and are given orally. Because citrate enhances absorption of toxic elements, including aluminum and sodium bicarbonate, it is the preferred drug.

Answers: 1. ophthalmic, otic; 2. the urine will turn reddish color.

What You NEED TO KNOW

Contraindications/Precautions

Sodium bicarbonate is contraindicated for patients with hypertension, heart disease, and peptic ulcer and those who are losing chlorides because of vomiting, diuresing, or through gastrointestinal suction.

Drug Interactions

Drug interactions with sodium bicarbonate include increased effects of anorexiants and sympathomimetics. There is an increased duration of action when sodium bicarbonate is given concurrently with amphetamines and ephedrine. Drugs that have decreased effects when given in combination with sodium bicarbonate include lithium, salicylates, tetracyclines, and sulfonylureas.

Adverse Effects

Adverse effects of systemic antacids include flatulence, gastric distention, electrolyte imbalance, metabolic alkalosis, sodium and fluid retention, dehydration, renal calculi, and milk-alkali syndrome. Because an increase in serum pH causes potassium to move into the cell from the extracellular fluids, hypokalemia may result. Severe tissue damage may follow infiltration of IV site. Rapid IV administration in neonates may cause hypernatremia, decreased cerebral spinal fluid pressure, and intracranial hemorrhage. Overtreatment of acidosis causes alkalosis, the evidence of which includes decreased consciousness from hypernatremia, tetany from hypocalcemia, dysrhythmias from hypokalemia, and seizures.

> ⚠ Sodium bicarbonate is contraindicated during pregnancy. Sodium bicarbonate is to be used cautiously in older adults and in patients with edema or who have sodium-retaining disorders.

What You DO

Nursing Responsibilities

When administering systemic antacids, the nurse should:

- Use a patent IV line to avoid extravasation of the drug into surrounding tissues
- Monitor serum electrolytes, carbon dioxide, arterial pH, and vital signs to determine the effectiveness of systemic antacid therapy and to monitor for complications of therapy.

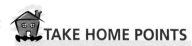

TAKE HOME POINTS

When sodium bicarbonate is given IV, the rate of administration should not exceed 50 mEq/hr.

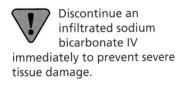
Discontinue an infiltrated sodium bicarbonate IV immediately to prevent severe tissue damage.

- Monitor cardiac rhythm carefully when the patient is receiving IV administration of systemic antacids.
- Instruct the patient who is taking long-term sodium bicarbonate that milk-alkali syndrome is likely to occur, the symptoms of which include headache, mental confusion, anorexia, nausea, vomiting, soft-tissue calcification, hypercalcemia, hypophosphatemia, renal and ureteral calculi, and metabolic alkalosis.

Do You UNDERSTAND?

DIRECTIONS: **Indicate in the space provided whether the statement is *true* or *false*. If the answer is false, correct the statement to make it true (using the margin space).**

_____ 1. The actions of lithium and tetracyclines are increased when given concurrently with sodium bicarbonate.

_____ 2. Administration of IV sodium bicarbonate should not exceed 50 mEq/hr.

References

Arcangelo VP: *Pharmacotherapeutics for advanced practice: a practical approach,* Philadelphia, 2001, Lippincott.

Black JM, Hawks JH: *Medical-surgical nursing: clinical management for positive outcomes,* ed 7, St Louis, 2005, Elsevier.

Gutierrez K, Queener S: *Pharmacology for nursing practice,* Philadelphia, 2004, Mosby.

Hardman JG, Limbird LE: *Goodman & Gilman's the pharmacological basis of therapeutics,* ed 10, New York, 2001, McGraw-Hill.

Johnson PH, editor: *Nurse practitioner's drug handbook,* ed 3, Springhouse, Pa, 2000, Springhouse.

Karch AM: *Focus on nursing pharmacology,* ed 3, Philadelphia, 2006, Lippincott.

Kee JL, Hayes ER, McCuistion LE: *Pharmacology: a nursing process approach,* ed 5, Philadelphia, 2006, Elsevier.

Khan MG: *Cardiac drug therapy,* ed 5, Philadelphia, 2000, WB Saunders.

Lehne R: *Pharmacology for nursing care,* ed 5, Philadelphia, 2004, WB Saunders.

Lewis SM, Heitkemper MM, Dirksen SR: *Medical-surgical nursing: assessment and management of clinical problems,* ed 6, St Louis, 2004, Mosby.

Answers: 1. false; the actions are decreased. 2. true.

Lilley L, Harrington S, Snyder J: *Pharmacology and the nursing process,* ed 4, St Louis, 2005, Mosby.

McCance K, Huether S: *Pathophysiology: the biologic basis for disease in adults and children,* ed 4, St Louis, 2002, Mosby.

McKenry LM, Salerno E: *Mosby's pharmacology in nursing,* ed 21, St Louis, 2003, Mosby.

Opie LH, Gersh BJ: *Drugs for the heart,* ed 6, Philadelphia, 2005, WB Saunders.

Smeltzer SC, Bare BG: *Brunner and Suddarth's textbook of medical-surgical nursing,* ed 10, Philadelphia, 2004, Lippincott.

Wilson BA, Shannon MT, Stang CL: *Nurses drug guide,* Upper Saddle River, New Jersey, 2006, Pearson.

NCLEX® Review

Section A

1. Adverse effects may occur following nitrofurantoin administration. These adverse effects include which of the following?
   1 Hemolytic anemia
   2 Extrapyramidal symptoms
   3 Stevens-Johnson syndrome
   4 Pseudomembranous enterocolitis

2. Which of the following is a life-threatening adverse effect of ofloxacin?
   1 Urticaria
   2 Agranulocytosis
   3 Seizures
   4 Dystonia

3. Which of the following is a common effect of phenazopyridine?
   1 CNS depression
   2 Increased seizure activity
   3 Orange-red urine
   4 Lens opacity

4. Oxybutynin and tolterodine are contraindicated in which of the following conditions?
   1 Hypertension
   2 Dysphonia
   3 Paraplegia
   4 Bowel obstruction

Section B

5. The diuretic action of spironolactone may be decreased when given with:
   1 aspirin.
   2 verapamil.
   3 amphotericin B.
   4 metolazone.

6. The nurse knows that the direct action of loop diuretics is in the:
   1 proximal tubule.
   2 distal tubule.
   3 ascending loop of Henle.
   4 descending loop of Henle.

7. A patient is taking furosemide (Lasix) and has a serum potassium level of 4.2. Which symptoms should the nurse monitor for in this patient?
   1 Hypotension and hyperkalemia
   2 Drowsiness and muscle flaccidity
   3 Hyperglycemia and hyperuricemia
   4 Diarrhea and hypertensive crisis

8. Which drug reduces potassium excretion while still decreasing edema?
   1 Metolazone
   2 Bumetanide
   3 Spironolactone
   4 Hydrochlorothiazide

9. Metolazone is contraindicated in patients who have:
   1 diabetes mellitus.
   2 renal dysfunction.
   3 congestive heart failure.
   4 concurrent blood administration

Section C

10. When the hematocrit level rises 5 points in 2 weeks for a patient who is taking erythropoietin, which of the following is the nurse's best course of action?
    1 Continue to monitor hematocrit levels daily.
    2 Call the health care provider and expect a dose reduction.
    3 Change the frequency of monitoring the hematocrit to every month.
    4 Take no action because a rise in hematocrit is the expected action of this drug.

11. Which of the following is true about iron supplements?
    1 Iron tablets may be crushed.
    2 Antacids increase iron absorption.
    3 Liquid forms should be given undiluted for greater efficacy.
    4 Liquid forms may stain teeth when not taken with a straw.

12. Which of the following is a major adverse effect of phosphate-binding drug such as calcitriol?
    1 Hypocalcemia
    2 Hypercalcemia
    3 Anemia
    4 Hypotension

13. Cation-exchange resins are used in which of the following conditions?
    1 Hypocalcemia
    2 Hypercalcemia
    3 Hypokalemia
    4 Hyperkalemia

14. Which of the following characteristics is true for systemic antacids?
    1 Systemic antacids are not absorbed well in the GI tract.
    2 Systemic antacids are used in the treatment of metabolic alkalosis.
    3 Systemic antacids are commonly found to decrease anorexiant effects when given concurrently.
    4 Systemic antacids are apt to lead to milk-alkali syndrome when given long-term.

NCLEX® Review Answers

Section A

1. 1 Hemolytic anemia is an adverse effect of nitrofurantoin. Extrapyramidal symptoms, Stevens-Johnson syndrome, and pseudomembranous enterocolitis are not adverse effects of nitrofurantoin.

2. 2 Agranulocytosis is a life-threatening adverse effect of ofloxacin. Urticaria, seizures, and dystonia are neither life-threatening nor adverse effects of ofloxacin.

3. 3 Orange-red urine is a common, distinctive effect of phenazopyridine use. Phenazopyridine does not cause CNS depression, an increase in seizures, or lens opacity.

4. 4 Oxybutynin and tolterodine are contraindicated in patients with bowel obstruction. Neither oxybutynin nor tolterodine is contraindicated in patients with hypertension, dysphonia, or paraplegia.

Section B

5. 1 The diuretic action of spironolactone is decreased when given concurrently with aspirin. There is no known drug interaction with verapamil, amphotericin B, or metolazone.

6. 3 The direct action of loop diuretics occurs primarily in the ascending loop of Henle. Thiazide and thiazide-like diuretics act primarily on the distal collecting tubules. Potassium-sparing diuretics have a direct action on the distal tubules.

7. 3 Furosemide is a loop diuretic, and 4.2 is a normal potassium level. Adverse effects for the nurse to monitor include hyperglycemia, hyperuricemia, hypokalemia, hypotension, muscle spasms, and constipation.

8. 3 Spironolactone reduces the excretion of potassium and reduces edema. Loop diuretics (e.g., bumetanide) and thiazide diuretics (e.g., metolazone, hydrochlorothiazide) promote potassium excretion.

9. 4 Metolazone is contraindicated for individuals with hypokalemia, anuria, and concurrent blood administration.

Section C

10. 2 When the hematocrit rises more than 5 points in 2 weeks, the best nursing action is to notify the health care provider and expect a dose reduction of epoetin alfa. When the hematocrit has not risen 5 points in 2 weeks and remains below the target range, the nurse should notify the health care provider and expect a dose increase. Monitoring hematocrit levels daily and every month are incorrect because frequent monitoring is considered to be twice weekly. Doing nothing because a rise in hematocrit is expected is incorrect because a rapid elevation of hematocrit may lead to seizures.

11. 4 Liquid iron preparations may stain the teeth when not taken with a straw. Iron tablets should not be crushed. Antacids decrease iron absorption. The liquid form should be adequately diluted.

12. 2 The primary adverse effect of phosphate binding drugs is hypercalcemia. Evidence includes headache, irritability, dizziness, tinnitus, metallic taste, GI distress, and weakness. Calcitriol is a vitamin D supplement that promotes absorption of calcium. Hypocalcemia is incorrect because the most common major adverse effect is hypercalcemia. Anemia is incorrect because it is a subsequent effect of hypercalcemia. Hypotension is incorrect because calcitriol does not appear to affect blood pressure.

13. 4 Cation-exchange resins act by releasing sodium in exchange for hydrogen ions in the acidic stomach environment. Hydrogen ion is exchanged for potassium ion in the colon to be eliminated in feces. Cation-exchange resins are therefore used in hyperkalemia to reduce high potassium levels; thus hypocalcemia, hypercalcemia, and hypokalemia are incorrect.

14. 4 Systemic antacids may lead to milk-alkali syndrome. Systemic antacids are thoroughly absorbed. Antacids are used to treat metabolic acidosis. Antacids increase the duration of anorexiant action when given concurrently.

Drugs Used to Treat Reproductive System Alterations

Estrogen, progestins, and androgens can be replaced with synthetic substitutions, alone or in combination. The goal of replacement hormones is to perform the function of naturally produced hormones and to treat certain medical conditions.

What You WILL LEARN

After reading this chapter, you will know how to do the following:

- ✔ Compare estrogens with progestins regarding their pharmacodynamics.
- ✔ Recall the indications of estrogen-based drugs.
- ✔ Explain the life-threatening adverse effects associated with estrogen therapy.
- ✔ Compare androgen drugs with estrogens and progestins.
- ✔ Identify the indications and adverse effects for patients taking an androgen drug.
- ✔ Discuss the role of uterine motility drugs during pregnancy and the related nursing responsibilities.

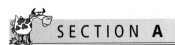

SECTION A

MALE AND FEMALE HORMONES

What IS an Estrogen Drug?

Noncontraceptive Estrogens	Trade Names	Uses
conjugated estrogens [ESS-troh-jenz]	Premarin	Reduces menopausal symptoms; prevents osteoporosis
estradiol [ess-trah-DYE-ohl]	Estraderm	Reduces menopausal symptoms; prevents osteoporosis

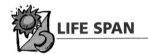

LIFE SPAN

Estrogen assists in retaining bone mass in postmenopausal women.

Action

Estrogen is a hormone that produces several physiologic actions. These actions involve developmental changes, suppression of androgen production, and alteration in mineral, carbohydrate, protein, and lipid metabolism. Estrogens, similar to other hormones, are thought to act primarily through gene expression. The hormones pass through the cellular membrane to bind with a receptor in the nucleus. Estrogen receptors are present in the female reproductive system, breasts, pituitary gland, hypothalamus, bone, and liver, as well as in numerous tissues in males. Estrogen also promotes the development of the uterine lining.

Estrogen blocks bone resorption while promoting the accumulation of minerals in bones. Estrogen decreases the low-density lipoprotein (LDL) and increases the high-density lipoprotein (HDL) cholesterol levels, thereby altering lipid metabolism. This factor is protective in nature because elevated LDL and decreased HDL levels predispose the patient to coronary artery disease (CAD) and resultant myocardial infarction (MI).

Uses

Estrogens are most commonly used as hormone replacement therapy (HRT) in postmenopausal women to decrease menopausal symptoms. HRT is usually lifelong for suppressing vasomotor symptoms (e.g., hot flashes, sweating) and for preventing urogenital atrophy (e.g., vaginal dryness), osteoporosis, and CAD. However, in recent years there is a recommendation that estrogens be taken for a period of 5 years at the lowest dosage possible that will treat menopausal symptoms.

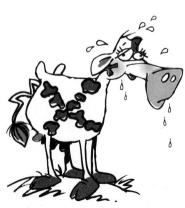

Estrogens can help.

HRT is also used to treat primary ovarian failure, hypermenorrhea, endometriosis, developmental delay or hypogonadism, and acne in adults. Because the growth of prostate cancer depends on the androgen hormone, the use of estrogen to suppress androgen provides a useful treatment for prostate cancer.

What You NEED TO KNOW

Contraindications/Precautions

Estrogen is contraindicated during pregnancy, unsuccessful abortions, and lactation, as well as for adolescents who have incomplete epiphyseal closure. Estrogen should be used with caution in multiparous women with irregular menses.

Estrogen is also contraindicated for patients with a history of thrombophlebitis, peripheral vascular disorders, thromboembolic disorders, breast or endometrial cancer, undiagnosed genital bleeding, cystic mastitis, cerebral vascular accident (CVA), CAD, MI, and hepatic dysfunction.

Cautious use of estrogen is necessary in patients who have depression, renal disease, hypertension, migraines, seizures, asthma, diabetes mellitus, obesity, gallbladder disease, systemic lupus erythematosus (SLE), and those who are heavy smokers (more than 15 cigarettes per day).

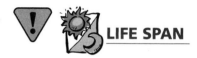

LIFE SPAN

Prolonged estrogen therapy in postmenopausal women may lead to an increased risk for uterine cancer. Excessive uterine development from estrogen may lead to uterine hyperplasia (excessive tissue growth) with prolonged exposure to estrogen alone.

Drug Interactions

Carbamazepine, barbiturates, and rifampin decrease estrogen effectiveness when taken concurrently. Estrogen can increase the effects of corticosteroids and hepatotoxic drugs such as dantrolene. The risk for cyclosporin toxicity increases when taken with estrogen. Concurrent use of estrogen therapy and an anticoagulant may cause a decrease in anticoagulation effects. Estrogen may interfere with the action of tamoxifen. Estrogen may increase caffeine levels when taken together. Estrogen may also increase cardiovascular adverse effects in smokers.

Adverse Effects

Common adverse effects of estrogen therapy involving gastrointestinal (GI) distress (e.g., nausea, vomiting, and abdominal cramps) usually decrease within 2 to 3 months with continued use. Low-dosage estrogen therapy reduces the risk for GI distress.

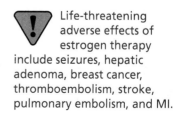

Life-threatening adverse effects of estrogen therapy include seizures, hepatic adenoma, breast cancer, thromboembolism, stroke, pulmonary embolism, and MI.

Adverse central nervous system (CNS) and cardiovascular effects include headache, dizziness, muscular twitching (chorea), depression, thrombophlebitis, hypertension, fluid retention, and weight gain. Worsening of myopia or astigmatism and intolerance to contact lenses has been reported.

Amenorrhea, cervical erosion, enlargement of uterine fibromas, vaginal candidiasis, nipple discharge, and changes in libido have occurred with estrogen. Edema, gynecomastia, testicular atrophy, and reversible impotence may occur in men.

When deprived of estrogen, the endometrium will bleed within 48 to 72 hours. Hypomenorrhea, midcycle breakthrough bleeding, and increased spotting are adverse effects of estrogen deficiency. The adverse effects of excess estrogen include nausea, vomiting, bloating, diarrhea, dysmenorrhea, brown skin discoloration (**melasma**), polyps, hypertension, migraines, breast fullness, and tenderness.

Other adverse effects include anorexia, increased appetite, jaundice, hyperglycemia, reduced carbohydrate tolerance, leg cramps, hair loss, urticaria, red nodules on the legs (erythema nodosum), dermatitis, colitis, acute pancreatitis, excessive thirst, and hypercalcemia.

What You DO

Nursing Responsibilities

The patient should have a thorough physical examination before estrogen therapy is initiated; including a Papanicolaou (Pap) smear when appropriate. Estrogen therapy may be administered orally, intramuscularly (IM), intravenously (IV), intravaginally, and as a transdermal patch. HRT may be given in a continuous-dosage regimen with the same dose every day, or on a cyclic schedule. With the cyclic schedule, the estrogen is taken for 21 days and stopped for 7 days. The discontinuation of estrogen will lead to menstrual bleeding. When administering estrogens, the nurse should:

- Instruct the patient to apply the transdermal patch to a clean, dry area on the body trunk. Tell the patient that if the patch falls off, to reapply it and return to the original treatment schedule.
- Teach the patient to rotate transdermal application sites and allow 1 week before reapplication to the previous site to avoid skin irritation.

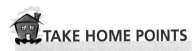

TAKE HOME POINTS

Avoid transdermal application on irritated skin or those areas with excessive oil production, such as the breast and waistline.

- Keep estrogen tablets in a dry container that is protected from light. Counsel the patient who is experiencing nausea to take estrogen with or immediately following solid food.
- Encourage the patient to avoid caffeine intake and smoking to reduce the risk for thromboembolism or an MI.
- Monitor the patient's weight and blood pressure for early detection of fluid retention, weight gain, and hypertension.
- Instruct the patient to direct the vaginal applicator of intravaginal estrogen back toward the sacrum when it is inserted.
- Suggest that the patient void before inserting the drug in the vagina to avoid having to ambulate after the medication is inserted.
- Instruct the patient to wash the hands before and after administration and report signs of irritation, such as redness, swelling, or excoriated skin in the perineal area.
- Teach the patient the breast self-examination technique for early detection of breast cancer and to keep appointments for annual mammograms after the age of 40 to 45.
- Monitor blood glucose levels regularly in patients with diabetes who are taking estrogen, because hyperglycemia may occur.
- Observe hepatic function and serum lipid levels for early detection of dysfunction.
- Teach patients the importance of ambulation and exercise to reduce vascular complications.
- Inform the patient that estrogen therapy should be stopped 4 weeks before procedures associated with prolonged immobilization (e.g., hip or knee replacement).
- Advise the patient to report immediately a suspected pregnancy, intermittent vaginal bleeding or discharge, unexplained or sudden abdominal pain, numbness, stiffness in legs, shortness of breath, chest pain or pressure, visual changes, flashing lights, severe headaches, vaginal bleeding or discharge, breast changes, swelling of extremities, yellow skin or sclera, dark urine, and light-colored stools.
- Reassure male patients who are taking estrogen therapy that impotence and estrogen-induced female characteristics will disappear after treatment is discontinued.

Do You UNDERSTAND?

DIRECTIONS: Complete the following statements with the appropriate terms from the italicized list provided.

1. Estrogen therapy is _____ for patients with a negative pregnancy test.

2. Estrogen therapy is _____ for patients with a history of thrombophlebitis.

3. Estrogen therapy with anticoagulants may cause a decrease in _____.

unknown   *indicated*   *contraindicated*
anticoagulation   *coagulation*

What IS a Progestin Drug?

Progestins	Trade Names	Uses
progesterone [proh-JESS-ter-one]	Progestasert	Treatment of amenorrhea or dysfunctional uterine bleeding
norethindrone [nor-eth-IN-drone]	Norlutin	Treatment of amenorrhea or dysfunctional uterine bleeding
medroxyprogesterone acetate [meh-DROX-ee-proh-JESS-ter-one]	Provera	Treatment of amenorrhea or dysfunctional uterine bleeding
norethindrone [nor-eth-IN-drone]	Micronor	Birth control; treatment of amenorrhea and endometriosis
norgestrel [nor-JESS-trell]	Ovrette	Birth control

Action

Progesterone is a steroid hormone synthesized and released in the testes, ovary, adrenal cortex, and placenta. This hormone maintains uterine development in the second half of the menstrual cycle, preparing it for implantation.

Progestins suppress the secretion of luteinizing hormone (LH), thereby controlling ovulation. With the suppression of LH, ovulation cannot occur, even with full develop rom implanting in the uterus and promotes the production of thick endometrial secretions. The thickened mucus of the cervix causes increased difficulty for the sperm to migrate and a less favorable uterine environment for egg implantation. Ultimately, these changes block ovulation and follicular maturation.

Similar to estrogens, progestins produce developmental changes and alterations in mineral, carbohydrate, protein, and lipid metabolism. Progestin also opposes estrogen-mediated uterine proliferation and reverses hyperplasia.

Uses

Progestin is used in the treatment of amenorrhea, dysfunctional uterine bleeding, cancer, endometriosis, and premenstrual syndrome. This drug is used as a progestin-only type of oral contraceptive, known as the "mini-pill." Progestin is also used to treat infertile women who have progestin deficiency. Progestin is usually given for 6 to 8 days to treat amenorrhea and given for 10 days to treat dysfunctional uterine bleeding.

What You NEED TO KNOW

Contraindications/Precautions

Progestins are contraindicated in patients with hypersensitivity, thrombophlebitis, vascular disorders, thromboembolism, stroke, or liver disease, as well as during pregnancy and lactation. Progestins are contraindicated in patients who have allergies to peanuts (the drug contains peanut oil) and in patients with undiagnosed vaginal bleeding, breast or genital malignancy, and unsuccessful abortion.

Drug Interactions

No drug interactions have been clinically reported.

Adverse Effects

Common adverse effects of progestins include dizziness, nausea, vomiting, abdominal cramps, breakthrough bleeding, and edema. Other adverse effects include migraines, somnolence, insomnia, hepatic disease, cholestatic jaundice, and hyperglycemia. Decreased libido, transient increase in sodium and chloride excretion, fever, itching, rash, urticaria, photosensitivity, hirsutism, alopecia, and pain at the injection site have also been reported.

When progestins are given within the first 4 months of pregnancy, birth defects (teratogenic effects) may occur.

Progestins should be used with caution for women who have had an abnormal Papanicolaou (pap) smear, as well as those with genital bleeding of unknown origin, previous ectopic pregnancy, sexually transmitted diseases, and previous pelvic surgery.

Progestins should be used cautiously in patients with anemia, diabetes mellitus, depression, suspected acute porphyria, salpingitis, and liver disease, as well as conditions in which fluid retention is a factor.

Life-threatening adverse effects include thrombolytic disorders and pulmonary embolism.

Gynecologic adverse effects include gynecomastia, galactorrhea, vaginal candidiasis, brown skin discoloration, vaginal dryness, cervical erosion, dysmenorrhea, and amenorrhea. Downward displacement of the eye, diplopia, papilledema, and retinal vascular lesions have been reported with progestin therapy.

Late menstrual cycle bleeding and amenorrhea are adverse effects of progestin deficiency. Hypomenorrhea, breast regression, vaginal candidiasis, depression, fatigue, weight gain, increased appetite, acne, oily scalp, hair loss are adverse effects of excess progestin.

What You DO

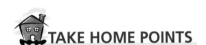

TAKE HOME POINTS

Inform the patient to expect withdrawal bleeding 48 to 72 hours after the dose and that bleeding ordinarily stops by the sixth day.

Nursing Responsibilities

Progestin may be administered orally, IM, intravaginally, and as a transdermal formulation. Progestin crystals may require dissolving in a vial under warm water before they are drawn into a syringe for IM injection. When administering progestins, the nurse should:

- Instruct the patient to have a thorough physical examination with a breast exam, Pap smear, and hematocrit level before progestin therapy is initiated and annually thereafter.
- Inform the patient to use an alternative form of birth control during the first 3 months to prevent contraception. Advise the patient who is undergoing progestin therapy to report suspected pregnancy immediately.
- Monitor the patient's blood pressure, weight, and intake and output for early detection of adverse effects.
- Monitor blood sugar levels regularly of the patient with diabetes.
- Monitor liver function studies. Because progestins affect the results of these tests, the results should not be considered definitive until the patient has stopped the therapy and waited at least 60 days.
- Inject IM formulations of progestin deeply into the tissues to avoid skin irritation. The administration sites should be rotated.
- Advise the patient who is undergoing progestin therapy to keep annual physical examination appointments.
- Advise the patient who is using the intrauterine progesterone contraceptive system (Progestasert) to expect spotting, cramping, and discomfort during the first 3 months.

- Encourage the patient to return to the health care provider to assess the efficacy and placement of the Progestasert device within 3 months of initial placement.
- Instruct the patient to check for the presence of the Progestasert threads on a regular basis to ensure placement, and warn the patient that pulling on the threads for any reason will harm the uterus.
- Warn the patient to expect a slightly heavier menstruation while the Progestasert device is in place.
- Warn the patient to avoid exposure to ultraviolet light, which may cause a severe photosensitive reaction or exaggerated sunburn.
- Advise the patient to use sunscreen as necessary.
- Instruct the patient who is taking progestins to report fever, acute pelvic pain, and unusual bleeding to the health care provider immediately for early detection of infection.

Do You UNDERSTAND?

DIRECTIONS: Indicate in the space provided whether the statement is *true* or *false*. If the answer is false, correct the statement to make it true (using the margin space).

_____ 1. Progestin is used for treat secondary amenorrhea, dysfunctional uterine bleeding, endometriosis, premenstrual syndrome, menopausal symptoms, and infertility in women with progestin deficiency.

_____ 2. Progesterone is a steroid hormone synthesized and released in the testes, ovary, adrenal cortex, and placenta.

_____ 3. Progestin is an intrauterine drug that also provides fertility control.

_____ 4. Progestin is a hormone that increases LH secretion.

Answers: 1. true; 2. true; 3. true; 4. false, progestin suppresses LH secretion.

What IS Combination Estrogen and Progestin?

Estrogen and Progestin Combinations	Trade Names	Uses
Hormone replacement therapy conjugated estrogens/ medroxyprogesterone acetate	Prempro	Treatment of menopausal symptoms
estradiol/norgestimate	Ortho-Prefest	Treatment of menopausal symptoms
Oral contraceptives ethinyl estradiol/levonorgestrel (monophasic)	Alesse	Prevention of pregnancy
ethinyl estradiol/norethindrone (biphasic 10/11)	Ortho-Novum 10/11	Prevention of pregnancy
ethinyl estradiol/norethindrone (triphasic 7/7/7)	Ortho-Novum 7/7/7	Prevention of pregnancy

Action

Estrogen and progestins control ovulation, the cyclical preparation of fertilization, and implantation. Estrogen reduces the release of the follicle-stimulating hormone (FSH) from the pituitary gland, thereby blocking follicle development. In turn, the ovum is less likely to travel through the fallopian tube to the uterus. Estrogen also inhibits contraception through a negative feedback system with the hypothalamus and pituitary gland.

Progestin in combination with estrogen promotes mammary gland development without causing lactation and increases body temperature during ovulation. A sudden decrease in progestin and estrogen levels causes bleeding.

Uses

Estrogen and progesterone are widely prescribed drugs, alone or in combination. The combination is most commonly prescribed for contraception measures and HRT in postmenopausal women to reduce menopausal symptoms. Estrogen and progesterone are also used to treat developmental delay or hypogonadism, primary ovarian failure, postcoital contraception, and acne in adults. The progestin portion of this drug combination is present to protect the patient against estrogen-induced uterine cancer.

What You NEED TO KNOW

Contraindications/Precautions

The contraindications and precautions are the same as those that are listed for estrogen and progestin in the previous discussion.

Drug Interactions

The drug interactions are the same as those listed above for estrogen and progestin. When used for contraception, estrogen also interacts with aminocaproic acid, barbiturates, anticonvulsants, antibiotics, and anti-fungals, causing an increase incidence of breakthrough bleeding and risk for pregnancy.

Adverse Effects

Estrogen therapy alone in women who have an intact uterus may lead to uterine cancer. When progestin is given in combination with estrogen, little or no risk for uterine cancer is present. However, the risk for breast cancer increases as a result of the addition of progestin. Women who are without a uterus may take estrogen alone with a 1% risk for breast cancer. Women with a uterus who are taking estrogen-progestin combination drugs increase the risk for breast cancer to 8%. Other adverse effects are the same as those listed for estrogen and progestin.

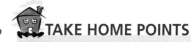

TAKE HOME POINTS

The risk for ovulation, spotting, bleeding, and pregnancy increases with each contraceptive pill not taken.

What You DO

Nursing Responsibilities

There are three basic regimens for combination estrogen and progestin drugs. *Monophasic* formulations have a fixed dose of estrogen-progestin, which remains constant throughout the menstrual cycle. *Biphasic* formulations have a constant amount of estrogen throughout the month, but the progestin dosage increases as the cycle progresses. *Triphasic* formulations have a varied amount of estrogen in two phases and varied amounts of progestin in three phases of the menstrual cycle.

HRT may be administered as one of five different regimens: (1) Continuous dosing provides a continuous dose of estrogen and progestin every day of the month. (2) Continuous sequential dosing provides for daily estrogen with the progestin taken only during the first 14 days of the cycle. (3) Cyclical sequential dosing provides for daily estrogen on days 1-25 and the progestin on days 1-25 or days 13-25. (4) Cyclical combined dosing means that both the combination estrogen and progestin are administered on days 1 through 25 only. (5) Women without a uterus may take only the estrogen component of HRT every day of the month. In addition to the nursing responsibilities that have been mentioned for estrogen and progestins, the nurse should:

- Instruct the patient to use an alternative form of birth control during the first 3 months to prevent contraception.
- Instruct the patient to wait 24 hours between doses when using contraceptive therapy.
- Tell the patient to take a missed dose as soon as possible or to take two tablets the next day. When two doses are missed, two tablets should be taken for the next 2 days; when three tablets are missed, the patient should start a new monthly cycle of tablets starting 7 days after the last tablet was taken.
- Instruct the patient that additional forms of birth control are recommended for a week after two missed doses or for 14 days after three missed doses.
- Inform the patient that when she does not experience ovulation within two cycles, pregnancy should be ruled out before continuing therapy.
- Warn the patient that after discontinuation of oral contraceptives, 1 to 3 months may pass before normal menstruation resumes.
- Advise the patient who is nursing to use an alternative form of birth control. When the mother is not nursing, oral contraception may be started immediately following the birth of the child.
- Inform the patient that she may experience spotting, cramping, and discomfort during the first 3 months of intrauterine progesterone contraception.
- Instruct the patient to discontinue HRT and start a new cycle after 5 days if she experiences intracyclic bleeding that resembles menstruation. Notify the health care provider if the problem persists for the early detection of endometrial cancer.
- Explain to the patient who is on cyclic HRT therapy that withdrawal bleeding may occur during the time the patient is not taking the drug, but that pregnancy cannot occur when fertility is not restored.

Do You UNDERSTAND?

DIRECTIONS: Provide appropriate responses for the following statements and questions.

1. When progestin is given with estrogen, what cancer risk is reduced?
   _____

2. When progestin is given with estrogen, what cancer risk is increased?
   _____

3. List the three basic contraceptive formulations: _____,
   _____, and _____.

4. List four HRT regimens: _____, _____,
   _____, and _____.

What IS an Androgen?

Androgens	Trade Names	Uses
danazol [DAN-ah-zole]	Cyclomen	Treatment of endometriosis and fibrocystic breast disease
nandrolone [NAN-droh-lone]	Durabolin	Treatment of metastatic breast cancer
testosterone [tess-TOSS-ter-one]	Testoderm	Treatment of delayed puberty and male hypogonadism

Action

An androgen is a steroid hormone that suppresses the pituitary output of FSH and LH, causing anovulation and amenorrhea. Testosterone, the male sex hormone, is the principle testicular androgen. In women, the ovary and adrenal gland produce minimal amounts of testosterone. Testosterone production is dependent on an intact hypothalamus, pituitary gland, and Leydig's cells in the testis.

Testosterone produces both androgenic and anabolic effects by binding to androgen receptors in skeletal muscle, the prostate gland, and the bone marrow. In some tissues, testosterone is initially converted to dihydrotestosterone in order to permit binding with androgen receptors.

Testosterone esters can cause an increase in plasma concentrations of estrogens; thus feminizing effects are observed. Androgens cause atrophy and interruption of normal and ectopic endometrial tissue, thereby stopping endometriosis.

Uses

Androgen therapy is most commonly used for male hypogonadism. The replacement of the androgen or testosterone will encourage all testosterone functions, except for spermatogenesis.

Other uses for androgens such as testosterone include refractory anemia, angioedema, mild and moderate endometriosis, fibrocystic breast disease, delayed puberty, palliation of breast cancer in women, breast cancer in postmenopausal women, cryptorchidism, and postpartum breast pain and engorgement. In the belief that these drugs will improve performance, athletes have also used androgens. However, this belief is proven to be false.

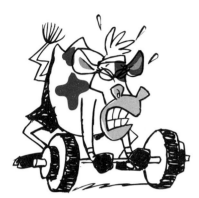

Androgens won't help.

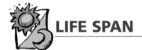

LIFE SPAN

Androgens are contraindicated for pregnant women and nursing mothers because they can cause development of male characteristics in the female infant. Androgens should be used with great care in children because profound masculinization may occur.

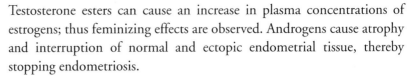

What You NEED TO KNOW

Contraindications/Precautions

Androgens are contraindicated for patients with a hypersensitivity to anabolic steroids, undiagnosed genital bleeding, porphyria, breast or prostate cancer, renal impairment, cardiac disorders, and hepatic dysfunction. Androgens should be used cautiously in patients with seizure disorders or migraine headaches.

Drug Interactions

Danazol when combined with carbamazepine may increase carbamazepine levels. Androgens increase the risk for nephrotoxicity. Combined with warfarin, androgens may cause a prolonged prothrombin time. Androgens may also affect the patient's insulin level, causing hypoglycemic response. The feminizing adverse effects of androgens include gynecomastia, which is significantly increased in children and adult males with liver disease.

Adverse Effects

An adverse effect of androgens is the presence of masculine secondary sex changes in adult women. Masculine sex changes include acne, facial hair growth, coarse voice, and menstrual irregularities. When androgen therapy is stopped immediately after symptoms are noticed, they will normally subside. Continued treatment may produce male-pattern baldness, body hair, and hypertrophy of the clitoris.

Androgen replacement in men may cause excessive erections when first initiated. Feminizing effects and toxic effects in adolescent and adult men depend on the dose and the length of exposure.

Additional adverse reactions of androgens include dizziness, headache, sleep disorders, fatigue, tremor, irritability, excitation, lethargy, sleep apnea, emotional lability, depression, paresthesia, elevated blood pressure, edema, and visual disturbances. GI and genitourinary adverse effects include nausea, vomiting, diarrhea, constipation, appetite changes, hematuria, vaginal bleeding, and testicular atrophy. Hepatic effects include irreversible jaundice, polycythemia, hepatitis, liver cell tumors, and hepatic dysfunction. Finally, muscle cramps, hypersensitive skin manifestations, hypercalcemia, chills, and allergic reactions have been noted.

 Patients taking androgens for prolonged periods may develop liver cancer.

Androgens increase the concentration of thyroid-binding globulin, thereby affecting thyroid function test results, plasma proteins, lipids, lipoproteins, urine tests, glucose tolerance test, cholesterol readings, and liver function test results.

What You DO

Nursing Responsibilities

When administering androgens, the nurse should:

- Instruct the patient to consume a high-calorie diet. Advise the patient to take the drug with food or meals if gastric upset occurs during therapy.
- Inject a parenteral androgen formulation deeply IM into the upper outer quadrant of the gluteal muscle.
- Teach the patient the proper way to apply the transdermal system, when appropriate. Avoid bony prominences and rotate transdermal sites for at least 1 week before returning to the same site. Inform the patient that the transdermal patch does not have to be removed during sexual intercourse.
- Remind the patient who is taking androgen that the buccal form can be stronger than other androgen forms.
- Encourage the patient to follow up with regular laboratory work and semen evaluation.
- Instruct the patient who is taking androgens for fibrocystic disease to perform breast self-examinations regularly for early detection of masses.

TAKE HOME POINTS

- Rotate IM injection sites to prevent atrophy. The transdermal patch should not be applied directly to the scrotum.
- Inform parents that children on androgen therapy require regular bone assessment to determine maturation.

- Advise the patient to use nonhormonal contraceptive methods while undergoing androgen therapy.
- Instruct the female patient to report masculinization adverse effects, such as acne, facial hair growth, coarse voice, sudden weight gain, and menstrual irregularities.

Do You UNDERSTAND?

DIRECTIONS: Provide the appropriate responses to the following questions from the italicized choices.

1. A negative feedback system influences testosterone; _____ *(increased, decreased)* testosterone suppresses the release of FSH and LH.
2. Athletes have also used androgens in the belief that they will improve performance, although this is _____ _____ *(indicated, contraindicated).*
3. In women, the ovary and adrenal gland produce testosterone in _____ *(moderate, minimal)* amounts.

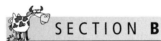

SECTION B

DRUGS AFFECTING UTERINE MOTILITY

Natural conditions of the reproductive system require drugs that promote and maintain pregnancy, induce or inhibit labor, promote or inhibit lactation, and terminate pregnancy. The drugs discussed in this section include tocolytics, oxytocics, prostaglandins, and ergot alkaloids.

What IS a Tocolytic?

Tocolytics	Trade Names	Uses
ritodrine [RYE-toe-dreen]	Yutopar	Stops premature labor
terbutaline [ter-BYOO-tah-leen]	Brethine	Stops premature labor
magnesium sulfate	$MgSO_4$	Treatment of seizures in preeclampsia and eclampsia

Action

Tocolytics (uterine relaxants) are β-adrenergic agonists that mimic the sympathetic nervous system effects at β_2 receptor sites. As such the intensity and frequency of uterine contractions is decreased and the gestational period lengthened. Terbutaline, although not approved by the FDA, is also used to stop preterm labor and lengthen the gestation period.

Uses

The tocolytics ritodrine and terbutaline have only one use: suppression of preterm labor which helps to maintain a pregnancy for additional days or weeks. Uterine contractions before 36 weeks are considered preterm or premature labor. Magnesium sulfate suppresses preterm labor but is used most frequently as an anticonvulsant to prevent or treat the complication of seizures in eclampsia and severe preeclampsia.

What You NEED TO KNOW

Contraindications/Precautions

Tocolytics are contraindicated for patients with hemorrhage, diabetes mellitus, hypovolemia, hypertension, dysrhythmias, heart disease, and chorioamnionitis. Tocolytics are used with caution in patients with hyperthyroidism.

Drug Interactions

When tocolytics are given with sympathomimetic drugs, the sympathetic effects are increased. Conversely, when tocolytics are combined with beta blockers, the sympathetic effects are decreased.

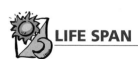 **LIFE SPAN**

Tocolytics are contraindicated for patients with a cervix that is dilated 4 cm or more, gestation of less than 20 weeks or greater than 36 weeks, severe preeclampsia, eclampsia, and intrauterine infection.

When corticosteroids are combined with tocolytics, the risk for potentially fatal postpartum pulmonary edema is increased.

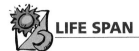

Fetal adverse effects include hypotension, tachycardia, hyperglycemia, and paralytic ileus.

Adverse Effects

The adverse effects of tocolytics are usually associated with IV administration but rare following oral administration. Maternal adverse effects of tocolytics include allergy, headache, tremor, anxiety, nervousness, restlessness, malaise, temporary hyperglycemia, rash, nausea, vomiting, palpitations, tachycardia, hypotension, hypertension, and widening pulse pressure. More serious adverse effects include chest pain, dysrhythmias, increased cardiac output, and pulmonary edema.

Magnesium intoxication effects include flushing, sweating, hypotension, hypothermia, cardiac and CNS depression, circulatory collapse, flaccid paralysis, depressed reflexes, and hypocalcemia with tetany.

What You DO

Nursing Responsibilities

Generally, tocolytics are administered IV and maintained for approximately 12 hours to quickly stop labor. These drugs are then continued by mouth to maintain suppression of labor. Oral therapy usually begins 30 minutes before termination of IV administration. Tocolytic therapy is restarted if uterine contractions reoccur. When administering tocolytics, the nurse should:

- Position the patient who is receiving tocolytics in the left lateral recumbent position throughout the infusion period to reduce the risk for hypotension.
- Use a micro-drip and infusion pump for tocolytic IV administration to prevent circulatory overload.
- Monitor the patient who is undergoing tocolytic therapy for pulmonary edema, particularly when the patient is taking corticosteroids. Continuously monitor maternal and fetal heart rate and maternal blood pressure for early detection of adverse effects.
- Administer oral tocolytics with food if GI distress occurs.
- Monitor the blood glucose levels of the patient who has diabetes for early detection of hyperglycemia.

Do You UNDERSTAND?

DIRECTIONS: Fill in the blanks with the appropriate responses.

1. Tocolytics act to _____ the uterus and _____ delivery.
2. Tocolytics are usually administered _____ (route) initially and then given _____.
3. Tocolytics are administered using a(n) _____ and _____ tubing.

What IS an Oxytocic?

Oxytocic	Trade Name	Uses
oxytocin [ox-eh-TOE-sin]	Pitocin	Initiates uterine contractions and stimulates letdown reflex in nursing mothers

What You NEED TO KNOW

Action

An oxytocic is a drug that functions similarly to the hormone oxytocin, which is produced in the hypothalamus and stored in the posterior pituitary gland. The uterus becomes progressively sensitive to oxytocin during the gestational period, peaking before delivery. Oxytocin increases the force, frequency, and duration of uterine contractions. Oxytocin also promotes the release of breast milk through the process of contracting cells that surround the alveoli of the breast. This action forces milk from the alveoli into the larger ducts and facilitates milk letdown in nursing mothers. Oxytocin also produces vasodilation of vascular smooth muscles to increase cerebral, coronary, and renal blood flow.

Answers: **1.** relax, delay; **2.** IV, orally; **3.** infusion pump, micro-drip.

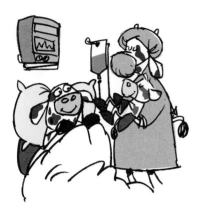

Inducing success.

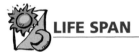

LIFE SPAN

Oxytocin is contraindicated during prematurity and fetal distress.

Oxytocin should not be used to induce labor when a vaginal delivery is contraindicated.

Uses

Oxytocin is used at term to stimulate or improve uterine contractions during labor, delivery, and the immediate postpartum period. Oxytocin is the drug of choice in the antepartum period to induce near-term labor after the cervix is dilated and presentation of the fetus has occurred. Oxytocin is also useful in managing inevitable, incomplete, or missed abortions. The stimulation of uterine contractions can also prevent or control postpartum hemorrhage and promote postpartum uterine involution (decrease in uterine size) to control bleeding. Oxytocin is also used as a diagnostic drug in the oxytocin challenge test to detect abnormal fetal heart rates.

Contraindications/Precautions

Oxytocin is contraindicated in patients with hypersensitivity and invasive cervical carcinoma. Oxytocin is also contraindicated for patients with borderline cephalopelvic disproportion, partial placenta previa, hydramnios, previous major surgery of cervix or uterus, uterine overdistension, grand multiparity, history of uterine sepsis or traumatic delivery, and severe toxemia.

Drug Interactions

When oxytocin is given with vasoconstrictors, severe hypertension may develop. Drug-drug interaction with cyclopropane anesthesia leads to hypotension, dysrhythmias, and maternal bradycardia.

With excessive doses of oxytocin or in sensitive patients, maternal adverse effects include amniotic fluid embolism, hyperstimulation of the uterus, prolonged tetanic uterine contractions, uterine rupture, cervical and vaginal lacerations, postpartum hemorrhage, and abruptio placentae. Fetal adverse effects include intracranial hemorrhage, deceleration of heart rate, hypoxia, hypercapnia, CNS impairment, and perinatal liver necrosis.

Adverse Effects

The adverse effects of oxytocin include hypotension, severe hypertension, headache, subarachnoid hemorrhage, uterine cramping, tachycardia, dysrhythmias, impaired renal flow, anaphylaxis, seizures, coma, and death. Severe water intoxication usually occurs with an excessive volume of IV solution without electrolytes, an IV rate that is too rapid, or prolonged IV administration.

What You DO

Nursing Responsibilities

Oxytocin is administered IV when stimulating uterine contractions, whenever possible. When delivery is eminent without time to initiate an IV, oxytocin is usually given IM after delivery. When given for milk letdown in lactation, oxytocin may be administered intranasally. When administering an oxytocin, the nurse should:

- Always administer oxytocin intravenous piggyback (IVPB) during the antepartum period in the smallest amount of fluid allowed and never in the main IV to prevent overdosing and water intoxication.
- Use a micro-drip and infusion pump for oxytocin IV administration to prevent water intoxication.
- Monitor uterine contractions, fetal and maternal heart rate, maternal blood pressure, and intrauterine pressure during oxytocin administration for early detection of adverse effects.
- Discontinue oxytocin immediately when uterine hyperactivity occurs to prevent adverse effects (e.g., uterine rupture) and fetal hypoxia.
- Instruct patients to report a sudden, severe headache immediately, which may indicate a hypertensive episode.

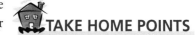

TAKE HOME POINTS

When inducing labor, administer the oxytocin IV rather than IM because IM administration is unpredictable to control. Never administer oxytocin via more than one route at a time.

Do You UNDERSTAND?

DIRECTIONS: Indicate in the space provided whether the statement is *true* or *false*. If the answer is false, correct the statement to make it true (using the margin space).

_____ 1. Oxytocin is given to promote milk letdown in nursing mothers.

_____ 2. During gestation, the uterus becomes progressively sensitive to oxytocin, peaking at delivery.

_____ 3. Initially, oxytocin is given IV in the antepartum period, then orally postpartum.

Answers: 1. true; 2. true; 3. false; IV initially then nasally because oxytocin is destroyed in the GI tract.

What IS a Prostaglandin?

Prostaglandins	Trade Names	Uses
dinoprostone *[dye-nah-PROS-tone]*	Cervidil Prepidil	Induction of labor, evacuation of uterus, and control of postpartum hemorrhage
carboprost tromethamine *[CAR-bo-prost]*	Hemabate	Induction of labor, evacuation of uterus, and control of postpartum hemorrhage

Action

Prostaglandins are hormones that are synthesized in all body tissues. The mechanism of action for many of the prostaglandins has yet to be determined, but these drugs are thought to stimulate the myometrium (e.g., the smooth muscle layer of the uterus). The contractions of the pregnant uterus are comparable to labor contractions of the full-term uterus and are usually adequate to evacuate the uterus. In the postpartum period, prostaglandins contract the myometrium to provide hemostasis (inhibit bleeding) at the placental attachment site.

Uses

Clinically, the use of prostaglandins is limited. In obstetrics, these drugs are used to induce abortion and cervical ripening, as well as to control postpartum hemorrhage. Dinoprostone and carboprost are used to induce abortion during the second trimester of pregnancy. Prostaglandins are usually given in conjunction with oxytocin to shorten the induction-to-abortion time and reduce adverse effects. These drugs are also used to evacuate the uterus in a missed abortion, benign hydatidiform mole, or for an intrauterine fetal death up to 28 weeks of gestation.

What You NEED TO KNOW

Prostaglandins should be used with caution in patients with hypotension, hypertension, diabetes mellitus, asthma, epilepsy, chorioamnionitis, or uterine scarring.

Contraindications/Precautions

Prostaglandins are contraindicated for patients who have acute pelvic inflammatory disease, uterine fibroids, cervical stenosis, and cardiac, pulmonary, renal, or hepatic disease.

Drug Interactions

Prostaglandins increase the action of oxytocic drugs. Recommendations are that these drugs should not be used concurrently.

Adverse Effects

Adverse effects of prostaglandins include headache, dizziness, fainting, flushing, hypertension, acute hypotension, chest pain, and dysrhythmias from the stimulation of vascular smooth muscle. Nausea, vomiting, and diarrhea may occur because of the stimulation of GI smooth muscles. Other adverse effects include fever, chills, shivering, bronchospasm, wheezing, and dyspnea. Sustained uterine contractility may cause cervical laceration and uterine rupture.

What You DO

Nursing Responsibilities

Prostaglandins are administered intravaginally. For cervical ripening, prostaglandin gel may be placed into the cervical canal immediately below the level of the internal mouth or opening of vagina via a prefilled syringe. When administering prostaglandins, the nurse should:

- Allow prostaglandin intravaginal suppositories to warm to room temperature before removing the foil wrapper.
- Insert the prostaglandin suppository high into the posterior vagina, and have the patient remain supine for 10 minutes.
- Be aware that a dilute IV oxytocin solution may be started 1 hour after the first dose of prostaglandin.
- Carefully monitor uterine activity and fetal status throughout administration of prostaglandins for early detection of hypertonic uterine contractility and fetal distress.

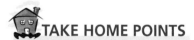

TAKE HOME POINTS

Carefully monitor uterine activity throughout prostaglandin administration. Beta adrenergic drugs may be used to halt uterine hypercontractility from prostaglandin therapy.

Do You UNDERSTAND?

DIRECTIONS: **Place a check mark next to the potential adverse effects of prostaglandin.**

_____ 1. Seizures
_____ 2. Dyspnea
_____ 3. Dysrhythmias
_____ 4. Coma

What IS an Ergot Alkaloid?

Ergot Alkaloids	Trade Names	Uses
ergonovine maleate [er-go-NOH-veen]	Ergotrate maleate	Treatment of postpartum hemorrhage
methylergonovine maleate [meth-ill-er-go-NOH-veen]	Methergine	Treatment of postpartum hemorrhage

Action

Ergot alkaloids stimulate adrenergic, dopaminergic, and serotonergic receptors, which in turn stimulate uterine contractions and constrict arterioles and veins, thereby affecting uterine and vascular smooth muscle. In small doses following delivery, uterine contractions are of moderate strength, with alternating uterine relaxation of a normal degree and duration. However, in large doses, uterine contractions are greatly increased in force and frequency, with reduced uterine relaxation. Sustained contractions are common with large doses and, when given during labor, can lead to maternal and fetal trauma. Sustained contractions result in a reduction of placental blood flow, leading to cervical laceration, uterine rupture, and fetal hypoxia.

Uses

The therapeutic use of ergot alkaloids in the postabortion and postpartum period is to increase uterine tone and decrease bleeding. The resulting sustained uterine contractions are desirable in this period. Because of the prolonged contractions, ergot alkaloids are not used to induce labor.

LIFE SPAN

Ergot alkaloids are contra-indicated for patients before delivery of the placenta, as well as those with threatened spontaneous abortion, uterine sepsis, and toxemia.

Answers: dyspnea; dysrhythmias.

What You NEED TO KNOW

Contraindications/Precautions

Ergot alkaloids are contraindicated for patients with hypersensitivity and hypertension.

Drug Interactions

Drug interactions of ergot alkaloids involve parenteral sympathomimetics and other ergot alkaloids. When these drugs are administered together, vasomotor action is increased, leading to hypertension.

> **!** Ergot alkaloids should be used with caution in patients with a history of cardiovascular, renal, or hepatic dysfunction.
> Severe overdose effects include seizures and gangrene.

Adverse Effects

The adverse effects of ergot alkaloids usually occur with IV administration. The most common adverse effects include severe hypertension, bradycardia, nausea, vomiting, allergic reaction, and shock. Other adverse effects include headache, dizziness, hallucinations, tinnitus, nasal congestion, dyspnea, foul taste, diaphoresis, palpitations, transient chest pain, thrombophlebitis, leg cramps, diarrhea, hematuria, and water intoxication. When IV methylergonovine is given undiluted, too rapidly, or in conjunction with regional anesthesia or vasoconstrictors, serious adverse effects may occur (e.g., particularly, severe hypertension, severe dysrhythmias, generalized headaches, stroke).

What You DO

Nursing Responsibilities

Because most adverse effects follow IV administration, IV use of ergot alkaloids is usually reserved for severe uterine bleeding or other life-threatening emergencies. When the situation necessitates the IV route, the drug is administered at a slow rate over a period of not less than 1 minute to avoid serious adverse effects. When administering ergot alkaloids, the nurse should:

- Discard ampules of methylergonovine that contain discolored solution or visible particles.
- Protect these drugs from light when in storage.

- Monitor vital signs and uterine response during and after parenteral administration of methylergonovine until the patient is stabilized, which is approximately 1 to 2 hours.
- Notify the health care provider in cases of sudden blood pressure increases or frequent periods of uterine relaxation.

Do You UNDERSTAND?

DIRECTIONS: Fill in the blanks with the appropriate responses.

1. _____ use of ergot alkaloids is usually reserved for severe uterine bleeding or other life-threatening situations.
2. IV solutions should be given at a _____ rate over a period of not less than _____ to avoid serious adverse effects.

References

Arcangelo VP: *Pharmacotherapeutics for advanced practice: a practical approach,* Philadelphia, 2001, Lippincott.

Gutierrez K, Queener S: *Pharmacology for nursing practice,* Philadelphia, 2004, Mosby.

Lehne R: *Pharmacology for nursing care,* ed 5, Philadelphia, 2004, WB Saunders.

Lewis SM, Heitkemper MM, Dirksen SR: *Medical-surgical nursing: assessment and management of clinical problems,* ed 6, St Louis, 2004, Mosby.

Lilley L, Harrington S, Snyder J: *Pharmacology and the nursing process,* ed 4, St Louis, 2005, Mosby.s

McCance K, Huether S: *Pathophysiology: the biologic basis for disease in adults and children,* ed 4, St. Louis, 2002, Mosby.

Answers: 1. IV; 2. slow, 1 minute.

NCLEX® Review

Section A

1. A woman who is on estrogen therapy should be advised to see her health care provider immediately if she experiences which of the following conditions?
   1 Osteoporosis
   2 Water retention
   3 Shortness of breath
   4 Diarrhea

2. Which of the following is not a contraindication for estrogen replacement therapy?
   1 Pregnancy
   2 Breast cancer
   3 Vascular disease
   4 Osteoporosis

3. Which of the following does *not* release the steroid hormone progestin?
   1 Testes
   2 Ovary
   3 Adrenal cortex
   4 Bone

4. Which of the following medications reduces the effectiveness of oral contraceptives with estrogen and progestin?
   1 Rifampin
   2 Theophylline
   3 Digoxin
   4 Cyclosporin

5. Your patient wants to know how oral contraceptives with estrogen and progestin prevent pregnancy. Which of the following is the principal explanation of this therapy?
   1 Blocks the passage of sperm
   2 Decreases progesterone levels
   3 Inhibits ovulation and implementation of the egg
   4 Decreases estrogen levels

Section B

6. The tocolytic magnesium sulfate is used to prevent which of the following complications of severe preeclampsia?
   1 Hypotension
   2 Seizures
   3 Depressed reflexes
   4 GI distress

7. What is the mechanism of action for tocolytic drugs?
   1 Induce ovulation
   2 Halt preterm labor
   3 Facilitate milk letdown
   4 Induce abortion

8. During oxytocic treatment, which of following is a serious adverse effect?
   1 Water intoxication
   2 Ovarian hyperstimulation
   3 Cephalopelvic disproportion
   4 Invasive cervical carcinoma

9. Which of the following statements about dinoprostone treatment is incorrect?
   1 The drug is administered intravaginally.
   2 The drug may cause bronchospasm and chest pain.
   3 The drug is contraindicated in patients with pelvic inflammatory disease.
   4 The nurse should remove the foil wrapper of the intravaginal suppository when it is chilled.

10. Which of the following statements about ergot alkaloid use during labor is correct?
    1 Large doses can lead to maternal and fetal trauma.
    2 Hypotension is a common adverse effect of ergot alkaloids.
    3 IV administration is the most common route.
    4 Ergot alkaloids are the drugs of choice in patients with renal disease.

NCLEX® Review Answers

Section A

1. **3** Life-threatening adverse effects of estrogen therapy include seizures, thromboembolism, stroke, pulmonary embolism, MI, hepatic adenoma, and an increased risk for endometrial and breast cancer. Shortness of breath may indicate pulmonary embolism and should be reported immediately. Estrogen decreases the risk for osteoporosis, and patients may be unaware that they are experiencing it anyway. Water retention and diarrhea are effects that need not be reported immediately.

2. **4** Estrogen replacement therapy is intended to prevent osteoporosis. Estrogen is contraindicated in women during pregnancy and in patients with breast cancer and vascular disease.

3. **4** Estrogen, not progesterone, is found in the bone. Progesterone is a steroid hormone synthesized and released by the testes, ovary, adrenal cortex, and placenta.

4. **1** When carbamazepine, phenobarbital, and rifampin are taken with estrogen, estrogen effectiveness is decreased. Theophylline and digoxin have no drug interaction with estrogen and progestin. Cyclosporine results in increased risk for toxicity when administered with estrogen, not reduced effectiveness.

5. **3** Estrogen suppresses secretion of FSH, thus blocking follicle development and subsequently inhibiting ovulation. With a depression of LH, ovulation cannot occur, even with full development of the follicle. Progestin also causes endometrium changes that may prevent an egg from being implanted in the uterus.

Section B

6. **2** Magnesium sulfate can suppress preterm labor but is used primarily as an anticonvulsant to prevent or treat the complication of seizures in severe preeclampsia or eclampsia. Magnesium sulfate is not used to prevent hypotension, depressed reflexes, or GI distress.

7. **2** Tocolytic drugs act on the reproductive system to stop preterm labor and thus maintain a pregnancy. Tocolytics are β-adrenergic agonists that mimic the sympathetic nervous system activity at β_2 sites, relax smooth muscle, and stop or slow uterine contractions. The action of tocolytics does not induce ovulation, facilitate milk letdown, or induce abortion.

8. **1** The nurse should monitor the patient for water intoxication during oxytocic therapy. Ovarian hyperstimulation and invasive cervical carcinoma are not adverse effects of oxytocics. Oxytocin is contraindicated in patients with cephalopelvic disproportion.

9. **4** Dinoprostone should be allowed to warm to room temperature before removing the foil wrapper. Dinoprostone is administered by intravaginal suppository, is contraindicated in patients with pelvic inflammatory disease, and may cause bronchospasm and chest pain.

10. **1** Large doses of ergot alkaloid during labor may cause maternal and fetal trauma. Hypertension, not hypotension, is a common adverse effect. IV ergot alkaloids are reserved for severe uterine bleeding or other life-threatening emergencies because most adverse effects follow IV administration. Ergot alkaloids are not the drugs of choice in patients with renal disease but should be used with caution in these individuals.

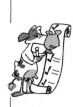

Notes

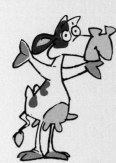

Chapter 13

Drugs Used to Treat Musculoskeletal System Disorders

What You WILL LEARN

After reading this chapter, you will know how to do the following:

✔ Compare the action of most nonsteroidal antiinflammatory drugs with COX-2 inhibitors.

✔ Describe the nursing responsibilities of disease-modifying antirheumatic drugs.

✔ Discuss the action and contraindications of antigout drugs.

✔ Describe the drug interactions and adverse effects of muscle relaxants.

 SECTION A

NONSTEROIDAL ANTIINFLAMMATORY AGENTS

This section reviews pharmacologic drugs that affect inflammatory conditions of the musculoskeletal system. Because antiinflammatory agents are the most widely used drugs of prescription and over-the-counter (OTC) use, the nurse must have a thorough understanding of these drugs to evaluate patient responses, identify adverse effects, and teach patients appropriately. This section discusses nonsteroidal antiinflammatory drugs.

What IS a First-Generation Nonsteroidal Antiinflammatory?

First-Generation Nonsteroidal Antiinflammatory Agents	Trade Names	Uses
acetylsalicylic acid [ah-SEE-till-sal-ih-SILL-ick]	Aspirin Ecotrin	Treatment of arthritis, gout, and SLE
ibuprofen [eye-byoo-PROH-fen]	Motrin Advil	Treatment of arthritis
naproxen [nah-PROX-en]	Naprosyn Aleve	Treatment of arthritis, gout, and ankylosing spondylitis
oxaprozin [ox-ah-PROH-zen]	Daypro	Treatment of acute and chronic osteoarthritis and rheumatoid arthritis
indomethacin [in-doe-METH-ah-sin]	Indocin	Treatment of arthritis, gout, and ankylosing spondylitis
ketorolac [key-TORE-oh-lack]	Toradol	Short-term management of mild to moderate pain
meclofenamate [me-kloh-fen-AM-ate]	Meclofen	Treatment of arthritis
piroxicam [peer-OX-ih-cam]	Feldene	Treatment of arthritis

Action

Nonsteroidal antiinflammatory drugs (NSAIDs) mimic the antiinflammatory effects of cortisone but are not chemically related. Therefore they are called nonsteroidal antiinflammatory drugs. First-generation NSAIDs are known as nonselective inhibitors because they inhibit prostaglandin synthesis by inhibiting both forms of cyclooxygenase (COX): COX_1 and COX_2. The antiinflammatory effects of first-generation NSAIDs include suppression of inflammation, pain relief, and fever reduction. The suppression of inflammation is achieved through the inhibition of COX, which is the enzyme responsible for the synthesis of prostaglandins. Prostaglandins are chemical mediators that are released at inflammatory sites, causing vasodilation, redness, warmth, increased capillary permeability, swelling, and sensitization of nerve cells to pain. Thus NSAIDs reduce inflammation by inhibiting the formation and release of prostaglandins.

Acetylsalicylic acid (aspirin) is a salicylate that not only decreases inflammation but also acts as an analgesic, antipyretic, and anticoagulant. Ibuprofen and naproxen provide stronger antiinflammatory effects than aspirin with less gastrointestinal (GI) irritation; however, they are more prone to drug interactions with other high protein-bound drugs. Piroxicam is convenient with once-a-day dosing and causes less GI distress than aspirin.

Uses

First-generation NSAIDs are used for their analgesic effect in mild-to-moderate pain and antiinflammatory effect in the treatment of arthritis, bursitis, tendonitis, ankylosing spondylitis, and systemic lupus erythematosus (SLE). These NSAIDs are also used to relieve pain for headaches and dysmenorrhea. Aspirin is also used in acute coronary syndrome (ACS), deep venous thrombosis (DVT), and transient ischemic attacks (TIAs) for suppression of platelet aggregation. NSAIDs are safer than opioids in older adults for short-term use.

What You NEED TO KNOW

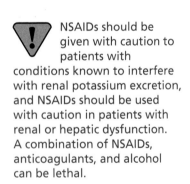

NSAIDs should be given with caution to patients with conditions known to interfere with renal potassium excretion, and NSAIDs should be used with caution in patients with renal or hepatic dysfunction. A combination of NSAIDs, anticoagulants, and alcohol can be lethal.

Contraindications/Precautions

All NSAIDs are contraindicated for patients with hypersensitivity. Salicylates are contraindicated for patients with viral illnesses, such as influenza or chickenpox, because this combination is associated with Reye's syndrome. Indomethacin is contraindicated for patients who are taking triamterene because the combination may increase the risk for nephrotoxicity. Generally, NSAIDs are contraindicated in people who have cardiovascular dysfunction, hypertension, peptic ulcer and those who are pregnant or lactating.

Drug Interactions

NSAIDs may exacerbate bleeding effects when given concurrently with warfarin. Prolonged use of NSAIDs and acetaminophen increases the risk for renal impairment. NSAIDs may induce lithium toxicity when these drugs are taken together. When phenytoin and NSAIDs are taken concurrently, drug levels may be altered, resulting in phenytoin toxicity.

Acetylsalicylic acid (ASA) inhibits valproic acid metabolism, thereby causing valproic acid levels to rise. Hypoglycemia may occur when oral hypoglycemics are used with NSAIDs. NSAIDs reduce the antihypertensive effect of beta blockers and angiotensin-converting enzyme (ACE) inhibitors. NSAIDs reduce the effects of loop and thiazide diuretics, which may lead to induced congestive heart failure (CHF). When NSAIDs and potassium-sparing diuretics are given together, hyperkalemia may occur.

Adverse Effects

The most common adverse effects of first-generation NSAIDs include GI irritation (e.g., anorexia, nausea, vomiting, diarrhea, and peptic ulcer formation), as well as sodium and water retention. Other common adverse effects include headache, drowsiness, dizziness, and fatigue. Renal adverse effects include reversible impairment of glomerular filtration, leading to chronic renal failure. Administering 1 to 2 g of salicylates per day decreases uric acid excretion. NSAIDs affect platelet aggregation and prolong bleeding time. Large doses of NSAIDs cause auditory and visual disturbances. Tinnitus is usually the first sign of toxicity. High doses of salicylate stimulate the respiratory center resulting in hyperventilation and respiratory alkalosis. Toxic doses depress the respiratory center and cause metabolic acidosis. Prolonged use of NSAIDs may lead to bone marrow depression.

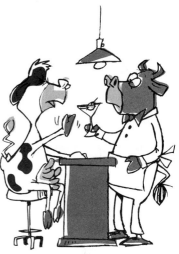

No thanks.

What You DO

Nursing Responsibilities

NSAIDs are taken orally. When administering first-generation NSAIDs, the nurse should:

- Instruct the patient to take first-generation NSAIDs with food or milk to decrease GI distress.
- Caution the patient to avoid the use of tobacco, alcohol, and other drugs that cause gastric irritation when taking first-generation NSAIDs.
- Advise the patient who is taking first-generation NSAIDs to avoid high-sodium foods because fluid retention may occur.
- Explain to the patient that some first-generation NSAIDs may take several weeks to produce maximal therapeutic effects. The normal

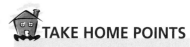

TAKE HOME POINTS

Instruct the patient to avoid crushing enteric-coated or extended-release tablets.

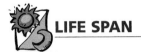

LIFE SPAN

Aspirin should be discontinued 3 to 7 days before elective surgery or dental procedures because of the decrease in platelet aggregation and the risk for hemorrhage.

therapeutic range of salicylates is 15 to 30 mg/dL, whereas toxicity is greater than 30 mg/dL.

- Warn the patient to avoid aspirin use in children younger than 19 years of age.
- Instruct the patient who is taking anticoagulant drugs concurrently with first-generation NSAIDs to observe for bleeding tendencies (e.g., black or tarry stools, bruising, nosebleeds).
- Monitor renal and hepatic function tests in patients who are undergoing long-term therapy for early detection of dysfunction.
- Inform the patient who is taking first-generation NSAIDs to notify the health care provider when pain or fever persists for 3 days or when tinnitus occurs.
- Counsel the patient who is taking first-generation NSAIDs to consult with the health care provider before taking OTC drugs.
- Instruct the patient to immediately report the following: blood in the urine or stool, abdominal pain, changes in hearing, tinnitus, and swelling.

Do You UNDERSTAND?

DIRECTIONS: **Match Column A with Column B.**

Column A	Column B
_____ 1. The most common adverse effects after ingesting first-generation NSAIDs.	a. To decrease inflammation
_____ 2. Primary reason for taking first-generation NSAIDs.	b. GI disturbances
_____ 3. Nursing implications with concurrent first-generation NSAID and oral anticoagulant.	c. Monitor bleeding and petechiae

Answers: 1. b; 2. a; 3. c.

What IS a Second-Generation Nonsteroidal Antiinflammatory?

Second-Generation Nonsteroidal Antiinflammatory Agents	Trade Names	Uses
celecoxib [CELL-ah-COX-ib]	Celebrex	Treatment of arthritis
nabumetone [nah-BU-meh-tone]	Relafen	Treatment of arthritis
meloxicam [meh-LOCKS-ih-cam]	Mobic	Treatment of osteoarthritis

Action

Second-generation NSAIDs are known as selective inhibitors and block only COX-$_2$, decreasing inflammation and pain. These drugs do not inhibit COX-$_1$. Therefore second-generation NSAIDs do not cause GI irritation as much as first-generation NSAIDs, nor do they affect platelet aggregation. Nabumetone and meloxicam are not true COX-$_2$ selective inhibitors but are more like second-generation NSAIDs than first-generation NSAIDs because they inhibit COX-$_2$ more than COX-$_1$.

Uses

Second-generation NSAIDs are used to relieve signs and symptoms of osteoarthritis and rheumatoid arthritis. Celecoxib is also used to relieve dysmenorrhea.

What You NEED TO KNOW

Contraindications/Precautions

All NSAIDs are contraindicated for patients with hypersensitivity. Celecoxib is contraindicated in individuals who have an allergy to aspirin or sulfonamides. Second-generation NSAIDs should be used cautiously in individuals with a history of GI ulcers, dehydration, renal or hepatic dysfunction, hypertension, heart failure, or concurrent use of anticoagulants, steroids, alcohol consumption, and smoking.

Drug Interactions

There are no known drug interactions with meloxicam. Celecoxib and nabumetone may increase the risk for lithium toxicity when given together; they may increase bleeding when given with anticoagulants.

Adverse Effects

Second-generation NSAIDs cause less GI distress than first-generation drugs. Adverse effects of celecoxib and nabumetone include headache, dizziness, dyspepsia, flatulence, diarrhea, constipation, peripheral edema, and rash. Meloxicam may also cause insomnia and photosensitivity.

What You DO

Nursing Responsibilities

NSAIDs are administered orally. When administering second-generation NSAIDs, the nurse should:

- Instruct the patient to take nabumetone with food or milk to decrease GI distress.
- Encourage the patient to avoid the use of tobacco, alcohol, and other drugs that cause gastric irritation when taking second-generation NSAIDs.
- Advise the patient who is taking NSAIDs to avoid high-sodium foods because fluid retention may occur.
- Warn the patient to avoid performing tasks requiring mental alertness (e.g., driving, operating heavy machines) until the effects of the medication are known.
- Instruct the patient to notify the physician of ringing in the ears, persistent abdominal cramping, unusual bruising or bleeding, swelling of the extremities, and chest pain.
- Monitor renal and hepatic function test results for potential impairment.

Do You UNDERSTAND?

DIRECTIONS: Indicate in the space provided whether the statement is *true* or *false*. If the answer is false, correct the statement to make it true (using the margin space).

_____ 1. Second-generation NSAIDs inhibit COX_1 more than COX_2.

_____ 2. Second-generation NSAIDs cause less GI distress than first-generation drugs.

_____ 3. Sodium and fluid retention is common with second-generation NSAIDs.

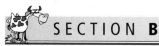

SECTION **B**

DISEASE-MODIFYING ANTIRHEUMATIC DRUGS

In the past, aspirin and other NSAIDs were used as first-line drugs in the early stages of rheumatoid arthritis. Because only the synovial membranes are inflamed with painful swelling in the early stages, NSAIDs controlled the symptoms adequately. Disease-modifying antirheumatic drugs (DMARDs) were reserved for severe cases of rheumatoid arthritis or cases in which NSAIDs were ineffective. Currently, some rheumatologists believe that aggressive therapy with DMARDs, initiated early in the disease, can interrupt joint degeneration. Recently, a combination of two or more DMARDs has been used for greater effectiveness in the treatment of rheumatoid arthritis.

This section reviews various DMARDs, which alter the disease process of arthritis. DMARDs include gold preparations, antimalarials, folic acid antagonists, glucocorticoids, and tumor necrosis factor blockers.

What IS a Gold Preparation?

Gold preparation	Trade Names	Uses
gold sodium thiomalate [thigh-oh-MAH-late]	Myochrysine	Treatment of rheumatoid arthritis
auranofin [au-RANE-eh-fin]	Ridaura	Treatment of rheumatoid arthritis
aurothioglucose [ah-row-thigh-oh-GLUE-cose]	Solganal	Treatment of rheumatoid arthritis

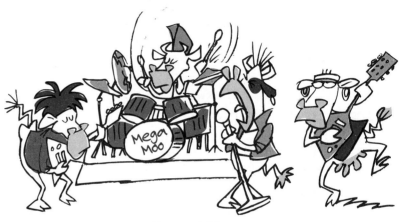

Heavy metal therapy.

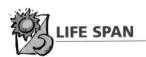

LIFE SPAN

Gold agents are contraindicated during pregnancy and lactation.

Action

Gold agents are DMARDs that relieve symptoms of rheumatoid arthritis. Gold compounds (**chrysotherapy** or **heavy metal therapy**) suppress prostaglandin synthesis and interrupt the progression of rheumatoid arthritis in the early synovitis stage. These drugs decrease synovial inflammation and delay the destruction of cartilage and bone. Gold therapy cannot reverse existing structural joint damage. Relief of symptoms may take 6 to 8 weeks to occur.

Uses

Gold agents are used effectively in the treatment of rheumatoid arthritis. These drugs reduce swelling and pain.

What You NEED TO KNOW

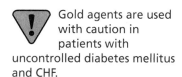

Gold agents are used with caution in patients with uncontrolled diabetes mellitus and CHF.

Contraindications/Precautions

Gold agents are contraindicated for patients with exfoliative dermatitis, colitis, eczema, SLE, blood dyscrasias, and severe hepatic or renal dysfunction.

Drug Interactions

When gold agents are given concurrently with other nephrotoxic, hepatotoxic, and bone marrow depressants, the toxicity may be increased. Penicillamine may increase nephrotoxicity and bone marrow depression when given with gold agents.

Adverse Effects

The most common adverse effects of gold agents include rash, itching, and oral ulcers (**stomatitis**). Other adverse effects include photosensitivity, redness, anorexia, dyspepsia, flatulence, abdominal cramps, diarrhea, hepatitis, and hair loss (**alopecia**). Unique adverse effects of gold therapy include a metallic taste, nitritoid reaction, and ocular gold deposits. Nitritoid reactions include dizziness, flushing, fainting, sweating, nausea, vomiting, headache, and weakness. Serious adverse effects include hematuria, bradycardia, severe blood dyscrasias, Stevens-Johnson syndrome, interstitial pneumonitis, nephrotoxicity, and anaphylactic shock.

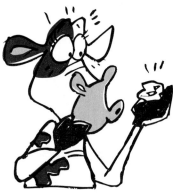

Gold agents can cause oral ulcers.

What You DO

Nursing Responsibilities

Gold agents are administered orally and injected intramuscularly (IM). When administering gold agents, the nurse should:

- Rule out pregnancy before initiating gold therapy.
- Counsel the patient to use birth control measures during gold therapy.
- Monitor complete blood count (CBC) and platelet count throughout therapy for early detection of bone marrow depression.
- Monitor the patient for hepatic and renal toxicities.

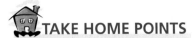

TAKE HOME POINTS

Exposure to sunlight may aggravate chrysiasis. The patient who is receiving gold injections should remain in a recumbent position at least 30 minutes to avoid a nitritoid resaction.

- Advise the patient to decrease exposure to sunlight and ultraviolet light when taking gold to prevent gray-blue skin pigmentation from gold deposits (**chrysiasis**).
- Instruct the patient who is taking gold agents to have eye examinations performed at least every 3 months.
- Instruct the patient who is taking gold agents to perform careful oral hygiene to decrease discomfort from stomatitis.
- Inform the patient to report yellow sclerae, metallic taste, sore mouth, weakness, bruising, unusual bleeding, tenderness, itching, skin eruptions, gray-blue discoloration of skin or mucous membranes, dark urine, and visual or hearing impairment to the health care provider.
- Inject gold agents into the gluteus muscle.

Do You UNDERSTAND?

DIRECTIONS: Fill in the blanks with the appropriate response.

1. Three examples of gold preparations are _____,
   _____, and _____.
2. Three adverse effects of gold preparations are _____,
   _____, and _____.
3. Instruct the patient taking gold agents to seek an eye exam every
   _____ months.
4. Inject gold agents into the _____ muscle.

What IS an Antimalarial?

Antimalarial	Trade Names	Uses
hydroxychloroquine [hye-drox-ee-KLOR-oh-kwin]	Plaquenil	Treatment of rheumatoid arthritis and SLE

Action

The antirheumatic action of hydroxychloroquine is unknown, but the drug is thought to inhibit prostaglandin, thereby reducing inflammation. The therapeutic effect may not occur for up to 6 months.

Uses

Hydroxychloroquine is typically used in combination with NSAIDs in the treatment of rheumatoid arthritis and SLE to reduce inflammation and initiate remission. Antimalarial drugs are used to treat an acute malarial attack as well.

What You NEED TO KNOW

Contraindications/Precautions

Antimalarial drugs are contraindicated for patients who are pregnant, lactating, have retinal or visual field changes, and porphyria. Hydroxychloroquine should be used cautiously in patients with hepatic dysfunction, alcoholism, blood dyscrasias, severe GI or neurologic disorders.

Drug Interactions

When penicillamine is combined with hydroxychloroquine, serious skin, hematologic, and renal toxicities may develop. Concurrent digoxin may increase the risk for digitalis toxicity. Aluminum and magnesium-containing antacids and laxatives decrease the absorption of hydroxychloroquine.

Adverse Effects

The most common adverse effects of antimalarials include headache, anorexia, abdominal cramps, nausea, vomiting, diarrhea, and retinopathy. Other adverse effects include visual disturbances, alopecia, dizziness, irritability, personality changes, seizures, itching, and weakness. Prolonged high-dose hydroxychloroquine therapy (which is frequently necessary for rheumatoid arthritis) may result in serious and, occasionally, irreversible toxicities, such as hematologic and hepatic toxicity, retinopathy, and cardiomyopathy.

What You DO

Nursing Responsibilities

Hydroxychloroquine is administered orally and should be given with food. When administering antiarthritic agents, the nurse should:

- Instruct the patient to take antacids or laxatives at least 4 hours before or after hydroxychloroquine.
- Monitor complete blood count (CBC) and platelet count throughout therapy for early detection of bone marrow depression.
- Monitor the patient who is receiving hydroxychloroquine for hepatic and renal toxicities.
- Instruct the patient to have eye examinations performed at least every 3 months.
- Inform patients to report any weakness, unusual bleeding, bruising, skin eruptions, and visual or hearing impairment.
- Warn the patient to avoid excessive exposure to the sun to prevent drug-induced dermatoses.

Do You UNDERSTAND?

DIRECTIONS: **Indicate in the space provided whether the statement is *true* or *false*. If the answer is false, correct the statement to make it true (using the margin space).**

_____ 1. The therapeutic effect of hydroxychloroquine (Plaquenil) usually occurs after 1 month of therapy.

_____ 2. Antimalarial drugs are to be used cautiously in patients with blood dyscrasias.

_____ 3. Retinopathy and visual disturbances may occur with antimalarials.

_____ 4. Instruct the patient to have an eye examination every 1 year.

Answers: 1. False; the therapeutic effect may take up to 6 months; 2. True; 3. True; 4. False; every 3 months.

What IS a Folic Acid Antagonist?

Folic Acid Antagonist	Trade Names	Uses
methotrexate [meth-oh-TREX-ate]	Mexate	Treatment of rheumatoid arthritis

Action

Folic acid antagonists are also known as antimetabolites or immunosuppressive agents. Because folic acid agents suppress cancer growth and proliferation, they are useful in suppressing the inflammatory process of rheumatoid arthritis. Methotrexate interferes with mitotic process of nucleic acid synthesis by blocking folic acid.

Uses

Folic acid antagonists have been effective in treating rheumatoid arthritis.

What You NEED TO KNOW

Contraindications/Precautions

Methotrexate is contraindicated for patients with severe hepatic or renal disease. Cautious use is indicated for patients who have peptic ulcers, ulcerative colitis, and bone marrow suppression.

Drug Interactions

Folic acid preparations may decrease the effectiveness of methotrexate therapy. Theophylline levels may be increased when given with methotrexate. When methotrexate is taken with sulfasalazine or alcohol, the risk for hepatotoxicity is increased. Increased methotrexate levels and toxicity may result when given with salicylates, NSAIDs, sulfonamides, sulfonylureas, phenytoin, tetracyclines, penicillin, and probenecid.

Adverse Effects

Adverse effects of methotrexate include GI ulceration (particularly of the oral mucosa), gingivitis, glossitis, stomatitis, anorexia, nausea, vomiting, and diarrhea. Other effects are headache, photosensitivity, hypotension,

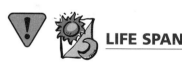

LIFE SPAN

- Methotrexate is contraindicated during pregnancy.
- Methotrexate should be used with caution in older adults.
- Methotrexate is given cautiously to patients with peptic ulcers, ulcerative colitis, infections, poor nutritional status, and bone marrow dysfunction.

> Fatal GI and hematologic toxicities have occurred when NSAIDs, penicillin, salicylates, sulfonamides, sulfonylureas, phenytoin, tetracyclines, and chloramphenicol are given with methotrexate.

drowsiness, alopecia, blurred vision, rash, pruritus, chills, fever, and muscle pain. More serious adverse effects include pulmonary toxicity, thromboembolism, bone marrow depression, nephrotoxicity, hepatotoxicity, and sudden death.

What You DO

Nursing Responsibilities

Methotrexate should be given 1 hour before or 2 hours after meals. When administering methotrexate, the nurse should:

- Monitor the patient receiving methotrexate for hepatic, renal, and pulmonary toxicities.
- Instruct the patient taking methotrexate to inspect the mouth daily and report any discomfort, patchy necrotic areas, bleeding, or overgrowth of black furry tongue to the health care provider.
- Monitor blood glucose periodically because methotrexate can precipitate diabetes mellitus.
- Warn the patient taking methotrexate that exposure to ultraviolet light or sunlight may increase the risk for dermatologic reactions.
- Caution the patient to take contraceptive precautions to prevent pregnancy for at least 12 weeks following methotrexate therapy.
- Counsel the patient taking methotrexate to avoid alcohol to prevent hepatotoxicity.
- Instruct the patient to avoid taking OTC drugs without consulting the health care provider because many of these medications contain folic acid, which alters methotrexate response.
- Instruct the patient to report any sore mouth, weakness, unusual bleeding, bruising, and skin eruptions.

Do You UNDERSTAND?

DIRECTIONS: For each drug listed below, identify the interaction if given with methotrexate.

Drug	Interaction with Methotrexate
1. Folic acid	_____
2. Theophylline	_____
3. Aspirin	_____
4. Penicillin	_____
5. Sulfonylureas	_____

What IS a Tumor Necrosis Factor Blocker?

Tumor Necrosis Factor Blockers	Trade Names	Uses
etanercept [ee-TAN-er-cept]	Enbrel	Treatment of rheumatoid arthritis
infliximab [in-FLICKS-ih-mab]	Remicade	Treatment of rheumatoid arthritis
adalimumab [ah-dah-LIM-you-mab]	Humira	Treatment of rheumatoid arthritis
leflunomide [lee-FLEW-no-mide]	Arava	Treatment of rheumatoid arthritis

Action

Tumor necrosis factor (TNF)–receptor antagonists (TNF blockers) bind to the TNF and block it from attaching to cell surface TNF receptors, thereby mediating the inflammatory response. These agents are also known as *immunomodulators*.

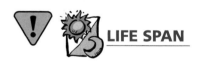 **LIFE SPAN**

- Etanercept is contraindicated for women during lactation and for children less than 4 years of age.
- Etanercept should be used cautiously during pregnancy.

Answers: **1. decreased effectiveness of methotrexate; 2. increased levels of theophylline; 3. increased methotrexate levels and toxicity; 4. increased methotrexate levels and toxicity; 5. increased methotrexate levels and toxicity.**

Uses

TNF blockers are ussed effectively in the treatment of rheumatoid arthritis. Infliximab is also used to treat moderate to severe Crohn's disease.

What You NEED TO KNOW

Contraindications/Precautions

TNF blockers are contraindicated for patients with sepsis and elderly or pregnant individuals. Adalimumab should be given cautiously to patients with cardiovascular disease or central nervous system demyelinating disorders. Leflunomide should be given cautiously to patients with renal or hepatic dysfunction, immunodeficiency, or bone marrow abnormalities. Etanercept should be used cautiously in patient prone to infection, such as older adults and patients with diabetes mellitus.

Drug Interactions

Adalimumab absorption is reduced when given with methotrexate. Leflunomide may increase bleeding effects of warfarin. Rifampin increases the concentration of leflunomide. Concurrent or recent use of etanercept with methotrexate, leflunomide, azathioprine, or cyclophosphamide may lead to pancytopenia.

Adverse Effects

Adverse effects of TNF blockers include headache, dizziness, depression, insomnia, demyelinating disorders, myocardial ischemia, hypotension, hypertension, heart failure, dyspepsia, abdominal pain, dyspnea, pharyngitis, sinusitis, cough, respiratory tract infection, rash, paresthesias, peripheral edema, and pancytopenia. Leflunomide may cause hypokalemia, hepatotoxicity, and Stevens-Johnson syndrome.

What You DO

Nursing Responsibilities

Etanercept, adalimumab, and anakinra are injected subcutaneously (Sub-Q). Infliximab is administered intravenously (IV) over at least 2 hours, and leflunomide is administered orally. When administering TNF blockers, the nurse should:

- Monitor complete blood count (CBC) and platelet count for early detection of bone marrow depression.
- Monitor the patient's potassium level for early detection of hypokalemia.
- Instruct patients to report weakness, bleeding, and difficulty breathing to the health care provider.
- Inject etanercept, adalimumab, and anakinra Sub-Q into thigh, abdomens, or upper arm, with a rotation of sites.
- Monitor the patient who is taking etanercept for signs of infection and immediately report these to the health care provider.

TAKE HOME POINTS

- Never inject etanercept into an old injection site or into an area that is tender, bruised, red, or hard.
- Never administer vaccinations, particularly live vaccines, to patients who are taking etanercept.

Do You UNDERSTAND?

DIRECTIONS: Match Column A with Column B.

Column A	Column B
_____ 1. TNF blockers treat _____.	a. diabetes mellitus.
_____ 2. Luflunomide is given cautiously to patients with _____.	b. rheumatoid arthritis.
_____ 3. Etanercept is given cautiously to patients with _____.	c. renal or hepatic dysfunction.

Answers: 1. b; 2. c; 3. a.

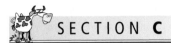

SECTION C

ANTIGOUT AGENTS

Antigout medications treat painful gouty attacks and prevent further attacks from occurring. A supersaturation of serum uric acid and crystal deposits that form in joints and surrounding tissue are characteristics of gout; thus antigout medications are focused on altering uric acid. Drugs are available that reduce uric acid production, increase renal uric acid excretion, treat acute gout, and prevent recurrent attacks (e.g., antimitotics, NSAIDs, analgesics, corticosteroids, xanthine oxidase inhibitors, uricosurics).

In the first stage of gout (**asymptomatic hyperuricemia**), drugs are rarely required. In the second stage (**acute gouty arthritis**), antimitotics are the drugs of choice for the first attack. NSAIDs (particularly indomethacin) are preferred for subsequent attacks. Glucocorticoids may be used for patients who fail to respond to other drugs. The third stage (**asymptomatic intercritical period**) is treated with antimitotics, xanthine oxidase inhibitors, or uricosurics. The final stage of gout (**chronic tophaceous**) is treated primarily with xanthine oxidase inhibitors. This section reviews uric acid inhibitors, uricosurics, and antimitotics.

What IS an Antimitotic?

Antimitotic	Trade Name	Use
colchicine [KOHL-chi-seen]	Colchicine	Treatment of acute gout

Action

Antimitotics (the oldest gout medication) are antiinflammatory drugs, the effects of which are specific for gout. Colchicine inhibits the phagocytic response to urate crystals and inhibits the migration of leukocytes to the inflamed site, thereby decreasing the inflammatory response. Colchicine causes neutrophils to block the release of the chemical mediators that are required in the inflammatory response, reduces mobility and adhesion of polymorphonuclear leukocytes, and inhibits production of leukotriene.

Colchicine inhibits the inflammatory response, thereby generally eliminating pain within 48 hours of the onset of an acute gout attack and decreasing gouty signs and symptoms both rapidly and dramatically.

Uses

Colchicine has three uses: treating acute gouty attacks, aborting an impending attack, and reducing the incidence of chronic gout attacks. Colchicine is the drug of choice to relieve acute gouty attacks.

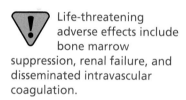

LIFE SPAN

Antimitotics should be used with caution in women during pregnancy and lactation and in older or debilitated patients.

What You NEED TO KNOW

Contraindications/Precautions

Colchicine is contraindicated for patients with severe GI, cardiac, hepatic, or renal disorders.

Drug Interactions

When cimetidine and erythromycin are given concurrently with colchicine, the risk for colchicine toxicity is increased. Colchicine may decrease absorption of vitamin B_{12}.

Adverse Effects

The common adverse effects of colchicines include nausea, abdominal cramping, vomiting, and diarrhea. Intravenous (IV) administration may lead to tissue necrosis from extravasation. Early signs of colchicine toxicity include nausea, anorexia, abdominal pain, vomiting, diarrhea, and paralytic ileus. Diarrhea may be severe and bloody. Other signs of colchicine toxicity include stomatitis, fever, malaise, rash, joint pain, hypocalcemia, dehydration, and oliguria.

Life-threatening adverse effects include bone marrow suppression, renal failure, and disseminated intravascular coagulation.

What You DO

Nursing Responsibilities

Usually joint pain and swelling decrease within 8 to 12 hours and disappear within 24 to 72 hours after oral colchicine therapy and 6 to 12 hours after IV therapy. Colchicine should be discontinued when an acute gouty attack is relieved. To avoid colchicine toxicity, therapy is not usually

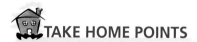

TAKE HOME POINTS

Take care to prevent IV extravasation of colchicine because severe tissue irritation and nerve damage may result. The patient with gout should have colchicine on hand.

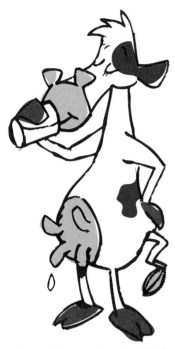

Take colchicine with milk or food.

repeated within 3 days. When administering antimitotics, the nurse should:

- Inform the patient that colchicine may be given with food or milk to decrease the risk for GI distress.
- Counsel the patient to avoid beer, ale, and wine because these substances may cause sudden, unexpected gouty attacks.
- Instruct the patient that colchicine is effective only when taken at the first warning sign of an acute gout attack, not several days later.
- Instruct the patient to discontinue colchicine and immediately report any nausea, vomiting, and severe diarrhea to the health care provider because these are the first signs of toxicity. IV administration of colchicine eliminates most GI adverse effects.
- Advise the patient to report fever, fatigue, bleeding gums, sore mouth or throat, or any unusual bleeding or bruising to the health care provider for early detection of bone marrow suppression.

Do You UNDERSTAND?

DIRECTIONS: **Circle the beverages that should be encouraged when undergoing colchicine therapy. Place a square around the beverages that should be avoided.**

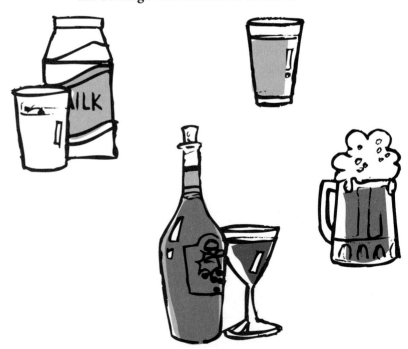

Answers: beverages to be encouraged: milk, water; beverages to be avoided: beer, wine.

What IS a Uric Acid Inhibitor?

Uric Acid Inhibitor	Trade Name	Use
allopurinol [al-oh-PURE-ih-nohl]	Zyloprim	Treatment of hyperuricemia in gout

Action

Uric acid inhibitors are also known as xanthine oxidase inhibitors because they inhibit the xanthine oxidase enzyme, thereby decreasing the serum uric acid level. Because the xanthine oxidase enzyme is responsible for converting hypoxanthine into xanthine and xanthine into uric acid, the inhibition of the xanthine oxidase enzyme blocks the production of uric acid.

Uses

This uric acid inhibitor is the drug of choice in the treatment of chronic tophaceous gout. Allopurinol reduces uric acid production and serum levels, which prevents tophus formation and promotes regression of preformed tophi. Allopurinol is frequently used prophylactically.

What You NEED TO KNOW

Contraindications/Precautions

Uric acid inhibitors are contraindicated for patients with hypersensitivity. These drugs should be used with caution in patients with a history of peptic ulcer disease, bone marrow depression, and hepatic or renal dysfunction.

Drug Interactions

Increased effects of ACE inhibitors, theophylline, warfarin, phenytoin, and oncology drugs occur when allopurinol is given concurrently. The risk for allopurinol toxicity is increased when given with thiazide diuretics, particularly in patients with renal dysfunction. Antacids decrease the absorption and action of allopurinol.

Adverse Effects

The adverse effects of allopurinol include drowsiness, headache, dizziness, metallic taste, rash, nausea, vomiting, abdominal discomfort, diarrhea,

Fatal hypersensitivity syndrome is the most serious (although rare) toxicity of uric acid inhibitors. Fever, rash, eosinophilia, and hepatic or renal dysfunction are characteristics of fatal hypersensitivity syndrome.

bone marrow depression, and hepatotoxicity. Cataracts and retinopathy may occur from prolonged allopurinol therapy.

What You DO

Nursing Responsibilities

Allopurinol should be taken with food to eliminate GI distress. Tablets may be crushed and mixed with food or taken with fluids. When administering xanthine oxidase inhibitors, the nurse should:

- Monitor serum uric acid levels at least every 1 to 2 weeks to verify dose adequacy and maintain uric acid levels at 6 mg/dL.
- Monitor baseline CBC before beginning therapy and monthly for early detection of toxicity.
- Monitor baseline renal and hepatic function tests before therapy and monthly for early detection of toxicity.
- Instruct the patient taking allopurinol to report the first sign of a rash immediately to the health care provider.
- Inform the patient that a therapeutic response to allopurinol is usually expected in 1 to 3 weeks.
- Initiate allopurinol 1 to 2 days before administrating an antineoplastic when given concurrently.
- Tell the patient that periodic ophthalmic examinations are required when undergoing long-term allopurinol therapy.
- Warn the patient to avoid alcohol, caffeine, and thiazide diuretics because these items increase uric acid levels.

TAKE HOME POINTS

Because acute gouty attacks are likely to occur during the first 6 weeks of therapy, antimitotics may be given in combination therapy for the first 3 to 6 months of allopurinol treatment. Allopurinol should be immediately discontinued at the first sign of a rash because of a potentially fatal hypersensitivity reaction. Therapeutic responses to allopurinol include normal uric acid levels, gradual decrease in tophi, joint pain relief, and increased joint mobility.

Do You UNDERSTAND?

DIRECTIONS: Provide appropriate responses to the following questions.

1. When undergoing allopurinol therapy, which laboratory tests require periodic monitoring? _____
2. When undergoing allopurinol therapy, what adverse effect should be reported immediately? _____

Answers: 1. CBC, hepatic, and renal function tests; 2. rash.

What IS a Uricosuric?

Uricosurics	Trade Names	Uses
probenecid [pro-BEN-ih-sid]	Benemid	Treatment of hyperuricemia in acute gout
sulfinpyrazone [sul-fin-PEER-ah-zone]	Anturane	Treatment of hyperuricemia in acute gout

Action

Uricosurics block renal tubular reabsorption, which promotes excretion of uric acid.

Uses

Uricosurics are used in the treatment of chronic hyperuricemia in gout to reduce the urate concentration in serum.

What You NEED TO KNOW

Contraindications/Precautions

Uricosurics are contraindicated for patients with hypersensitivity, blood dyscrasias, or uric acid kidney stones and for those who are taking β-lactam antibiotics or low-dose salicylates.

Uricosurics should be used cautiously in patients with a history of peptic ulcer disease and renal dysfunction.

Drug Interactions

Probenecid increases the therapeutic effects of indomethacin and other NSAIDs. Salicylates counteract the action of uricosuric. Uricosurics inhibit the metabolism of tolbutamide, leading to hypoglycemia, and they inhibit the metabolism of warfarin, causing a bleeding tendency. Uricosurics also increase the concentrations of penicillins, cephalosporins, and other β-lactam antibiotics. Alcohol increases serum urate levels when taken with uricosurics.

Adverse Effects

Uricosurics are usually well tolerated and have a low incidence of adverse effects. Common adverse effects of uricosurics include headache, dizziness, flushed skin, rash, sore gums, anorexia, nausea, vomiting, alopecia, peptic ulcer aggravation, urinary frequency, renal calculi, and blood dyscrasias. Hypersensitivity (e.g., itching, fever, sweating, hypotension, anaphylactic reaction) may also occur.

What You DO

Nursing Responsibilities

The goal is to reduce the uric acid level to 5 to 6 mg/dL, which depletes urate body storage, prevents the formation of tophi, and prevents renal damage. When gouty attacks have been absent for at least 6 months and serum urate levels are controlled, daily doses of uricosurics may be reduced to the lowest effective dose that maintains gout control. When administering uricosurics, the nurse should:

- Instruct the patient taking uricosurics to increase fluid intake to at least 3000 mL/day to promote uric acid excretion and prevent renal calculi.
- Tell the patient to take uricosurics in divided doses with meals, milk, or antacids to prevent gastric distress.
- Advise the patient taking uricosurics to avoid alcohol to prevent GI distress and increased serum urate levels.
- Inform the patient taking uricosurics that the frequency of acute gouty attacks may increase during the first 6 to 12 months of uricosuric treatment; thus the health care provider may prescribe another concurrent prophylactic drug.
- Monitor blood glucose for patients who are taking uricosurics and concurrent sulfonylureas because these patients may require a dose adjustment to prevent hypoglycemia.
- Instruct the patient to take uricosurics as ordered and to avoid discontinuing the medication without consulting the health care provider.
- Caution the patient taking uricosurics to avoid taking aspirin or OTC drugs without consulting the health care provider.

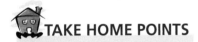

TAKE HOME POINTS

When gastric distress continues, a dose reduction may be required. An irregular dose schedule, such as skipped doses, may drastically increase serum urate levels and lead to gout attacks. Salicylates decrease uric acid excretion, which counteracts the uricosuric action.

Do You UNDERSTAND?

DIRECTIONS: **Provide appropriate responses to the following questions.**

1. What drugs counteract the uricosuric action when given concurrently? _____

2. What are four of the most common adverse effects of a uricosuric? _____

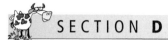

SECTION **D**

MUSCLE RELAXANTS

What IS a Centrally Acting Muscle Relaxant?

Central Muscle Relaxants	Trade Names	Uses
cyclobenzaprine *[SIGH-kloe-BEN-zuh-preen]*	Flexeril Cycoflex	Treatment of muscle spasms
baclofen *[BACK-low-fen]*	Lioresal	Treatment of muscle spasms
carisoprodol *[car-eye-so-PRO-dole]*	Soma	Treatment of muscle spasms and rigidity
tizanidine *[tih-ZAN-ih-deen]*	Zanaflex	Treatment of muscle spasms and rigidity
methocarbamol *[meth-oh-CAR-buh-mahl]*	Robaxin	Treatment of muscle spasms

Action

The exact action of centrally acting muscle relaxants is unknown. However, these drugs are thought to produce CNS depression of the thalamus, brain stem, basal ganglia, and spinal cord. These agents may also block nerve impulses that lead to increased skeletal muscle tone and contraction. Tizanidine increases inhibition of spinal motor neurons to relieve spasticity.

Answers: 1. salicylates; 2. headache, loss of appetite, nausea, vomiting.

Uses

Centrally acting muscle relaxants are used primarily to reduce muscle spasms. Baclofen inhibits neurotransmission at the spinal level and is used in the management of detrusor sphincter incoordination associated with spinal cord disease and reduction of severe spasticity of multiple sclerosis or cerebral palsy.

What You NEED TO KNOW

Contraindications/Precautions

Centrally acting muscle relaxants are contraindicated for patients with porphyria (a rare inherited disorder of porphyrin metabolism).

Drug Interactions

When alcohol, antihistamines, CNS depressants, or MAOIs are taken concurrently with central muscle relaxants, the interaction intensifies CNS depression. Intensified CNS depression increases the risk for hepatotoxicity. Drug interaction with MAOIs and centrally acting muscle relaxants may also lead to a hypertensive crisis. When orphenadrine and propoxyphene are taken together, the patient may experience increased confusion, anxiety, and tremors. An increased hypotensive effect occurs when centrally acting muscle relaxants are taken with antihypertensives.

Adverse Effects

Adverse effects of centrally acting muscle relaxants include visual disturbances, headache, dizziness, hypotension, weakness, fatigue, drowsiness, ataxia, nervousness, irritability, dry mouth, taste alterations, anorexia, nausea, vomiting, diarrhea or constipation, urinary frequency, urgency, and urinary retention. The adverse effects of tizanidine include hallucinations, bradycardia, and prolonged Q-T intervals. Baclofen may cause nasal congestion, slurred speech, confusion, tinnitus, nystagmus, anorexia, abdominal pain, dysuria, muscle stiffness, urgency, and male sexual dysfunction.

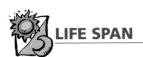 **LIFE SPAN**

Centrally acting muscle relaxants are contraindicated for children under 12 years of age and for women during pregnancy or lactation.

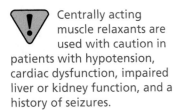 Centrally acting muscle relaxants are used with caution in patients with hypotension, cardiac dysfunction, impaired liver or kidney function, and a history of seizures.

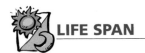 **LIFE SPAN**

Older patients are especially sensitive to centrally acting muscle relaxants and may develop confusion, depression, and hallucinations.

What You DO

Nursing Responsibilities

Centrally acting muscle relaxants should be discontinued over a 2-week or longer period. Abrupt withdrawal after prolonged administration leads to anxiety, agitation, tachycardia, seizures, hallucinations, and exacerbation of spasticity. When administering centrally acting muscle relaxants, the nurse should:

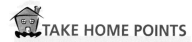

TAKE HOME POINTS

Assist with or supervise ambulation because the initial loss of spasticity may affect the patient's ability to stand or walk.

- Administer the drug with food or milk if patient experiences GI distress.
- Institute safety measures to compensate for the potential of causing drowsiness in the patient.
- Warn the patient to avoid driving or operating hazardous equipment until the response to the drug is known.
- Teach patient to change positions slowly.
- Warn the patient that CNS depression is intensified by alcohol.
- Monitor liver function for early detection of hepatotoxicity.
- Instruct the patient to report drowsiness, dizziness, ataxia, delusions, or hallucinations because most of these adverse effects can be decreased by dose reduction.
- Inform the patient that centrally acting muscle relaxant drugs may elevate blood glucose levels, necessitating dose adjustments in oral hypoglycemics and insulin.
- Taper baclofen slowly over 1 to 2 weeks when discontinuing to prevent development of psychoses and hallucinations.

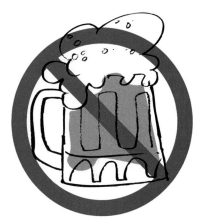

Do You UNDERSTAND?

DIRECTIONS: Indicate in the space provided whether each statement is *true* or *false*. If the answer is false, correct the statement to make it true (using the margin space).

_____ 1. Centrally acting muscle relaxants are used in the treatment of spasticity in patients with multiple sclerosis or cerebral palsy.

_____ 2. Alcohol exacerbates this drug class and relaxes muscles but stimulates the CNS.

_____ 3. When centrally acting muscle relaxants are discontinued, they should be tapered over a 4-day period.

Answers: 1. true; 2. false; alcohol exacerbates CNS depression; 3. false; taper over 2 weeks or more.

What IS a Peripheral Muscle Relaxant?

Peripheral Muscle Relaxants	Trade Names	Uses
dantrolene [dan-troe-LEEN]	Dantrium	Treatment of spasticity associated with spinal cord injury, CVA, cerebral palsy, and multiple sclerosis
quinine [KWIE-nine]	Quinamm Quiphile	Prevention and treatment of nocturnal leg cramps

Action

Peripherally acting muscle relaxants exert their actions by different methods. Dantrolene inhibits calcium release from sarcoplasmic reticulum, thereby reducing muscle contractility. Quinine acts similarly to salicylates and exerts a curare-like skeletal muscle relaxation.

Uses

Dantrolene is used in the management of spasticity from upper motor neuron (UMN) disorders, spinal cord disorders, or cerebral disease, as well as perioperative management of malignant hyperthermia. Quinine is used primarily in the treatment of nocturnal leg cramps.

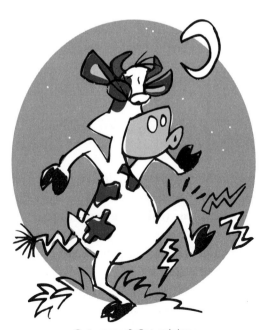

Got cramps? Get quinine.

What You NEED TO KNOW

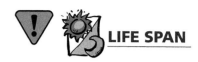 **LIFE SPAN**

Contraindications/Precautions

Peripherally acting muscle relaxants are contraindicated for patients with hepatic dysfunction.

Drug Interactions

CNS depression is intensified when alcohol and CNS depressants are taken concurrently with dantrolene. The interaction of estrogens and dantrolene leads to an increased risk for hepatotoxicity. When calcium channel blockers are taken with dantrolene, an increased risk for ventricular fibrillation occurs. Quinine increases the effects of oral anticoagulants, digoxin, anticholinergics, and neuromuscular blockers. Anticonvulsants, barbiturates, and rifampin increase the metabolism of quinine, reducing its effectiveness. Conversely, sodium bicarbonate, carbonic anhydrase inhibitors, and antacids decrease quinine excretion, increasing the risk for toxicity.

Adverse Effects

Adverse effects of peripherally acting muscle relaxants include headache, dizziness, euphoria, blurred vision, confusion, abnormal sweating, chills, tachycardia, severe itching, hives, abnormal hair growth, nausea, vomiting, abdominal cramps, and diarrhea. The specific adverse effects of dantrolene include nervousness, insomnia, weakness, speech disturbances, photosensitivity, urinary frequency or retention, nocturnal diuresis, erectile dysfunction, depression, and seizures. Prolonged high doses of dantrolene can lead to hepatotoxicity. Specific adverse effects of quinine use include anxiety, fever, rash, tinnitus, ototoxicity, angina, acute asthmatic episodes, blood dyscrasias, hypothermia, cardiovascular collapse, coma, and death.

- Peripherally acting muscle relaxants are contraindicated for women during pregnancy and lactation and for children under 5 years of age.
- Peripherally acting muscle relaxants are used with caution in patients with impaired cardiac or pulmonary function and those over the age of 35, particularly women.

What You DO

Nursing Responsibilities

When administering peripherally acting muscle relaxants, the nurse should:
- Monitor IV administration carefully to avoid extravasation because the IV solution is extremely irritating to the tissues.
- Observe liver function studies for early detection of hepatotoxicity.

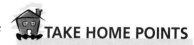 **TAKE HOME POINTS**

Carefully monitor digoxin levels in the patient who is concurrently taking quinine.

- Monitor coagulation studies resulting from the interaction with warfarin.
- Instruct the patient who is concurrently taking oral anticoagulants to report increased bruising or bleeding.
- Monitor digoxin levels resulting from a drug interaction with quinine.
- Instruct the patient to report severe diarrhea because the dose may need to be reduced to prevent dehydration and electrolyte imbalance.
- Teach the patient to avoid tasks that require alertness and motor skills until response is known.
- Instruct the patient not to discontinue drug abruptly, or hallucinations or seizures may occur.

Do You UNDERSTAND?

DIRECTIONS: Provide appropriate responses to the following questions.

1. Peripherally acting muscle relaxants might be used as a treatment for what spasticity disorders? _____
2. Quinine therapy is used to treat what disorder? _____

References

Abrams AC Pennington SS, Lammon CB: *Clinical drug therapy: rationales for nursing practice,* ed 8, Philadelphia, 2007, Lippincott.

Black JM, Hawks JH: *Medical-surgical nursing: clinical management for positive outcomes,* ed 7, St. Louis, 2005, Elsevier.

Gutierrez K, Queener SF: *Pharmacology for nursing practice,* St Louis, 2003, Mosby.

Hardman JG, Limbird LE: *Goodman & Gilman's the pharmacological basis of therapeutics,* ed 10, New York, 2001, McGraw-Hill.

Johnson PH, editor: *Nurse practitioner's drug handbook,* ed 3, Springhouse, Pa, 2000, Springhouse.

Karch AM: *Focus on nursing pharmacology,* ed 3, Philadelphia, 2006, Lippincott.

Kee JL, Hayes ER, McCuistion LE: *Pharmacology: a nursing process approach,* ed 5, Philadelphia, 2006, Elsevier.

Lehne RA: *Pharmacology for nursing care,* ed 5, Philadelphia, 2004, WB Saunders.

Lilley LL, Harrington S, Snyder JS: *Pharmacology and the nursing process,* ed 4, St Louis, 2005, Mosby.

McKenry, LM, Salerno, E: *Mosby's pharmacology in nursing,* ed 21, St Louis, 2003, Mosby.

Smeltzer SC, Bare BG: *Brunner and Suddarth's textbook of medical-surgical nursing,* ed 10, Philadelphia, 2004, Lippincott.

Wilson BA, Shannon MT, Stang CL: *Nurses drug guide,* Upper Saddle River, New Jersey, 2006, Pearson.

Answers: 1. UMN disorders, spinal cord disorders, or cerebral disease; 2. nocturnal leg cramps.

NCLEX® Review

Section A

1. Which of the following is a type of NSAID?
   1 Oxicam
   2 Uricosuric
   3 Immunosuppressive
   4 Gold agent

2. Which represents the action of an NSAID?
   1 Reduces serum urate levels
   2 Inhibits formation of prostaglandins
   3 Inhibits destructive lysosomal enzyme activity in joints
   4 Reduces xanthine oxidase enzyme production

3. The COX-2 form of cyclooxygenase is associated with the reduction of which adverse effect?
   1 Pain
   2 Fever
   3 GI distress
   4 Constipation

4. A patient is taking naproxen (Naprosyn). Which should the nurse teach the patient to monitor?
   1 Ankle edema
   2 Constipation
   3 Increased appetite
   4 Deep vein thrombosis

5. A patient is taking aspirin and has a serum blood level of 32 mg/dL. Which symptom would the nurse observe the patient for?
   1 Fever
   2 Tinnitus
   3 Headache
   4 Stevens-Johnson syndrome

Section B

6. Which DMARD requires periodic eye examinations?
   1 Gold agents
   2 Methotrexate
   3 Etanercept
   4 Hyaluronic acid

7. Which DMARD may cause a nitritoid reaction?
   1 Gold agents
   2 Antimalarials
   3 Glucocorticoids
   4 Tumor necrosis factor blockers

8. A patient is taking etanercept (Enbrel). By which route should the nurse should administer this drug?
   1 Orally
   2 Subcutaneously
   3 Intramuscularly
   4 Sublingually

9. A patient taking auranofin (Ridaura) asks the nurse why she is getting this drug because she heard it was a "heavy duty drug." The nurse explains that aggressive therapy with DMARDs is given to:
   1 control the painful swelling.
   2 interrupt joint degeneration.
   3 promote prostaglandin synthesis.
   4 inhibit the phagocytic response to urate crystals.

10. A patient is taking infliximab (Remicade). The nurse knows to monitor:
    1 oral ulceration.
    2 potassium for hyperkalemia.
    3 potassium for hypokalemia.
    4 gray-blue discoloration of mucous membranes.

Section C

11. The goal of antigout therapy is to maintain which of the following serum uric acid levels?
    1 2 mg/dL
    2 4 mg/dL
    3 6 mg/dL
    4 10 mg/dL

12. A 24-year-old female patient is taking antigout medication. Which antigout drug should be used with caution for this patient?
    1 Colchicine
    2 Probenecid
    3 Allopurinol
    4 Sulfinpyrazone

13. A patient is taking allopurinol for treatment of gout. The nurse should inform the patient to prevent increased uric acid levels by avoiding all of the following except:
    1 wine.
    2 beer.
    3 coffee.
    4 orange juice.

14. The nurse knows to monitor the blood glucose of the patient taking:
    1 colchicine.
    2 probenecid.
    3 allopurinol.
    4 cyclopentolate.

15. A patient is taking probenecid. The nurse should instruct the patient to:
    1 maintain fluid intake to at least 1500 mL/day.
    2 avoid taking concurrent aspirin for pain.
    3 have eye examinations at least every 3 months.
    4 keep acetylcysteine on have for potential toxic overdose.

Section D

16. Which laboratory values are important to monitor when administering peripheral-acting muscle relaxants?
    1 Sodium level
    2 Phenytoin levels
    3 Potassium level
    4 Liver function studies

17. Baclofen is used primarily to treat which of the following disorders?
    1 Leg cramps
    2 Hyperactivity
    3 Narcolepsy
    4 Muscle spasms

18. Methocarbamol (Robaxin) is prescribed for a patient. The nurse knows that methocarbamol is contraindicated for patients with:
    1 seizures.
    2 porphyria.
    3 diabetes mellitus.
    4 hepatic dysfunction.

19. A patient is awakened by leg cramps during the night and asks the nurse which of her ordered medicines would help her. The nurse knows that _____ is used for nocturnal leg cramps.
    1 quinine (Quinamm)
    2 carisoprodol (Soma)
    3 dantrolene (Dantrium)
    4 cyclobenzaprine (Flexeril)

20. A patient is taking tizanidine (Zanaflex). The nurse plans to teach him to:
    1 prevent CNS depression by avoiding alcohol.
    2 report headaches as an early sign of hypertension.
    3 report IV infiltration to avoid extravasation of tissues.
    4 periodically discontinue drug for 2 to 4 days for greater effectiveness.

NCLEX® Review Answers

Section A

1. 1 An oxicam is a type of NSAID, along with salicylates, propionic acid derivatives, acetic acid derivatives, pyrazolones, anthranilic acids, and COX-2 inhibitors. Uricosurics are antigout drugs. Immunosuppressives and gold agents are DMARDs.

2. 2 The action of NSAIDs inhibits the formation of prostaglandins but does not reduce serum urate levels (action of antigout drugs), inhibit destructive lysosomal enzyme activity in joints (action of gold compounds), or reduce xanthine oxidase enzyme production (action of allopurinol, a xanthine oxidase inhibitor).

3. 3 GI distress is reduced because without COX-1 inhibition, the protection of the stomach lining is preserved. Pain and fever reduction are desired effects, not adverse effects. Constipation is not an adverse effect from COX-2 inhibitors; diarrhea would be a more common adverse effect.

4. 1 Naproxen may cause an adverse effect of ankle edema from sodium and water retention, diarrhea, anorexia, and prolonged bleeding time.

5. 2 The normal therapeutic range of salicylates is 15 to 30 mg/dL and toxicity occurs above 30 mg/dL. Tinnitus is usually the first sign indicative of toxicity. Fever, headache, and Stevens-Johnson syndrome are not toxic effects of salicylates.

Section B

6. 1 Gold agents may cause corneal gold deposits and retinopathy. Methotrexate, etanercept, and hyaluronic acid do not cause adverse effects that require periodic eye examinations.

7. 1 Gold agents may cause a nitritoid reaction. Antimalarials, glucocorticoids, and tumor necrosis factor blockers do not cause this adverse effect.

8. 2 Etanercept should be given subcutaneously, not orally, intramuscularly, nor sublingually.

9. 2 Auranofin interrupts joint degeneration in patients with arthritis. It is not given to control swelling or inhibit phagocytic response to urate crystals. Auranofin suppresses prostaglandin activity rather than promote prostaglandin synthesis.

10. 3 Infiximab may cause hypokalemia but is not associated with oral ulceration, hyperkalemia, or gray-blue discoloration of mucous membranes.

Section C

11. 3 The goal of antigout therapy is to maintain serum uric acid levels between 5 and 6 mg/dL. The remaining options (2 mg/dL, 4 mg/dL, and 10 mg/dL) are incorrect serum uric acid levels in gout prevention.

12. 1 Colchicine should be used with caution during pregnancy. Probenecid, allopurinol, and sulfinpyrazone do not have this precaution.

13. 4 Alcohol and caffeine should be avoided when taking allopurinol. Therefore orange juice is acceptable, but wine, beer, and coffee are not.

14. 2 The nurse should monitor the blood glucose for uricosurics, such as probenecid. Colchicine, allopurinol, and cyclopentolate are not known to affect the blood glucose.

15. 2 Aspirin concurrent with probenecid should be avoided. Fluid intake should be maintained at 3000 mL/day when taking probenecid. Eye examinations and acetylcysteine are not associated with probenecid.

Section D

16. 4 It is important to monitor the liver function studies when taking direct-acting muscle relaxants. These drugs are not known to affect sodium, potassium, or phenytoin levels.

17. 4 Baclofen is used primarily to treat muscle spasms not leg cramps, hyperactivity, nor narcolepsy.

18. 2 Methocarbamol is contraindicated for patients with porphyria. This drug should be used with caution for those with a history of seizures or hepatic dysfunction. There is no contraindication for diabetics.

19. 1 Quinamm is used for nocturnal leg cramps. Carisoprodol treats muscle spasms and rigidity. Dantrolene is used for to treat spasticity associated with SCI, CVA, cerebral palsy, and multiple sclerosis.

20. 1 Tizanidine may lead to CNS depression when combined with alcohol. Tizanidine is given orally, should be tapered off over 1 to 2 weeks when discontinued, and may cause hypotension as adverse effect not hypertension.

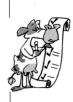

Notes

Drugs Used to Treat Sensory System Alterations

What You WILL LEARN

✔ Contrast the drugs used in the treatment of increased intraocular pressure.
✔ Explain the meaning of a mydriatic, a miotic, and a cycloplegic drug.
✔ Identify the indications for patients taking an otic drug.
✔ Recall the nursing responsibilities for patients taking an otic drug.
✔ Discuss the role of an antipruritic, emollient, keratolytic drug for the patient with a skin disorder.
✔ Explain the nursing responsibilities for a patient who is receiving drug therapy for acne or burns.

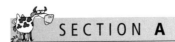

SECTION A

OPHTHALMIC AGENTS

Visual disorders present a danger to patients, largely because vision is one of the most cherished senses. Although many eye disorders are correctable with eyeglasses or contact lenses, others require drugs to control or treat. This section reviews selected drugs used in the treatment of eye disorders, including ocular lubricants, decongestants, miotics, carbonic anhydrase inhibitors, mydriatics, and cycloplegics.

What IS an Ocular Lubricant?

Ocular Lubricants	Contents
artificial tears	White petrolatum, mineral oil, and anhydrous lanolin
tyloxapol (Enuclene)	Benzalkonium chloride

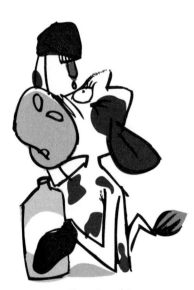

Keep it moist.

Action

Ocular lubricants include single-ingredient formulations, such as benzalkonium chloride, sodium chloride, and polyvinyl alcohol. Combination formulations include petrolatum, mineral oil, and lanolin. Ocular lubricants keep the eyes moist with isotonic solutions and wetting agents. The most important action of artificial tear formulations is that they stabilize the tear film while preventing tear evaporation.

Uses

Ocular lubricants are used for their local effects in the eye. They alleviate dry eyes and provide lubrication for patients with an artificial eye. These drugs offer lubrication and protection for exposure-related inflammation of the cornea (keratitis), decreased corneal sensitivity, corneal erosions, dry cornea (during or following eye surgery), and removal of a foreign body. Lubricants with high thickness (viscosity) alone do not necessarily provide relief for all dry eye conditions.

What You NEED TO KNOW

Contraindications/Precautions

Ocular lubricants should be used with caution in patients with sensitivities to the ingredients.

Drug Interactions

Ocular lubricants may alter the effects of other concurrently administered drugs used in the eye.

Adverse Effects

Ocular lubricants generally cause no irritation or toxicity to eye tissues. Adverse effects of ocular lubricants include photophobia, lid edema, stinging, temporarily blurred vision, and eye discomfort.

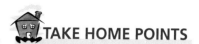

TAKE HOME POINTS

Some contact lenses may absorb the drugs or their additives.

What You DO

Nursing Responsibilities

Because nearly all ocular lubricants are available without a prescription, the health care provider and pharmacist frequently carry the primary responsibility of assisting and counseling the patient regarding their selection and proper use. When administering ocular lubricants, the nurse should:

- Advise the patient to consult with the health care provider regarding the concurrent use of ocular lubricants and contact lenses.
- Inform the patient that no single formulation of natural tears has been identified that universally improves the signs and symptoms of dry eyes while maintaining patient comfort and acceptance.

Do You UNDERSTAND?

DIRECTIONS: Fill in the blanks with the appropriate responses.

1. List five ingredients that are common in ocular lubricants:

   _____, _____,

   _____, _____,

   and _____.

2. Ocular lubricants are indicated for patients with _____

   or _____.

3. High _____ alone does not provide relief for all dry eye problems.

What IS an Ocular Decongestant?

Ocular Decongestants	Trade Names
naphazoline *[naf-AZ-oh-leen]*	Allerest
oxymetazoline *[ox-ih-met-AZ-oh-leen]*	OcuClear
tetrahydrozoline *[tet-ra-high-DROZ-ah-leen]*	Visine Murine

Action

Ocular decongestants stimulate α-receptors on the vascular smooth muscle of the eye and nasal mucosa. The result is local vasoconstriction and a decrease in ocular congestion. Strong solutions of an ocular decongestant also dilate the pupil **(mydriasis).** The drug's effects are noted in about 10 minutes with a duration of action of 2 to 6 hours.

Uses

Ocular decongestants are typically used for the short-term local treatment of ocular congestion, itching, minor irritation, and red eyes (hyperemia).

Answers: 1. sodium chloride; polyvinyl alcohol, petrolatum, mineral oil, lanolin; 2. dry eyes; an artificial eyes; 3. viscosity.

What You NEED TO KNOW

Contraindications/Precautions

Ocular decongestants should be used cautiously in patients with hyperthyroidism, heart disease, hypertension, diabetes mellitus, eye disease, infection, and injury.

Drug Interactions

When ocular decongestants are given concurrently with monoamine oxidase inhibitors (MAOIs) or inhalation anesthetics, a greater adrenergic response and hypertensive crisis may occur. When absorbed systemically, oxymetazoline can increase the effect of tricyclic antidepressants. Local ophthalmic anesthetics increase the absorption of oxymetazoline. Beta blockers increase the systemic effects of oxymetazoline when given together.

Adverse Effects

Adverse effects of ocular decongestants include transient burning, stinging, dryness, blurred vision, pupillary dilation, and increased or decreased intraocular pressure (IOP). Rebound congestion and eye redness may occur when the drug is overused. The adverse effects from systemic absorption include headache, nervousness, dizziness, weakness, hypertension, chest pain, and dysrhythmias.

What You DO

Nursing Responsibilities

When administering ocular decongestants, the nurse should:
- Explain to the patient that systemic absorption of ocular decongestants from conjunctival membranes can occur.
- Advise the patient to remove contact lenses before applying an ocular decongestant.
- Instruct the patient to contact the health care provider when the ocular decongestant provides no relief after using the drug for 2 days.

Ocular decongestants should be used cautiously in patients with hyperthyroidism, heart disease, hypertension, diabetes mellitus, and eye disease, infection, or injury. Caution should also be used in patients prone to ketoacidosis and in those with eye redness of an unknown cause.

TAKE HOME POINTS

- Instruct the patient to contact the health care provider before using an over-the-counter ocular decongestant.
- Applying pressure to the inner canthus of the eye for 3 to 5 minutes is useful in preventing systemic absorption of all eye drugs.
- Advise the patient to use the ocular decongestant sparingly to avoid rebound redness and congestion.

- Warn the patient that the drug should be used only in the prescribed dose when needed and to avoid sharing the drug with family members or others.
- Instruct the patient to report any systemic reactions (e.g., dizziness, chest pain) to the health care provider. The drug may be discontinued.
- Warn the patient that oxymetazoline may cause bradycardia, hypotension, dizziness, and weakness with excessive use.
- Store ocular decongestants away from heat, light, and humidity (not in the bathroom medicine cabinet) and out of children's reach.
- Instruct the patient to avoid using the drug when the solution is brown or contains a precipitate.

Do You UNDERSTAND?

DIRECTIONS: Fill in the blanks with the appropriate responses.

1. Ocular decongestants should be used with caution in patients with

    _____, _____,

    _____, _____,

    and _____.

2. The brand of the ocular decongestant tetrahydrozoline commonly used to clear red eyes is _____.

3. In susceptible individuals, systemic absorption of an ocular decongestant may cause _____ and _____

    _____.

Answers: 1. acute-angle glaucoma, diabetes mellitus, hypertension, cardiac disease, eye disease; 2. Visine; 3. chest pain, dizziness.

What IS an Ocular Miotic Drug?

Miotics	Trade Names
Anticholinesterase miotics	
demecarium [dem-ee-CARE-ee-um]	Humorsol
echothiophate [ek-oh-THIGH-oh-fate]	Phospholine Iodide
Cholinergic miotics	
carbachol [CAR-ba-coal]	Isopto-carbachol
pilocarpine [pie-low-CAR-peen]	Pilocar
Beta-Blocker miotics	
betaxolol [be-TAX-oh-lole]	Betoptic
timolol 0.25% [TIE-moe-lole]	Timoptic

Action

The classes of ocular miotics include cholinergic miotics, anticholinesterase miotics, and beta blockers. Each class of ocular miotics produces miosis through different mechanisms. Anticholinesterase miotics inhibit the breakdown of acetylcholine (ACh), a parasympathetic nervous system transmitter, by the enzyme cholinesterase. This action allows ACh to accumulate. The additional ACh acts on the ciliary muscles and the sphincters of the iris, causing ciliary muscles to contract and pupils to dilate.

Cholinergic miotics enhance the action of ACh. Contraction of the sphincter of the iris, contraction of ciliary muscles, and a deepening of the anterior chamber occur. The filtration angle is made larger, which increases outflow of aqueous humor, thus decreasing IOP.

The exact action of beta blockers is unknown, although all ocular formulations antagonize circulating catecholamines on β_2-receptors in the ciliary epithelium. Thus a fall in the production of aqueous humor and IOP takes place.

Uses

Anticholinesterase miotics and cholinergic miotics are used to treat chronic, open-angle glaucoma. However, beta blockers are now preferred for initial therapy. Miotics may also be used to treat conditions that obstruct the outflow of aqueous humor.

What You NEED TO KNOW

Cholinergic miotics should be used with caution in patients with peptic ulcer disease, Parkinson's disease, seizures, and hyperthyroidism.

Contraindications/Precautions

Generally, ocular miotics are contraindicated for patients with hypersensitivity, severe bradycardia, greater than first-degree heart block, cardiogenic shock, uncontrolled heart failure, asthma, and chronic airflow limitation.

Drug Interactions

Epinephrine, cyclopentolate, belladonna alkaloids, and ocular anticholinesterase drugs decrease the effectiveness of ocular miotics. Echothiophate increases the effects of succinylcholine, organic insecticides, cholinesterase inhibitors, and systemic anticholinesterase drugs. When cholinergic drugs are given together with physostigmine, additive toxicity is the result. Anticholinesterase miotics decrease the effects of cholinergic miotics. A greater reduction in IOP occurs when pilocarpine is given concurrently with epinephrine and timolol.

When ocular beta blockers are given with systemic beta blockers or reserpine, systemic effects are increased. Pilocarpine, epinephrine, and carbonic anhydrase inhibitors enhance the lowering of IOP when given with ocular beta blockers. Systemic absorption may result in additive bradycardia and hypotension when ocular miotics are used concurrently with antihypertensives and antiarrhythmics.

Adverse Effects

Adverse effects of anticholinesterase miotics generally include decreased visual acuity, ocular burning, and rash. These drugs produce accommodative myopia and can be problematic in young patients because pupillary constriction and eyelid twitching interferes with vision. Other adverse effects of anticholinesterase miotics include brow ache, headache, eye pain, ciliary and conjunctival congestion, and tearing. Long-term use of these drugs can cause thickening of the conjunctiva and obstruction of the nasolacrimal canals.

Pilocarpine is better tolerated than are other miotics. The adverse effects of cholinergic miotics include irritation, conjunctivitis, and blepharitis. Allergic reactions and systemic effects are uncommon. With prolonged use, cholinergic miotics may cause tolerance, resistance, retinal detachment, obstruction of tear ducts, cysts on the iris, and cataracts.

Ocular beta blockers are usually well tolerated. The adverse effects are most noticeable during the first 2 weeks of therapy and include mild eye irritation, conjunctival redness, eye pain, headache, decreased corneal sensitivity, transient dry eye syndrome, and blurring of central vision. Refractive changes resulting from withdrawal of miotics may be responsible for some reports of blurred vision. Occasionally, ocular beta blockers mask the symptoms and increase the frequency of hypoglycemic episodes in patients with diabetes mellitus.

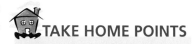

TAKE HOME POINTS

A miotic may cause blurred vision; thus taking the drug at bedtime is preferable to any other time of day.

What You DO

Nursing Responsibilities

When administering ocular miotics, the nurse should:
- Obtain a current drug history because many systemically administered drugs affect the eyes.
- Ask the patient specifically about chronic, systemic diseases that are associated with eye disorders (e.g., diabetes mellitus, arthritis, hypertension, thyroid disease).
- Determine when the patient's last eye examination was performed and when the eyeglass prescription was last changed. Encourage the patient to have regular eye examinations.
- Inquire specifically about nearsightedness (**myopia**), farsightedness (**hyperopia**), glaucoma, and uncontrollable eye deviation (**strabismus**).
- Teach the patient taking ocular miotics the importance of washing hands before drug administration.
- Instruct the patient that pressure on the inner canthus of the eye after ocular drug administration will help prevent systemic absorption.
- Assess for redness, swelling, or other irritation and systemic effects that were not present before treatment was started.
- Inform the patient that only ocular formulations are to be used in the eye.
- Advise the patient that eye drops that have changed color or become cloudy should be discarded.
- Warn the patient to move about carefully until the full effect of the drug is known.

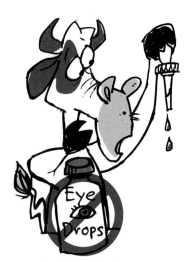

Caution: color change.

Do You UNDERSTAND?

DIRECTIONS: **Match Column A with Column B.**

Column A	Column B
_____ 1. Inhibits the breakdown of ACh by the enzyme cholinesterase, thereby allowing ACh to accumulate.	a. Beta blocker miotics
_____ 2. Enhances the effects of ACh, the parasympathetic nervous system neurotransmitter.	b. Anticholinesterase miotics
_____ 3. Antagonizes circulating catecholamines on β_2-receptors in the ciliary epithelium.	c. Cholinergic miotics

What IS an Ocular Osmotic?

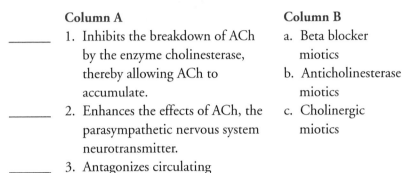

Ocular Osmotics	Trade Names
glycerin [GLI-sir-in]	Ophthalgan
isosorbide [eye-so-SORE-bide]	Isomotic
mannitol [MAN-ih-tole]	Osmitrol
urea [your-EE-ah]	Ureaphil

Action

The ocular osmotics are "diuretics for the eye." These drugs cause the plasma to be hypertonic compared with IOP fluid. By increasing osmolarity, osmotics cause fluid to be drawn from the corneal epithelium to the tear film for elimination from the eye. Ocular osmotics also decrease the production of aqueous humor by acting on hypothalamic osmoreceptors.

Uses

Osmotics are used for short-term reduction of intraocular fluid and IOP in patients with glaucoma, corneal edema, and corneoscleral lacerations. Osmotics are used for preoperative and postoperative surgical repair of a detached retina, cataract extraction, and surgical repair of the cornea. Ocular osmotics are also used to interrupt an acute attack of glaucoma before laser or surgical intervention.

- Osmotics should be used cautiously in patients with cardiac disease, renal or hepatic dysfunction, and diabetes mellitus.
- Ocular isosorbide should be used with caution in patients with diseases that are associated with sodium retention, such as heart failure.

What You NEED TO KNOW

Contraindications/Precautions

Ocular osmotics are contraindicated for patients with hypersensitivity, anuria, and severe dehydration. Ocular isosorbide is contraindicated in patients with acute pulmonary edema and hemorrhagic glaucoma. Mannitol and urea are contraindicated in patients with heart failure, progressive renal or hepatic dysfunction, active intracranial bleeding, or sickle cell disease with central nervous system involvement.

Drug Interactions

Systemic diuretics enhance the IOP-lowering effects of glycerin. Mannitol increases the risk for digoxin toxicity when given concurrently. Urea and mannitol decreases lithium levels when given together.

Adverse Effects

The adverse effects of ocular osmotics include a pounding headache (because of a decrease in cerebrospinal fluid volume), nausea, vomiting, and occasional diarrhea. The shift in body fluids increases the workload on the heart and may precipitate heart failure. Glycerin may cause hyperglycemia and glycosuria.

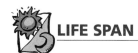
LIFE SPAN

The oral form of glycerin is used cautiously in older or dehydrated patients. Osmotics should be used with caution during pregnancy and lactation.

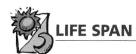
LIFE SPAN

Confusion and amnesia are adverse effects of ocular osmotic use in older adults. Monitor older adults who are taking glycerin for disorientation or seizure activity.

- Lying down during and after administration of glycerin helps prevent or relieve headache.

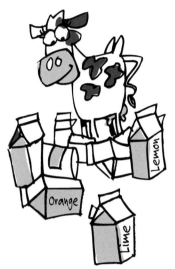

Give me glycerine with citrus.

What You DO

Nursing Responsibilities

The ocular osmotics, glycerin and isosorbide, are given orally, whereas mannitol and urea are given intravenously (IV). When administering ocular osmotics, the nurse should:

- Wash hands before administering an eye drug.
- Avoid administering a hypotonic IV solution following the administration of an osmotic drug because these fluids cancel the effect of the osmotic.
- Ensure that the IV line is patent before administering the drug to avoid extravasation of the drug and subsequent tissue necrosis.
- Administer oral glycerin with lemon, lime, or orange juice, or use the commercially prepared flavored solution to improve taste and minimize nausea and vomiting. The drug may also be mixed with unsweetened fruit juice. Pour over cracked ice and sip through a straw to increase palatability.
- Monitor the patient for 5 to 10 minutes after oral glycerin administration for evidence of persistent or increased eye pain and decreased visual acuity.
- Inform the patient that glycerin or ocular isosorbide may cause thirst.
- Advise the patient to call the health care provider if a severe headache develops.
- Monitor patients with diabetes who are taking glycerin for alterations in serum glucose levels.

Do You UNDERSTAND?

DIRECTIONS: Fill in the blanks with the appropriate responses.

1. The four ocular osmotic drugs used in the treatment of increased IOP are _____, _____, _____, and _____.

2. Patients with an acute attack of glaucoma may receive an osmotic drug that acts to _____ _____.

3. Necrosis may result when extravasation of urea occurs. Thus the most important nursing intervention is to be certain the patient has a _____.

What IS a Carbonic Anhydrase Inhibitor?

Carbonic Anhydrase Inhibitors	Trade Names
acetazolamide [ah-set-ah-ZOLE-ah-mide]	Diamox
brinzolamide [brin-ZOL-ah-mide]	Azopt
dichlorphenamide [dye-klor-FEN-ah-mide]	Daranide
dorzolamide [dor-ZOL-ah-mide]	Trusopt
methazolamide [meth-ah-ZOL-ah-mide]	Neptazane

Action

Carbonic anhydrase is an enzyme that promotes the conversion of carbonic acid to carbon dioxide and water. Carbonic anhydrase inhibitors block the enzyme activity in ciliary epithelium, thereby decreasing the production of aqueous humor and IOP. The reduction in pressure usually results in pupillary constriction (**miosis**) and opening of the anterior chamber of the eye.

Uses

Carbonic anhydrase inhibitors are used for the long-term treatment of open-angle glaucoma and other glaucoma that is refractory to cholinergic miotics, beta blockers, and epinephrine. Emergency treatment of acute closed-angle glaucoma includes use of beta blockers and osmotics, in addition to carbonic anhydrase inhibitors. Carbonic anhydrase inhibitors are also used to decrease IOP for preoperative and postoperative eye surgery patients.

What You NEED TO KNOW

Contraindications and Precautions

Acetazolamide and methazolamide should be used cautiously in patients with respiratory acidosis, emphysema or pulmonary obstruction, or diabetes mellitus.

Acetazolamide and methazolamide are contraindicated in patients with acute-angle glaucoma, decreased sodium or potassium levels, kidney or liver disease, adrenal gland dysfunction, or acid-base imbalance characterized by hyperchloremic acidosis.

Drug Interactions

Acetazolamide decreases the elimination of methenamine, procainamide, and quinidine when given together. Diflunisal increases the therapeutic, as well as the toxic, effects of acetazolamide. Methazolamide decreases elimination of amphetamines, procainamide, quinidine, and flecainide. Conversely, methazolamide increases the elimination of salicylates and phenobarbital. Additionally, methazolamide augments the effects of thiazide diuretics when given concurrently; it exacerbates hypokalemia when given with glucocorticosteroids.

Adverse Effects

The adverse effects of carbonic anhydrase inhibitors include transient myopia, alteration in taste, anorexia, nausea, vomiting, diarrhea, malaise, fatigue, weakness, nervousness, and loss of libido. Lethargy and depression are common but frequently go unnoticed until the drug is discontinued.

What You DO

Nursing Responsibilities

When administering carbonic anhydrase inhibitors, the nurse should:

- Wash hands before administering an eye drug.
- Realize that dorzolamide is a sulfonamide drug that is absorbed systemically; therefore the same adverse effects of sulfonamides may occur.
- Administer the correct drug to the correct eye.
- Discourage the patient from using an eye cup because of the risk for contamination and spreading disease.
- Crush oral formulations of acetazolamide tablets and mix with highly flavored syrup, such as raspberry, cherry, or chocolate. Tablets can also be softened in hot water and added to honey or syrup.
- Monitor older adults and debilitated patients for drug-induced diuresis because diuresis promotes rapid dehydration, hypovolemia, hypokalemia, and hyponatremia and may cause circulatory collapse. Reduced doses may be indicated for these patients.
- Warn the patient who is taking carbonic anhydrase inhibitors to use caution when driving or performing tasks that require alertness, coordination, or physical dexterity because the drug may cause drowsiness.
- Instruct the patient to discard drugs that have changed color or become cloudy.

Do not administer two or more carbonic anhydrase inhibitors concurrently. Two or more oral carbonic anhydrase inhibitors increase the risk for additive effects. Do not open or crush sustained-release capsules.

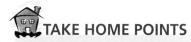

TAKE HOME POINTS

Containers of ophthalmic and otic drugs are similar in appearance in many cases. Ear formulations should not be used in the eye. Similarly, eye drugs should not be used in the ear.

Do You UNDERSTAND?

DIRECTIONS: Provide the appropriate answers to the following questions.

1. Are the actions of ocular carbonic anhydrase-inhibiting drugs used for reducing IOP different from that observed when the drug is used for other purposes (e.g., epilepsy, overdose)? _____

   _____

2. Why or why not? _____

Answers: 1. No differences exist, except in the use of the drugs; 2. The action of the drug is the same.

What ARE Mydriatic and Cycloplegic Drugs?

Mydriatic and Cycloplegic Drugs	Trade Names
Ocular anticholinergics	
homatropine [hoe-MA-troe-peen]	AK-Homatropine
cyclopentolate [sye-kloe-PEN-toe-late]	Cyclogyl
Adrenergics	
dipivefrin [dye-PI-ve-frin]	Propine
phenylephrine [fen-ill-EH-frin]	AK-Dilate

Action

The autonomic nervous system plays an important role in controlling the amount of light entering the eye and in focusing on images. The size of the iris controls the amount of light penetrating the eye, which contains two sets of muscles: the sphincter muscles and the dilator muscles. The pupil is constricted when the sphincter muscles contract; thus only a small amount of light passes through the pupil. The dilator muscles contain α-receptors that are innervated by the sympathetic nervous system. As the name implies, the pupil is dilated when these radial muscles contract after stimulation of the α-receptors. A mydriatic drug dilates the pupil without affecting accommodation.

Mydriatics and cycloplegic drugs dilate the pupil (**mydriasis**); thus the inner workings of the eye are visualized and diagnosis of eye problems can be made. Either anticholinergic or adrenergic drugs can be used to dilate the pupil.

Ocular anticholinergics block parasympathetic nervous system response to stimulation. Paralysis of ciliary muscles and relaxation of the muscles of the iris occurs, resulting in dilation of the pupil and loss of accommodation (**cycloplegia**).

Adrenergic drugs activate β_2-receptors in the canal of Schlemm, thereby increasing the outflow of aqueous humor. Epinephrine, when used alone, produces a 30% to 35% decrease in the rate of aqueous humor production. The duration of mydriasis and cycloplegia differs. Cycloplegia lasts a shorter period than does mydriasis, with recovery of accommodation taking several days. The outflow of aqueous humor is decreased with all of the ocular anticholinergics because of the miotic effect.

Uses

Ocular anticholinergic and adrenergic drugs (**mydriatics** and **cycloplegics**) are used to dilate the pupil for refraction and other diagnostic purposes. These drugs can be used in the treatment of anterior uveitis and keratitis, as well as secondary forms of glaucoma. These drugs also facilitate pupillary dilation during eye surgery and help decrease postoperative complications.

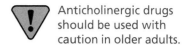

Anticholinergic drugs should be used with caution in older adults.

What You NEED TO KNOW

Contraindications/Precautions

Ocular anticholinergics are contraindicated in patients who have a shallow anterior chamber, closed-angle glaucoma, and hypersensitivity to the drug or to belladonna alkaloids. These drugs are also contraindicated for patients with scar tissue between the iris and the lens. Topical epinephrine and its analogs are contraindicated before removal of a piece of the iris (iridectomy) in closed-angle glaucoma because they may precipitate an acute attack.

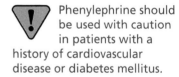

Phenylephrine should be used with caution in patients with a history of cardiovascular disease or diabetes mellitus.

Drug Interactions

Anticholinergics cause additive effects when given together with atropine. When anticholinergics are given concurrently with amantadine, the anticholinergic adverse effects are increased. CNS depression is intensified when anticholinergics are given with alcohol, antianxiety drugs, or sedative-hypnotics. The risk for tachycardia and hypertension is increased when anticholinergics are given together with ocular adrenergic drugs. Indomethacin inhibits the action of epinephrine when given concurrently. The effects of phenylephrine are enhanced when given with atropine and tricyclic antidepressants.

Adverse Effects

The adverse effects of ocular anticholinergic and adrenergic drugs include blurred vision, photophobia, and precipitation of closed-angle glaucoma. Chronic use of adrenergics causes rebound congestion of the conjunctiva. Absorption of the drug through the tear ducts and blood

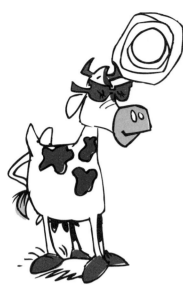

Protect your eyes.

vessels of the eye causes systemic effects, including dry mouth, constipation, fever, tachycardia, and central nervous system effects.

What You DO

Nursing Responsibilities

When administering mydriatics and cycloplegics, the nurse should:

- Wash hands before administering an eye drug.
- Double-check the drug order.
- Retract the lower lid gently with your thumb or index finger against the cheek bone to expose the lower conjunctival sac with the patient looking upward. Rest your hand holding the dropper or tube of ointment on the patient's forehead. Without touching the dropper to the eye structures, instill the prescribed number of drops into the conjunctival sac.
- Apply an ointment evenly in a thin stream along the inside edge of the entire lower eyelid from the inner to the outer canthus. Instruct the patient to gently close the eyes. Using a clean tissue, gently wipe away excess drug, moving from the inner canthus to the outer canthus.
- Record drug administration, noting which eyes received the drug.
- Advise patients to wear sunglasses to reduce the discomfort of photophobia caused by mydriatic-cycloplegic drugs.

Do You UNDERSTAND?

DIRECTIONS: Provide appropriate answers to the following questions.

1. What are the first two steps in administering mydriatic-cycloplegic drugs?

   _____

2. What is the last step in administering a mydriatic-cycloplegic drug?

   _____

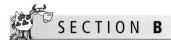

SECTION **B**

OTIC AGENTS

Hearing and balance disorders interfere with the patient's involvement in social activities, constructive use of leisure time, and ability to communicate, leading to social isolation. Removing earwax (cerumen) helps the patient avoid problems associated with impaired sound reception. This section reviews selected drugs used in the treatment of ear disorders including ceruminolytic drugs.

What IS a Ceruminolytic Drug?

Ceruminolytic Drugs	Trade Names
carbamide peroxide	Debrox Ear Drops
triethanolamine, polypeptide oleate, condensate	Cerumenex Ear Drops

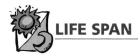

LIFE SPAN

Ceruminolytic drugs should not be administered to children less than 12 years of age.

Action

A ceruminolytic contains glycerin to soften cerumen and carbamide peroxide to loosen debris through the action of oxygen effervescence. These drugs help to emulsify and disperse excess or impacted cerumen.

Uses

Removal of cerumen is frequently necessary for otoscopy examination, audiometry, and tympanometry or when the patient experiences discomfort or hearing loss from excessive or dry cerumen. Additionally, ceruminolytic provides antiseptic protection.

What You NEED TO KNOW

Contraindications/Precautions

Ceruminolytic drugs are contraindicated for patients with a perforated eardrum, swimmer's ear, and itching of the ear canal, as well as those with an allergy to preservatives (e.g., benzethonium chloride, sulfites, and thimerosal) because many otic drugs contain these ingredients.

Drug Interactions

No known drug interactions have been noted with ceruminolytic drugs.

Adverse Effects

Ceruminolytic drugs are irritating to the ear and may cause an allergic reaction, particularly with prolonged exposure.

What You DO

Nursing Responsibilities

When administering a ceruminolytic drug, the nurse should:
- Inform the patient that ceruminolytic drugs should be used over a 2- to 3-day period to soften the wax.
- Inform the patient that holding the drug in the hand before use will warm the otic solution.
- Teach the patient the correct way to use and administer ceruminolytic drugs.
- Fill the ear canal with the drug while the patient's head is tilted at a 45-degree angle.
- Straighten the ear canal using one hand. Rest your hand holding the drug dropper 1 cm ($^1/_2$ inch) above the ear canal. Place the ceruminolytic directly in the affected ear without touching the dropper to the ear or ear canal. Apply gentle pressure on the tragus (cartilage projection anterior to the external ear opening) or gently massage the tragus with your finger. Instruct the patient to remain in a side-lying position for 2 to 3 minutes.
- Remove the cerumen mechanically using a soft rubber otic bulb syringe and warm water to gently irrigate the ear.
- Warn the patient to avoid using the otic preparation for more than 4 consecutive days and to avoid contact with the eyes. Accidental ocular exposure causes immediate pain and irritation; however, severe injury is rare.
- Inform the patient that some individuals have a continual problem with cerumen impaction and to avoid Q-tips or other implements to remove cerumen.

TAKE HOME POINTS
- Instill drops alongside the auditory canal, allowing them to flow in without falling directly on the eardrum (tympanic membrane). When drops are ordered for the other ear, wait 15 minutes and repeat this procedure with the other ear. Ceruminolytic drugs may be used once a week to prevent recurrence of the problem.
- Pull the auricle (pinna) down and back gently for children under 3 years of age or up and back for children over 3 years of age and adults.

- Advise the patient to contact the health care provider if inflammation or irritation persists after using a ceruminolytic drug.

Do You UNDERSTAND?

DIRECTIONS: **Indicate in the space provided whether the statement is** ***true*** **or** ***false.*** **If the answer is false, correct the statement to make it true (using the margin space).**

_____   1. Ceruminolytic drugs are safe for children under 10 years of age.

_____   2. Patients can experience hearing loss because of excessive earwax.

_____   3. A patient with a perforated eardrum can safely receive ceruminolytic drugs.

SECTION **C**

DERMATOLOGICS

The skin is the body's largest organ, the primary goal of which is to act as a barrier against the influences of the outside environment. The functions of the skin include protection, temperature regulation, immune responsiveness, biochemical synthesis, and improved appearance. Dermatologic drugs correct dysfunction of the skin topically and systemically.

This section reviews the use of pharmacologic methods to treat common skin diseases. Dermatologic complaints are frequently treated on an outpatient basis. This section also provides information about drugs that are used for the treatment of burns, poison ivy, and acne. Emulsions, lotions, creams, ointments, antipruritics, and keratolytics are also discussed.

Answers: 1. false; ceruminolytic drugs should not be administered to children less than 12 years of age; 2. true; 3. false; ceruminolytic drugs are contraindicated for patients with a perforated eardrum.

What IS an Emollient?

Emollients	Trade Names
Lanolor Cream; Desitin Ointment; Lubriderm Cream; Zinc Oxide Ointment; Nivea Moisturizing Lotion; Vitamin E Lotion, Oil, and Cream; Neutrogena Body Lotion; Vitamin A and D Ointments; Alpha Keri Emollient; Retinol Cream	None listed

Action

Topical emollients are agents that soften, lubricate, moisturize, and soothe skin surfaces. These agents promote hydration through topical absorption and remove excess keratin in dry skin.

Uses

Topical emollients, frequently offered in more than one formulation, provide temporary relief of discomfort resulting from skin irritation, itching, minor burns, sunburns, diaper rash, chapped or dry skin, and poison ivy.

What You NEED TO KNOW

Contraindications/Precautions

Emollients are contraindicated for patients with an allergy to the drug.

Drug Interactions

Emollients have no known drug interactions.

Adverse Effects

Adverse effects include local irritation, stinging, burning, and redness.

What You DO

Nursing Responsibilities

Emollients are available as emulsion, lotion, cream, gel, oil, ointment, or bath formulations. These agents are applied topically for external use only. When administering emollients, the nurse should:

• Avoid contact of emollients with the patient's eyes and open wounds.

- Instruct the patient to report increased irritation, allergic reaction, or worsening of the condition.
- Document all irritation, stinging, burning, redness, and swelling.

Do You UNDERSTAND?

DIRECTIONS: Indicate in the space provided whether the statement is *true* or *false*. If the answer is false, correct the statement to make it true (using the margin space).

_____ 1. Eye contact must be avoided.

_____ 2. Avoid open wounds.

_____ 3. Report increased irritation, allergic reaction, or worsening condition.

What IS an Antipruritic Drug?

Antipruritic Drugs	Trade Names
benzocaine [BEN-zo-cane]	Americaine
crotamiton [kroh-TAM-ih-ton]	Eurax
dyclonine [DYE-kloh-neen]	Dyclone
pramoxine [prah-MOX-een]	Tronothane

 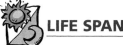

LIFE SPAN

- Antipruritics are contraindicated during pregnancy and for children less than 2 years of age. Antipruritic use is discouraged in children under 6 years of age and should be used cautiously in older adults.
- Antipruritics should be used cautiously in patients with denuded skin, severely traumatized mucosa, or sepsis.

Action

Antipruritic agents are surface anesthetics that inhibit the conduction of the nerve impulses from the sensory nerve endings and thus stop discomfort and itching.

Uses

Antipruritic drugs are used for temporary relief of pain and discomfort of minor burns, sunburn, wounds, insect bites, toothache, sore throat pain, canker sores, hemorrhoids, rectal fissures, and itching of the anus or vulva.

Answers: 1. true; 2. true; 3. true.

Some of these drugs are used for catheter and endoscope insertion. Systemic antipruritic drugs can relieve allergic conditions associated with allergic dermatoses.

What You NEED TO KNOW

Contraindications/Precautions

Antipruritics are contraindicated for patients with hypersensitive or allergic reaction to the drug or any components.

Drug Interactions

Antipruritics have no known drug interactions.

Serious adverse effects of benzocaine include toxicity, anaphylaxis, and methemoglobinemia in infants.

Adverse Effects

Adverse effects of antipruritics include allergic reactions, burning, rash, and redness. Skin irritation may occur, particularly with prolonged use. Adverse effects following systemic absorption of dyclonine include dizziness, drowsiness, blurred vision, nervousness, tremors, depression, seizures, hypotension, bradycardia, and cardiac or respiratory arrest.

What You DO

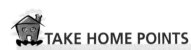

Nursing Responsibilities

Antipruritic preparations are available in gels, creams, sprays, and lotions. When administering antipruritics, the nurse should:
- Clean and dry the affected area thoroughly before application.
- Apply lotions and creams with a gloved hand, and wash hands thoroughly before and after treatment.
- Massage crotamiton gently into the skin. Application is usually effective for 6 to 10 hours.
- Teach the patient to hold a spray formulation at arms length to avoid eye contamination.
- Advise the patient to avoid eating for 1 hour after the drug is sprayed into the mouth because the numbing affect may impede swallowing.
- Instruct the patient to contact the health care provider and stop treatment when the condition worsens, fails to improve, or when signs of sensitivity, irritation, or infection occur.

TAKE HOME POINTS
- Flush the eyes with water for 15 minutes if an antipruritic drug accidentally comes in contact with the eyes.
- Test the return of the gag reflex by gently touching the soft palate with a cotton-tipped applicator while holding the tongue down with a depressor. If the patient does not swallow or gag, then wait another hour before allowing the patient to drink or eat to prevent aspiration.

Do You UNDERSTAND?

DIRECTIONS: Name four problems or complications that antipruritics drugs treat or procedures for which antipruritics may be used.

1. _____

2. _____

3. _____

4. _____

What IS a Keratolytic Drug?

Keratolytic Drugs	Trade Names
podophyllum resin [pode-oh-FILL-um]	Pod-Ben-25
podofilox [poh-DAHF-ih-lox]	Condylox
masoprocol [mah-SOH-proh-kol]	Actinex

Action

Keratolytic drugs directly affect epithelial cell metabolism, causing degeneration and a pause in mitosis, a slow disruption of cell movement, and an erosion of tissue. This action is caustic, affecting embryonic and tumor cells selectively before they develop into adult cells. The caustic action promotes shedding of the horny layer of skin, ranging from skin peeling to an extensive shedding of the epidermal layer of the skin.

Uses

Keratolytic drugs are used to treat benign growths including warts (genital and perianal), papillomas, and fibroids. Keratolytic drugs are also clinically used to treat hyperkeratotic skin disorders, verrucae, xerosis,

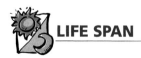

LIFE SPAN

Keratolytics are contraindicated during pregnancy and lactation and for children.

Answers: 1. otic preparation available for otitis itching; 2. gels, creams, and lotion preparations available for toothaches, sore throat pain, and canker sores; 3. preparations available for hemorrhoids, rectal fissures, itching of the anus or vulva, and as genital desensitizers; 4. anesthetic lubricants for catheter insertion and endoscopes.

ichthyosis, and photoaging. Irritated, friable, and bleeding skin fails to respond to treatment.

What You NEED TO KNOW

Contraindications/Precautions

Keratolytic drugs are contraindicated in patients with birthmarks, moles, warts with hair growth, as well as oral, cervical, or urethral warts. They should not be used on normal skin and mucous membranes that surround affected areas. Keratolytic drugs are also contraindicated in patients with hypersensitivity to the drug, impaired circulation, diabetes mellitus, or an allergy to sulfites.

Drug Interactions

Keratolytics have no known drug interactions.

Adverse Effects

The adverse effects of keratolytics include skin irritation, burning, itching, tingling, blistering, wrinkling, flaking, dryness, and peeling. Other adverse effects include bleeding, crusting edema, leather-like skin, and painful intercourse. Systemic adverse effects include vomiting, diarrhea, insomnia, peripheral neuropathy, coma, seizures, respiratory and renal failure, and bone marrow depression.

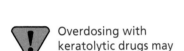

TAKE HOME POINTS

Protect the surrounding skin or tissue with petrolatum. When keratolytics are spilled on the skin, wipe off with alcohol, acetone, or tape remover. Proper disposal of all used applicators is important to prevent contamination of other areas.

Overdosing with keratolytic drugs may cause toxicity.

What You DO

Nursing Responsibilities

Because of the potency of podophyllum resin, the health care provider is usually responsible for application. When administering keratolytics, the nurse should:

- Caution the patient that drug application over a large area is discouraged.

- Teach the patient the proper technique of drug self-administration. Instruct the patient to remove the last drug application thoroughly from the affected area with soap and water before the next application.
- Instruct the patient to apply the drug to the lesion, allow the area to dry, apply a loose bandage to cover the site, cover with tape, and remove as per the prescribed frequency instructions.
- Warn the patient that when contact with the eyes occurs, flush with warm water for 15 minutes, remove film that is precipitated by flush, and report the incident to the health care provider.
- Caution the patient to avoid applying the drug to normal body tissue, and when it occurs, wipe the area with alcohol to remove.
- Avoid applying the drug when the wart is inflamed or irritated.
- Inform the patient that when application causes extreme pain, pruritus, or swelling, remove the application with alcohol and notify the health care provider.
- Inform the patient to store podophyllum resin in an airtight, light-resistant container and to avoid exposure to heat.
- Warn the patient that keratolytics may cause itching, burning, discomfort, and tenderness of the affected site and surrounding area for 2 to 6 days.
- Inform the patient that the wart will become blanched, then necrotic within 24 to 48 hours. Sloughing begins at 72 hours, with no scarring. A mild antiinfective can be applied until fully healed.
- Advise the patient that the sexual partner should be referred for examination when the keratolytic treatment is intended for treatment of genital warts.
- Use the minimal amount of drug to avoid excess systemic absorption.
- Counsel the patient to call the health care provider immediately when symptoms of toxicity occur (e.g., seizures, peripheral neuropathy, and respiratory depression).
- Emphasize adverse effects of keratolytic drugs to the patient because the danger of misuse and systemic toxicity is high.
- Warn the patient who is using masoprocol to protect clothing and linen because the drug may cause staining.
- Instruct the patient to avoid exposure to sunlight and cosmetics while using keratolytic drugs.

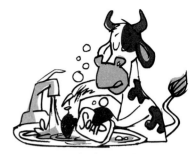

Wash, then apply.

Do You UNDERSTAND?

DIRECTIONS: Fill in the blanks in the following statements.

1. Keratolytic drugs directly affect _____ _____ metabolism, causing degeneration and a pause in _____.
2. When applying keratolytics, protect the surrounding skin or tissue with _____.
3. Avoid keratolytic application when the wart is _____ or _____.

What IS a Burn Treatment Drug?

Burn Treatment Drugs	Trade Names
mafenide [meh-FEN-ide]	Sulfamylon
nitrofurazone [nye-troh-FYOOR-ah-zone]	Furacin
silver sulfadiazine [sul-fah-DYE-ah-zeen]	Silvadene

Action

Drugs used in the treatment of burns prevent bacterial growth, thereby assisting with the healing of burned tissue. Mafenide interferes with bacterial cellular metabolism and reduces bacteria in burns, which allows for spontaneous healing of deep burns. Nitrofurazone inhibits the aerobic and anaerobic cycles of carbohydrate metabolism in bacteria. Silver sulfadiazine exerts a bactericidal action on the bacterial cell membrane and cell wall to reduce bacteria. Nitrofurazone and silver sulfadiazine are bactericidal drugs that exert broad-spectrum antibacterial action on gram-positive and gram-negative microorganisms.

Answers: 1. epithelial cell, mitosis; 2. petrolatum; 3. inflamed, irritated.

Uses

These drugs are useful in the prevention and treatment of bacterial infections in burns, skin grafts, and donor sites.

> ⚠ Burn drugs should be used cautiously in patients with renal impairment and acid-base imbalance. Mafenide acetate should be used cautiously in patients with asthma.

What You NEED TO KNOW

Contraindications/Precautions

Burn drugs are contraindicated in patients with atrophy or hypersensitivity to the drug or sulfites. Sulfite sensitivity tends to be more prevalent in patients with asthma compared with the general population. Silver sulfadiazine is contraindicated in patients with glucose-6-phosphate dehydrogenase (G6PD) deficiency.

Burn drugs are contraindicated during pregnancy and lactation, as well as for premature infants, neonates, and children because these agents may increase the risk for bilirubin infiltration into the spinal cord and brain (kernicterus).

Drug Interactions

Silver sulfadiazine may cause inactivation of enzymes when used with topical proteolytic enzymes.

Adverse Effects

Topical burn drug interactions generally cause few life-threatening crises, except when the patient experiences an allergic reaction. Allergic reactions include skin irritation, rashes, pruritus, burning, hives, blisters, redness, skin discoloration, and swelling of the lips or face.

Mafenide may cause tachypnea, diarrhea, G6PD deficiency, bone marrow suppression, and disseminated intravascular coagulation. Mafenide also inhibits carbonic anhydrase, leading to metabolic acidosis, which is usually compensated through hyperventilation.

Nitrofurazone has a polyethylene glycol base, which may be absorbed through denuded skin. Impaired kidneys may not adequately eliminate nitrofurazone and may lead to metabolic acidosis and progressive renal impairment.

Photosensitivity and an increased risk for kernicterus may occur with silver sulfadiazine. When extensive systemic absorption occurs, silver sulfadiazine administration may result in a decreased neutrophil count.

Prolonged use of these drugs may result in superinfections, including overgrowth of other microorganisms, such as *Candida albicans*.

What You DO

Nursing Responsibilities

To avoid allergic reactions, culture and sensitivity tests are recommended before applying burn drugs. When administering burn drugs, the nurse should:

- Teach the patient to use the drug only as prescribed and to avoid sharing the drug with others.
- Discard the drug when the color is incorrect, according to the package.
- Store drugs in tight containers to avoid exposure to direct sunlight, prolonged heat, and alkaline materials.
- Adhere strictly to sterile technique and gloved hands to avoid wound contamination.
- Flush the wounds with sterile saline as appropriate to facilitate dressing removal.
- Inspect patient's skin daily, noting any changes.
- Monitor signs of rash, infection, and toxicity continuously.
- Use burn drugs only on the affected areas; keep the burn medicated at all times.
- Apply burn drugs to a clean, debrided wound to enhance absorption.
- Protect skin around the wound with zinc oxide as appropriate when using a wet dressing.
- Document marked discomfort, acidosis, and fungal infections.
- Monitor renal function studies and acid-base balance for patients who are undergoing nitrofurazone therapy.
- Report signs of metabolic acidosis to the health care provider because mafenide will usually be discontinued for 24 to 48 hours to allow restoration of acid-base balance.
- Monitor the complete blood count of patients who are undergoing silver sulfadiazine therapy for early detection of leukopenia.
- Instruct the patient to report rash, irritation, swelling, or other evidence of an allergic reaction to the health care provider.
- Caution the patient to report to the health care provider when no improvement occurs, the condition worsens, or systemic and adverse reactions occur.

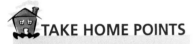

TAKE HOME POINTS

Sterile technique and gloved hands help avoid wound contamination. Dressings are not always necessary, but when used, they should be nonocclusive and light.

Do You UNDERSTAND?

DIRECTIONS: Match Column A with Column B.

Column A

_____ 1. Careful use with patients who are diagnosed with renal failure and asthma.

_____ 2. Used cautiously when patient has renal insufficiency.

Column B

a. Silver sulfadiazine

b. Mafenide acetate

What IS an Acne Treatment Drug?

Acne Treatment Drugs	Trade Names
isotretinoin [eye-so-TREAT-ih-noyn]	Accutane
azelaic acid [ah-zih-LAY-ick]	Azelex
tetracycline [te-trah-SIGH-clean]	Topicycline
erythromycin [eh-RIH-throw-MY-sin]	Akne-Mycin
clindamycin [klin-dah-MY-sin]	Cleocin

Action

Acne treatment drugs decrease the sebaceous gland size and inhibit sebaceous gland differentiation, thereby causing a decrease in oil secretion. Acne treatments may also inhibit follicular keratinization. Antibiotics used to treat acne disrupt bacterial protein synthesis.

Uses

Broad-spectrum antibiotics are frequently used to treat acne vulgaris. Topical treatment is usually prescribed first, and when no clinical improvement takes place, systemic therapy is then introduced.

Answers: 1. b; 2. a.

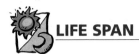

LIFE SPAN

Acne drugs are contraindicated during pregnancy and lactation. Clindamycin is contraindicated for infants. Tetracycline is contraindicated in children less than 11 years of age.

Isotretinoin can cause CNS and facial and cardiac anomalies in the fetus. Inform the female patient that a pregnancy test and contraceptive use is required with prior to using isotretinoin.

What You NEED TO KNOW

Contraindications/Precautions

Acne drugs are contraindicated for patients with hypersensitivity. Isotretinoin is also contraindicated for patients with allergies to isotretinoin, parabions, or combinations of these products, and tetracycline is contraindicated for patients with sensitivity to sodium bisulfate. Alcohol, soap, and cosmetics should be used cautiously when undergoing acne therapy.

Isotretinoin must be used cautiously in patients with diabetes mellitus, coronary artery disease, obesity, alcoholism, pancreatitis, hepatitis, renal or hepatic impairment, retinal disease, and rheumatology disorders. Azelaic acid should be used with caution in children under 12 years old and in patients with dark complexions. Tetracycline must be used cautiously in patients with myasthenia gravis and asthma.

Adverse Effects

Adverse effects of acne drugs include temporary stinging or burning on application, tingling, itching, yellow discoloration of skin, redness, irritation, swelling, and peeling. Tetracycline interacts with isotretinoin, causing dryness or oiliness and excessive skin irritation. Intolerance to contact lenses and photosensitive reactions may occur. Prolonged use may cause overgrowth of bacterial or fungal infections can cause major birth defects.

What You DO

Nursing Responsibilities

Acne drugs are usually topical formulations, but some may be taken orally when necessary. When administering acne drugs, the nurse should:

- Apply lotions and creams with a gloved hand; wash hands thoroughly before and after treatment.
- Instruct patients to wash their hands before applying a generous amount of drug to the affected area.
- Warn the patient that medicated soaps, cleansers, and other acne treatments contain peeling agents.

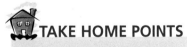

TAKE HOME POINTS

Adhere strictly to the use of gloves and thorough handwashing before and after treatment. Avoid applying acne drugs in the mouth, nose, and eyes.

- Remind the patient that the application may cause stinging, local irritation, or dryness.
- Warn the patient taking tetracycline drugs to avoid exposure to direct sunlight to prevent photosensitivity reactions.
- Caution the patient to avoid sharing the drug with others.
- Inform the patient that topical drugs may stain clothes.
- Advise the patient to report to the health care provider if no improvement occurs, if the condition worsens, or adverse effects occur.
- Encourage patients with diabetes who are taking isotretinoin to monitor blood glucose levels regularly.

Do You UNDERSTAND?

DIRECTIONS: Provide appropriate responses to the following questions.
1. How does a broad-spectrum antibiotic assist in clinically improving acne? _____
2. What route is the first-line defense against acne? _____
_____

References

Gutierrez K, Queener S: *Pharmacology for nursing practice*, Philadelphia, 2004, Mosby.

Lehne R: *Pharmacology for nursing care*, ed 5, Philadelphia, 2004, WB Saunders.

Lewis SM, Heitkemper MM, Dirksen SR: *Medical-surgical nursing: assessment and management of clinical problems*, ed 6, St Louis, 2004, Mosby.

Lilley L, Harrington S, Snyder J: *Pharmacology and the nursing process*, ed 4, St Louis, 2005, Mosby.

McCance K, Huether S: *Pathophysiology: the biologic basis for disease in adults and children*, ed 4, St Louis, 2002. Mosby.

Answers: 1. antibiotics disrupt bacterial protein synthesis; 2. topical treatment is usually prescribed first, and systemic therapy is then introduced when no clinical improvement occurs.

NCLEX® Review

Section A

1. The health care provider may recommend which of the following products to a patient who complains of dry eyes?
   1 Naphazoline
   2 Polyvinyl alcohol
   3 Timolol
   4 Demecarium

2. The use of carbachol for a patient with glaucoma would have which of the following effects?
   1 Dilation of the iridic sphincter and subsequent reduction in IOP
   2 Increased outflow of aqueous humor and subsequent decrease in IOP
   3 Mydriasis
   4 Vasoconstriction of collecting channels

3. Which of the following adverse effects is most commonly associated with pilocarpine?
   1 Iridic cysts
   2 Eye irritation
   3 Lacrimal system obstruction
   4 Retinal detachment

Section B

4. The health care provider is teaching a parent the proper way to administer an ear drug to a child. Which of the following points is important to include in the teaching?
   1 Pull the pinna down and back.
   2 Pull the pinna up and back.
   3 Pull the pinna down and forward.
   4 Pull the pinna up and forward.

5. A patient who is learning to take an otic drug should be taught to do which of the following?
   1 Keep the cap to the solution loosely closed.
   2 Hold the drug in the hands to warm it.
   3 Administer an otic drug at cold temperatures.
   4 Warm the drug in a microwave oven before use.

Section C

6. Which of the following agents helps to prevent bacterial growth, thereby helping to heal burned tissue?
   1 Silver sulfadiazine
   2 Antipruritic
   3 Tetracycline
   4 Keratolytic

7. Which of the following is *not* a primary function of the skin?
   1 Protection
   2 Support colonization of bacteria
   3 Immune responsiveness
   4 Thermoregulation

8. Which of the following techniques would *not* be used when applying silver sulfadiazine to a burned area of skin?
   1 Cover the burned area with airtight dressing.
   2 Keep the burned area covered with drug at all times.
   3 Apply the drug in a thin layer over the burned area.
   4 Use a sterile technique when applying the drug.

9. Which of the following statements about crotamiton, an antipruritic dermatologic drug, is correct?
   1 It should be administered using a sterile technique.
   2 It should be gently massaged into the affected area.
   3 When an antipruritic comes into contact with the eyes, immediately close eyes and bandage for 2 hours.
   4 When given for endoscope insertion, the patient may eat immediately after the procedure.

10. Silver sulfadiazine is associated with which of the following adverse effects?
    1 Discoloration of skin
    2 Peeling of skin layers
    3 Elevated blood glucose
    4 Fetal anomalies

NCLEX® Review Answers

Section A

1. 2 Drugs are ocular lubricants that relieve dry eyes and are composed of sodium chloride, polyvinyl, petrolatum, mineral oil, and lanolin. Naphazoline is an ocular decongestant. Timolol is an ocular beta blocker. Demecarium is an anticholinesterase miotic used for the treatment of glaucoma.

2. 2 Carbachol is a cholinergic miotic that contracts the sphincter of the iris and ciliary muscles. By deepening the anterior eye chamber, the larger filtration angle causes an increased outflow of aqueous humor and decreased IOP. Carbachol contracts, not dilates, the iridic sphincter. Carbachol causes miosis (pupil constriction), not mydriasis (pupil dilation). Carbachol does not cause vasoconstriction of the collecting channels.

3. 2 Pilocarpine is an ocular cholinergic that commonly causes ocular burning and tearing adverse effects. Pilocarpine does not cause iridic cysts, obstruction of the lacrimal system, or retinal detachment.

Section B

4. 1 When administering an otic drug to a child, the mother should pull the pinna down and back for a child who is under 3 years of age. Pulling the pinna up and back should be performed for children over age 3 and for adults. Pulling the pinna forward is an inappropriate action.

5. 2 When teaching an adult about eye drug administration, the nurse should instruct the patient to hold the container in the hand, thereby warming the otic solution. The patient should keep the solution cap tightly, not loosely, closed. Otic drugs should be administered at a warm, not cold, temperature. The microwave oven would warm the drug excessively, possibly cause a burn.

Section C

6. 1 Silver sulfadiazine is designed to prevent bacterial growth of burned tissue. An antipruritic is used to relieve itching. Tetracycline is used as an acne treatment. A keratolytic is a caustic agent that promotes shedding of the horny layer of skin.

7. 2 Primary functions of the skin include protection, immune responsiveness, and thermoregulation. Supporting colonization of bacteria is not a primary function of the skin.

8. 1 Covering the area with airtight dressing is an inappropriate intervention. Burned areas should not be covered with occlusive dressings because healing would be impeded. Keeping the burn area covered with drug at all times, applying drug in a thin layer over the burned area, and using sterile technique are appropriate interventions.

9. 2 Crotamiton should be gently massaged into the affected area. A clean technique is acceptable; it need not be sterile. When an antipruritic comes into contact with the eyes, the eyes should be thoroughly and immediately flushed with water for 15 minutes, not closed and bandaged. The patient should avoid eating for 1 hour after an antipruritic spray of the throat. The nurse must check for the return of the gag reflex before allowing the consumption of food or fluid.

10. 1 Discoloration of skin is an adverse effect associated with silver sulfadiazine. Silver sulfadiazine is not associated with peeling of skin layers (action of keratolytic) or elevated blood glucose levels (adverse effect of isotretinoin). Silver sulfadiazine is not associated with fetal anomalies.

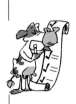

Notes

Drugs Used for Pain Relief

This chapter reviews pharmacologic control of pain. Harmful effects of unrelieved pain include confusion, prolonged stress response, depressed immune response, tumor growth, and increased hypercoagulation. Because they are the primary pain managers, nurses must have a thorough understanding of analgesics to provide adequate pain relief for patients. Nonnarcotic, narcotic, and antimigraine agents are discussed in this chapter.

What You WILL LEARN

After reading this chapter, you will know how to do the following:

- ✔ Compare the adverse effects of nonnarcotic and narcotic analgesics.
- ✔ Discuss the nursing responsibilities of narcotic administration.
- ✔ Compare the action of various types of antimigraine agents.

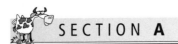

SECTION **A**

NONNARCOTIC ANALGESICS

What IS a Nonnarcotic Analgesic?

Nonnarcotic Analgesic	Trade Name	Use
acetaminophen [ah-SEAT-ah-MIN-ah-fen]	Tylenol	Relief of pain

Action

Acetaminophen, a nonprostaglandin derivative, has an unknown analgesic action but is thought to inhibit prostaglandin synthesis and block pain impulse at pain receptor sites in the peripheral nervous system, thereby elevating the pain threshold. Acetaminophen also acts on the hypothalamic heat-regulating center to dissipate heat through the process of vasodilation and sweating, thereby reducing fever. Acetaminophen has weak antiinflammatory activity because of the minimal inhibition of peripheral prostaglandins.

Uses

Acetaminophen is used in the treatment of pain and fever associated with a variety of conditions, including influenza and the relief of arthritic musculoskeletal pain. Acetaminophen is also used for patients who are receiving immunizations or those with viral illnesses because salicylates may cause Reye's syndrome.

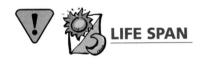

LIFE SPAN

- This agent should be used cautiously
  in patients with renal and hepatic dysfunction or chronic alcoholism.
- Acetaminophen should be used cautiously during pregnancy and lactation

What You NEED TO KNOW

Contraindications/Precautions

Acetaminophen is contraindicated for patients with renal dysfunction, hypersensitivity, and anemia.

Drug Interactions

Alcohol exacerbates the effects of acetaminophen, increasing the risk for hepatotoxicity when taken together. Long-term concurrent administration of barbiturates, carbamazepine, rifampin, or phenytoin with acetaminophen can increase the risk for hepatotoxicity. Cholestyramine decreases the absorption of acetaminophen. An increased risk for bleeding may occur when given concurrently with oral anticoagulants.

Adverse Effects

Adverse effects of acetaminophen include headache, fever, skin rash, hemolytic anemia, and renal dysfunction.

Hepatotoxicity is a potentially fatal adverse effect that is associated with prolonged use or overdose. Acute hepatic necrosis occurs when doses of 10 to 15 g are administered. Doses greater than 25 g are fatal. Acetaminophen toxicity is defined as a plasma concentration of 200 mcg/mL.

What You DO

Nursing Responsibilities

Acetaminophen may be administered either with food or on an empty stomach. When administering acetaminophen, the nurse should:

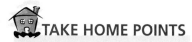**TAKE HOME POINTS**

Warn patients that psychologic dependence can occur with acetaminophen.

- Advise the patient to avoid alcohol when taking more than one to two doses of acetaminophen per day.
- Instruct the patient who is taking acetaminophen and oral anticoagulants to report any increased bleeding, bruising, and nosebleeds.
- Counsel the patient who is taking acetaminophen to consult the health care provider when fever lasts longer than 3 days or is over 103° F.
- Inform the patient that acetaminophen is available as chewable tablets, granules, extended-release tablets, solutions, liquids, elixirs, and suppositories.
- Instruct the patient to avoid acetaminophen use for more than 10 days for adults and 5 days for children without consulting the health care provider because abuse potential is high.
- Empty the patient's stomach contents and immediately administer acetylcysteine (Mucomyst) to minimize liver damage when an acetaminophen overdose occurs.

Do You UNDERSTAND?

DIRECTIONS: Provide appropriate responses to the following questions.

1. Acetaminophen toxicity is defined as a plasma concentration of what amount? _____

2. What symptoms should the patient who is taking acetaminophen report? _____

3. What organ is damaged by an acetaminophen overdose? _____

_____

What IS a Nonsteroidal Antiinflammatory Drug?

Refer to pages 519 and 523 for the discussion of nonsteroidal antiinflammatory drugs (NSAIDs).

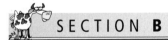

SECTION B

NARCOTIC ANALGESICS

Many types of receptor sites are present in body cells. Analgesics bind to certain receptors in the cells that influence the perception of pain. Narcotic (**opiate**) analgesics are classified as agonists and agonist-antagonists. Agonists are drugs that mimic the regulatory function of the body and have an affinity for their respective receptor sites. Antagonists may either block interaction at certain receptor sites or compete for those receptor sites. Agonists-antagonists have some characteristics of both agonists and antagonists. This section discusses opioid agonists, agonists-antagonists, and antagonists.

What IS a Narcotic Analgesic?

Narcotic Analgesic	Trade Names	Uses
morphine sulfate [MOR-feen]	Duramorph MS Contin	Relief of severe acute or chronic pain
fentanyl [FEN-tah-nil]	Sublimaze Duragesic	Management of chronic pain
meperidine [meh-PER-ih-deen]	Demerol	Relief of moderate to severe pain
oxycodone [OX-ee-KOH-doan]	Percodan	Relief of mild to moderately severe pain
codeine sulfate [KOH-deen]	Paveral	Relief of mild to moderate pain

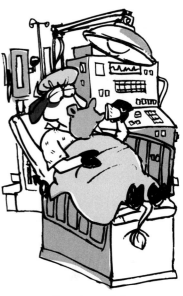

Conscious relief.

Action

Narcotic analgesics (opiate agonists) relieve pain without loss of consciousness. These drugs bind with opioid receptors at specific receptor-binding sites (e.g., limbic system, thalamus, hypothalamus, midbrain, spinal cord) in the central nervous system (CNS). Agonist activity at the receptor site can result in analgesia, euphoria, depression, hallucinations, miosis, sedation, decreased body temperature, decreased gastrointestinal (GI) motility, cardiac stimulation, and respiratory depression. Narcotic analgesics alter pain at the spinal cord and higher levels in the CNS, as well as the patient's emotional response.

Uses

Narcotic analgesics are used to relieve mild to severe pain or as a preoperative medication. These drugs are usually given when nonnarcotic analgesics are unsuccessful. Low-dose narcotic analgesics are generally safer than are nonsteroidal antiinflammatory drugs (NSAIDs) for long-term use in older adults. The first choice of severe pain control via the patient-controlled analgesia (PCA) pump is morphine. MS Contin is a recommended choice for oral controlled-release pain medication. Meperidine has been used for the pain of myocardial infarction (MI) but is not as effective as is morphine. Some sources state that meperidine is not recommended for use other than the GI laboratory and for the treatment of shivering. Fentanyl transdermal relieves severe chronic pain. Oxycodone relieves moderate-to-severe pain. Codeine sulfate relieves mild-to-moderate pain.

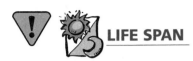

LIFE SPAN

- Caution should be used in older patients, as well as in those who are very young, debilitated, pregnant, or in labor.
- Caution should be used in patients with dysrhythmias and emphysema.

What You NEED TO KNOW

Contraindications/Precautions

Narcotic analgesics are contraindicated for patients with hypersensitivity, increased intracranial pressure, suspected head injuries, seizures, asthma, severe respiratory depression, hepatic and renal dysfunction, acute alcoholism, biliary tract surgery, and acute ulcerative colitis. Meperidine is contraindicated for patients with renal insufficiency because dysfunctional kidneys cannot eliminate the toxic metabolite (normeperidine) that this drug produces.

Drug Interactions

CNS effects are increased when narcotic analgesics are given concurrently with sedatives, barbiturates, benzodiazepines, tricyclic antidepressants, and alcohol. When narcotic analgesics are given with monoamine oxidase inhibitors (MAOIs), seizures, hypertensive crisis, hyperpyrexia, and respiratory depression may occur. Phenothiazines may antagonize analgesic effects when given with narcotic analgesics.

Adverse Effects

The adverse effects of narcotic analgesics include rash, itching, anaphylaxis, euphoria, dizziness, fainting, sweating, confusion, seizures, visual disturbances, drowsiness, palpitations, bradycardia, flushing of neck and face, orthostatic hypotension, and decreased respirations. Other adverse effects affecting the GI system include anorexia, dry mouth, nausea, vomiting, constipation, urinary retention, and decreased libido. Overdose effects include bronchoconstriction, severe respiratory depression or arrest, skeletal muscle flaccidity, coma, and cardiac arrest. Meperidine produces a toxic metabolite (normeperidine) that may remain in the body for 8 to 21 hours. In patients with renal dysfunction, normeperidine may accumulate more than 30 hours in the body, leading to an increased risk for neurotoxicity.

What You DO

Nursing Responsibilities

Narcotics are among the "scheduled" drugs, which are strictly regulated because of their potential for abuse. Narcotics require strict documentation because they are considered to be controlled substances. Documentation is required on the institution's narcotic sheet and on the nurses' notes. Additionally, two nurses at set intervals count the narcotics to validate the narcotic sheet. Any waste of narcotics must be witnessed and documented.

Multiple routes of administration are available: oral, transdermal, subcutaneous (Sub-Q), intramuscular (IM), IV, and rectal. Anesthetists may also use spinal, epidural, inhalation, and transmucosal routes. When administering narcotics, the nurse should:

- Assess the nature of the patient's pain, status, and vital signs before and after drug administration. Opioid naives (patients who are receiving their first opioid dose) are more likely to develop respiratory depression than are patients who have been receiving daily doses.
- Administer narcotics before the patient's pain becomes too severe to enhance effectiveness.
- Document the intensity of the patient's pain, medication administered, route, dose, and response.
- Instruct the patient to avoid crushing or chewing controlled-release tablets.
- Inform the patient that immediate-release capsules may be swallowed intact or that the contents may be sprinkled on food or mixed in juice to decrease the bitter taste.
- Aspirate before IM injections to avoid inadvertent IV administration.
- Advise the patient who is taking opiate agonists to breath deeply, cough, and turn from side to side frequently to decrease the risk for atelectasis.
- Provide safety and protect the patient from falls because opiate agonists may cause dizziness and drowsiness.
- Monitor the patient's pupil changes and reaction, urine output, and bowel sounds for early detection of adverse effects.
- Notify the health care provider when the opiate-agonist is ineffective. The dose may need to be increased or the drug may be discontinued and another opiate-agonist ordered until the pain is relieved.

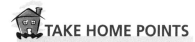

TAKE HOME POINTS

- The nurse must sign out each narcotic before administration.
- Pain is typically undertreated.
- Agonist-antagonists should not be administered when the patient has a respiratory rate less than 12 respirations per minute, shallow respirations, constricted or dilated pupils, or CNS hyperactivity.
- Monitor the patient who is taking narcotic analgesics for respiratory depression.
- Check doses carefully, particularly in children, and follow agency protocols for documentation.
- Describe the nature of pain before giving the drug and the degree of relief after the drug's onset of action.
- Intravenous (IV) injection of undiluted narcotic analgesics may lead to tachycardia and fainting.
- Provide side rails and assistance with ambulation after administering opiate agonists.
- Discontinuation of morphine and meperidine abruptly may lead to withdrawal effects (e.g., nausea, vomiting, diarrhea, dilated pupils, muscle twitching, nervousness, restlessness).

- Instruct the patient to avoid alcohol and other CNS depressants when taking opiate agonists.
- Have emergency equipment (ambu bag and mask for ventilation, oxygen, naloxone). Several hours of observation in narcotic overdosing may be required.
- Inform patients that opiate agonists should be tapered during discontinuation.

Do You UNDERSTAND?

DIRECTIONS: Indicate in the space provided whether the statement is *true* or *false*. If the answer is false, correct the statement to make it true (using the margin space).

_____ 1. Monitor patients who are taking opioid agonists for respiratory depression.

_____ 2. Meperidine is contraindicated for patients with renal dysfunction.

_____ 3. Controlled-release tablets should be crushed or chewed for better pain control.

What IS an Agonist-Antagonist?

Agonist-Antagonists	Trade Names	Uses
butorphanol [byoo-TOR-fah-nole]	Stadol	Control of moderate to severe pain
nalbuphine	Nubain	Control of moderate to severe pain
buprenorphine	Buprenex	Control of moderate to severe pain

Action

Agonist-antagonists are narcotics with a narcotic antagonist or blocker added. Agonist-antagonists act as an opioid agonist on one type of receptor and as a competitive antagonist on other receptors. Theories suggest that these agents produce analgesia at a subcortical level in the limbic system by binding at opiate receptor sites and reducing the intensity of pain stimuli from sensory nerve endings.

Answers: 1. true; 2. true; 3. false; controlled-release tablets should not be chewed or crushed.

Uses

Agonist-antagonists are used for moderate to severe pain or as a preoperative medication. These drugs are useful to treat pain for patients with renal colic, burns, and cancer.

What You NEED TO KNOW

Contraindications/Precautions

Agonist-antagonists should be used with caution in patients with a head injury, increased intracranial pressure, acute MI, coronary insufficiency, hypertension, biliary tract surgery, hepatic or renal dysfunction, respiratory depression, or chronic obstructive pulmonary disease (COPD) and in those who have a history of drug dependency.

Drug Interactions

When agonist-antagonists are given with other CNS depressants or alcohol, both CNS and respiratory depression are increased.

Adverse Effects

Adverse effects of agonist-antagonists are similar to those of opioid agonists, including rash, itching, headache, drowsiness, dizziness, fainting, sweating, euphoria, confusion, palpitations, bradycardia, nausea, flushing, difficulty urinating, and respiratory depression. Because these agents have agonist and antagonist actions, acute withdrawal effects can develop in opiate-dependent individuals. Opioid withdrawal effects peak 48 hours after drug discontinuation. Withdrawal effects include nausea, vomiting, anorexia, abdominal cramps, restlessness, fainting, and increased blood pressure. These agents have habit-forming potential because they contain narcotics.

Agonist-antagonists should be used with caution in patients with head injury, increased intracranial pressure, acute MI, coronary insufficiency, hypertension, biliary tract surgery, hepatic or renal dysfunction, respiratory depression, or COPD, as well as in those who have a history of drug dependency.

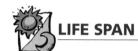

LIFE SPAN

Safe use in pregnant women before labor and during lactation and in children under 18 years of age has not been established.

What You DO

Nursing Responsibilities

Agonist-antagonists may be administered orally, Sub-Q, IM, and IV. For frequent long-term injections, IM is the preferred route over Sub-Q. When administering agonist-antagonists, the nurse should:

- Monitor the patient who is taking agonist-antagonists for respiratory depression.
- Instruct the patient to avoid combining agonist-antagonists with alcohol or other CNS depressants.
- Instruct patients to avoid activities that require alertness (e.g., driving) when taking opioid agonist-antagonists.
- Advise the patient that abrupt discontinuation may cause withdrawal effects, including nausea, vomiting, anorexia, abdominal cramps, restlessness, chills, fainting, and increased blood pressure. Opioid withdrawal effects peak 48 hours after drug discontinuation.

TAKE HOME POINTS

Do not administer opioid agonist-antagonists when the patient's respiratory rate is less than 12 respirations per minute. Agonist-antagonists may cause dizziness and drowsiness.

Do You UNDERSTAND?

DIRECTIONS: **Indicate in the space provided whether the statement is *true* or *false*. If the answer is false, correct the statement to make it true (using the margin space).**

_____ 1. Agonist-antagonists should be administered when the patient's respiratory rate is less than 10 respirations per minute.

_____ 2. Opioid withdrawal effects peak 48 hours after drug discontinuation.

What IS an Opiate Antagonist?

Opiate Antagonists	Trade Names
naloxone [nal-OX-ohn]	Narcan
nalmefene [NAL-meh-feen]	Revex
naltrexone [nal-TREX-ohn]	Revia

Answers: 1. false; respirations should be 12 or greater before giving agonist-antagonists; 2. true.

Action

Opiate antagonists block (or antagonize) receptor sites from narcotics or displaces opiates at opiate-occupied receptor sites inhibiting the action of the narcotic. These agents are antidotes to opiate agonists and agonist-antagonists.

Uses

Opiate antagonists are used to reverse the opiate effects of narcotic overdose. These agents are also used to reverse respiratory depression.

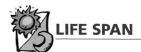

LIFE SPAN

Safe use of opiate antagonists during pregnancy and lactation has not been established.

What You NEED TO KNOW

Contraindications/Precautions

Opiate antagonists are contraindicated for patients with respiratory depression resulting from nonopioid agents.

Drug Interactions

When flumazenil is given with nalmefene, seizures may result.

Adverse Effects

The adverse effects of opiate antagonists include slight drowsiness, hypertension, hyperventilation, tremors, and reversal of analgesia. When reversal is too rapid, the patient may develop sweating, nausea, vomiting, elevated partial thromboplastin time (PTT), and tachycardia.

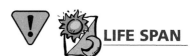

LIFE SPAN

- Opiate antagonists should be used with caution in neonates and children.
- Opiate antagonists should be used with caution in patients with a suspected narcotic dependency or cardiac irritability.

What You DO

Nursing Responsibilities

Opiate antagonists are given IV because of the urgency of the situation of overdose and respiratory depression. When administering opiate antagonists, the nurse should:
- Monitor the patient's vital signs and respiratory status because the duration of the narcotic analgesics may be longer than that of the opiate antagonist and respiratory depression may reoccur. Administer repeated doses of opiate antagonists as required.

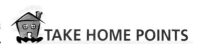

TAKE HOME POINTS

Monitor vital signs, particularly respirations, after administering opiate antagonists.

- Check the patient for development of sweating, nausea, vomiting, and tachycardia for detection of too rapid reversal of opiate antagonists.
- Monitor the patient for bleeding, particularly in surgical and obstetric patients because opiate antagonists may alter coagulation.
- Evaluate the patient's liver function tests for early development of hepatotoxicity.

Do You UNDERSTAND?

DIRECTIONS: Fill in the blanks in the following statements by selecting the appropriate response from the italicized choices.

1. Duration of opiate antagonist is usually _____ *(longer, shorter)* compared with narcotic analgesics.
2. Evidence of an excessive opiate antagonist administration is _____ _____ *(bradycardia, tachycardia)*.

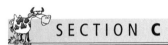

SECTION C

ANTIMIGRAINE AGENTS

Antimigraine agents control severe periodic headaches that usually have throbbing or stabbing pain as characteristics. Because migraines are a result of a dysfunction in the neurotransmitter serotonin and low serotonin levels, pharmacologic migraine control focuses on altering the serotonin concentration. Antimigraine agents are used to terminate an acute attack and prevent further attacks from occurring. Agents that are used to treat an acute migraine attack include aspirin-like analgesics, opioid analgesics, ergot derivatives, and triptans. Agents that are used to prevent migraine attacks include β-adrenergic blockers, amitriptyline, methysergide, and valproic acid. Explanations of many of these drug categories are provided in other chapters of this text. This section contains information regarding ergot derivatives and triptans.

Answers: 1. shorter; 2. tachycardia.

What IS an Ergot Alkaloid?

Ergot Alkaloid	Trade Names	Uses
ergotamine tartrate [er-GOT-ah-meen]	Ergostat	Prevent and abort acute migraine and cluster headaches
ergotamine tartrate with caffeine	Cafergot	Prevent and abort acute migraine and cluster headaches
dihydroergotamine [dye-high-droh-er-GOT-ah-meen]	Migranal DHE 45	Prevent and abort acute migraine and vascular headaches
methysergide maleate [meth-ih-SIR-jide]	Sansert	Prevent recurrent migraine, cluster, and other vascular headaches

Action

Ergot derivatives block or alter α-adrenergic, dopaminergic, and serotonin receptor sites in the brain and depress the vasomotor center, causing constriction of cranial blood vessels, decrease in the pulsation of cranial arteries, and decrease in basil artery perfusion. Because serotonin is a vasoconstrictor, ergot derivatives reduce the hyperperfusion of the dilated basilar artery and vascular bed. Methysergide is a semisynthetic ergot derivative that inhibits serotonin at postsynaptic receptors. Methysergide acts as a competitive antagonist of serotonin peripherally and may act as a serotonin agonist in the CNS. The antiserotonin effects of methysergide are greater compared with other ergot derivatives and result in inhibiting the peripheral vasoconstrictor effects of serotonin and serotonin-induced inflammation.

Uses

Ergot derivatives are used to prevent or treat acute migraine or vascular headache. Ergot derivatives are the drugs of choice in the treatment of an acute migraine attack. Dihydroergotamine is the drug of choice for rapid treatment of severe, refractory migraine, and cluster headaches. Combinations with ergot derivatives include an anticholinergic (e.g., belladonna), a sedative (e.g., pentobarbital), or an antihistamine (e.g., diphenhydramine) to prevent nausea and vomiting, which usually accompany migraines.

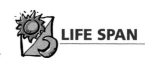 **LIFE SPAN**

Ergot derivatives are contraindicated during pregnancy and lactation because these agents are potent uterine stimulants and decrease uterine blood flow. Methysergide is also contraindicated for children and older adults.

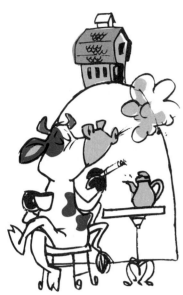

Cut out the coffee and smoking.

What You NEED TO KNOW

Contraindications/Precautions

Ergot derivatives are contraindicated for patients with angina, coronary artery disease, peripheral vascular disease, hypertension, hypersensitivity, malnutrition, sepsis, and hepatic or renal dysfunction. Methysergide is also contraindicated for patients with peptic ulcers, collagen diseases, debilitation, or severe infection.

Drug Interactions

When ergot derivatives are given in combination with beta blockers and other vasoconstrictors, the risk for peripheral ischemia and gangrene is increased. Examples of vasoconstrictors include cocaine, epinephrine, norepinephrine, metaraminol, methoxamine, phenylephrine, and tobacco. Therefore smoking increases the risk for vasoconstriction when it is concurrent with an ergot derivative. Antibiotics, troleandomycin, and erythromycin may lead to ergot toxicity when given with ergotamine. When ergotamine is combined with caffeine (Cafergot), GI absorption is enhanced.

Adverse Effects

The most common adverse effects of ergot derivatives are nausea and peripheral ischemia. Transient cold fingers and toes accompanied by tingling and numbness are indicative of peripheral ischemia from vaso-constriction. Other adverse effects include vomiting, tachycardia or bradycardia, diminished or absent pulses, dysrhythmias, edema, itching, leg weakness, muscle pain, paresthesia, and chest pain. Other adverse effects from methysergide include visual changes, drowsiness, insomnia, restlessness, depression, euphoria, and peripheral edema. A rare adverse effect after prolonged therapy is fibrosis in cardiac, pulmonary, retroperi-toneal, or penile tissue. When methysergide is discontinued abruptly, rebound headaches may occur. Because methysergide is chemically related to the hallucinogen lysergic acid diethylamide (LSD), overdose symptoms include visual changes, excitement, thought impairment, unsteadi-ness, dissociation, nightmares, hallucinations, convulsions, and impaired respirations.

Serious toxicity from an excessive amount of ergot agents is called ergotism and may lead to peripheral ischemia (e.g., cold, pale, numb extremities, gangrene). Because continuous excessive doses of ergot agents can cause physical dependence, rebound headache, increased frequency of headaches, dilated pupils, mental depression, restlessness, thirst, nausea, vomiting, diarrhea, and convulsions are among the withdrawal symptoms. Dihydroergotamine causes little nausea and vomiting and no physical dependence, but diarrhea is a common adverse effect.

What You DO

Nursing Responsibilities

Ergot derivatives may be given orally, IV, sublingually, rectally, or via inhalation. When administering ergot derivatives, the nurse should:

- Instruct the patient that ergot derivatives should be taken at the first symptoms of a headache. The patient should then lie down and relax in a quiet, darkened room for 2 to 3 hours for the medication to be most effective.
- Advise the patient to take methysergide with food to decrease GI distress. Inform the patient that intranasal and IV routes usually relieve migraines in less than 5 minutes.
- Counsel the patient to avoid chewing or swallowing sublingual tablets; instead, the medication should be allowed to dissolve completely.
- Advise the patient that methysergide should be taken for no longer than 6 months. After 6 months of methysergide therapy, allow 3 to 4 weeks to pass without taking the drug.
- Instruct the patient that when no response to methysergide therapy appears within 3 weeks, treatment should be discontinued and the health care provider should be notified.
- Monitor the patient's drug level for early detection of toxicity. The normal peak of methysergide is 60 ng/mL, and the normal trough level is 17 ng/mL.
- Inform patients that although migraine relief is achieved from dihydro-ergotamine, the headache usually returns in approximately 18% of patients within 24 hours.
- Instruct the patient to avoid increasing the dose without consulting the health care provider because overdosing is the leading cause of ergotamine adverse effects.

TAKE HOME POINTS

- Teach the patient that ergot derivatives should be taken at the first warning or aura of a migraine.
- Instruct the patient that intranasal and rectal routes of antimigraines are usually preferred over oral therapy when nausea or vomiting is present.
- Discontinue methysergide gradually over a 2- to 3-week period, never abruptly.
- Warn the patient that prolonged use or excessive doses may lead to ergotism and gangrene.

- Instruct the patient who is taking ergot derivatives to report shortness of breath, persistent paresthesia, leg muscle pain or weakness, cold or numb fingers or toes, pain in the chest, edema, abdomen, or muscles, and irregular heartbeat to the health care provider immediately.

Do You UNDERSTAND?

DIRECTIONS: **Provide appropriate responses to the following questions.**

1. What are two routes of administration that relieve migraine headaches? _____
2. What is added to ergotamine to facilitate GI absorption? _____
3. What type of tablets should not be chewed or swallowed but allowed to dissolve completely? _____

What IS a Triptan?

Triptans	Trade Names	Uses
sumatriptan [soo-mah-TRIP-tan]	Imitrex	Treat acute migraine and cluster headaches
naratriptan [nar-ah-TRIP-tan]	Amerge	Treat acute migraine headaches
rizatriptan [rye-za-TRIP-tan]	Maxalt	Treat acute migraine headaches
zolmitriptan [zole-mih-TRIP-tan]	Zomig	Treat acute migraine headaches
almotriptan [al-moe-TRIP-tan]	Axert	Treat acute migraine headaches
frovatriptan [fro-vah-TRIP-tan]	Frova	Treat acute migraine headaches
eletriptan [el-eh-TRIP-tan]	Relpax	Treat acute migraine headaches

Action

Triptans, the newest migraine agents available, are also known as serotonin 5-HT$_1$ receptor agonists. These agents bind to serotonin receptors 5-HT$_1$B or 5-HT$_1$D, or both, to cause vasoconstriction of cerebral blood vessels and inhibit the release of pain-producing inflammatory neuropeptides.

Uses

Triptans are used to relieve acute migraine attacks. Sumatriptan is usually more effective than is ergotamine for treating acute cluster headache attacks.

What You NEED TO KNOW

Contraindications/Precautions

Triptans should be used with caution in patients with coronary artery disease.

Drug Interactions

The major drug interaction of triptans involves severe vasoconstriction when they are given with ergot derivatives within 24 hours of each other. MAOIs decrease absorption of sumatriptan when they are given together or within 2 weeks of each other. Weakness, incoordination, and hyper-reflexia have been reported when triptans are taken with selected serotonin reuptake inhibitors (SSRIs).

Adverse Effects

Most of the adverse effects of triptans are mild and transient, usually occurring within 1 hour after oral or Sub-Q administration and subsiding within 1 hour after onset from an oral dose and 10 to 30 minutes after an Sub-Q dose. The adverse effects include hypersensitivity, weakness, fatigue, nausea, hearing deficit, ocular irritation, visual disturbance, dizziness, drowsiness, edema, polyuria, urgency, tachycardia, palpitations, hypertension, and dysrhythmias. Angina has occurred in rare instances after sumatriptan administration. An overdose can lead to a reduced respiratory rate, tremors, seizures, cyanosis, reddened extremities, muscular incoordination, and pupil dilation.

What You DO

Nursing Responsibilities

Triptans may be administered orally, intranasally, or Sub-Q. Although food does not appear to affect absorption, it delays peak concentration

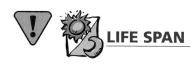

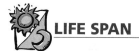

LIFE SPAN

- Triptans should be used with caution in patients with coronary artery disease.
- Triptans should be used with caution in children and older adults.

LIFE SPAN

Triptans are contraindicated for women during lactation and pregnancy and in those who may become pregnant.

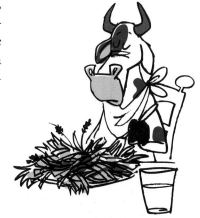

Food delays the peak concentration of triptans.

by approximately 30 minutes. When administering triptans, the nurse should:

- Administer the first dose of sumatriptan Sub-Q and under medical supervision.
- Inform the patient that when the first dose of oral naratriptan is ineffective, the dose may be repeated in 4 hours. When required, a second dose of rizatriptan may be repeated in 2 hours. With zolmitriptan administration, repeated doses may be taken every 2 hours for 24 hours. However, when no response to naratriptan, rizatriptan, or zolmitriptan is forthcoming, the health care provider should be consulted before taking another tablet.
- Instruct patients to report tingling, flushing, or dizziness to the health care provider.
- Inform the patient that although migraine relief is achieved from sumatriptan in all stages of an acute attack, the headache usually returns in approximately 40% of patients within 24 hours.
- Advise patients that while taking triptans, they should immediately report wheezing, facial swelling, rash, hives, chest pain, or tightness in the throat or chest to the health care provider.
- Warn patients that sumatriptan should be taken as soon as possible after migraine onset.
- Instruct the patient to use safety precautions when taking triptans when visual alterations and unsteadiness occur (e.g., when driving).
- Monitor the patient for severe acute depression and suicidal ideation.
- Monitor the patient's liver function tests for early detection of adverse effects.

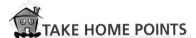

TAKE HOME POINTS

Monitor for unexpected cardiovascular responses following the first dose of sumatriptan.

Do You UNDERSTAND?

DIRECTIONS: **Indicate in the space provided whether the statement is *true* or *false*. If the answer is false, correct the statement to make it true (using the margin space).**

_____ 1. A major drug interaction of triptans, when given with ergot, is severe vasoconstriction.

_____ 2. Migraines usually diminish within 30 minutes after administering oral triptans.

Answers: 1. true; 2. false; migraine headache should diminish in 2 hours.

References

Baker B: Avoid triptans for migraine in pregnant patients, *Ob Gyn News* 35(17):9, 2000.

Bateman N: Triptans and migraine, *Lancet* 355(9207):860, 2000.

Gutierrez K, Queener SF: *Pharmacology for nursing practice*, St Louis, 2003, Mosby.

Hardman JG, Limbird LE: *Goodman & Gilman's the pharmacological basis of therapeutics*, ed 10, New York, 2001, McGraw-Hill.

Johnson PH, editor: *Nurse practitioner's drug handbook*, ed 3, Springhouse, Pa, 2000, Springhouse.

Karch AM: *Focus on nursing pharmacology*, ed 3, Philadelphia, 2006, Lippincott.

Kee JL, Hayes ER, McCuistion LE: *Pharmacology: a nursing process approach*, ed 5, Philadelphia, 2006, Elsevier.

Lehne RA: *Pharmacology for nursing care*, ed 5, Philadelphia, 2004, WB Saunders.

Lewis SM, Heitkemper MM, Dirksen SR: *Medical-surgical nursing: assessment and management of clinical problems,* ed 7, St Louis, 2004, Mosby.

Lilley LL, Harrington S, Snyder JS: *Pharmacology and the nursing process*, ed 4, St. Louis, 2005, Mosby.

McKenry LM, Salerno E: *Mosby's pharmacology in nursing*, ed 21, St Louis, 2003, Mosby.

Wilson BA, Shannon MT, Stang CL: *Nurses drug guide*, Upper Saddle River, New Jersey, 2006, Pearson.

NCLEX® Review

Section A

1. A patient is taking acetaminophen. The nurse should warn the patient that _____ is the maximum dose per day.
   1 2 g
   2 4 g
   3 10 g
   4 25 g

2. Which liquid should the patient be instructed to avoid when taking acetaminophen?
   1 Wine
   2 Milk
   3 Coffee
   4 Grapefruit juice

3. The patient who is taking phenytoin concurrently with acetaminophen is in danger of:
   1 hepatotoxicity.
   2 renal toxicity.
   3 gastric ulceration.
   4 Stevens-Johnson syndrome.

4. The nurse warns the patient taking acetaminophen that adverse effects of this medication include:
   1 headache.
   2 hypotension.
   3 bradycardia.
   4 hypoglycemia.

5. The nurse knows that the antidote for acetaminophen overdose is:
   1 naloxone (Narcan).
   2 naltrexone (Revia).
   3 buprenorphine (Buprenex).
   4 acetylcysteine (Mucomyst).

Section B

6. Which opiate is responsible for producing toxic metabolites?
   1 Codeine sulfate
   2 Fentanyl
   3 Meperidine
   4 Oxycodone

7. Which adverse effect of opiates is the most serious?
   1 Dilated pupils
   2 Seizures
   3 Orthostatic hypotension
   4 Respiratory depression

8. A patient is receiving IV morphine following severe chest pain. The nurse knows the IV morphine should be diluted to prevent:
   1 tachycardia.
   2 hypertension.
   3 respiratory stimulation.
   4 skeletal muscle rigidity.

9. A patient is receiving nalbuphine (Nubain). Forty-eight hours after drug discontinuation, the nurse should monitor for:
   1 hypotension.
   2 increased appetite.
   3 abdominal cramps.
   4 skeletal muscle flaccidity.

10. A patient is given a dose of naloxone (Narcan). The nurse knows that:
    1 the patient must be monitored for bradycardia.
    2 IM administration is preferred.
    3 only one dose of IV naloxone is given.
    4 the patient's vital signs and respiratory status must be monitored.

Section C

11. Which of the following migraine preparations has increased GI absorption?
    1 Dihydroergotamine
    2 Ergotamine tartrate
    3 Methysergide maleate
    4 Ergotamine tartrate with caffeine

12. Which adverse effects are the most common with ergot derivatives?
    1 Vomiting and diarrhea
    2 Tachycardia or bradycardia
    3 Itching and rebound headache
    4 Nausea and cold fingers and toes

13. The onset of action for intranasal dihydroergotamine occurs within which of the following time frames?
    1 5 minutes
    2 30 minutes
    3 2 hours
    4 4 hours

14. A patient is taking ergotamine tartrate with caffeine. The nurse knows that an excessive amount of this drug may lead to ergotism, which means:
    1 tinnitus.
    2 gangrene.
    3 penile fibrosis.
    4 peripheral edema.

15. A patient is taking ergotamine tartrate. The nurse knows that concurrent use of _____ may lead to ergot toxicity.
    1 tobacco
    2 belladonna
    3 erythromycin
    4 methysergide maleate

NCLEX® Review Answers

Section A

1. **2** The maximum dose of acetaminophen per day is 4 g.

2. **1** Avoid concurrent alcohol when taking more than 1 to 2 doses of acetaminophen per day.

3. **1** When long-term phenytoin is concurrent with acetaminophen, the risk for hepatotoxicity is increased.

4. **1** Headache may be an adverse effect of acetaminophen. Hypotension, bradycardia, and hypoglycemia are not known adverse effects of acetaminophen.

5. **4** The antidote for acetaminophen overdose is acetylcysteine.

Section B

6. **3** Meperidine is responsible for producing the toxic metabolite normeperidine, which may lead to neurotoxicity. Codeine, fentanyl, and oxycodone produce no toxic metabolites.

7. **4** The most serious adverse effect of opiates is respiratory depression. Breathing oxygen is more essential to life than are dilated pupils, seizures, and orthostatic hypotension.

8. **1** IV morphine should be diluted to prevent tachycardia and fainting. Morphine dilates vessels and may lead to hypotension not hypertension, respiratory depression not respiratory stimulation, and skeletal muscle relaxation and flaccidity, not rigidity.

9. **3** Abdominal cramps should be monitored 48 hours after discontinuation of nalbuphine, indicating opioid withdrawal effects. Other withdrawal effects include hypertension not hypotension and anorexia not increased appetite. Skeletal muscle flaccidity is not associated with nalbuphine.

10. **4** Vital signs and respiratory status should be monitored after a dose of naloxone because they may decrease again after the duration of action of naloxone is completed. Tachycardia usually occurs when reversal of opiate antagonists is too rapid. Naloxone is given IV not IM. More than one dose may be required to reverse opiate toxicity.

Section C

11. 4 When caffeine is combined with ergotamine tartrate (Cafergot), GI absorption is increased. Dihydroergotamine, ergotamine tartrate alone, and methysergide maleate do not increase GI absorption.

12. 4 The most common adverse effects of ergot derivatives are nausea and peripheral ischemia, which is evidenced by cold fingers or toes. Vomiting and diarrhea, tachycardia or bradycardia, and itching or rebound headache are not common adverse effects of ergot derivatives.

13. 1 The onset of action for intranasal and IV ergot derivatives is rapid, less than 5 minutes. The remaining options (30 minutes, 2 hours, and 4 hours) are incorrect onsets of action for intranasal and IV ergot derivatives.

14. 2 Ergotism means peripheral ischemia evidenced by cold, pale, numb extremities and gangrene. Tinnitus is not associated with ergotamine. Peripheral edema is an adverse effect, and penile fibrosis is a rare adverse effect of ergotamine, but neither of these effects are included in the definition of ergotism.

15. 3 Concurrent erythromycin and ergotamine may lead to ergot toxicity—not concurrent use of tobacco, belladonna, or methysergide maleate.

Notes

Drugs Used for Nutritional Imbalances

Vitamins and minerals are essential to the body's metabolic activities and necessary in maintaining the dynamic equilibrium required for good health. These substances are generally obtained from the diet. However, when the intake of vitamins or minerals is inadequate, deficiencies may occur and the health of the individual is affected. Factors that affect the dietary requirement and function of minerals and vitamins are lifestyle, environmental, genetic predisposition, hormone balance, growth, other drugs, and disease processes. Vitamins and minerals that are used for nutritional imbalances are discussed in this chapter.

What You WILL LEARN

After reading this chapter, you will know how to do the following:

✔ Identify the indications for patients taking a vitamin or mineral.

✔ Contrast fat-soluble vitamins with water-soluble vitamins.

✔ Identify the drug interactions associated with fat-soluble vitamins

✔ Discuss the contraindications and precautions for the patient taking a water-soluble vitamin.

✔ List the uses for mineral-based drugs, such as calcium, potassium, and iron.

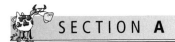

SECTION A

VITAMINS

What IS a Fat-Soluble Vitamin?

Fat-Soluble Vitamins	Trade Names
vitamin A	Aquasol A
vitamin D (calcitriol)	Rocaltrol
vitamin E	Aquasol E
vitamin K (phytonadione)	Aqua-Mephyton

Action

The fat-soluble vitamins—A, D, E, and K—are found in the oil or fats of foods. Fat-soluble vitamins bind with specific plasma proteins and are then stored in the fat areas of the body. An excess accumulation in storage may cause toxicity. For the body to absorb fat-soluble vitamins, fat or bile salts are required.

Uses

Vitamin A is used in the growth and development of bones, teeth, retina, and epithelial and embryonic tissue. Vitamin A is also used in the synthesis of hydrocortisone.

Vitamin D prevents and treats rickets; promotes calcium, magnesium, and phosphorus absorption and metabolism; and controls parathyroid hormone levels.

Vitamin E is an antioxidant that prevents formation of free radicals that damage cell membranes. Vitamin E also promotes the growth and development of muscles, increases fat metabolism, aids the body's use of vitamin A, and prevents the formation of blood clots.

Vitamin K is necessary for the synthesis of blood coagulation factors II (**prothrombin**), VII, IX, and X in the liver. Vitamin K is also the antidote for an oral anticoagulant overdose.

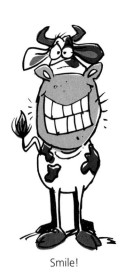

Smile!

What You NEED TO KNOW

Contraindications/Precautions

Vitamin D should be used with caution in patients with coronary disease, renal dysfunction, arteriosclerosis, asthma, or hypoparathyroidism and in those undergoing dialysis. Vitamin E has no contraindications.

Drug Interactions

Mineral oil decreases the absorption of vitamins A, D, E, and K. Oral contraceptives increase levels of vitamin A.

Use of vitamin D in patients on chronic renal dialysis may lead to hypomagnesemia. Concurrent use of digoxin or verapamil with vitamin D may precipitate dysrhythmias. Concurrent administration of phenobarbital and phenytoin may decrease vitamin D levels. Corticosteroids counteract vitamin D effects.

Sucralfate decreases the absorption of vitamins E and K. Vitamin E may also enhance the action of oral anticoagulants. Vitamin K antagonizes the effect of warfarin.

Adverse Effects

Excess vitamin A may cause inflammation of the skin, conjunctiva, and lips; dry mucus membranes; baldness; and peeling of the palms of hands and soles of feet. Overdosing of vitamin A causes malaise, anorexia, abdominal discomfort, lethargy, and vomiting (**hypervitaminosis syndrome**). Overdosing of vitamin A also causes headache, dizziness, irritability, increased intracranial pressure, dry cracked skin, edema, jaundice, hypomenorrhea, blurred vision, and irreversible bone demineralization.

Early adverse effects of excessive vitamin D include headache, dizziness, weakness, nausea, vomiting, dry mouth, constipation, diarrhea, metallic taste, and muscle and bone pain. Late adverse effects of vitamin D include anorexia, irritability, polyuria, polydipsia, photophobia, itching, and decreased libido.

Vitamin E is generally considered nontoxic. However, prolonged use of excessive doses of vitamin E causes skeletal muscle weakness, headache, blurred vision, nausea, diarrhea, abdominal cramps, and fatigue.

Adverse effects of vitamin K include transient flushing and alteration in taste. Excessive amounts of vitamin K alter coagulation factors, thus contributing to blood clots.

- Vitamin A should be used with caution during pregnancy and lactation. Vitamin D should be used with caution in older adults. Vitamin K should be used with caution in women during pregnancy and lactation and in children.
- Vitamin A should be used with caution in patients with renal dysfunction, in women who are taking contraceptives, and in cases of prolonged administration. Anaphylactic shock and death have been reported following the IV administration of vitamin A. Vitamin K should be used with caution in those with hepatic impairment and in patients taking oral anticoagulants.

What You DO

Nursing Responsibilities

Fat-soluble vitamins are generally given orally. Vitamin K may also be given Sub-Q or IM. When administering fat-soluble vitamins, the nurse should:

- Advise the patient to avoid concurrent use of mineral oil with fat-soluble vitamins because it decreases absorption of the vitamins.
- Instruct the patient to take vitamins A and E on an empty stomach. When the patient has gastrointestinal distress, vitamins A and E may be taken with food or milk. Vitamins D and K may be taken without regard to food.
- Tell the patient that food sources of vitamin A include liver, butter, cheese, whole milk, egg yolk, meat, fish, dark-green leafy vegetables, carrots, squash, sweet potatoes, and cantaloupe.
- Advise the patient that food sources of vitamin D include fish, liver, and oils.
- Tell the patient that food sources of vitamin E include wheat germ, vegetable oils, green leafy vegetables, dairy products, nuts, meat, liver, eggs, and cereals.
- Teach the patient that food sources of vitamin K include cauliflower, spinach, fish, liver, eggs, meats, cereal grain products, dairy products, and fruits.
- Advise the patient to swallow oral vitamin D whole and to avoid chewing or crushing the vitamin.
- Counsel the patient to avoid magnesium antacids when taking vitamin D.
- Instruct the patient to obtain sufficient exposure to sunlight to help satisfy vitamin D requirements.
- Protect vitamin K from the light.
- Instruct the patient who is taking vitamin K to avoid alcohol, ibuprofen, and aspirin and to report any bleeding.
- Warn the patient to report hypervitaminosis (e.g., malaise, anorexia, nausea, vomiting, diarrhea, headache, dizziness, irritability, dried and cracked skin, edema, jaundice, hypomenorrhea, blurred vision) to the health care provider.

TAKE HOME POINTS

- Monitor calcium and phosphorus levels at least twice weekly, then once weekly for 12 weeks until the patient with chronic renal failure who is taking vitamin D stabilizes; monitor monthly thereafter.
- Heparin is the antidote for vitamin K overdose.

Do You UNDERSTAND?

DIRECTIONS: Fill in the blanks in the following statements by selecting the appropriate response from the italicized choices.

1. Vitamins A, D, E, and K are _____ (*fat-soluble, water-soluble*) vitamins.
2. Vitamin K should be used with caution in patients taking _____ _____ (*anticoagulants, corticosteroids*).
3. Vitamin E is considered a(n) _____ (*antioxidant, procoagulant*).
4. Vitamin A is used in the synthesis of _____ (*hydrocortisone, clotting factors*).

What IS a Water-Soluble Vitamin?

Water-Soluble Vitamins	Trade Names
vitamin B_1 (thiamine) [THIGH-ah-min]	Betalin
vitamin B_2 (riboflavin) [RYE-bow-fly-vin]	None listed
vitamin B_3 (niacin) [NYE-ah-sin]	Nicobid
vitamin B_6 (pyridoxine) [peer-ih-DOX-een]	Hexa Betalin
vitamin B_9 (folic acid) [FOE-lick]	Folvite
vitamin B_{12} (cyanocobalamin) [sye-ANN-oh-koh- BAL-ah-min]	Cyanabin
vitamin C (ascorbic acid) [ah-SKOR-bic]	Ascorbicap

Action

Vitamin C and the B-complex vitamins are water-soluble and found in the watery portion of foods. The B-complex vitamins include vitamins B_1, B_2, B_3, B_6, B_9, and B_{12}. These vitamins are readily excreted in the urine with small amounts stored in the body; therefore water-soluble vitamins rarely cause toxicity, and regular daily intake is required.

Answers: 1. fat-soluble, 2. anticoagulants, 3. antioxidant, 4. hydrocortisone.

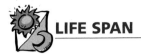

LIFE SPAN

Folic acid helps prevent neural tube defects in the fetus. Niacin is contraindicated during pregnancy and lactation.

Uses

Vitamin B_1 promotes carbohydrate and aerobic metabolism, transmission of nerve impulses, maintenance of normal growth and development, and synthesis of acetylcholine. Vitamin B_2 acts as a catalyst in oxidation-reduction reactions of glucose and amino acid. It is also responsible for the metabolism of fatty acids.

Vitamin B_3 acts as a catalyst in oxidation-reduction reactions of cholesterol and fatty acids. Vitamin B_3 also causes vasodilation and prevents and treats pellagra.

Vitamin B_6 promotes protein, fat, and carbohydrate metabolism; facilitates release of glucose from liver and muscles; promotes formation of neurotransmitters; and treats neuropathy.

Vitamin B_9 helps in protein synthesis and erythropoiesis. It also stimulates the production of red blood cells, white blood cells, and platelets.

Vitamin B_{12} is essential for growth, cell reproduction, hematopoiesis; synthesis of nucleic acid and myelin; and treatment of vitamin B_{12} deficiency and pernicious anemia.

Vitamin C is an antioxidant that promotes collagen formation, tissue repair, wound healing, gastrointestinal absorption of iron, and synthesis of peptide and epinephrine. Vitamin C also prevents and treats scurvy.

Contraindications/Precautions

Vitamin B_1 should be used with caution in patients with hypersensitivity. Vitamin B_3 should be used with caution in patients with a history of gallbladder disease, liver disease, glaucoma, angina, gout, diabetes, and coronary artery disease. Vitamin B_3 is contraindicated for patients with liver impairment, severe hypotension, active peptic ulcer or bleeding, and hypersensitivity. Vitamin B_9 is contraindicated for the treatment of pernicious anemia and other megaloblastic anemias when vitamin B_{12} is deficient. Vitamin B_{12} is contraindicated for patients with hypersensitivity. Vitamin C should be used with caution in patients with diabetes and those who are prone to renal calculi, on a sodium restricted diet, or those taking anticoagulants.

Drug Interactions

Vitamins B_1, B_2, and B_{12} have no known drug interactions. Vitamin B_3 enhances the effects of antihypertensive drugs, causing hypotension. Concurrent use of isoniazid, hydralazine, penicillamine, or oral contraceptives decreases the therapeutic effects of vitamin B_6. Vitamin B_6 may reverse or antagonize the effects of levodopa. Concurrent use of sulfasalazine, methotrexate, trimethoprim, oral contraceptives, and aminosalicylic acid with vitamin B_6 decreases vitamin B_9 levels. Folic acid decreases hydantoin concentrations.

Large doses of vitamin C may decrease the response to oral anticoagulants and disulfiram. Vitamin C requirements may be increased with concurrent use of salicylates, oral contraceptives, and smoking. The absorption of iron is increased when vitamin C is taken with iron-rich foods.

Adverse Effects

Adverse effects of vitamin B_1 include a warm feeling, itching, weakness, sweating, restlessness, nausea, angioedema, pulmonary edema, hypersensitivity, anaphylactic shock, and death. Vitamin B_2 is nontoxic but may cause yellow discoloration of urine when taken in large doses. Adverse effects of vitamin B_3 include transient headache, generalized flushing, feeling of warmth, nausea, vomiting, flatulence, bloating, dry skin, itching, tingling of extremities, jaundice, and elevated hepatic function tests. Adverse effects of vitamin B_6 include a slight flushing and warm feeling. Although rare, vitamin B_6 causes paresthesia and seizures, usually with large parenteral doses. Adverse effects of vitamin B_9 include hypersensitivity reactions, decreased vitamin B_{12} serum levels, altered sleep patterns, difficulty concentrating, irritability, excitement, overactivity, mental depression, confusion, anorexia, impaired judgment, bitter taste, and flatulence. Adverse effects of vitamin B_{12} include allergic reactions and hypersensitivity.

Vitamin C is usually nontoxic, except when excessive doses are taken. Adverse effects include transient soreness at IM and Sub-Q injection sites, temporary dizziness, and faintness following rapid IV administration of vitamin C. Overdosing with vitamin C causes nausea, vomiting, diarrhea, gout attacks, and renal stones.

Nursing Responsibilities

Most water-soluble vitamins are given orally. Vitamin B_1 may also be given IM or IV. When GI absorption is severely impaired, vitamin B_9 may be given Sub-Q, IM, or IV. Parenteral vitamin B_{12} should be given IM or deep Sub-Q. When administering water-soluble vitamins, the nurse should:

- Instruct the patient to take oral vitamins C, B_1, B_3, and B_{12} with food. Large doses of vitamins C and B_3 should be given in small, divided doses because the body will excrete excessive amounts beyond the current requirement. Vitamin B_6 may be given without regard to food.

- Teach patients that the need for vitamin B_1 and B_6 is increased when the diet is high in carbohydrates.
- Instruct the patient to taper vitamin C dosages when discontinuing. Abrupt discontinuation of large doses may lead to bleeding gums, gingivitis, and loosened teeth (**rebound scurvy**).
- Rotate IM injection sites of vitamin B_1 and apply cold compresses to relieve pain at injection site.
- Tell the patient that food sources of vitamin C include citrus fruits, such as oranges, limes, lemons, strawberries, tomatoes, leafy vegetables, melons, and cabbage.
- Teach the patient that food sources of vitamin B_1 include brewer's yeast, beef, pork, milk, liver, nuts, legumes, whole grains, enriched flour, and cereal.
- Advise the patient that food sources of vitamin B_2 include meat, fish, poultry, dairy products, broccoli, asparagus, spinach, mushrooms, grains, cereal, and bakery products.
- Instruct the patient that food sources of vitamin B_3 include organ and lean meats, brewer's yeast, poultry, fish, and peanuts.
- Tell the patient that food sources of vitamin B_6 include yeast, whole-grain cereals, liver, legumes, green vegetables, and bananas.
- Teach the patient that food sources of vitamin B_9 include liver, oranges, broccoli, Brussels sprouts, spinach, beets, whole-wheat products, peas, dried beans, and lentils. The best source is asparagus.
- Advise the patient that food sources of vitamin B_{12} include liver, fish, dairy products, clams, oysters, and crab.

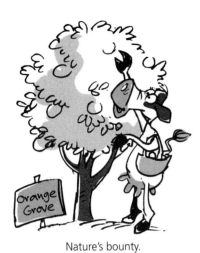

Nature's bounty.

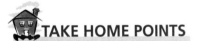

TAKE HOME POINTS

Warn the patient to take the oral vitamin B_{12} dose promptly when it is mixed with juice because ascorbic acid affects the stability of vitamin B_{12}.

Do You UNDERSTAND?

DIRECTIONS: **Match each vitamin in Column A with its corresponding term in the list of scrambled words in Column B.**

Column A	Column B
_____ 1. Vitamin B_3	a. incain
_____ 2. Vitamin B_6	b. dificaolc
_____ 3. Vitamin B_9	c. doxiprieny
_____ 4. Vitamin B_{12}	d. manboaycilocan

Answers: 1. niacin; 2. pyridoxine; 3. folic acid; 4. cyanocobalamin.

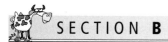

SECTION **B**

MINERALS

What IS a Mineral?

Minerals	Trade Names
sodium (sodium bicarbonate)	None listed
potassium (potassium chloride)	K-Dur Micro-K
calcium (calcium citrate)	Citra Cal
phosphorus	K-Phos Neutro-Phos
magnesium (magnesium oxide)	Mag-Ox 400
iron (ferrous gluconate)	Fergon
zinc	None listed

Action

Minerals function as structural components, forming bones, teeth, and nails and acting as components of enzymes. Minerals are essential for the body's regulation of water metabolism, blood volume, cell membrane permeability, tissue excitability, and the maintenance of acid-base balance. The body excretes minerals; thus they must be replaced through the intake of food or supplements.

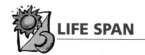

LIFE SPAN

Calcium is used to treat tetany of the newborn.

Uses

Sodium regulates fluids, tissues, water, and acid-base balance and conducts electrical impulses of muscles and nerves. Sodium also prevents or treats extracellular volume depletion and dehydration or sodium depletion. Sodium prevents heat prostration.

Potassium is the principal intracellular cation of most body tissues. Potassium maintains intracellular tonicity, cell metabolism, transmission of impulses, acid-base balance, and renal function. Potassium also maintains contraction of cardiac, skeletal, and smooth muscles, as well as prevents and treats hypokalemia.

Calcium maintains the integrity of nervous and muscular systems, normal cardiac function, cell permeability, and blood coagulation. Calcium promotes bone growth and the activity of endocrine and exocrine glands. Calcium also treats calcium deficiency, end-stage renal failure (calcium acetate), hypoparathyroidism, osteoporosis, rickets, and osteomalacia.

Phosphorus functions at the intracellular level for energy transport and energy production (adenosine diphosphate [ADP] and adenosine triphosphate [ATP]). Phosphorus aids calcium transport, acts with phospholipids in cell membranes, is a component of deoxyribonucleic acid (DNA) and ribonucleic acid (RNA) molecules, lowers urinary calcium levels, and increases urinary phosphate levels.

Magnesium aids in sodium and potassium transport, phosphate transfer, muscular contraction, nerve conduction, enzyme systems, energy release with conversion of ATP to ADP, and treats hypomagnesemia, preeclampsia, and dysrhythmias.

Iron, a component of hemoglobin, myoglobin, and enzymes, maintains heat production, aids in muscle and catecholamine metabolism, and prevents and treats iron deficiency. Iron supplements are needed in chronic renal failure to correct the iron deficiency anemia, which is a major abnormality in renal failure.

Zinc promotes the growth and repair of tissue, is an integral part of enzymes that are required for protein and carbohydrate metabolism, and controls copper absorption in the long-term treatment of Wilson's disease.

What You NEED TO KNOW

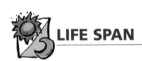

LIFE SPAN

Potassium and calcium should be used cautiously during pregnancy. Phosphorus should be used cautiously during pregnancy and lactation.

Contraindications/Precautions

Potassium is contraindicated in patients with severe renal impairment, crushing injuries, Addison's disease, hyperkalemia, severe hemolytic reactions, acute dehydration, anuria, heat cramps, and in those who are receiving potassium-sparing diuretics or angiotensin-converting enzyme (ACE) inhibitors.

Calcium is contraindicated for patients with hypercalcemia, hypophosphatemia, and renal calculi. Calcium should be used cautiously in patients with hypoparathyroidism who are also receiving high doses of vitamin D and in those who have aspirin hypersensitivity (because some calcium products contain tartrazine that may cause allergic reactions, including bronchial asthma).

Phosphorus is contraindicated for patients with hyperkalemia, Addison's disease, severe renal impairment, hyperphosphatemia, or hypercalcemia. Phosphorus should be used cautiously in patients who are on a sodium- or potassium-restricted diet or those with cardiac disease, acute dehydration, renal and hepatic dysfunction, edema, hypernatremia, or hypertension.

Magnesium is contraindicated for patients who are experiencing abdominal pain, nausea, vomiting, diarrhea, fecal impaction, intestinal obstruction, or heart block following delivery. Iron is contraindicated for patients with hemolytic anemia, hemosiderosis, cirrhosis of the liver, peptic ulcer, hemochromatosis, or ulcerative colitis.

Drug Interactions

Sodium has no known drug interactions. Concurrent use of potassium with potassium-sparing diuretics or ACE inhibitors may cause hyperkalemia.

Calcium enhances the inotropic and toxic effects of digoxin. It also decreases the absorption and effects of verapamil, tetracycline, quinolone antibiotics, iron, atenolol, and zinc. Concurrent use of calcium with thiazide diuretics may result in hypercalcemia. When hypocalcemic drugs are taken concurrently with antacids that contain magnesium, hypermagnesemia may occur. Reduced absorption may occur when hypocalcemic drugs are taken with cholestyramine or mineral oil.

Phosphate absorption and action are decreased when given concurrently with vitamin D and antacids with magnesium, aluminum, or calcium. When phosphates and potassium-containing drugs are given together, hyperkalemia may occur. Magnesium salts decrease the absorption of quinolones, digoxin, nitrofurantoin, penicillamine, and tetracyclines. When given concurrently with iron, antacids lower iron absorption.

Ascorbic acid and chloramphenicol enhance the absorption of iron. Iron decreases the absorption of tetracyclines, ofloxacin, penicillamine, and ciprofloxacin and may delay the effects of chloramphenicol. Drugs that may have a decreased absorption or effectiveness when given with iron include levodopa, levothyroxine, methyldopa, penicillamine, quinolones, and tetracyclines. The absorption and effectiveness of fluoroquinolones and tetracyclines are decreased when these drugs are given concurrently with zinc.

Sodium should be used cautiously in patients with kidney dysfunction, preeclampsia, and peripheral or pulmonary edema. Potassium should be used cautiously in patients with severe burns and cardiac or renal disease, preeclampsia, acute pancreatitis, hypoparathyroidism, osteomalacia, or renal calculi. Magnesium should be used cautiously in patients with renal disease.

Parenteral iron should be given only in the upper-outer quadrant of the buttocks using the Z-track technique.

Adverse Effects

Sodium overdosing causes electrolyte imbalances, gastrointestinal irritation, anorexia, nausea, vomiting, diarrhea, abdominal cramps, restlessness, confusion, weakness, irritability, convulsions, coma, hypertension, tachycardia, and pulmonary edema.

Potassium's adverse effects include nausea, vomiting, diarrhea, abdominal pain, and oliguria. Hyperkalemia (e.g., a potassium level greater than 5.5 mEq/L) can cause muscle weakness, paresthesias, nausea, diarrhea, hypotension, bradycardia, dysrhythmias, and cardiac arrest.

Calcium's adverse effects include mild hypercalcemia (e.g., a calcium level greater than 10.5 mg/dL), which can be asymptomatic or appear as headache, anorexia, nausea, vomiting, abdominal pain, constipation, dry mouth, thirst, metallic taste, and polyuria. Severe hypercalcemia (e.g., a calcium level greater than 12.5 mg/dL) causes neuromuscular irritability, confusion, delirium, and coma. Hypercalcemia occurs more frequently with calcitrate and calcium carbonate compared with calcium acetate.

The common adverse effects of phosphorus include nausea, vomiting, abdominal pain, and diarrhea. Less frequently, phosphorus causes headache, dizziness, weakness, confusion, muscle cramps, numbness, tingling, pain, shortness of breath, swelling of lower extremities, weight gain, thirst, and bone and joint pain.

A magnesium overdose causes hypermagnesemia and is manifest as weakness, hypotension, bradycardia, ECG changes, nausea, vomiting, urinary retention, and hyporeflexia. Hypermagnesemia is a serum magnesium level greater than 3.0 mg/dL.

The common adverse effects of iron include nausea, vomiting, diarrhea, constipation, and dark-colored stools. Liquid iron preparations may stain teeth. Iron overdosing may also produce lethargy, abdominal pain, weak thready pulse, hypotension, fever, hyperglycemia, decreased tissue perfusion, leukocytosis, dyspnea, metabolic acidosis, coma, convulsions, shock, vascular congestion, pulmonary edema, anuria, and death.

Zinc's adverse effects include nausea and vomiting. An overdose of zinc causes nausea, severe vomiting, dehydration, and restlessness.

TAKE HOME POINTS

- Use caution when giving a calcium formulation to a patient on digoxin because of an increased risk for digoxin toxicity.
- To enhance absorption of iron, administer this mineral with citrus juice or fruits.
- To prevent staining of the teeth, administer adequately diluted liquid iron through a straw; then have the patient rinse the mouth with water immediately after taking the drug.
- Warn the patient that tarry black stools may result from iron therapy.

What You DO

Nursing Responsibilities

Mineral supplements are generally given orally, but they may be administered IV in acute situations. When administering mineral supplements, the nurse should:

- Give sodium tablets with 8 ounces of water up to 10 times a day in the treatment of heat cramps and dehydration.
- Inform patients that excessive consumption of sodium chloride may lead to acidosis and hypokalemia. Report to the health care provider serum sodium levels exceeding 146 mEq/L.
- Inform the patient that good sources of potassium in foods are milk, bananas, raisins, prunes, dates, avocado, beef, lamb, chicken, turkey, veal, watermelon, cantaloupe, apricots, pears, broccoli, Brussels sprouts, spinach, potatoes, and lentils.
- Give potassium with an 8-ounce glass of water or fruit juice to ensure that drug is swallowed and does not cause esophagitis by dissolving and irritating the mucous membranes. Instruct the patient to avoid chewing any extended-release or long-acting potassium preparation.
- Instruct the patient to report signs and symptoms of potassium toxicity (e.g., muscle weakness, paresthesias, nausea, diarrhea, hypotension, and bradycardia) because potassium toxicity can occur with therapeutic doses.
- Administer calcium with meals containing fats and carbohydrates to increase absorption of calcium. Sources of calcium include milk, milk products, and dark green vegetables.
- Instruct the patient to drink an 8-ounce glass of water when taking calcium and to report any anorexia, nausea, vomiting, constipation, abdominal pain, polyuria, thirst, or dry mouth (signs and symptoms of hypercalcemia) to the health care provider.
- Inform the patient foods high in fiber decrease calcium absorption because of decreased transit time.
- Monitor serum calcium levels two times a week initially after beginning therapy and periodically thereafter.
- Advise the patient that swallowing phosphorus capsules should be avoided. Rather, the capsule should be opened and the powder inside dissolved in water.

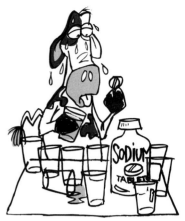

I'm thirsty.

- Inform patients who are on sodium- and potassium-restricted diets that phosphate products contain high amounts of these minerals.
- Monitor serum phosphorus, calcium, potassium, sodium levels (because phosphate products contain high amounts of potassium and sodium), and renal function tests.
- Tell the patient that food sources of magnesium include nuts, meats, legumes, fish, whole-grain cereals, milk, and green leafy vegetables.
- Monitor the pulse and blood pressure every 15 minutes or at more frequent intervals as indicated when giving IV magnesium sulfate. Check the patient's patellar reflex before each repeated doses of parenteral magnesium. Signs of early magnesium toxicity include depressed or absent reflexes.
- Tell the patient that food sources of iron include red meat, liver, dark-green leafy vegetables, carrots, raisins, prunes, and apricots.
- Advise the patient that iron therapy is usually continued for 2 to 3 months after the hemoglobin level returns to normal. As a rule, iron therapy should not last longer than 6 months.
- Monitor hemoglobin and reticulocyte values for drug effectiveness.
- Tell the patient that absorption of iron may be decreased when taken with milk, eggs, and caffeine-containing drinks.
- Inform the patient that iron formulations should not be crushed or the contents of the capsule emptied.
- Administer iron and calcium 2 hours before or after tetracyclines, fluoroquinolones, or other drugs affecting iron absorption. When gastrointestinal distress occurs from iron, the drug may be taken with meals. However, iron should not be taken within 1 hour of bedtime.
- Administer zinc tablets 1 hour before or 2 to 3 hours after meals. If gastrointestinal distress occurs, zinc may be taken with food.
- Advise patients to avoid taking zinc concurrently with coffee because it reduces zinc absorption by 50%.
- Counsel the patient to avoid foods that are high in copper (e.g., liver, pork, tofu, shellfish, nuts, dried beans, mushrooms, broccoli, avocado, cocoa, chocolate), calcium, and phosphorus when taking zinc.

Do You UNDERSTAND?

DIRECTIONS: Fill in the blanks in the following statements by selecting the appropriate response from the italicized choices.

1. _____ *(folic acid, vitamin C)* is an antioxidant essential for collagen formation and tissue repair.

2. Taking zinc concurrently with a cup of coffee reduces the absorption of zinc by _____ *(50%, 75%)*.

3. Calcium should be taken _____ *(with food, on an empty stomach)*.

4. Iron commonly causes _____ *(black, red)* stools.

References

Gutierrez K, Queener S: *Pharmacology for nursing practice*, Philadelphia, 2004, Mosby.

Lehne R: *Pharmacology for nursing care*, ed 5, Philadelphia, 2004, WB Saunders.

Lilley L, Harrington S, Snyder J: *Pharmacology and the nursing process*, ed 4, St Louis, 2005, Mosby.

Maham K, Escott-Stump S: *Krause's food, nutrition, and diet therapy*, ed 10, Philadelphia, 2000, Saunders.

Answers: 1. vitamin C; 2. 50%, 3. with food, 4. black

NCLEX® Review

NCLEX® Review

Section A

1. Which of the following vitamins is essential for the synthesis of blood coagulation factors in the liver?
   1 Vitamin B
   2 Vitamin C
   3 Vitamin D
   4 Vitamin K

2. Vitamin C is used for the treatment or prevention of which of the following conditions?
   1 Thiamine deficiency
   2 Scurvy
   3 An overdose of anticoagulants
   4 Chapped or dry skin

Section B

3. Sodium is used in the treatment and prevention of which of the following conditions?
   1 Beriberi
   2 Scurvy
   3 Heat prostration
   4 Anemia

4. To evaluate the effectiveness of iron therapy, the nurse should monitor which of the following tests?
   1 Renal function studies
   2 Hepatic function studies
   3 Sodium and potassium levels
   4 Hemoglobin and reticulocyte levels

5. Which of the following is the best food source of vitamin B_9 (folic acid)?
   1 Fish
   2 Milk
   3 Asparagus
   4 Strawberries

NCLEX® Review Answers

Section A

1. 4 Vitamin K is essential for the synthesis of blood coagulation factors. Vitamins B, C, and D are not associated with blood coagulation.

2. 2 Vitamin C is used for the prevention and treatment of scurvy. Vitamin C is not used for the treatment and prevention of thiamine deficiency, overdose of anticoagulants, or chapped or dry skin.

Section B

3. 3 Sodium is used in the prevention and treatment of heat prostration. Sodium is not used in the treatment and prevention of beriberi, scurvy, or anemia.

4. 4 The nurse should monitor hemoglobin and reticulocyte levels to evaluate the effectiveness of iron therapy. Iron therapy is usually continued for 2 to 3 months after the hemoglobin level returns to normal. Renal and hepatic function studies or sodium and potassium levels do not indicate the effectiveness of iron therapy.

5. 3 The best food source that is listed for vitamin B_9 is asparagus. Fish, milk, and strawberries are not the best food sources of vitamin B_9.

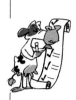

Notes

Index

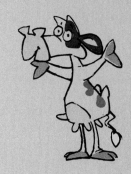